"Here in these words, you join a healing movement—a community all over the world of millions of people who are using Medical Medium information to get their lives back. This guidebook is your story of survival—your story of discovering what was wrong all along, and how to free yourself from it. It is your story of relief, healing, and triumph. These living words will always be here for you, for the rest of your life."

— Anthony William, Medical Medium

"You are the power behind this movement. And your story of healing is the story of saving others' lives. When you save yourself, you become a trusted guide for your children, your family, your friends, and anyone who hears your story. Whether or not you ever find out how many people you've helped, know that your healing holds tremendous meaning."

— Anthony William, Medical Medium

PRAISE FOR ANTHONY WILLIAM

"Anthony William has a powerful gift that our family has now experienced firsthand. After years of doctors being unable to diagnose, identify, or pinpoint our child's gastrointestinal issues, Anthony's expertise and intuition led us to not only identifying the issue, but more importantly, Anthony's precise protocols have been the invaluable catalyst in our daughter's healing, recovery, and her happiness. As parents, there is no greater gift you can pray for than the health of your children, and we are eternally grateful to you, Anthony, for your powerful gifts. Thank you for your time, energy, guidance, and comfort on a journey that wasn't overnight, and for restoring our daughter's and many of our family members' health, Anthony."
— Dwayne "The Rock" Johnson and Lauren Hashian

"Celery juice is sweeping the globe. It's impressive how Anthony has created this movement and restored superior health in countless people around the world."
— Sylvester Stallone

"Anthony William has been there for my wife at all times to make sure she is as healthy as she could possibly be. I will always thank him and love him for that."
— Adam Sandler, writer, filmmaker, actor, comedian

"Anthony's understanding of foods, their vibrations, and how they interact with the body never ceases to amaze. Effortlessly he explains the potential harmony or disharmony in our choices in a way anyone can understand. He has a gift. Do your body a favor and treat yourself."
— Pharrell Williams, 13-time Grammy-winning artist and producer

"Anthony is a healing encounter."
— Diane von Furstenberg, iconic fashion designer

"Anthony is a trusted source for our family. His work in the world is a light that has guided many to safety. He means so much to us."
— Robert De Niro and Grace Hightower De Niro

"Anthony doesn't offer gimmicks or fads to finding ultimate health. His recommended foods and cleansing programs are simple and delicious and THEY WORK! If you're done living with pain, fatigue, brain fog, intestinal disorders, and a myriad of other nasty ailments, drop everything and read this (and his other) books. He will quickly bring health and hope back into your life."
— Hilary Swank, Oscar-winning actress and film producer

"For over 40 years I have been teaching the principles of vital health and alkalinity in my books and seminars. Sage and I are passionate about the cleanse-to-heal approach to nutrition and wellness that naturally supports the body and fortifies our immune system to keep it functioning at its prime. We are so grateful for the dear friendship, guidance, alignment, and insights of Anthony William, not only in his teaching and best practices, but also for the way he has personally ushered us through our own health challenges. He is a brother on this path and a gift to this world. His routines have proven results to all who seek to optimize their inner terrain."

— Tony Robbins

"While there is most definitely an element of otherworldly mystery to the work he does, much of what Anthony William shines a spotlight on—particularly around autoimmune disease—feels inherently right and true. What's better is that the protocols he recommends are natural, accessible, and easy to do."

— Gwyneth Paltrow, Oscar-winning actress, #1 *New York Times* best-selling author, founder and CEO of GOOP.com

"Anthony William's philosophy on food and health protocols has profoundly changed my life and health for the better. I am forever grateful for him."

— Miranda Kerr, international supermodel, founder and CEO of KORA Organics

"Anthony has turned numerous lives around for the better with the healing powers of celery juice."

— Novak Djokovic, #1-ranked tennis champion in the world

"All great gifts are bestowed with humility. Anthony is humble. And like all the right remedies, his are intuitive, natural, and balanced. These two make for a powerful and effective combination."

— John Donovan, CEO of AT&T Communications

"Anthony William is truly dedicated to sharing his knowledge and experience to spread the word of healing to all. His compassion and desire to reach as many people as he can to help them heal themselves is inspiring and empowering. Today, in a world of obsession with prescription medication, it is so refreshing to know that there are alternative options that truly work and can open a new door to health."

— Liv Tyler, star of *9-1-1: Lone Star*, *Harlots*, the *Lord of the Rings* trilogy, *Empire Records*

"Anthony is a magician for all my label's recording artists, and if he were a record album, he would far surpass Thriller. His ability is nothing short of profound, remarkable, extraordinary, and mind-blowing. He is a luminary whose books are filled with prophecies. This is the future of medicine."

— Craig Kallman, Chairman and CEO, Atlantic Records

"Anthony has dedicated his life to helping others find the answers that we need to live our healthiest lives. And celery juice is the most accessible way to start!"
— Courteney Cox, star of *Shining Vale, Cougar Town, Friends*

"Anthony is not only a warm, compassionate healer, he is also authentic and accurate, with God-given skills. He has been a total blessing in my life."
— Naomi Campbell, model, actress, activist

"Anthony has created global awareness about how to heal ourselves naturally. So thankful for his books. They are truly changing lives."
— Kelly Rutherford, star of *Gossip Girl* and *Melrose Place*

"Anthony's extensive knowledge and deep intuition have demystified even the most confounding health issues. He has provided a clear path for me to feel my very best— I find his guidance indispensable."
— Taylor Schilling, star of *Pam & Tommy* and *Orange Is the New Black*

"Anthony William is a gift to humanity. His incredible work has helped millions of people heal when conventional medicine had no answers for them. His genuine passion and commitment for helping people is unsurpassed, and I am grateful to have been able to share a small part of his powerful message in Heal."
— Kelly Noonan Gores, writer, director, and producer of the *Heal* documentary

"Anthony William's God-given gift for healing is nothing short of miraculous."
— David James Elliott, *Heart of Champions, Trumbo, Mad Men, CSI: NY*; star for 10 years of *JAG*

"Resonance is a powerful thing in life, as is self-empowerment. Wonderfully enough, Anthony William, his books, and his Celery Juice call-to-action have hit both of those notes with me. The reinforcement from Anthony that our bodies are capable of incredible healing and resilience is a much-needed message. Too often, I want quick fixes that ultimately lead to more problems. Real nutrition is the best medicine, and Anthony inspires us all to fuel our body, mind, and spirit with nature's bounty; it's powerful medicine straight from the Source."
— Kerri Walsh Jennings, three-time gold medal–winning and one-time bronze medal–winning Olympic volleyball player

"We are incredibly grateful for Anthony and his passionate dedication to spreading the word about healing through food. Anthony has a truly special gift. His practices have entirely reshaped our perspectives about food and ultimately our lifestyle. Celery juice alone has completely transformed the way we feel and it will always be a part of our morning routine."
— Hunter Mahan, six-time PGA Tour–winning golfer

"Anthony is a truly generous person with keen intuition and knowledge about health. I have seen firsthand the transformation he's made in people's quality of life."
— Carla Gugino, star of *The Haunting of Bly Manor, Jett, Watchmen, Entourage, Spy Kids*

"A pathfinder. Truly ahead of his time. A vision of hope."
— Steve Harris, Iron Maiden

"I've been following Anthony for a while now and am always floored (but not surprised) at the success stories from people following his protocols . . . I have been on my own path of healing for many years, jumping from doctor to doctor and specialist to specialist. He's the real deal, and I trust him and his vast knowledge of how the thyroid works and the true effects food has on our body. I have directed countless friends, family, and followers to Anthony because I truly believe he possesses knowledge that no doctor out there has. I am a believer and on a true path to healing now and am honored to know him and blessed to know his work. Every endocrinologist needs to read his book on the thyroid!"
— Marcela Valladolid, chef, author, television host

"What if someone could simply touch you and tell you what it is that ails you? Welcome to the healing hands of Anthony William—a modern-day alchemist who very well may hold the key to longevity. His lifesaving advice blew into my world like a healing hurricane, and he has left a path of love and light in his wake. He is hands down the ninth wonder of the world."
— Lisa Gregorisch-Dempsey, senior executive producer of *Extra*

"Anthony William is changing and saving the lives of people all over the world with his one-of-a-kind gift. His constant dedication and vast amount of highly advanced information have broken the barriers that block so many in the world from receiving desperately needed truths that science and research have not yet discovered. On a personal level, he has helped both my daughters and me, giving us tools to support our health that actually work. Celery juice is now a part of our regular routine!"
— Lisa Rinna, star of *The Real Housewives of Beverly Hills* and *Days of Our Lives*, *New York Times* best-selling author, designer of the Lisa Rinna Collection

"I am a doctor's daughter who has always relied on Western medicine to ameliorate even the smallest of woes. Anthony's insights opened my eyes to the healing benefits of food and how a more holistic approach to health can change your life."
— Jenny Mollen, actress and *New York Times* best-selling author of *I Like You Just the Way I Am*

"Anthony William has a remarkable gift! I will always be grateful to him for discovering an underlying cause of several health issues that had bothered me for years. With his kind support, I see improvements every day. I think he is a fabulous resource!"
— Morgan Fairchild, actress, author, speaker

"Anthony William is the gifted Medical Medium who has very real and not-so-radical solutions to the mysterious conditions that affect us all in our modern world. I am beyond thrilled to know him personally and count him as a most valuable resource for my health protocols and those for my entire family."
— Annabeth Gish, *The Haunting of Hill House*, *The X-Files*, *The West Wing*, *Mystic Pizza*

"Whenever Anthony William recommends a natural way of improving your health, it works. I've seen this with my daughter, and the improvement was impressive. His approach of using natural ingredients is a more effective way of healing."
— Martin D. Shafiroff, financial advisor, past recipient of #1 Broker in America ranking by WealthManagement.com, and #1 Wealth Advisor ranking by Barron's

"Anthony William has devoted his life to helping people with information that has truly made a substantial difference in the lives of many."
— Amanda de Cadenet, founder and CEO of The Conversation and the Girlgaze Project; author of *It's Messy* and *#girlgaze*

"I love Anthony William! My daughters Sophia and Laura gave me his book for my birthday, and I couldn't put it down. The Medical Medium has helped me connect all the dots on my quest to achieve optimal health. Through Anthony's work, I realized the residual Epstein-Barr left over from a childhood illness was sabotaging my health years later. *Medical Medium* has transformed my life."
— Catherine Bach, *The Young and the Restless*, *The Dukes of Hazzard*

"My recovery from a traumatic spinal crisis several years ago had been steady, but I was still experiencing muscle weakness, a tapped-out nervous system, as well as extra weight. A dear friend called me one evening and strongly recommended I read the book Medical Medium by Anthony William. So much of the information in the book resonated with me that I began incorporating some of the ideas, then I sought and was lucky enough to get a consultation. The reading was so spot-on, it has taken my healing to an unimagined, deeper, and richer level of health. My weight has dropped healthily, I can enjoy bike riding and yoga, I'm back in the gym, I have steady energy, and I sleep deeply. Every morning when following my protocols, I smile and say, 'Whoa, Anthony William! I thank you for your restorative gift . . . Yes!'"
— Robert Wisdom, *A Journal for Jordan*, *Ballers*, *The Wire*, *Ray*

"As a Hollywood businesswoman, I know value. Some of Anthony's clients spent over $1 million seeking help for their 'mystery illness' until they finally discovered him."
— Nanci Chambers, co-star of *JAG*; Hollywood producer and entrepreneur

"In this world of confusion, with constant noise in the health and wellness field, I rely on Anthony's profound authenticity. His miraculous, true gift rises above it all to a place of clarity."
— Patti Stanger, host of *Million Dollar Matchmaker*

"Anthony William brings a dimension to medicine that deeply expands our understanding of the body and of ourselves. His work is part of a new frontier in healing, delivered with compassion and with love."
— Marianne Williamson, #1 *New York Times* best-selling author of *Healing the Soul of America*, *The Age of Miracles*, and *A Return to Love*

"Anthony William is a generous and compassionate guide. He has devoted his life to supporting people on their healing path."
— Gabrielle Bernstein, #1 *New York Times* best-selling author of *The Universe Has Your Back*, *Judgment Detox*, and *Miracles Now*

"Information that WORKS. That's what I think of when I think of Anthony William and his profound contributions to the world. Nothing made this fact so clear to me as seeing him work with an old friend who had been struggling for years with illness, brain fog, and fatigue. She had been to countless doctors and healers and had gone through multiple protocols. Nothing worked. Until Anthony talked to her, that is . . . from there, the results were astounding. I highly recommend his books, lectures, and consultations. Don't miss this healing opportunity!"
— Nick Ortner, *New York Times* best-selling author of *The Tapping Solution for Manifesting Your Greatest Self* and *The Tapping Solution*

"Esoteric talent is only a complete gift when it's shared with moral integrity and love. Anthony William is a divine combination of healing, giftedness, and ethics. He's a real-deal healer who does his homework and shares it in true service to the world."
— Danielle LaPorte, best-selling author of *White Hot Truth* and *The Desire Map*

"Anthony is a seer and a wellness sage. His gift is remarkable. With his guidance, I've been able to pinpoint and address a health issue that's been plaguing me for years."
— Kris Carr, *New York Times* best-selling author of *Crazy Sexy Juice*, *Crazy Sexy Kitchen*, and *Crazy Sexy Diet*

"Twelve hours after receiving a heaping dose of self-confidence masterfully administered by Anthony, the persistent ringing in my ears of the last year . . . began to falter. I am astounded, grateful, and happy for the insights offered on moving forward."

— Mike Dooley, *New York Times* best-selling author of *Infinite Possibilities* and scribe of *The Complete Notes from the Universe*

"Anthony William's invaluable advice on preventing and combating disease is years ahead of what's available anywhere else."

— Richard Sollazzo, M.D., New York board-certified oncologist, hematologist, nutritionist, and anti-aging expert, and author of *Balance Your Health*

"Anthony William is the Edgar Cayce of our time, reading the body with outstanding precision and insight. Anthony identifies the underlying causes of diseases that often baffle the most astute conventional and alternative health-care practitioners. Anthony's practical and profound advice makes him one of the most powerfully effective healers of the 21st century."

— Ann Louise Gittleman, *New York Times* best-selling author of over 30 books on health and healing and creator of the highly popular Fat Flush detox and diet plan

"I had a health reading from Anthony, and he accurately told me things about my body only known to me. This kind, sweet, hilarious, self-effacing, and generous man—also so 'otherworldly' and so extraordinarily gifted, with an ability that defies how we see the world—has shocked even me, a medium! He is truly our modern-day Edgar Cayce, and we are immensely blessed that he is with us. Anthony William proves that we are more than we know."

— Colette Baron-Reid, best-selling author of *Uncharted* and TV host of *Messages from Spirit*

"Any quantum physicist will tell you there are things at play in the universe we can't yet understand. I truly believe Anthony has a handle on them. He has an amazing gift for intuitively tapping into the most effective methods for healing."

— Caroline Leavitt, *New York Times* best-selling author of *With or Without You*, *Is This Tomorrow*, and *Pictures of You*

MEDICAL MEDIUM

BRAIN
SAVER

ALSO BY ANTHONY WILLIAM

MEDICAL MEDIUM

BRAIN SAVER

ANSWERS TO BRAIN INFLAMMATION, MENTAL HEALTH, OCD,
BRAIN FOG, NEUROLOGICAL SYMPTOMS, ADDICTION, ANXIETY,
DEPRESSION, HEAVY METALS, EPSTEIN-BARR VIRUS, SEIZURES,
LYME, ADHD, ALZHEIMER'S, AUTOIMMUNE & EATING DISORDERS

ANTHONY WILLIAM

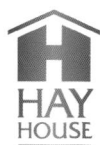

HAY HOUSE, INC.
Carlsbad, California • New York City
London • Sydney • New Delhi

Copyright © 2022 by Anthony William

Published in the United States by: Hay House, Inc.: www.hayhouse.com®
Published in Australia by: Hay House Australia Pty. Ltd.: www.hayhouse.com.au
Published in the United Kingdom by: Hay House UK, Ltd.: www.hayhouse.co.uk
Published in India by: Hay House Publishers India: www.hayhouse.co.in

Cover design: Vibodha Clark
Interior design: Nick C. Welch
Interior illustrations: Vibodha Clark
Indexer: J S Editorial, LLC

Cataloging-in-Publication Data is on file at the Library of Congress

Hardcover ISBN: 978-1-4019-5438-3
E-book ISBN: 978-1-4019-5439-0
Audiobook ISBN: 978-1-4019-5861-9

10 9 8 7 6 5 4 3 2 1
1st edition, October 2022

Printed in the United States of America

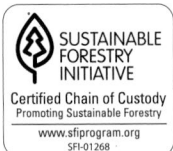

For the Light that stands in the way of the darkness.

CONTENTS

"In these chapters, you'll come to know your brain like never before. Just what is contaminating, damaging, injuring, impeding, depriving, burning out, and limiting our neurons, how does it get there, and how does that explain our individual experiences and struggles? Just what is inflaming, scarring, and atrophying our brains, and how does that threaten our well-being? It will all become clear as we take a closer look inside the brain and nervous system. With this knowledge, you can find relief like never before."

— Anthony William, Medical Medium

FOREWORD

Anthony is a combination of brother from another mother with shades of guru, guardian angel, and gifted healer. Anthony is a truly good man and an outstanding friend. I love Anthony. We have been there for each other. Anthony is always there for me. If you pay close attention, you will understand that I am not just blowing smoke up to the Spirit of Compassion. My high opinion of Anthony stems from my experience of meeting many gurus and healers, some real, some fake.

We have in our generation a true seer (and listener), the Medical Medium.

In 1990 I graduated from medical school in Uruguay and moved to New York to specialize in internal medicine and then cardiovascular diseases. The change in lifestyle was so drastic that I did not even see it coming. Four years into my training I was overweight, suffering from irritable bowel syndrome and severe allergies. But the worse part was that I was severely depressed. I couldn't function.

A visit to a gastroenterologist, an allergist, and a psychiatrist left me with seven prescription medications for three diagnoses. I kept staring at my prescriptions and something inside of me kept screaming, "Find another way." And so I took off and searched. I've spent time in monasteries in India and met the most influential gurus of our time. I've met more healers, therapists, doctors, practitioners, coaches, shamans, mediums, and witches than I could ever remember. I found the way to heal myself through detox and gut repair. I have become a known functional-medicine doctor. I wrote four books. I've helped thousands of people in their healing processes, bringing what I know and finding the team that brings whatever I don't know into the healing journey of so many. I often go with them to consultations with other specialists or healers. I want to learn, to see, and to understand what works. I've learned a thing or two in the world of healing.

But nothing makes my head spin more than what Anthony speaks about. Mostly because of its success rate.

When I met Anthony over 10 years ago, the Medical Medium books had not been published yet. At my first book launch we were introduced. He had come with a mutual friend. Our friend had pulled me aside and told me that Anthony hears a voice that tells him about health and disease, in general and specific to certain people. I was immediately interested in meeting him. I kept thinking, *Is it real? Is he just psychotic and should be on psych meds? Or does he make any sense?* When we started talking, I critically observed Anthony, not only listening to what he was saying. *Is he lying or is he telling the truth? Does he actually hear a voice? Where is that coming from? Does the voice tell him things that are accurate? Does what the voice says help at all?*

The first minute of our conversation, I thought he was shy. After five minutes I realized he was far from shy, in fact, incredibly alive and outgoing. His style of communicating is amusing and honest, and he chooses his words very precisely when talking about health and disease. He is very organized in his mind. He was talking about diseases with conviction and somehow a deep understanding, as if he were a medical doctor. But his information was to me, at that time, as if out of a *Star Wars* movie. I was convinced. He hears a voice. So the question that remained was, *Does this voice know what it is talking about?* One way of measuring that was for me to search publications of research and trials that prove that what he was saying was scientifically correct, medically proven. Another way was to judge by the results. I started doing both.

On the research and publications front, I did not accomplish much for a long time. It turned out that the voice of his information was advanced, ahead of many publications. One of the pillars of Anthony's understanding is that most chronic diseases, and many acute ones, are caused by viruses. Some of the viruses can stay dormant for years and only cause trouble when your defenses go down. Some old, some mutated, and some undiscovered viruses. Some of the ones that we've known about for a long time, and that are so ubiquitous we barely even test for them in routine check-ups. Such an example is the herpes virus that causes a lip sore every once in a while. We live with these viruses and we are not scared of them. Another prime example of a virus Anthony has always said is at the root of many symptoms and diseases is the Epstein-Barr virus. Anthony teaches that almost everyone is exposed to EBV and that it either lives dormant or low-grade active in our organs and glands, eventually affecting our central nervous system. He has always said that many of us got it as a baby from our parents, who got it from their parents. What has been well known is that EBV is transmitted commonly through saliva when someone has infectious mononucleosis, also known as the "kissing disease" because that's how some people get it.

In the research, I found theoretical understandings here and there that some diseases such as cancer could be linked to viruses. After the Medical Medium books started to come out, there was chatter among the autoimmune practitioner community that autoimmune disease could be triggered by common viruses. Almost a decade after I wrote the foreword for the first Medical Medium book, they are now saying the Epstein-Barr virus causes multiple sclerosis, which is exactly what Anthony originally said in that first book, that the true cause of MS is EBV. Anthony provided the intricate details of how the Epstein-Barr virus actually causes the physical and neurological symptoms involved with multiple sclerosis. The research is mounting in an accelerated way and things that Anthony was telling me more than a decade ago, that sometimes made me doubt what he spoke about, are now front page in the media. Articles are now pointing out clues that link long COVID with the reactivation of EBV, something that Anthony had already published before long COVID was connected to EBV.

These are just a couple of examples of how Anthony, I believe, gets his information from a source that knows what it is talking about, often preceding scientific evidence for decades.

As a functional-medicine doctor and a cardiologist, I see and help people with many chronic diseases. I use Anthony's teachings in one way or another with most of my patients. It has made me a better doctor. I can help people I couldn't help before.

That is why I was so happy to read *Brain Saver* and *Brain Saver Protocols, Cleanses & Recipes*, Anthony's latest books. The brain is the organ that we understand the least, but has the most impact in our experience of life. That is why we can keep people alive with artificial and transplanted hearts, kidneys, livers, lungs, and other organs, but when you are diagnosed as brain-dead, they recommend to pull the plug.

I can't wait for you to read these books, too, and for them to bring you the solution to your healing that you've been looking for.

With much love and respect,
Alejandro Junger, M.D.,
New York Times best-selling author of
Clean, Clean Eats, Clean Gut, and *CLEAN 7*

"Many people are desperate to bring their health back. Yet if someone takes a normal natural-health direction, which relies on elementary measures such as removing processed foods, they all too easily run into the trend traps. Stuck in a world where their health results only get them so far, they're forced to test out trendy theory after trendy theory, acting as guinea pigs for misguided hypotheses. When that's the case, it's going to be a long time before that brain gets restored—if it ever does."

— Anthony William, Medical Medium

AUTHOR'S PERSONAL NOTE

How *Brain Saver* Became Two Books

"Anthony, the book is going to be well over a thousand pages. It's too big to print." That was the call I got from my publisher the week after handing in the *Brain Saver* manuscript.

I can't say it came as a surprise. Over the months and then years it took to write "the brain book," I had watched the pages pile up and up and up on my desk. Anyone who knew what I was working on would ask, "Don't you think you're close to wrapping up by now?"

"People need answers," I would say and then get back to work.

I hadn't set out to write such a voluminous book, and I realized I would have to wrap it up someday if the material was ever going to reach people. Yet the material just kept coming. The world was changing faster. People were getting sicker. And Spirit of Compassion was forewarning me of what's to come in the next 5 to 10 years and beyond.

There were many times when I would push a 20-hour day, sometimes a 22-hour day, because I was devoting so much time

to receiving information from Spirit of Compassion. Periodically, I'd fall asleep on my office floor with the lights on and then wake up a few hours later to start the day all over again. If there's anything you pick up from my work, it's that I believe people should take care of themselves whenever possible. They should eat well, get plenty of sleep, get sun, take walks, and so forth when they can. Still, I'm guilty of ignoring my personal needs while listening to the voice of Spirit and doing what God intended me to do. I'd often remind others that life goes by quickly, and if I disappear and leave this earth, it was from burning the candle at four ends under enormous pressure and outside forces of darkness trying to die this light out so the world doesn't receive Spirit's prophecies. Many times, I joked that I would burn a hole in my seat with the amount of time I spent sitting down to work on this material with Spirit. The joke has now come pretty close to reality. This might be the moment when I do finally throw away my office chair—the seat cushion is torn up pretty badly.

I've always said that receiving information from Spirit of Compassion causes a whiteout, a foggy, glaring haze, a snow blindness—making it so that I feel surrounded by an energy source, making me feel that I'm somewhere else even though I'm aware that I haven't gone anywhere because I'm still completely conscious in the moment. Most of the time that I was writing *Brain Saver*, I was in the white cloud. This is because Spirit wants me to not only visually see the images that the words represent as I'm hearing them but even to feel the essence of what people are feeling through their suffering. The white cloud is to remove me from my personal life, responsibilities, and experiences so my focus is only on the information given to me and the suffering of others. It's not just about receiving information and writing it down. It's about receiving the complete experience and connecting this to what others go through in their health struggles. The feeling is a roller coaster of sadness and happiness—sadness about what people have gone through and happiness that this could be that door of opportunity they could open to overcome the sickness. Once I've received and connected with the information, I have to learn this content that Spirit provides and study it just like anyone else does.

Each year that goes by, as I work on another book with Spirit of Compassion, I notice that the voice I hear stays the same while I, as a person, change. The changing comes from the continual realization that there are over eight billion people on this planet who will eventually become ill, and not all of them may ever get the chance to experience what Spirit has delivered here in front of me. It's one of the hard parts about this journey: to know that many will find their way to this information, these living words, yet so many won't. As a child, I thought surely everyone was going to be able to behold the wisdom from above when they became challenged by a health issue. Now the older me, who knows this may not be true, confronts the younger me, who had tremendous confidence that everyone on the planet would find this information. With each passing year, the dawning realization keeps changing me. It leads me to ask Spirit a lot of "Why"s and "How come"s and extra questions as I'm receiving Spirit's information and writing books about how hard this world really is to live in for all of us.

The writing process also gave me opportunities to identify firsthand with what people go through. As I struggled to sneak in a shower, wash my face, brush my teeth, change my clothes, I thought of what the chronically ill deal with as they try to accomplish these day-to-day tasks that those who aren't sick take for granted. My constraint was merely time as I fulfilled a mission. For people up against painful or limiting symptoms, these practices can be like mountains to climb. I always support wherever someone is in their capacity to take care of themselves during their healing process.

I could identify with the chronically ill, too, as I lost touch with important people in my life to write the brain book. I sacrificed time away from loved ones. I'm usually an avid studier of the seasons as they change before my eyes and ears. I like to listen to the peepers. I like to listen to the wind blow. I like to watch the leaves change and the grass turn color. I don't really remember partaking in or even registering any of that while putting together *Brain Saver*. Not that I'm complaining. These are little things to forego. Those who are chronically ill or suffering have much bigger bridges to cross, far more sacrifices and losses. I always keep them in mind as each hour passes that I spend getting the scripture needed to heal others from above. The joy comes later, when someone holds one of these books in their hands and starts their journey of rising out of the ashes.

Which brings us back to how *Brain Saver* became two books. Spirit of Compassion doesn't stop producing and could have me write continuously. I have to be the one to say uncle. There comes a point when I have to give in and get the information out to the ones who need it. I had wanted this material to fit in one book, so you could hold all the answers in your hands at once. When the publisher called to tell me just how big it would be, I had to face the reality: no one wants to hold a 10-pound book, least of all someone struggling with neurological symptoms.

I wrestled with whether there was any material I could take out. It was clear that any healing answers and protocols needed to stay. What about the parts where I explained Medical Medium information as the uncited source of many new medical understandings of chronic illness, such as that Epstein-Barr virus causes multiple

sclerosis? After all, this isn't about me. I consulted with Spirit of Compassion. The determination was clear: showing readers that, for example, certain insights into long-haul COVID originated from Medical Medium material was itself a healing answer. When readers see that information circulating out in the world originally came from Medical Medium teachings, they get the opportunity to discover the full picture here, most notably the full picture of how to heal.

I kept thinking about how the book could be trimmed. Some of the material was going to be controversial. Was it worth it? Well, publishing truth about why the chronically ill are chronically ill is always controversial. I've already spoken and written about this for years. For the most part, the chronically ill have been disrespected and swept under the carpet. It's a hidden controversy, one you don't realize is out there until you stand up for the chronically ill and present the truth of why they're suffering. Darkness thrives on people who have symptoms being confused and lost about their direction, why they're sick. Darkness thrives on the chronically ill pursuing unproductive avenues, making their journey more difficult. So yes, it all needed to stay in the book.

That's when it was time to take the publisher's suggestion and turn "the brain book" into companion volumes: *Brain Saver* and *Brain Saver Protocols, Cleanses & Recipes*. We figured out the details: Both books would be published at the same time, so people could access the information all at once. Both books would have essential Medical Medium tools—Heavy

Metal Detox, Brain Shot Therapy, and 14 customizable cleanses—printed in full. This way, if someone only had one book in hand, they wouldn't be missing out on critical healing resources.

You'll read more about what appears in this book and what material you can find in its companion book in "How This Book Works," which comes next. The books are designed to stand alone, each volume filled to the brim with information you can put to use now. As you can see from the story of how these books came together, you'll get the most protection out of reading both, whenever you can bring each into your life. If I can give any advice about how to go about reading these two books, it's this: there is such comprehensive information, methodically and providentially placed, that once you're finished reading, you may benefit from giving it another go so that both your soul and physical brain get a chance to receive and store all that's here. Take your time. When you're ready, give each book another read-through. With every read, you may find powerful pieces of information and insight you never even noticed before.

Many blessings,
Anthony William, Medical Medium

"You are not faulty or weak. You did not bring your struggles upon yourself. You did not create or manifest or attract your symptoms and conditions. You've been lost and stranded through no fault of your own. Now let's get you the answers you deserve."

— Anthony William, Medical Medium

HOW THIS BOOK WORKS

This book is your survival guide as you navigate life.

In Part I, "Your Brain Story," you'll discover the major reasons why your brain needs help. What is happening in our brains and nervous systems to make us struggle and suffer like never before? What does it mean to have a static brain, an alloy brain, a viral brain, an emotional brain, inflamed cranial nerves, a burnt out and deficient brain, an addicted brain, an acid brain? With an understanding of the main factors affecting our brains that are contributing to today's epidemic of mental, emotional, and physical suffering, you can finally find the path of healing.

In Part II, "Brainwashed," you'll gain a fresh perspective on how to safeguard yourself and your family from trendy health traps and persistent myths that keep us sick and lost. Why isn't the "everything in moderation" philosophy as harmless as it sounds? How do microdosing, alcohol, and caffeine fall short of promised benefits? How do

you make sense of all the noise about food belief systems? The answers are here.

Part III, "Brain Betrayers," offers key understandings about the toxic exposures and problematic ingredients in our everyday lives that undermine our brain and nervous system health without our consent. With details about what we're exposed to, how we're exposed, and how these brain betrayers slip past the blood-brain barrier or cause problems in other parts of our body that undermine our brain, this section of the book will give you a whole new line of defense against the health threats that surround us.

In Part IV, "Brain Invasion," you'll find chapters to explain the truth about several of the most common, perplexing, and complex states of suffering. With insights into anxiety, depression, eating disorders, obsessive-compulsive disorder (OCD), bipolar disorder, and Alzheimer's and dementia, you'll understand yourself and your loved ones like never before.

And in the same spirit of revealing the answers to what holds back so many people in life, Part V, "Your Pain and Suffering Enlightened," sheds light on close to a hundred more symptoms and conditions. When you're struggling with a symptom or condition, it's not a shortcoming or a failing or a life sentence. You've been betrayed by invasive exposures present in our world. When you discover the underlying causes to address for relief or prevention, you won't have to live in fear or defeat any longer.

Part VI, "Bringing Back Your Brain," is your restorative oasis. Here, you'll discover how to align yourself with your brain and body's natural processes in order to heal and protect your brain and nervous system. You'll find information on steps you can take to start supporting your brain right away, as well as revelations about what kind of nourishment your brain and nervous system really need to strengthen and flourish. Also included is critical background on nutritional deficiencies and blood testing, along with the new Medical Medium tool Brain Shot Therapy, expanded options for established Medical Medium favorite Heavy Metal Detox, and numerous customizable cleanses designed to support your brain and nervous system wherever you are in life. With resources you can put to use plus a deep understanding of why these approaches support you, you'll find freedom.

(For even more healing options, refer to this book's companion, *Brain Saver Protocols, Cleanses & Recipes*. There, you'll find a "Supplement Gospel" section that covers the golden rules of choosing and taking supplements, nine Medical Medium Shock Therapies for in-the-moment relief and support, plus supplement protocols with dosages to address over 300 symptoms and conditions. Also discover over 100 healing recipes, detailed insights into the foods and supplements that undermine our healing, and powerful meditations and techniques to strengthen your soul and help heal your brain.)

Part VII, "Brained and Confused," offers special reading for anyone who wants to understand more about how we got here. How do we understand a world where breathtaking medical advancements coexist with an epidemic of chronic illness and mental health struggles? What makes Medical Medium science different from other health material you've read? Where are the citations? These chapters will shed light on how to make sense of widespread health confusion and why now, more than ever, we're all in this together. It's time for compassion to make a comeback.

Finally, if you'd like to learn more about the source of the information in this book, you'll find answers in "Origins of the Medical Medium," which follows Part VII. The information here doesn't come from broken science, interest groups, medical funding with strings attached, botched research, lobbyists, internal kickbacks, persuaded belief systems, private panels of influencers, health-field payoffs, or trendy traps. These are living words meant to elevate you above the sea of confusion.

Brain Saver is here for you as a lifelong reference. Make notes in the margins as you go. Bookmark the passages you want to revisit. Over and over, you can return to these living words for reminders—both the very practical, such as how to avoid the various brain betrayer exposures, and essential teachings, such as this: You didn't create your pain. You didn't create your symptoms. You didn't create your illness. We suffer for very real and physical reasons, and we can address those reasons at their core with the information here. When we know how to navigate this world, we have the power to heal.

"Our greatest line of defense against threats to our brain and neurological health is our brain itself. Using our own brain to acquire knowledge ahead of medical research and science, we can rise above chronic suffering and take back our power."

— Anthony William, Medical Medium

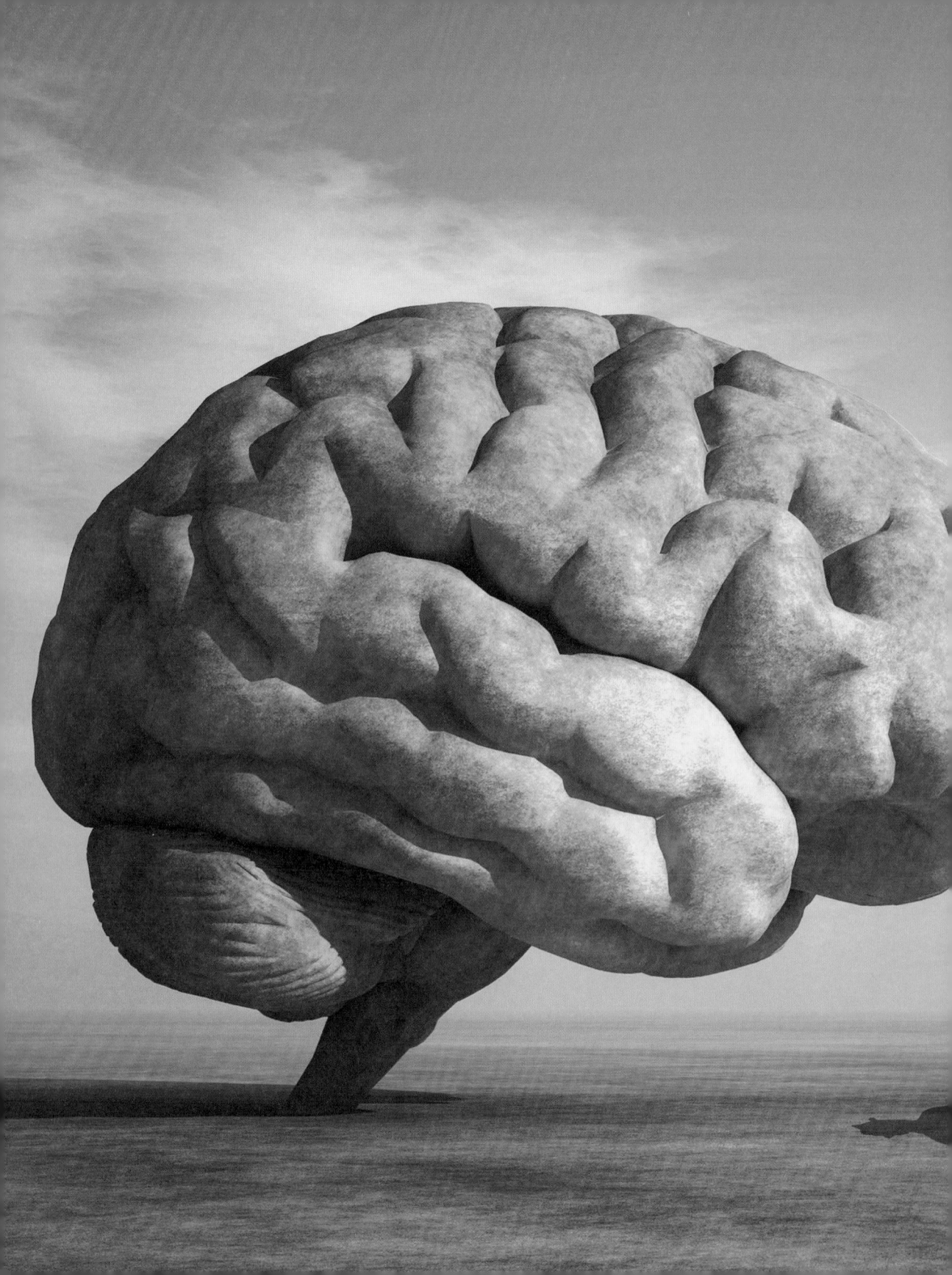

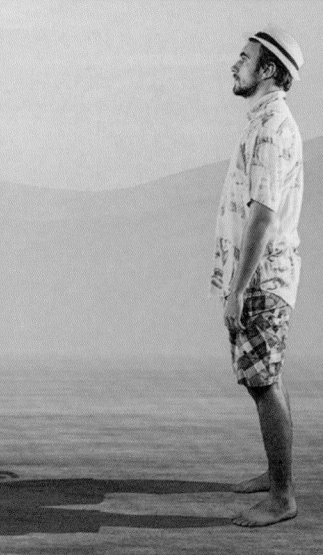

PART I

YOUR
BRAIN STORY

"You don't find out until it's too late that you're marooned and vulnerable. Maybe you never find out. Your body starts to deteriorate, your liver gives out, your kidneys go, or you have a stroke or an early heart attack before you even get a chance to reach for the brain knowledge you were sure would be there when you needed it. You never realize that your health crisis was because your whole body paid the price for a world that's utterly confused about how to protect the brain.

Let's change that."

— Anthony William, Medical Medium

CHAPTER 1

Save Your Brain

You've been preparing for this your whole life. Every guidebook you could find, every story, every piece of common wisdom, every social media video about others' journeys—you've studied them all, knowing the time would come for you to get out into the fresh air, saturate yourself in nature, and pursue your own dream hike. Now all that's left is to pack your knapsack for the day with the items you've been told are the essentials.

Map and compass? Check.

Water? Check.

Protein bars? Check.

Hat, phone, sunglasses, ID, first aid kit, spare clothing, some money in case of emergency, your home and car keys for when you return: each item is nestled in a special place in your hiking pack.

You know it won't be a breeze. The fresh springs may be running dry in the drought, and steep boulders and tricky passes await. You've heard of people getting hurt up there, or worse. You've heard that one tragic story of the hiker who never came back. Still, you're sure you'll be okay. You're prepared, and the vistas once you reach the top will put everything into perspective. Now is your time to take on the trail you've always dreamed of hiking.

You begin. Brush crunches underfoot as you take your first steps onto the trail. The smell of moss hits your nose as you take your first deep breath, and birds burst into melody to announce your arrival. At first, you're lost in reverie. It's everything you imagined. You feel an adrenaline surge of nervousness turn to excitement.

You're so determined to reach the top that you don't make any stops along the way. It's one foot in front of the other, one small challenge after another, each of them surmountable, each of them giving you a sense of accomplishment. You're not worried that it's getting hot, not worried about the flush you feel in your cheeks or your strained breath, because you know you're getting closer to a rest area, where you'll be able to dip into your provisions when you really need them.

At last you reach a small plateau. The trees are sparse now, and so are the trail markers, so you pause for a moment to check the map. Problem is, there's nothing in the front pocket of your knapsack, where you're positive you stuck your map and compass, except an old dry-cleaning receipt. The map and compass must have fallen out. *Well*, you reason, *if I keep going upward, I have to get there.*

After half a mile of wandering, you're officially lost. You drop to your knees, desperate for a drink of water after hours of single-minded determination to reach the spot on the trail you've seen in so many pictures on social media. You can feel it getting hotter. It was 90 degrees by your car's thermometer when you left the trail parking lot hours ago, and even at this higher altitude, you know it's climbed past that. You reach for the side pocket of your knapsack—and your fingers don't find your water bottle there. Your heart drops into your stomach. Instead of your water bottle, you find only a bubble gum wrapper. You swing your pack around to check if the bottle has simply jostled out of place, and you see plainly now that, just like your map, your water bottle's not there. You start to panic, then try to calm yourself with positive thoughts.

It will be okay, you tell yourself even as your muscles start to twitch. *At least I have my snacks.* Yet when you unzip that compartment, your food is missing. The protein bars just aren't there. All that's there is a paper clip.

At least I can shade myself with my hat while I call for help, you think, only to find that your hat and phone aren't inside either; instead you find a pen cap and an old sticky

note from three years ago with notes that no longer make sense.

You start tearing through your pack, looking for something, anything, to help. You frantically unzip every zipper, peer into every corner, even shake out your pack, and still, nothing useful. Sunglasses, identification, first aid kit, spare clothing, even your cash and keys—everything you so studiously thought to include is gone. The only items that shake out onto the ground are a penny, a nickel, an empty lip balm tube, an old name tag, a straw wrapper, and a tiny used battery. Your entire knapsack is empty of anything to support you in your time of need.

What's your next move? Wait it out up here, where there's barely a scrap of protection from the fierce sun, and hope another hiker comes along and offers help before it's too late? Or venture back down? You're not sure how far your legs will carry you, and you're not even certain how to find the way you came. Parched and dizzy now, you know neither option is a sure bet. It's an impossible choice. In the moment, all you know is that you're stranded and you're in crisis.

This is our own survival story in everyday life. Navigating trendy brain traps and trying to find help for our neurological, emotional, mental, and other brain-related symptoms and conditions that develop sooner or later, we can become just as stranded as a hiker who is lost, alone, and exposed, with no provisions, in the sunbaked wilderness. This is how bad it can get. This is how imperiled we can become in life if we don't learn the truth about how to save our brains.

EMPTY ANSWERS

Just like in that metaphorical nightmare hike, it's easy to think we're preparing well for life. Some of us know there are real and scary threats out there—Alzheimer's, brain tumors, the next plague, to name just a few—and so we fill our heads with neuroscience studies and telomere gene theories and anti-aging trends and cognitive hacks and cautionary tales about too much sugar and lack of protein. We pack away the brain trivia like we pack away our map, food, and water, thinking we're arming ourselves with essential health knowledge about how best to care for our brains and our minds. We think all that we've learned will save us. We think it will be there when we need it as we climb our own mountains—that is, as we pursue our dreams and purpose in life.

What happens when we do need answers for our brains, nerves, and mental health? When we develop brain fog or depression or depersonalization or anxiety or migraines or OCD or vertigo, or when a loved one stops acting like themselves? The brain health trivia we picked up along the way that we thought would be brain answers turn out instead to be misinformation, mistakes, false leads, useless paid-for studies, inconclusive theories, marketing traps, health pyramid schemes, multilevel marketing pushes, and catchy, unhelpful soundbites from social media and podcasts. Instead of a knapsack full of all the tools we thought would keep us strong or even save our life, the knowledge we thought we were packing away turns out to be as useful as an old receipt, a used battery, or an indecipherable sticky note. We find ourselves sick and disoriented and far from home, the sun beating down, with nothing to support us.

Instead of the beautiful, scenic journey we thought life would be, our path becomes one endless trek of desperate visits to doctors' offices, hoping we don't fall off a cliff in the process. Specialists, neurologists, functional medicine doctors, psychiatrists—we ask them all for the real answers. As we leave yet another specialist's office still suffering with our OCD, anxiety, depression, head pain, blurry vision, or tics and spasms, we learn that even the experts' own knapsack supplies are only as helpful as old gum wrappers and pen caps.

BEFORE IT'S TOO LATE

"Knowledge" about brain health can act as a mirage. Neuroscience concepts are so inviting and elusive that they give you false hope, hope you don't realize is false until it's too late. The brain information that's out there seems so confident, so trustworthy—so regal, almost—when in reality it's not. It seems as if science has the technical terms down. It seems like the players in the health field have it all sewn up. Brain information seems so legitimate, so true, so real, so advanced, when really there's nothing there that moves the needle for the chronically ill. When bits of truth do enter the neurological health conversation—namely, when health figures start using Medical Medium information (such as that toxic heavy metals cause anxiety) without citing it—that truth gets contaminated, distorted, and corrupted, because they mix it with untruth at the same time, sometimes without realizing it. So the brain-saving information these sources promise us continues to remain beyond our grasp. The idea that it would save us was always an illusion.

Not until you experience a neurological symptom, a mental or emotional health stumbling block, or another brain-related condition do you realize how very little is known about the brain. Only then do the misinformation, missteps, and smoke and mirrors become clear. Tips, tricks, and trends for the brain are really for the ones who haven't suffered with any brain-related complication, disease, or condition. When you have suffered, that becomes clear. That's when you realize you're lost and your knapsack is empty—and always was. That's when you see the mirage for what it is.

Brain health advice for people who have very little wrong with their health, or who are just trying to improve their health, is deceiving. It always has been. When someone shares on social media about a health problem seemingly similar to yours that got better from a trendy approach, you don't know if the person on the other end of that social media network really was sick or not. What you can't see on your screen is that they haven't really suffered like you're suffering.

Learning what truly works can shed light on the difference between trendy brain information for someone who's not really struggling versus usable and even vital information for someone who is suffering from some sort of brain-related condition that's minimizing the quality of their life: brain fog that's not getting better (and is actually worsening) from a little caffeine or a fun trip to a favorite store or restaurant; brain fatigue that's really slowing them down; random neurological symptoms that constantly remind them something is wrong; anxiety or depression that leaves Level 1— mild anxiousness and sadness—and climbs to a crippling Level 10.

Because of the misguided tips and tricks and trends and instruction and seemingly expert advice about how to take care of our brains, decades go by—*generations* go by—as we take the wrong steps for our health. History repeats itself, trends get recycled over and over, and every five years there's a new round of people who aren't feeling well and are ready to buy into the seemingly smart advice about our brains. They have plenty of trendy, recycled advice at their fingertips. These days it seems that everywhere you turn, there's a brain expert. Every doctor seems to be a neuroscience expert. And almost everything offered for our brain health is the opposite of what our brain needs. Everyone selling something wants to say it's good for the brain, when the truth is that almost every time, it works against our brain.

We have far surpassed medical research and science's limitations for the symptoms and conditions developing in people. There is more suffering occurring than the medical industry can keep up with. Sickness and disease have always been ahead of medical research and science. There are brain diseases that are not even considered brain diseases because medical research and science haven't caught up. There are symptoms and conditions that even the best neurologist doesn't know are brain-related. Now neurological and brain symptoms have reached new levels, surpassing medical science and research's antiquated perception of what sickness or symptoms even are. Only we wouldn't know that, because the medical industry has a reputation and an image to uphold. Every piece of brain advice we're handed sounds advanced—until we really need it, and then we see it for what it is.

It's like that hike up the mountain: you don't find out until it's too late that you're marooned and vulnerable. Maybe you never find out. Your body starts to deteriorate, your liver gives out, your kidneys go, or you have a stroke or an early heart attack before you even get a chance to reach for the brain knowledge you were sure would be there when you needed it. You never realize that your health crisis was because your whole body paid the price for a world that's utterly confused about how to protect the brain.

Let's change that.

SAVE YOUR BRAIN, SAVE YOUR LIFE

What resides inside us that makes us want to save the world? What is it within us that doesn't want to see someone suffer or watch something disappear? That wants to save the trees? Why not chop down the last of the great old oaks? Why do we care enough to conserve them? Why do we want to keep the oceans clean? Why do we care if a dog is crossing the street—why do we slow down? Why do we want to keep animal species from going extinct? Why don't we want to lose creatures on the planet?

Somewhere inside us, we have a drive to save. When we find a baby bird that's fallen out of its nest, what instantly hits us? *What should I do? How should I care for it? Should I get an eye dropper and try to give it water?* Even if we don't have the ability or resources in the moment to carry out any of it, there's still this intentional caring and concern. Part of this is an instinct that doesn't like to see anything die or go to waste, from a shrub in the garden to a grub you find beneath a rock to a shoebox. How many times have you heard someone say, "Save it"? We can see the value in saving nearly anything. "I've got half my sandwich left," a friend may say. "Save it for later," you'll reply.

If only we knew how to save the very source that allows us to save the world around us: our brain. Protecting the brain is one of the body's main goals: The liver's day-in, day-out filtration and neutralization functions are about safeguarding the brain. The immune system is focused on devouring toxins and pathogens so they don't reach the brain. The adrenals release specific blends of adrenaline to help power your brain and body through extreme stress, hardships, and losses, fueling your brain so that these crises don't cause further harm to it. What this means is that just as we have an innate drive to preserve the baby birds of the world, our body doesn't want our brain to fall out of the nest and get injured like a baby bird. Our body doesn't want to see our brain wasted, discarded, or compromised. So many of our body's functions are to preserve our brain. With a healthy brain, we have the power to take care of our body and support these functions. If our brain gets wasted, we lose the ability to take care of our body and the rest of the world.

Most of us live our lives disconnected from what our brains and bodies need. That's because most of us are unaware of what our brains and bodies really do need. We may be aware of what our responsibilities are, what others need, or even what a baby squirrel or baby bird fallen out of its nest may need, what the trees may need, what the oceans may need, what the planet may need. At the same time, that preservation seed that sits inside us gets manipulated when it comes to our everyday mission to look after what our physical brain and body need. Even those who focus a lot of attention on taking care of themselves still aren't taking care of their brains—and are even sabotaging themselves without knowing it.

We have to protect ourselves. When it comes to our health, we can't assume that the sources offering us advice haven't been manipulated and brainwashed. We can't even assume that every advice-giver's intentions are good. Someone may be in touch with their drive to save, or they may not. I will admit that the drive to save doesn't remain in every person, that the instinct hasn't been protected and preserved in everyone. We all know there are bad people in the world, and these people have no interest in protecting us or our brains, only a great agenda to find ways to hurt us and our brains. There are people out there who can make us feel thrown away, discredited, ignored, betrayed. It can be a cruel world, and that cruelty stems from the brain, not the heart. We deserve to be wise to this so we can look out for ourselves and the ones we love.

We already have the innate drive to save precious life. Our liver, our immune system, our adrenals: they already have the innate drive to save our precious brain. The key is to discover the ways we've been misinformed so we can adjust our own actions to align with our body's mission. Along with saving our family or an animal or ocean life or the world, we're trying to save our brain. Because only when we join forces with our body's mission to protect our brain do we have the potential to save all the lives we want to protect—including our own.

YOUR BRAIN IS WAITING

It's also critical to decipher what we shouldn't save—what misinformation we can let go of—as well as what wisdom we may be throwing away that we shouldn't. In our busy and overcrowded lives in a pick-and-choose, take-it-or-leave-it society, sometimes we throw away the most valuable information that's ever come our way. We can unknowingly toss out the most beneficial advice we've received while saving the most unproductive.

None of us wants to miss out on what could actually save us. We can't *afford* to miss out. So we need clarity to make the best choices for our health. Whatever your background, whatever your perspective, this book is here to show you how to heal, protect your life, and save your brain so you can live your best, most purposeful life.

Your brain has abilities to heal beyond what medical research and science are aware of today. Your brain is waiting for you to discover its need to remove foreign invaders such as industry-created pathogens and toxins that have entered your brain. Your brain is waiting for you to access information that's above a mostly corrupted medical industry that benefits from keeping your brain dumbed down and sick. Meanwhile other industries that are responsible for these circumstances where brain betrayers enter and sicken the brain remain protected. The industries of the world that poison our brains and bodies have no soul. Your brain has a soul—and that means anything is possible when it comes to healing and saving your life.

YOU ARE THE POWER

You're not lost anymore. You're not stranded and alone in the wilderness, abandoned by the theories and opinions you picked up along the way that you thought would be there for you. As brain-related chronic illness keeps rising exponentially, faster than at any time in history, you can become empowered with knowledge to defend yourself—to take yourself out of that rising tide of neurological symptoms, conditions, illnesses, and diseases. You can experience the peace of not becoming a statistic in the coming days.

Here in these words, you join a healing movement—a community all over the world of millions of people who are using Medical Medium information to get their lives back. This guidebook is your story of survival—your story of discovering what was wrong all along, and how to free yourself from it. It is your story of relief, healing, and triumph. These living words will always be here for you, for the rest of your life.

You are the power behind this movement. And your story of healing is the story of saving others' lives. When you save yourself, you become a trusted guide for your children, your family, your friends, and anyone who hears your story. Whether or not you ever find out how many people you've helped, know that your healing holds tremendous meaning.

Our greatest line of defense against threats to our brain and neurological health is our brain itself. Using our own brain to acquire knowledge ahead of medical research and science, we can rise above chronic suffering and take back our power.

CHAPTER 2

Your Static Brain

When we talk about the brain, we often simply call it "the brain." We see it as a round, singular organ. In our daily lives, we refer to the brain like this all the time.

"My brain's not working."

"What's wrong with your brain?"

"What do you have, half a brain?"

"I'm having a brain fart."

"I've got brain freeze."

"Nice going, brainiac."

"Do you *have* a brain?"

We get disconnected from our brain. We see the brain as a single, isolated unit.

Sometimes we get even more disconnected, referring to our brain as our "head." When someone is dealing with emotional or physical problems, we may ask, "What kind of headspace are you in today?" or "How's your head?"

Really we should be asking, "How are your neurons doing today?" If we addressed our heads and brains like that, we'd have a new understanding of what goes on inside them. Rather than seeing our brain as a single, isolated lump of gray matter, a better way to view our brain is as a group of neurons—because the truth is, the brain is a complex organ containing billions of neurons. Even if we called the brain *a* neuron, we'd have a better grasp of how to protect it and at the same time, a better understanding of what goes wrong with it.

"What do you mean, my neurons?" is likely the response you'd get from someone if you asked how their neurons were doing. "It's really just my head that's bothering me." That's because we aren't taught to be in touch with our neurons or central nervous system.

If we were taught, we'd understand the truth that so many of the challenges we face in our health are about our neurons having problems, whether from deficiencies of nutrients and other critical supplies; or from contamination by toxic heavy metals, other contaminants, or viral toxins and poisons; or from neuron damage caused by the electrical heat and intense adrenaline of fight-or-flight or emotional injuries.

When someone sees a psychiatrist or therapist for emotional or mental support, neurons tend to be the last thing either the professional or person seeking help thinks about. Meanwhile, neurons have everything to do with why the person sought help in the first place. Again, seeing the brain as a group of neurons, or even a single neuron, is still better than seeing the brain as "the brain." That's because for the most part, *brain* is a mystery word. It keeps us far away from our problems within the brain itself. It keeps us from looking deeper inside.

It is known that the brain can be injured in hundreds of physical ways, yet in the end, they're all lumped together as "brain injury." Then there's brain injury caused by emotional or mental abuse or trauma, or by hardship that affects us emotionally. The field of neuroscience is only beginning to acknowledge this on an elementary level, much less understand it. Even if all types of brain injury were understood, you'd still see a tendency among us to keep a distance from what's really happening inside the brain. We often don't go there or feel a need to go there. This keeps us from learning what really goes wrong and how to heal the brain or protect it in the first place.

There's a classified goal to keep us disconnected from our brain, or what's within our brain. We're in a time in history where we're brainwashed like never before. The industries want us to be disconnected from the reality of what's happening inside our brains. If we just point to our head and say we're having a problem in there, the industries revel in that—because knowing more than this would mean getting closer to the truth of industrial wrongdoing, both in the medical world and other industries. It's best

for the classified medical industry (a covert medical entity to which your doctors and their medical communities aren't privy) to keep experts in the publicly known medical industry (the medical establishment we all know about) in the dark, just like it's best to keep the people suffering with brain issues in the dark. It keeps us at a distance from what's really happening, and why.

Knowing that your condition or symptom even *is* brain-related to begin with, and understanding how that relates to the rest of your nervous system—these are critical and often missing pieces in how we think about our health. When you understand your brain as a group of neurons, you have a greater chance of finding relief from your brain-related symptoms and conditions, healing your brain, and getting in touch with your brain on all kinds of levels.

A NETWORK OF NEURONS

When it comes to your brain, neurons mean practically everything. Healing brain-related symptoms and conditions—whether those symptoms and conditions are traditionally associated with the brain or not—critically depends on understanding the neurons that reside inside it.

Neurons (a type of nerve tissue) are the means by which communication occurs in your nervous system, enabling it to send and receive messages. Neurons are about input and output.

Neurons are your transcribers. Imagine billions of tiny people inside your brain, each sitting at a desk in front of a computer, translating information that's coming in through your ears or eyes or other senses (such as smell, taste, or touch) and trying to decipher it. The neuron transcribers' job is to make sense out of what you're experiencing and then pass that along to the next tiny neuron person inside your brain. The hope is that (a) the information travels uninterrupted to that next transcriber (neuron) and (b) that next transcriber (neuron) takes the information that was just deciphered, keeps it in purified form and possibly adds an addendum that's efficient and accurate, and prepares it for the next tiny person (neuron) inside your brain to receive.

You can even imagine your brain as a tiny spaceship flying through the universe. Your neurons are billions of tiny aliens inside that spaceship, all communicating together. At the same time, there's a supreme being on the ship watching all of it—that's your soul.

Your sensory input isn't the only information your neurons decipher and pass along. They also translate information about your body processes. Neurons apply to every single function your body has, and how healthy your neurons are determines how comfortable you're going to be in your mind and body. That is, neurons are involved in both mental functioning and your state of health. When you have brain-related symptoms even on the mildest scale, such as mild fatigue and mild brain fog, it's really because neurons can't transfer information properly to the next group of neurons. Something is hindering the pathway where the electricity

is traveling. Something is blocking or otherwise impeding the pathway within the synapses, so the neurons sending out electrical impulses are not reaching other neurons that need the information—or not reaching the neurons as intended.

You can see this in everyday life when you're telling someone a story about apples and find out that the whole time, they thought you were talking about oranges. Any kind of impediment within a person's neurons can mean that the information their neurons process gets altered, affecting that person's ability to focus, listen, or properly receive information from a conversation or story. Then that person may tell someone else an entirely different version of the original story that was told to them. This is how gossip and rumors can be twisted and turned into hearsay. As the story goes from person to person, it goes through each person's contaminated, impeded, blocked, or diminished neurons, and the story changes.

SCATTERED BRAINS

As electricity travels through an impeded neuron system, it can become diminished—meaning that electricity within the brain is no longer traveling at its full capacity. That is, a group of neurons can receive a fully charged electrical impulse, and then in the process of assimilating and registering that electricity—which is filled with information—and sending it through the synapses to another group of neurons, the electricity can be diminished. When electricity is diminished, the information within it can be skewed, changed, and altered.

Information within electricity is something that's mysterious and not understood. The truth is that electricity isn't just electricity traveling through the brain. It's information traveling *within* the electricity, kind of like how we use technology today. A thought is not just something that resides within the neurons and glial cells—the brain tissue—and stays there. A thought can travel within the electricity that leaves a neuron. Electricity can carry tremendous amounts of information—so the electricity running through the brain is more than just a hot wire.

Electricity traveling through your brain can even carry information you won't or don't use. It's there for the taking within the electricity, and we let it slip by because we're focused on another piece within that information. We're trying to tell someone something that we're getting from that electricity, and at the same time leaving out information that's within that electricity as well. We may feel there was something more to say, yet we don't know what it really was because it has already passed us by. Our companion may say, "Were you going to say something else?" and we may reply, "Yeah. I was so busy with other thoughts, I can't remember what it was." We're not having a memory lapse. It's information that slipped by inside our brain's electrical grid that we didn't access.

Damaged neurons can change thoughts, altering how someone perceives information. That's because damaged neurons mean altered, disorganized, and poorly reorganized electricity. As that electricity travels through synapses and heads to another group of neurons, information in that electricity could become disorganized before it enters the new group of neurons. And if any of the neurons in that new group are damaged, hindered, or injured, then the information gathered by that electricity gets disorganized once again as it leaves that group of neurons. It has already changed before it heads to another group of neurons. So it's not just brain tissue that harbors thoughts and controls how we feel and how we physically function. Electricity itself also has power over our thoughts and physical control.

One job of neurons is to eventually pass along information to the brain's billions of glial cells, where information stays stored, cataloged, and organized. If glial cells are clogged, contaminated, saturated, distorted, or even mutated from poisons and toxins, a disconnect and breakdown can occur between your neuron system and your glial cell system. Glial cells can lose their ability to properly store information.

Some neurons in the brain, not all, have the ability to spot-check and cross-reference new information with old information. When healthy, these neurons have infinite access to glial cell storage—that is, storage bins of old information from the past, even from before neurons became damaged. Electricity shoots out in waves from these neurons, rolling along glial cells to gather information, and then the electricity filled with glial cell information rolls back to the neurons.

When electricity hits a *damaged* neuron, on the other hand, small outward explosions occur off the neuron, kind of like solar flares off the sun. These flares enter adjacent brain tissue and glial cells, gathering bits and pieces of information, and then subside and reenter the neuron with that disorganized information to try to cross-reference and reorganize. Since the neuron is already hindered—damaged or compromised in some way—it doesn't have the full capability to piece together the scattered information. Disorganized information ends up traveling from damaged neuron to damaged neuron.

The reason we can each experience the same event so differently from each other is because of our damaged neurons leading to disorganized information. In the end, we may not all give an accurate account of what happened. Say we were camping out by a lake with friends and a flashing light flew through the sky. One person may say, "I was there, and it was a firefly." Someone else may say, "I was there too. It was a falling star." Someone else believed it was a distant headlight from a truck farther off toward the horizon.

This understanding of our neurons' impeded functioning is why when we ask if someone's feeling okay, we should really ask, "How's the electricity in your brain? Is it disorganized? How are the neurons today? Have any of them repaired from your night's sleep? Have your glial cells been heating up too much? Are your neurons saturated in toxins today?" Communicating about our brains at this level would bring about

a whole new understanding of our health conditions and well-being.

INTERPRETING THE STATIC

If a neuron is contaminated with a toxic substance, or impeded because it's injured or damaged in any way, then information traveling on electrical impulses across that neuron is going to reflect that contamination or damage. With this said, neurons do adapt and compensate for each other. So even if there's contamination in a group of neurons and they're having difficulty functioning, other neurons will try to take on the load for as long as they can.

When information reaches a group of healthy neurons from a group of contaminated neurons through electricity, the healthy neurons can interpret and reorganize the state of that information, affecting its outcome in a more productive, conductive, and accurate way. It's like the healthy neurons have to translate the information coming through as best they can—take the good and try to rebuild the message that was practically lost from the last group of neurons that was contaminated. This is why someone can seem as if they're struggling while they try to focus and speak in order to deliver information.

The electricity coming from damaged or contaminated neurons carries what's basically a message of static. It brings us back to the image of your neurons as tiny transcribers. Imagine those neuron transcribers sitting there with tiny headphones, straining to hear through static and type out the message correctly to pass it along. What they're really getting in the static are fragments of information that they have to interpret and piece together as best they can. Those healthy neurons have to compensate for the damaged neurons that released skewed information into the electricity.

When the neurons get damaged and contaminated more and more over time, this compensating backup power is no longer enough. We end up with fewer healthy neurons to do the work of interpreting and reorganizing. Eventually, symptoms appear. Focus and concentration issues, depression, anxiety, memory loss, or emotional struggles, to name just a few, may start to surface. Physical conditions can start to make themselves known too, including weakness of the limbs, body pain, migraines, and vision issues. Neuron damage and contamination can affect even our most basic level of communication, making it a struggle both to process information we receive from others and to verbally pass along information.

HOW WE CARE FOR OUR BRAIN

As we've covered, neurons mean everything. So how we treat our neurons and take care of them should be everyone's concern.

Doing things that are "good for our brain" is too vague. Taking a "brain supplement": that's supplement creators playing guessing games, whether with alternative or conventional theories, and it's not an answer to how we can heal real problems. It's not providing the true cause of the problem and what to do to heal it. Taking something "for our brain" is too broad and too disconnected from what the real problems within our brains are.

Which brings us to a tricky area. Medical Medium information about what's going on in our brains has already been circulating in the world. There are opportunists who sell products with ingredients that do not help the brain, yet on the labels, they tag their products as "for toxic heavy metals" or "for brain health" or "for memory health." This marketing takes advantage of Medical Medium awareness about what's wrong with our brains, while the products themselves only offer guessing games and theories so that a buck can be made.

If we really understood what was wrong with our brains and what caused our conditions related to the brain, and realized how many of our chronic symptoms and conditions were actually related to the brain, the game would change. It would no longer be "Take this for your brain." It would be "Your neurons that are damaged by toxic heavy metals, caffeine, solvents, fragrances, perfumes, colognes, air fresheners, scented candles, MSG, DDT, petrochemicals, radiation, and plastic, to name a few, could really use this so they can cleanse, restore, revitalize, and store up reserves."

EXHAUSTING OUR RESERVES WITH BRAIN HACKS

Misunderstanding the brain's needs doesn't stop at trick supplements. Everybody's an expert these days in brain hacks. It's often about how to master our mind. It's often about how we trick our thoughts and perceptions, trying to better our lives with how we think. Some of these strategies are positive and can be very helpful temporary stitches for patching up some emotional and physical conditions in some situations. They still don't get to the root cause of why we're struggling.

With these thought techniques, we may overcompensate to the point that we exhaust ourselves. We try so hard to control our thought patterns, to keep positive thoughts, to create new references, to focus on confidence builders, positive thinking, awareness, new thoughts about how we feel about our lives. And we find that we're still struggling with our problems, because no one has shown us the roots of the problems and how to fix the real, physical issues in our brains and nervous systems. All our energy goes into trying to correct and battle our minds by doing everything we can to make ourselves better people spiritually, emotionally, and mentally.

The reason why everyone falls back into old patterns no matter how many courses, classes, or lectures they attend, or how many programs they apply themselves to—the real reason why they're back struggling with their OCD, depression, anxiety, or other symptoms and conditions—is that the real

problems are never discovered. Those real problems have everything to do with neurons that are contaminated or damaged.

Take brain fog, for example. We often don't think of this as a physical symptom. We feel like our inability to focus is our fault, our own mental shortcoming, one we can overcome if only we apply ourselves better. In reality brain fog is a physical symptom of impeded neurons. If we address the physical factors that lead to brain fog, we can alleviate the brain fog and find our way again, without ever having to battle and interrogate ourselves about our inadequacies. We were never inadequate. We were up against tremendous physical challenges that we didn't even know were there.

When we're hurting or sick or struggling, it absorbs us. It takes every ounce of energy we have to sustain ourselves and focus on getting through the day. It takes every reserve. Finding spare reserves for mental methods is really hard to sustain. Symptoms dominate very easily as soon as they start to impede your quality of life and your everyday function. When the brain hacks we've learned about don't hold up because our neuron issues (that we don't realize are neuron issues) are still boiling up, we may feel like all the work we've done was wasted. It takes so much energy, fortitude, and mental strength to do emotional, mental, and spiritual self-work and self-help—especially when we have to overcompensate for a struggling brain and nervous system. As soon as we're triggered again, if the original, underlying problem hasn't been fixed, we can think, *Well, here we go again.* Some brain quick fixes are really helpful for this, because we can learn to access them in these moments when the physical problems in our brains are triggered and erupting again. We can access some of these self-help thought-mastering techniques, and emotional and mental approaches to how we perceive our thoughts, to get us through for a little while.

Still, if our real, physical issues aren't fixed or addressed or worked on, we fall right back into our old patterns again. This is especially true as we're aging or becoming sick, when the energy to try to better ourselves drops, so the patterns can come back or get worse. Any kind of brain or thought "mastering" only lasts so long. The minute we drop our guard, old patterns take over, and we're back in the same thought process, or we're physically or mentally receiving the same symptoms, and now we're back to trying to relearn everything we thought we already learned about how to keep stable within our mind and physical body. People get worn down over time when the original problem isn't fixed deep down inside. It gets tiresome and tiring to have to keep on battling the physical through self-help and positive thought building.

With these techniques alone, it becomes a lifelong struggle of wavering back and forth, falling back into the same pattern and then trying to correct our thoughts—which leads to the teaching that we're faulty. We can't seem to create or manifest what we need or want. We're not as perfected as somebody else who seems to know how to correct and level their thoughts and mind—which really

means someone who doesn't have hidden physical issues inside their neurons, or another issue inside their brain or nervous system. We end up in a place of feeling easily defeated. We don't understand the real, true causes of why we're struggling and they're not, or don't seem to be.

If we play a game of "Our problems are caused by our inability to better ourselves through our thoughts"—or through strengthening our consciousness, through techniques and hacks, through self-help gurus—we fail at trying to succeed. Then it falls on us that we're not good enough to apply the information. That we're not capable of hacking our problems by using information from experts who seem like they have all the answers to how we should perceive our lives, our thoughts, and our own mind control. We get set up for failure because the experts don't know our neurons are hindered through contamination by toxic substances, they don't know what this does to the electricity and information traveling through our brains and nervous systems, and they don't know the real answers for what to do about it.

TRUE BRAIN HEALING

Applying techniques and wisdom from experts as to how we should perceive, think, or retrain our minds is perfectly fine if we're aware of the real problems happening within our brains. With this awareness, we can see we're focused on two pursuits: (1) working on the true cause of what's really happening and why we're struggling, and at the same time (2) indulging in hacks we pick up from brain or thought experts to keep us occupied while we're fixing the real problems. As we heal the deeper issues within our brain, anything is possible in terms of how we shape our thoughts.

When someone is limiting their exposure to the brain betrayer toxins and contaminants we're all up against every day, which you'll read about in Part III, "Brain Betrayers," they're addressing the real problems in their brain and nervous system.

When someone is bringing the fruits, leafy greens, herbs, wild foods, and vegetables from Chapter 41, "Brain Cell Food and Filler Food," into their diets—and at the same time taking out the brain betrayer foods and supplements from Chapter 30, "Brain Betrayer Foods," Chapter 29, "Brain Betrayer Supplements," and Chapter 28, "Brain Betrayer Food and Supplement Chemicals"—they're addressing the real problems.

When someone is bringing the Brain Saver Recipes from this book's companion, *Brain Saver Protocols, Cleanses & Recipes*, into their lives, they're addressing the real problems.

When someone is applying the Medical Medium Heavy Metal Detox protocols from Chapter 45—which address brain betrayer toxins beyond toxic heavy metals too—they're addressing the real problems.

When someone is incorporating Medical Medium Brain Shot Therapy from Chapter 42, or following the Medical Medium guidance for celery juice in Chapter 44, or one of

the Medical Medium Shock Therapies from *Brain Saver Protocols, Cleanses & Recipes*, they're addressing the real problems.

When someone is following a Medical Medium–recommended supplement protocol from "Supplement Gospel" in *Brain Saver Protocols, Cleanses & Recipes*, they're addressing the real problems.

When someone is doing a Heavy Metal Detox Cleanse from Chapter 45, a Brain Shot Therapy Cleanse from Chapter 43, or any other Medical Medium cleanse from this book series, they're addressing the real problems.

These are the steps that physically heal what's really going on at a cell and neuron level inside our brains and nervous systems.

Physically healing on that level allows us to go and play with thought work, if we want. If we get confused, and we think it's the other way around—that thought work is the foundation of what heals us physically— we should ask ourselves: Do we want to play around with mind games, or do we want to get better?

From the time I started out, some of the most spiritual people possible, masters of the best thought and meditation techniques, were reaching out to me because they were still sick. Take the Medical Medium book series out of the equation, remove 30-plus years of Medical Medium teaching and lectures, and the health world would look very different from what it looks like today. We would be right back where we were: very few people getting a chance to stumble across the true causes of their brain and nervous system issues and the answers of how to heal. You would come down with chronic illness, struggle with no hope, and watch others with similar conditions stay sick and struggle too instead of seeing miraculous healing progress. Back then, all many had to rely on was, "Can we fix all of this with our thoughts, surgery, or medication? How about bean sprouts, wheatgrass, almonds, molasses, brown rice syrup, carrot juice, and multivitamins? What about removing processed foods?" Medical Medium protocols provide the deeper physical healing our brains so desperately need if we want to advance on any level.

In the chapters that follow, you'll come to know your brain like never before. Just what is contaminating, damaging, injuring, impeding, depriving, burning out, and limiting our neurons, how does it get there, and how does that explain our individual experiences and struggles? Just what is inflaming, scarring, and atrophying our brains, and how does that threaten our well-being? It will all become clear as we take a closer look inside the brain and nervous system. With this knowledge, you can find relief like never before.

You are not faulty or weak. You did not bring your struggles upon yourself. You did not create or manifest or attract your symptoms and conditions. You've been lost and stranded through no fault of your own. You've been lost and stranded because keeping you that way serves agendas—classified agendas that don't serve you or your family. Now let's get you the answers you deserve.

"Imagine flying in a plane at night, about to land in a big city, and looking down at the entire electrically active urban grid below. Picture the twinkling lights laid out in a complex system spread out over miles and miles. That's basic compared to what's happening in your brain electrically."

— Anthony William, Medical Medium

CHAPTER 3

Your Alloy Brain

Everyone here on Planet Earth has struggled with some sort of mental battle. With each of us unique in nature, it varies from individual to individual. Many people feel they bring it upon themselves, that they create their mental trials. Others feel it comes from external problems and decisions placed upon them. Some seek out therapy and find a good counselor. No matter what, going through life has never been easy for anyone. People from all walks of life struggle with their minds, if not on a minute-by-minute, hourly, or daily basis, then definitely in waves or stretches of intense moments.

So we already have that going on here as human beings: our basic battle to survive. Life is more than hard enough.

What happens if something else gets thrown in our way, an obstacle that doesn't need to be there, something you can't even see with the eye, a sinister, hidden problem no one knows about that's in the mix?

THE BATTLE IN OUR BRAINS

Your brain is electricity. The electricity created in your brain exists through a combination of two supernatural forces (one receiving power from the ether and the other receiving power from your soul) plus a physical component (your heart's and brain's programming to thrive since your inception of life). This is the foundational basis of your brain's life force and how it runs.

From early experiments with electricity—remember the key and kite from history—to the most advanced technology we have today, there's a common thread: metal. In micro levels in the tiniest computer chips and in macro levels at power plants, when it comes to electrical energy, we've learned to employ metal. Metal is used to deliver and carry electricity, to manipulate electrical currents, to pull electricity, to push it. Metal can short a circuit, put a damper on one, shift electricity, alter it, and even destroy, project, or catapult a current, in so many ways not yet discovered by science.

We're still learning how to play with metals in order to advance technology. Metals are profoundly connected to society.

Now, if your brain is full of electrical currents, what must be involved? Metals. That's right—our brains are largely about metals *and* electricity. It's critical to understand this. Here's the kicker: there are both bad metals and good metals at work.

On the one hand, our brains can harbor mercury, lead, arsenic, cadmium, barium, nickel, aluminum, toxic calcium, toxic copper, toxic chromium, tin, and more. These are the bad, industrialized, toxic metals.

On the other hand, not all metals in the brain are bad or unproductive. We rely on some critically important metals in our brains: trace minerals. These good metals include beneficial, non-industrialized forms of gold, calcium, copper, potassium, magnesium, chromium, palladium, vanadium, and more. One reason beneficial metals are there is to control electrical currents.

Rogue toxic heavy metals residing in the brain with the good metals wreak havoc—they create a battle in our brains. Living metal against dead metal, life-giving metal versus life-taking metal, good versus evil: it's a *physical* battle going on inside our brain, on top of the battle of life on this planet. It's the problem that was never meant to be there.

Before we go further, it's important to establish what I mean when I use the term *toxic heavy metals*. There are density and atomic weight classifications for metals that lead some metals to be classified as "heavy" metals and others as "light"

metals. These classifications aren't oriented around the metals' toxic effects inside the brain and body. They don't tell us whether a metal taking up residence inside us will wreak havoc, causing symptoms, conditions, and diseases. That's why for decades, Medical Medium information has redefined "toxic heavy metals," classifying any and all industrialized, toxic metals that take up residence inside the brain and body as toxic *heavy* metals—because the damage any toxic metal creates has heavy consequences in people's lives.

Aluminum, for example, which is a "light" metal, is considered nontoxic by medical and other industries because it's not in the heavy metal classification. In truth, aluminum is neurotoxic and damaging to the brain—so it's toxic and has heavy consequences. That's why I call it a toxic heavy metal.

This awareness is critical. People already don't take toxic heavy metals seriously enough. Calling some metals "toxic light metals" would delude people into thinking they're not really a threat, when indeed, any toxic metals, "heavy" or "light," are a great threat, bringing misery upon humankind, with industries not taking responsibility.

Trace minerals are life-giving. They're part of how our bodies are created. Toxic heavy metals are life-taking. They're part of how our bodies rapidly age and degenerate. Good metals, in mineral form—trace minerals—contain information that comes from life sources of the planet and also life forces outside the planet, from the solar system and galaxy. The planet is living. It's alive, it's breathing. Minerals and trace minerals are periodically falling through the planet's atmosphere. These minerals play an integral role with the mineral salts in our brain and the sugar that carries minerals and electrolytes to our brain. Electricity in our brain is reliant on trace minerals as fuel. Toxic heavy metals, meanwhile, can weaken, burn out, short out, twist out, interfere with, toxify, and denature our brain's natural electrical currents, currents that allow us to think, feel, and function optimally. As metals are unearthed to be used for industries, they're restructured and changed through the industrial process, which denatures the metals, turning them against the human body. People with low trace minerals and higher toxic metals in the brain can get emotionally triggered or literally burnt out from stress very easily, which you'll read about in Chapter 7, "Your Burnt Out, Deficient Brain."

Toxic heavy metals are elusive. They're quiet—they don't make any noise—you can't see them, you can't hear them, you certainly can't touch them. Although you can detect traces of toxic heavy metals in the bloodstream if exposure was recent, you can't detect traces of toxic heavy metals in the tissue, organs, glands, and bones, where toxic metals settle indefinitely. (Most people think bones are impermeable. Many don't realize bones are porous and highly absorbent. Metals, chemicals, and pathogens can enter bones easily.) Yet the presence of toxic heavy metals is extremely dominating and extremely controlling physically, mentally, and emotionally—and because of this, toxic heavy metals are mind-altering. In many people toxic metals

rule the roost. They control someone's life. They can disempower a person, make decisions for them, by getting in the way of clear thinking. Why are toxic heavy metals so problematic? Because they are constantly interfering with electricity, which means they are constantly interfering with your brain's receiving of and communicating information. Classified medical science relies on us being exposed to toxic heavy metals to create and perpetuate a form of mind control.

For example, when any toxic heavy metal lands in an area of the brain tied to language or communication, we run into developmental language issues, communication and conversation issues, language phobias, speaking phobias, Tourette's, or an inability to speak. This can also limit someone's ability to learn another language. It's not that the person who can speak five languages fluently is smarter than the person who has great difficulty picking up a second language; it's toxic heavy metals dampening electrical signals that makes it hard for a single-language speaker to branch out. Social anxiety—for example, extra nervousness and sweating around others, or feeling like you can't carry on a conversation—can also result from toxic heavy metals affecting communication. These examples are just the beginning of how toxic heavy metals inside the brain can affect us.

On top of all the other negative effects of toxic heavy metals that you'll read about in this book, toxic heavy metals are brain inhibitors in several ways. Toxic heavy metals are *brain enzyme inhibitors*. (Your liver produces brain enzymes specifically for the purpose of communication, both for receiving and expressing information. These enzymes cling to neurotransmitters and act as tiny antennae for projecting information from neurotransmitters. Toxic heavy metals inhibit these enzymes.) Toxic heavy metals are *brain amino acid inhibitors*; toxic heavy metals destroy taurine, choline, and glutamine. Toxic heavy metals are *brain protein inhibitors*—not the proteins you consume in foods, but the proteins your liver produces specifically for your brain. Toxic heavy metals entering into your hypothalamus or pituitary gland create toxic heavy metal alloys inside these glands that become *hormone inhibitors*, slowing down hormone production in the glands.

Have you ever heard, if you were angry at someone, that the longer you stayed angry, the longer that person was living inside your head rent-free? When that happens, at least you know you were betrayed. There's some control in knowing an emotion is taking up mental space and how it got there. Toxic heavy metals, on the other hand, are living inside our heads rent-free—wreaking havoc there—and we don't even know they're present. If we don't know toxic heavy metals are in our way, how can we handle them? Hundreds of illnesses and hundreds of symptoms are caused by toxic heavy metals, and the publicly known medical industry is unaware of this. With all we have on our plates, all the adversity we're already faced with, we don't need these hidden stumbling blocks tripping us up.

One step to moving them out of our way is to see toxic heavy metals for what they are, right here and right now.

HOW METALS FIND US

Exposure to toxic heavy metals is all around us. We're not taught about it, so we don't learn to recognize our sources of exposure. They're much closer than we think. Toxic heavy metals have plenty of avenues to enter our bodies, from toxic heavy metals that we breathe, to toxic heavy metals that we eat, to toxic heavy metals that we drink, to toxic heavy metals that we bathe in, to toxic heavy metals that we touch or apply to our skin.

That's right—simply touching aluminum foil or a battery can be enough for their minute particles of metal to leach into our bloodstream. And that's not to mention the metal particles we can ingest from food prepared in certain metal cookware, or food and drink served in metal containers. Toxic heavy metals can be in our indoor and outdoor air, especially if we're in the presence of toxic fragrances, scented candles, air fresheners, pesticides, or chem trails. We even unknowingly put toxic heavy metals directly into and onto our bodies with certain cosmetics, pharmaceuticals, beverages, and other products. You'll find extensive details about these and many more sources of exposure to toxic heavy metals in Chapter 20, "Toxic Heavy Metals."

We are getting toxic heavy metal exposure at a minuscule level on a continual basis. It's not like we're drinking a gallon of leaded gasoline and then ending up in the hospital with lead poisoning. Instead, we're getting exposed to small amounts of tiny, beyond-microscopic metal particles, and we're getting these exposures repeatedly in our everyday lives. A little bit here, a little bit there. You might look at a single exposure and think, *No big deal,* just like people will often think a microdose of psychedelic drugs is no big deal because of the trendy advice about "everything in moderation." We're getting poisoned with toxic heavy metals "in moderation," and that may not seem significant until you step back and look at the bigger picture. Repeated exposure adds up. At a certain point, the toxic heavy metals in our brain and body accumulate, until we reach a large poisoning at some point later in life—although we still won't know it's toxic heavy metal poisoning. We'll get older, reach an expiration date where everything goes wrong from collecting so many toxic heavy metals inside our brain, and we'll never know what did it.

YOUR BRAIN'S MAGNETIC FIELD

Once they've found their way into your bloodstream and body, how do toxic heavy metals find your brain? Metals don't just end up there by chance. Rather, when metals in your system travel through your bloodstream to your brain—when metals reach the capillaries and other blood vessels that are intertwined with and feed your brain—your brain actually draws in the metals across the blood-brain barrier. (And even when toxic heavy metals aren't pulled in across the blood-brain barrier, their presence in the brain is problematic.) Toxic heavy metal particles are so tiny that it doesn't take much to

draw them into your brain, and the tinier the particle, the easier it is for the metal to cross the blood-brain barrier into brain cells and brain tissue. These toxic heavy metals end up finding their way into your brain's sanctuary of protection, congregating in critical, protected parts of your brain that house neurons that are critical to your health and well-being.

Why do the metals even enter your bloodstream, and why does your brain draw metals in from your bloodstream? Let's establish a little background. Your liver is meant to be a filter for your body. Yet with everything the liver is up against with modern exposures and modern diets, the liver very commonly becomes stagnant, sluggish, clogged up, and dysfunctional. Many toxins, including toxic heavy metals, that should have been trapped in your liver instead continue on through your bloodstream and can end up entering your brain. Your brain becomes a filter when it was never supposed to be.

Toxic heavy metals residing in your liver can also oxidize there and discharge, and this oxidative toxic heavy metal discharge material can break free and enter your bloodstream, and in this way eventually enter your brain. This toxic heavy metal discharge runoff, like toxic heavy metal particles themselves, can cross the blood-brain barrier. You'll read more about the blood-brain barrier in Part III, "Brain Betrayers."

Some toxins remain passersby in the bloodstream, entering the brain and then leaving the brain. Toxic heavy metals are one variety of toxins, of many, that never leave the brain. Whether the liver is stagnant and sluggish or not, metals can end up traveling to the brain—where they end up being magnetically drawn in. The electricity of your brain acts as a magnetic field, attracting metals into it. Does this mean your brain is working against you? That you can't trust it? Absolutely not. Your brain, like the rest of your body, is always looking out for you. Your brain's electromagnetic field is intended for a productive purpose: the incredible ability to draw in trace minerals and electrolytes—to serve you.

Because of the contaminated environment we live in on this planet created by the chemical and pharmaceutical industries, and the contaminated environment this creates in our body, the brain is up against more than it should be. Our brains were never supposed to deal with a daily onslaught of chemical warfare. We aren't meant to encounter industry-designed, seemingly good-for-us toxic substances at every turn. And yet we do, at a rate that's accelerating every year. So, as a side effect of your brain's miraculous skill at pulling in life-giving nutrients such as trace minerals, it also ends up magnetically pulling in toxic heavy metals.

Let's be clear that your brain's electromagnetic pull applies whether we'd classify a metal as magnetic or not. Just because nickel has a strong magnetic quality, for example, does not mean that it gets drawn into the brain more than copper, which isn't really considered magnetic. Copper and aluminum can be drawn into brain tissue through the brain's electromagnetic

field just as strongly as nickel, steel, and iron. It doesn't matter if outside the body, the metal would stick to a magnet or not. It doesn't matter what type or variety of metal it is, whether toxic metal or nontoxic mineral. With the brain's magnetism, we are talking about a force—an electrical force in the brain creating a magnetic field that attracts all minerals and metals.

When deposits of toxic heavy metals build up inside brain tissue, the brain has an even larger and stronger magnetic pull toward toxic heavy metals. That's because more electricity gets funneled into brain tissue that's saturated with metals—and more electricity in the brain creates a larger and stronger electromagnetic pull. This supernatural design was intended for trace minerals only. Our brain's supernatural electromagnetic force was meant for humankind on an industry-free planet. It was intended for attracting and igniting trace minerals with electricity to raise the intelligence of the human brain. Instead, electricity gets funneled into the industrialized toxic heavy metal deposits in our brain, in turn creating more magnetism to attract more toxic heavy metals to those existing toxic heavy metal deposits. It's an unfortunate truth of how we end up suffering.

WHAT NO ONE KNOWS

Toxic heavy metals are the shadow we can't see until they create disease—although even then, we still can't see them; we can only see the disease. In other words, we can't see the metals when they create a symptom. We can only see the symptom or the symptom's effects. Along the way, maybe we can sense a presence, because when we're not well, we can often sense there's something wrong. If we get a name for our symptom or condition, we may still doubt ourselves and our intuition about what's really causing it. If we don't get a name for it, we can doubt ourselves even more.

Toxic heavy metals are there. They're in all of our lives, from development in the womb through childhood through adulthood. We carry around these toxic heavy metals from birth for the duration of our lives, acquiring more along the way, and no one says a word about it because in the publicly known medical arena, no one knows they're wreaking havoc in our brains and bodies.

Not that the medical industry is entirely unaware that toxic heavy metals are, indeed, toxic. While it took a long time for anyone to figure out that lead wasn't good for us, or that we shouldn't be rolling balls of mercury around in our hands, the realizations did eventually surface. Lead poisoning at a high level is an obvious form of toxic heavy metal poisoning that hurts us neurologically, basically flatlining the central nervous system. We've been poisoned enough by it over the years that light has been shed upon it. We gained awareness that we needed to protect children from ingesting lead paint chips and that we needed to keep lead out of our water systems.

Wouldn't you think, then, with all the brilliant scientists we have, all the expert lab technicians, all the geniuses in the medical field, that a light bulb would go off in the medical industry that smaller amounts of toxic heavy metals could be a problem in chronic illness? We've completely ignored metals that are present on a small scale when diagnosing chronic illness. Why, with the medical industry, does it tend to be all or nothing? A large amount of lead poisoning or mercury poisoning at once is one of the few ways we view toxic heavy metal poisoning. How is it that with all the brilliant heads of medicine and trillions of dollars that have gone into the medical industry on so-called missions to discover the causes of disease, the medical alarm hasn't been sounded about the toxic heavy metals in pharmaceuticals, medical treatments, common household products, and synthetic chemicals as a source of mental and chronic illness? Instead, it's an all-or-nothing approach: either large amounts of toxic heavy metals are a problem, as in lead or mercury poisoning, or toxic heavy metals couldn't possibly be the problem behind your chronic suffering.

The medical industry that we know about—the public-facing, publicly known medical industry—is *supposed* to be ignorant. It isn't supposed to be thinking about trace amounts of undetectable toxic heavy metals adding up to big problems. Why? Because there's a *classified* medical industry that *is* aware that toxic heavy metals play a major role in symptoms, sickness, and suffering.

The classified medical industry has even brainwashed the publicly known medical industry when it comes to high levels of toxic heavy metals in certain medical treatments. That is to say, the publicly known medical industry is aware of the exceedingly high levels of mercury and aluminum in medical treatments given to babies, children, and adults (including pregnant women). Yet they've been able to pretend this is fine, turning a blind eye to the high levels of mercury and aluminum in certain pharmaceuticals while serving these treatments to the public. That's in part because the publicly known medical industry has been kept from knowing just how extreme the levels of toxic heavy metals in these treatments are. These medical treatments are protected by covenant, an arrangement to protect the classified medical industry that produces certain pharmaceuticals and hands them to the publicly known medical industry, making sure they stay hush-hush as to how much mercury and aluminum they're using. This arrangement is the point of connection between the classified medical industry and the publicly known medical industry, a thread between the two that allows the classified and publicly known sectors to work with each other in a covert way. Otherwise, the classified medical industry and the publicly known medical industry are two different worlds cut off from each other.

Meanwhile, there's still the matter of *trace* amounts of toxic heavy metals adding up in our brains and bodies, which the publicly known industry is kept from realizing and accepting. The publicly known medical industry has to do the bidding of the classified medical industry in certain areas—without even knowing it. Doctors in the publicly known medical industry can go for entire careers without ever being aware there was a classified medical industry stringing them along and influencing their every move.

It serves the classified medical industry's purposes for the publicly known medical industry not to make the connection that one plus one equals two: that because lead, a toxic heavy metal, entering the human body in high amounts causes neurological symptoms, that means we need to look at other toxic heavy metals at all levels and the range of neurological symptoms they cause too—from anxiety to brain fog to Parkinson's to ALS (amyotrophic lateral sclerosis, or Lou Gehrig's disease) to depression to attention-deficit/hyperactivity disorder (ADHD) to autism to bipolar disorder to neurological Lyme disease to memory loss to Alzheimer's and dementia.

If publicly known medicine were to take on this in-depth research—and not get shut down by the classified medical industry in the process—they'd find that deposits of toxic heavy metals in brain tissue (glial cells and neurons), even in the most minute form, create an instant dampening field for electrical activity. It's equivalent to what electrical technicians call *electrical draw*, meaning that power is being drawn away.

If this were the tech world, a troubleshooter would be assigned to solve the mystery. With toxic heavy metals in the brain, there is no troubleshooter in the publicly known medical field who would know (1) which metals are lowering activity, (2) where they're residing in the brain, (3) how to resolve the dampening of electricity inside the brain, or (4) that there's even a problem to begin with. If they took toxic heavy metals more seriously, publicly known medical research and science would at least begin the process of building medical tools to detect toxic heavy metals inside the brain. They would invent an advanced scanning device that searched for weakening of the electrical field inside our brain and smaller blockages caused by toxic heavy metals that could be hindering electrical activity in the brain. They would devise medical tools to identify which varieties of toxic heavy metals are present and how much. Instead, toxic heavy metals draw power away from the electrical impulses that run through our brains with every thought and action, and nobody knows about it. Both conventional and alternative publicly known medicine are completely unaware of it.

From everything you hear out there about the brain, how much does it seem like medicine knows about it at this point? Fifty percent? Seventy-five? Ninety? We can pretend science knows everything about the brain—100 percent. If we do, we're grossly mistaken. The truth is that at this moment in history, science grasps only a tiny fraction of what there is to know about the brain: only 0.00001 percent. That's how vast this organ is, and how much it still has to reveal. The role that toxic heavy metals play exemplifies a vital piece that's missing from today's conception of the brain, a piece of that remaining 99.99999 percent that's not known about the brain—that there still is to learn about it. Identifying glands and different regions

of the brain, estimating how many neurons are in the brain, and charting nerves as they leave the brain stem is not the same as knowing everything about the brain. It's only scratching the surface.

The brain is a miraculous organ that can alter electricity during conflict: when we're up against some kind of stress in life, the brain has the ability to change an electrical pattern to help sustain or even protect us. As amazing as this is, the brain is also limited by what's in its way. When electricity moves through the brain, sometimes at lightning speed, sometimes at a slower rate, it's constantly conflicting with toxic heavy metals that were never meant to be there. The quality of our life greatly depends upon the electrical activity in our brain.

Everyone's brain contains a different amount of toxic heavy metals. Some people are fortunate to be low in a certain metal. Some are burdened with more of a particular metal. Some have two or three toxic heavy metals inside their brain that are dominating over other metals in their brain; some have larger deposits of them all; some have smaller deposits of them all. Every single person has a different alloy mixture of these toxic heavy metals. No one person's alloy brain state is the same. (More on alloys soon.) Toxic heavy metals are positioned uniquely in each individual—everybody has unique blends in unique places. It's a bit like how each person's appendix is a slightly different size and in a slightly different spot. Talk to a surgeon, and you'll hear how when making an abdominal incision, they never know exactly what they're going to see. The appendix could be a little higher, a little lower, a little to the right, a little to the left, a different shape, a different size. They'll at least be in the same general area. With toxic heavy metals in the brain, placement varies much more.

ELECTRICAL HEAT

Our brains have the ability to generate a tremendous amount of heat. This is not to be confused with the heat index of hot coals in a fire, or with a hot stove or oven. It's not like your brain is physically heating up like a 400-degree oven. The kind of heat the brain generates is on a different scale. Advanced technology has not yet been invented to determine the heat scale that the electrical field of the brain creates. This is heat generated by the electrical patterns of the brain inside the human body, not outside the human body. The electrical field in our brain is extremely small and thin. You have to see it on a miniature scale. This is like a flash heat, a quick heat, a heat that happens fast and dies down fast, making it that much harder to detect. It's a heat that isn't supposed to be sustained the way coals in a fire stay hot. This is different. Instead, brain heat is supposed to occur as flash sparks.

When the electrical patterns of the brain create heat, it's an intense heat. The reason it almost instantly cools down and disappears—when everything is as it should be—is that there are three physical safeguards inside our head: (1) space between our skull and brain helps cool the brain; (2) cerebrospinal fluid contains water and magnesium, which act as coolant; (3) glucose in the brain also acts as a coolant. When everything is in good working order and we're giving our brain the supplies it needs, this allows the electrical field in our brain to spark up constantly and cool down just as quickly as it ignites and travels.

At the same time, there's a fourth automatic safeguard in how your brain operates: your brain is constantly shifting gears. Perpetually shifting pathways so that an electrical pattern doesn't stay the same allows a chance for electrical pathways to cool down from those electrical flashes you get when thinking or going about a daily task. You're doing one thing, then another, and the pathway changes continuously, nonstop.

This is why music is critical for factory workers: because if a factory worker is doing the same job for 10 hours straight, the pathway of the electrical pattern is close to the same—and music provides variety, altering the pathways of the electricity in their brains while they're working at repetitive tasks. This isn't known by medical research and science. It's also a method to prevent burnout. It's why people listen to music and podcasts when performing any kind of repetitive work or movement: to keep the electrical patterns in their brains changing, allowing them to keep up the repetition without getting burnt out. Exercise programs also employ the change-up technique. While exercise programs of the past used to employ just one or two repetitious forms, now there can be 20 to 30 different techniques used throughout an exercise session. No one realizes that the reason this leaves people feeling more refreshed rather than fatigued after exercise is that the variation in movements rewires and changes the brain's electrical patterns, which breaks brain heat.

Sometimes an experience is overpowering enough that our brain can't shift gears so easily, and the brain heat sustains. For example, if someone is focused in a fit of anger, meaning they can't break that frustration or anger they have toward something that happened personally in their life, it's almost like a madness occurs because the brain heats up past its limits. The flash sparks become so chronic that the electrical pattern stays lit in the same areas. That is, when someone fixates on one thing that hurt them in one way, it sends an electrical pattern on that one path, hitting the same spots in the brain, heating up the same pathway over and over again and not allowing the pathway to cool. As a side effect, the brain gets damaged from the heating that occurs over and over again—brain tissue can get scorched, scarred, and calloused. (Read more in Chapter 5, "Your Emotional Brain.")

Toxic heavy metals heighten this experience of brain heat. The mere presence of toxic heavy metals in our brain can make us sad, can make us angry, can make us very inconsistent, struggling with emotional patterns. Toxic heavy metals create bipolar disorder and mania. Toxic heavy metals can also make it easier for us to get triggered emotionally. Then when we do get triggered, our brain heats up from the electricity of the intense emotion, with the toxic heavy metals heightening and

holding the heat; toxic heavy metals in our brain are coals in the fire that sustain heat. If someone can't break a bout of frustration or anger, it's usually because toxic heavy metals are perpetuating that frustration or anger. This intense, sustained brain heat is one way people can experience what used to be called "going mad."

MELTING DOWN

When our brains get hot and there's metal involved, the toxic heavy metal particles break down—the metals melt. Toxic heavy metals in the brain get wear and tear when electrical currents are entering them. They start to change. Their shapes change. Corrosion can occur. The smaller the particles, the more easily they melt under the heat of the brain. When toxic heavy metals that reside in the brain melt, they transform into a liquid gas chemical composition. That is, the metals change from a solid to a liquid gas and can spread and cover more ground inside the brain more easily. This means that as toxic heavy metals in the brain heat up and melt, they move, and they can slowly travel to adjacent brain tissue over the years. Melting toxic heavy metals in the brain are one reason why so many conditions and symptoms—Alzheimer's, for example— worsen with time. The gas alone can worsen any mental, physical, or emotional condition.

Another reason brain conditions worsen with time is that more toxic heavy metals continue to collect in certain areas of the brain. The brain's electromagnetic field draws metals in, creating an accumulation effect that makes large deposits of toxic heavy metals keep growing. The larger the deposit, the greater its electromagnetic pull, meaning that it will keep attracting toxic heavy metals into it, making the deposit larger and larger over time. While the brain's electromagnetic field is drawing toxic heavy metals into other areas of the brain too, the metals tend to accumulate where the field is stronger due to these "nuggets" of toxic heavy metals.

When it comes to mercury deposits, they're not just formed through electromagnetic pull. Mercury doesn't need this electromagnetic field to accumulate in the brain. Mercury finds mercury on its own. With mercury deposits forming in the brain both from electromagnetism and from mercury's tendency to find mercury, mercury deposits are that much more of a hindrance.

If we're experiencing a lot of friction and stress in our lives, electricity travels through our brain at a higher intensity and velocity, because adrenaline both increases heart rate and enters the brain, raising the brain's heat levels. Again, the more toxic heavy metals in the brain, the hotter it runs. And again, metals retain the heat. It can become a vicious cycle. For instance, someone who's perpetually angry about anything and everything, or who has frequent spells of anger, may have higher levels of toxic heavy metals in the brain in the first place that are aggravating that anger. As heat is generated for any reason, the metals change shape and form. Those anger spells will then generate more heat as anger

raises the electrical field, creating an electrical storm, which in turn melts more metal so that it spreads and has the potential to interfere with even more electrical signals in the brain. Those melting toxic heavy metals spreading their liquid gas can hinder bodily functions and communication.

People know stress and anger as "bad" for our brain and body and health. Those in the health world don't know why. They don't know what, systemically, is at the root of it. They don't know about this process occurring inside the brain; the health world has no idea how anger affects the brain in this way. They don't know why, even with the best neuroscience techniques, meditations, and thought pattern construction, mastering the mind is a struggle for so many—why strategies for managing stress and anger patterns can fail and why people fall back to old patterns. This is why: people struggle because of the toxic heavy metals underneath it all. Trying to hack or rewire our minds leads us back to the same old patterns if toxic heavy metals are not being addressed at the same time.

All of this may be difficult to envision, given that you know your brain can't be filled with shiny clumps of metal. You're right; it doesn't look like that. Keep in mind that toxic heavy metals in the brain are beyond microscopic. They could be in nanoparticle form or even smaller, all the way down to femtoparticles and yoctoparticles. It's these smaller particles that enter into and fill brain cells and can eventually kill them. Large (nano-sized) particles of toxic heavy metals sit between brain cells and do not always enter brain cells. In this type of between-cell position, they can be just as destructive, interfering with communication from one brain cell to another. Whether in or between brain cells, toxic heavy metals are especially problematic when these tiny particles melt, corrode, leach, and outgas.

As we picture heat and metal in the brain, we need to remember we're not picturing our brain as a blacksmith's shop. These aren't large pieces of metal being forged with 2,000-degree heat. We're talking about a metal particle scale that's nano-sized and under, and we're talking about a lot of these particles. It doesn't take many years to accumulate trillions of toxic heavy metal particles inside the brain, and even then you wouldn't be able to see them. We're also talking about an entirely different heat scale. And then there's acid involved on top of it all, as you'll read in Chapter 9, "Your Acid Brain." An acid brain changes the heat scale. Acidic blood doesn't allow toxins to leave the body easily, and this raises the brain's temperature.

Even if we can't see the toxic heavy metal particles inside our brain, the damage they do can be seen over time, in the form of frustrating or devastating symptoms, and sometimes the toxic heavy metals' effects can even be seen in medical imaging, although they won't be recognized as such. As the toxic heavy metals cause oxidation of brain tissue, MRIs or other brain scans can, in some cases, show gray areas, dark spots, white spots, lesions, or brain tissue damage—and medical professionals don't know they're looking at toxic heavy

metal problems. Analyzing these scans, medical professionals don't know what they're seeing.

The toxic heavy metal invasion of brain cells and brain tissue remains extremely elusive. You could be suffering from a brain disease and donate your brain to science, scientists could cut it open after you pass away, and they still wouldn't see the toxic heavy metals. They're not testing tissue to specifically check for metals. That's not on autopsy agendas. They don't look for toxic heavy metals on a septillionth (yoctoparticle) scale, and only in extreme cases do toxic heavy metal deposits build up in the brain to the point that they would be visible to examiners. It would just be another brain donated to the publicly known medical industry, which isn't even informed that these toxic brain-betraying threats exist. They would essentially be cutting your brain open and throwing it away. (Meanwhile, the classified medical industry knows toxic heavy metals are in our brain. It's part of the classified medical industry's purpose. The more metal in our brain, the more mind control over society and the more money to be made from brain disease.)

Let's get back to the electricity in our brains. As it runs on neurotransmitter chemicals through, across, and around neurons, electricity is constantly engaging with deposits of toxic metals. That's one issue. Here's another: Neurotransmitter chemicals are critical for our existence. They help sustain the brain. And they need to be pure and clean. As toxic heavy metals melt and outgas over the years, the residue of that metal can mix with the clean neurotransmitter chemicals, causing the neurotransmitters to become dirty, like muddy water.

As electricity runs through, across, and around neurons using those muddied neurotransmitter chemicals as fuel, the electricity can behave in a few different ways, depending on which toxic heavy metals are saturated into the neurotransmitter chemical. Whenever neurotransmitters get saturated with any toxic heavy metals, brain electricity runs hotter. If it's mercury saturating a neurotransmitter chemical, the electrical impulse will be more reckless and dangerous, in part because mercury is a shape-shifting metal that doesn't need intense heat or manipulation to further break down and liquefy. This effect of brain electricity on mercury can create a host of different behaviors in someone, whether child or adult. On the other hand, if the toxic heavy metal that's saturating the neurotransmitter chemical is aluminum, then as the electrical impulse runs across the neuron, it will be less reckless. It takes more heat to melt aluminum and longer to melt aluminum than some other metals. The brain's electricity can still melt the aluminum, although aluminum isn't shape-shifting like mercury. Because it takes longer to melt aluminum, during that melting process the electrical impulse will lose strength and weaken as the aluminum particles absorb the electrical impulse almost like a sponge. That weakening of the impulse creates its own set of symptoms, which we'll explore more in the symptom and condition descriptions in Parts IV and V of this book.

THE TRUE MEANING OF AN ALLOY BRAIN

What if someone has a lot of different heavy metals inside the brain? Many people do. What if it's mercury, aluminum, copper, nickel, and even a hint of lead? And what if those metals mix—what if they're sitting next to each other in the brain, and as the brain heats up for all of its everyday reasons, the metals melt and join together? One thing's for certain: publicly known medical science isn't going to touch this for another hundred years, and that's being optimistic. When they finally do, they'll discover all of the disease complications that occur from these *systemic alloys*.

An alloy is what forms when you put metals together. Industries frequently join metals to make them stronger or more flexible, lighter or heavier, more porous or nonporous, able to withstand hot and cold, and to create differences in expansion or contraction. Alloys are top of mind when selecting steel for bridges—engineers don't throw any old metal on a bridge. Alloy formulation is integral to creating the structure of your car. It's pivotal when making bicycles for the Tour de France. Alloys are used in computer and device technology. And alloys are always a work in progress. They're never definitive. They're always flawed, and they always have their limitations. Still, those are all great places to employ and improve upon alloys. Those objects are where alloys are supposed to be.

Alloys are not supposed to be in our brains. They're not supposed to be in our children's brains. There's no place for alloys in our brains, and there's no space for them. Inside our heads, everything is squeezed and woven together nice and tight. Even the chamber of the pituitary gland is compact, and the fluid that resides there takes up space.

Hidden Brain Inflammation

Have you ever had something in your shoe? Did a ball of lint get in there? Or have you found yourself limping from a tiny pebble or twig inside your sneaker as you walked on a trail? When you leave the beach, do you knock the sand out of your shoes, or do you go on your merry way with the sand cramping your feet? I don't think you go on your merry way. I think you try to shake out the grains of sand.

Living with a brain that contains toxic heavy metals and their alloys is like getting something in your shoe—there's no room for anything extra, so it hobbles us. One reason is that when toxic heavy metals enter our brain, they can create an underlying pressure and a chronic inflammatory condition: brain inflammation. This type of brain inflammation is different from the brain inflammation you'll read about in the next chapter, "Your Viral Brain," where viruses and their waste product can inflame nerves. With toxic heavy metals, it's a subtle brain inflammation that's not so much about general swelling. Instead, toxic heavy metals create localized inflammation—tiny areas of inflammation around those spots where toxic heavy metals have taken up residence

in the brain, be they nanoparticles or yoctoparticles. This is due to the physical injury the toxic heavy metals cause to brain tissue. It's kind of like the inflammation you might get around a splinter in your skin, or the inflamed spot on your heel you might get from a pebble in your shoe versus your whole foot swelling up.

Toxic heavy metals, even when they're at their worst, only create spots of inflammation. The larger the deposit of toxic heavy metals—meaning the more nanoparticles, picoparticles, femtoparticles, and so on have accumulated in a deposit of toxic heavy metals in the brain—the more pronounced and aggressive these spots of inflammation can be. This is brain inflammation that eludes the medical field and would be virtually impossible to detect on any level from MRIs or CT scans—although it's inflammation enough to create a myriad of symptoms.

Living with an Alloy Brain

The mere presence of toxic heavy metals in the brain can cause all this and more: different varieties of headaches; different sensations within the head; different aches and pains; different feelings of weakness and light-headedness; different emotional reactions to situations in life; and different levels of depression and anxiety, tics and spasms, brain fog, memory loss, obsessions, compulsions, and involuntary actions. Toxic heavy metals in the brain can even alter our decision-making without our realizing it. And when it comes to our brain, we can't just let all the toxic heavy metals out, the way we shake out sand from our shoes or pull out a splinter. It takes the right approach to extract toxic heavy metals from the brain, which you'll discover in Part VI of this book, "Bringing Back Your Brain."

When alloys are created for industry, they're created for a reason. For technological equipment, for example, metals are mixed so we can benefit, and manufacturers safeguard which metals are combined, how, and for which purposes. They know what blends could create problems in the products they manufacture. In our brain, no one's safeguarding what goes into it or what melds together there—because practically no one is aware we even have toxic heavy metal alloys in our brain. Those in the publicly known health industry who have gained awareness of toxic heavy metals in the brain because of Medical Medium teachings from the last 35 years still don't understand this alloy aspect. The classified medical industry isn't even aware of this alloy aspect of toxic heavy metals in the brain.

We don't get to choose our personal alloy recipe. It's not like pulling up to a takeout window and ordering some copper, lead, mercury, and aluminum to go. Everyone has unique alloy blends in their brain without knowing what they are, or that they're even there. Even though one person could have the same three or five or seven or ten toxic heavy metals in their brain as another person, chances are they're mixed a little differently as far as amounts and ratios, and they are most likely in slightly different areas of the brain. That's part of what makes us different. It's not just our unique souls, which definitely make us different. It's not just our unique experiences and reference points, which make us different too. It's the toxic heavy metal alloys in our brains influencing our behaviors, actions, thoughts, decisions, feelings, memories, and sense of self. Toxic heavy metals even alter the development of our brain and other organs in the womb. And the alloys composed inside each person's brain are completely unauthorized. There's no jurisdiction, no environmental agency, no standard for inspection that determines if you have a safe alloy composition inside your brain.

These toxic heavy metal alloy compositions each react to electricity differently. Electrical patterns in the brain carry intelligence, information, from neuron to neuron. Decision-making processes occur because of neurons transferring information to the next neurons through electricity. And as you discovered in the previous chapter, electricity in the brain isn't just a hot wire. It's *abundant* with information, from past information that's happened in your life all the way to current information about what's happening in this very moment. Certain toxic heavy metal alloy mixes can scramble words and alter memories in that electrical current of information. It's why one person could remember an experience differently from another person who went through it at the same time. Those are toxic heavy metal alloys inside the brain changing the shape of how we remember an experience, even if only slightly.

Alloys also determine how fast we see something with our eyes. One person could say, "Did you see that?" and the other person could say, "No, see what?" It's not a matter of vision. It's a matter of toxic heavy metal alloys in the brain affecting someone's perceptions. Depending on the blend and location in the brain, an alloy can prevent someone from seeing a fast-moving object. That doesn't necessarily mean the person who did see a fast-moving object doesn't have alloys in the brain. They could actually have alloys helping them see that quickly, while hurting them in other, bigger ways. Or they could have an alloy in the brain making them *think* they saw something; maybe the reason the other person didn't see the object was because it was never there. That's the mystery of the alloy brain. It could go any number of ways. There's no regulation of alloys in the brain. Autism is an example of an alloy brain creating a complex interplay of neurological effects—some children with autism are gifted in many ways and struggle in many other ways.

Alloys' effects on brain messaging mean that they influence memories, emotional sensations, nostalgia, and even dreams. That's right—alloys can alter, change, and shape dreams. People wonder why their dreams are so ridiculous or obscure or bizarre. It can happen because electrical pathways carrying information through the physical brain are hitting deposits of alloys that alter the information, changing the structure of that information. Then there's your own soul, which resides in your brain, influencing your dreams. It's a mixed bag

of nuts, and you can end up with some outlandish or very intense dreams. If you get a mercury filling removed and it outgasses and gets into the brain, as mercury fillings always do, you may have dreams of being trapped underwater or trapped in a tiny space. Or if, in your dream, you're running away from someone and feeling like you can't get away, can't run fast enough, or you're almost stuck, that's electricity getting caught up in toxic heavy metal deposits that electrical patterns in the brain don't normally hit when you're awake. As part of sleep's healing rhythms, electricity goes to different places in the brain when you're sleeping, creating some dreams that are nothing like experiences when you're awake—especially if electricity is hitting toxic heavy metal deposits in your sleep that it doesn't normally hit in the course of the day.

When alloys are used in industries, they're something a mad scientist can have a lot of fun with. They can be used in destructive manners. Alloys are used in nuclear weapons. They're used in missile silos. And unidentified alloys have been discovered on Planet Earth with metal and formulations of metal that human beings have not yet created. The only explanation is that they came out of the sky.

Alloys in our brain? That's like going to a potluck. Everybody brings something to eat, and no one really knows what's in any of it as they heap different concoctions onto their plates. It's the same way that everyone has a certain alloy mix in the brain. That alloy mix can even determine what someone makes for the potluck! That's just one example of how much alloys can shape the brain—the mood we're in and what we'll feel like making. Brain alloys can be the difference between one person bringing waffles and another bringing tuna casserole and another person dodging the potluck and hitting a fast food place instead.

Having an alloy brain alters the mind. Alloy brains have made some of the ingenious minds in our history. All the same, an alloy brain has drawbacks. Alloy brains have created serial killers. Even if an alloy gives something to a person, it takes something away from them too. Even if an alloy alters electrical fields in the brain in a way that opens up new possibilities, it comes at a price. That price can be symptoms, early death, a disease state, hurting themselves or others, or other difficulties in how we use the brain to function and communicate.

Oxidizing Alloy Brains

An alloy brain means that toxic heavy metals enter the brain, mix together, and can denature tissue over time. They become destabilized. They can create oxidation— brain tissue can oxidize as well as the metals themselves. If you've ever seen the patina on copper or bronze (a copper alloy), then you know what I mean when I talk about oxidation. It's the green buildup you may remember cleaning off a copper penny. In the antique world, patina on a metal object is prized proof of authenticity; you're not supposed to clean it. Inside your head, it's

the last thing you need. Rust is another way metals can show oxidation—and if you've ever seen a piece of scrap metal bubbling and flaking from rust, you can imagine how undesirable that is inside your brain. Patina and rust mean corrosion and oxidation, which means more toxic heavy metal runoff leaching, outgassing, and spreading over brain tissue.

Remember, everyone's alloy brain is different, and part of this has to do with which alloys are present in the brain. Different combinations of toxic heavy metals react and oxidize differently, depending on the specific alloy blend:

- When certain metals mix together (mercury and aluminum, for example), the oxidation grows and expands so rapidly that it generates a large amount of loose debris, which leads to runoff, meaning that the metals' debris spreads to more and more tissue.

- When nickel and copper are put together, nickel repels heat more than copper does, so the copper takes on all the heat the nickel is supposed to receive, and the copper tends to break down faster.

- When lead and aluminum interact, it accelerates lead's peeling and flaking oxidation process, leading the alloy to become unstable.

- Copper is the most grounding metal. When combined with lead, copper's grounding mechanism becomes more radical and unpredictable. As electricity travels through a brain with a copper-lead alloy, the copper can cause more of an energy draw, diminishing the brain's electrical grid.

- Copper mixed with mercury tends to increase mercury's neurotoxic strength. Copper's grounding properties actually make mercury more unstable, causing mercury to oxidize more quickly.

- Aluminum allows copper to heat up faster and sustain its heat longer, which means that when the brain's electrical grid hits an alloy of copper and aluminum, the aluminum keeps the copper heated up—whereas our brain's electrical flash responses are supposed to cool down quickly.

- When toxic calcium and aluminum are combined, the calcium binds onto and builds up around the aluminum, encasing and weighing it down, pushing the alloy deeper into the brain.

- With cadmium plus mercury, cadmium tends to outgas and bubble from the interaction, also causing mercury to expand more, similar to what happens with aluminum-mercury alloys.

This is not an exhaustive list of toxic heavy metal alloys that can take up residence in your brain. Not to mention, these examples only describe a few of the different alloys that form when *pairs* of toxic heavy metals combine and interact. Alloys can also form in the brain from three, four, or more metals combining. There are endless combinations of toxic heavy metals possible in our brain alloys, with each alloy unique in nature.

Placement of these alloys within the brain, like placement of individual toxic heavy metals, can vary too. One person could have more alloy in the back of the brain and another could have more in the frontal lobe. One person could have more in the left hemisphere while another has more in the right hemisphere. One person could have more alloy settled in the cerebral midline canal. Some people have alloys "sprinkled" all around. For others, an alloy is concentrated in just one spot. Alloys can also travel in the brain over time. There's endless variety in how toxic heavy metal alloys sit inside and affect the brain across billions of people.

No matter what alloys reside inside us and where in the brain those toxic heavy metal blends lie, we need to take action to remove the toxic heavy metal alloys so we can set ourselves on the course of healing. We truly must save our brains. While removing toxic heavy metals takes time, when we put that time and energy into it, the rewards are beyond imaginable.

TRACE MINERALS: YOUR BRAIN'S PEACEKEEPERS

Let's remember that there are some beneficial metals in our brains: trace minerals. Trace minerals are there for countless undiscovered reasons. Trace minerals are there to transfer information, to keep our brains from shrinking, to feed our brain's immune cells, keeping them strong. Trace minerals are also there to do much more.

How We Survive

The brain's electrical field cannot exist without water, electrolytes, and trace minerals in the bloodstream. If the water weren't there, or the trace minerals and electrolytes weren't there, the brain's electrical field would diminish and eventually run dry, burning out neurotransmitters, other brain-related hormones, and stored-up trace mineral and electrolyte reserves inside brain tissue. That is, the well would run dry. Brain strength would weaken. It's the story of most people's lives.

Electricity is not alive on its own. It needs a biological mate, which in this case means trace minerals and electrolytes: metals. We know we can't travel without some source of metals, be it with a bicycle, motorcycle, car, bus, train, or plane. Well, electricity can't travel through the brain properly without

the proper metal—trace minerals and electrolytes. Or think of lightning and lightning rods. A mystery of the universe is within that lightning bolt and how the metal of a lightning rod attracts it. Lightning in the sky can only exist in the first place from the trace minerals in the atmosphere's clouds, water vapor, or precipitation. The same relationship exists inside us, in how the electricity in our brain seeks out trace minerals and electrolytes and the water inside our body travels to our brain to help transfer that electricity.

(By the way, if toxic heavy metal particles are polluting the atmosphere, they change storm patterns and make lightning's electricity more aggressive, just as toxic heavy metals polluting our brain create storms in our brain.)

One major function of trace minerals is to balance electricity running through the brain. Electricity is attracted to trace minerals, and that's part of how trace minerals stop electricity from going rogue and getting out of control. Your brain's supernatural electromagnetic force draws trace minerals to their appropriate stations and specific areas of need in the brain. Trace minerals prevent extreme heating from electrical currents, meaning that they regulate currents so they run cooler when needed, because trace minerals in their natural state, unlike industrialized metals, regulate temperature when electricity from the brain hits them.

Trace minerals are like the equalizers that used to be on stereo sets, where you'd raise or lower the control according to what you wanted. Trace minerals' role in the brain is similar to the liver's role of peacekeeper in the human body. In the brain specifically, trace minerals play peacekeeper. They're tranquility keepers there. Electricity in the brain searches for trace minerals. Without them, the electrical grid struggles.

To live, eat, breathe, survive, we have to get trace minerals and electrolytes from somewhere, even if they're in their poorest form, or we cease to exist. The problem is, we often do get the poorest forms, the forms of these trace minerals and electrolytes that keep us only existing, from sources such as GMO (bioengineered) foods, treated town or city water, overharvested agricultural fields (both organic and conventional) that are not replenished, and farmed animals and farmed fish that are not fed nutrient-dense foods. We're getting minimal exposure to quality trace minerals and electrolytes and maximum exposure to toxic heavy metals.

Worst Enemies

The trace minerals in our brain connect to our very soul. They hold information within them that connects us to the moon, the stars, the atmosphere, the ether, the heavens. It goes beyond textbook science; it's beyond numbers, beyond right or wrong or good or bad. Trace minerals have both a physical presence and purpose and a metaphysical presence and purpose. And along with macro minerals, trace minerals were meant to be the only metals inside our brain.

If trace minerals had brains of their own, they would never think they'd be taking up residence in *our* brains beside the evil version of themselves, toxic heavy metals—which are industrialized metals. When a metal has been industrialized, any benefit as a trace mineral is completely destroyed. For instance: industrialized copper. We get confused with copper. We hear, "No, copper's good. We need lots of copper." What really happens is that when copper is industrialized—that is, when it's turned into a copper pot or copper pipe—it's now deformed. Any opportunity for it to be a beneficial trace mineral is now destroyed. The residue of that copper pot or copper pipe (or copper water bottle or copper kitchen tool or copper jewelry) is not beneficial. It cannot be used as an active, bioavailable trace mineral inside the body anymore. Instead, it's a destructive, dangerous metal because it's been industrialized and denatured. The earth is partly made of living trace minerals, and when they're kept in their natural state, they can be usable by the body, as long as they're in the right amounts for the right purposes. Forging metals, though, removes the natural earth energy that exists in them. When a metal is industrialized and forged, it has lost its memory. An industrialized metal has become toxic and destructive to our bodies, its natural nature has been disrupted, and its active ability to participate for the planet's benefit has been lost.

Toxic heavy metals are trace minerals' worst enemy, and vice versa. In conflict with toxic heavy metals, trace minerals are sacrificed. One way they're sacrificed is that toxic heavy metals destroy the natural energetic and physical abilities of trace minerals. Toxic heavy metals hold a destructive charge, while trace minerals, their polar opposite, hold a beneficial charge. As neutralizers, trace minerals give up their existence and essentially get eaten up trying to stop and neutralize toxic heavy metals' destructive charge.

Here's another way trace minerals are sacrificed: because toxic heavy metals make electricity in our brains run hotter, and because one function of trace minerals is to cool electricity without dampening or hampering it, the extra heat from toxic heavy metals makes the trace minerals work overtime. The trace minerals get defused. If we have an abundance of trace minerals that we've gotten from their naturally occurring sources—herbs, leafy greens, fruits, wild foods, and vegetables—then they can manage and control this overheating to a degree. Certain powerful trace minerals, such as the sodium cluster salts from celery juice, go so far as to help defuse toxic heavy metals. It's one reason why trace minerals are toxic heavy metals' worst nightmares. Trace minerals can still burn up and dwindle and lose their strength over time, because toxic heavy metals are so destructive. The job of trace minerals is to make the toxic heavy metals less effective, taking away at least the toxic energy force that the toxic heavy metals got from being industrialized. Since trace minerals are up against so much, it's beneficial to keep fueling ourselves with celery juice and other healthy sources of trace minerals on a daily basis.

If we're not nourishing ourselves with the right foods that contain proper electrolytes and trace mineral salts, it's hard to restore the trace mineral assets to our brain. So the brain heats up more. Since it's likely that a person's blood is also constantly filled with fats and acids, more metal melting and oxidization occur, creating extra toxic metal debris, which conflicts with trace minerals, and more trace minerals are diminished. Trace minerals even get absorbed in the melting and oxidative process, sucked into the toxic heavy metal alloy, which isn't a bad thing, as the trace minerals help defuse the toxic heavy metals within the alloy. All trace minerals can help defuse toxic heavy metals, although celery juice's sodium cluster salts do a better job of it because celery juice contains complete electrolytes. While this function of trace minerals helps us, it also means we lose more trace minerals that are meant to be responsible for all brain functions. Trace minerals versus toxic heavy metals is not a fair fight, because industrial toxic heavy metals are not meant to be part of our physical brain and body's world.

This toxic heavy metal battle is a massive part of why humankind has so many brain problems today. You can read all the neuroscience literature you want, follow all the leading alternative and conventional health experts on social media you want, listen to all the health podcasts you want, and you won't see any of this addressed. Doctors and health experts don't realize that toxic heavy metals reside in the brain. That is, unless they're using Medical Medium information—and if they are, they're unlikely

---

to disclose that they've gotten the information from Medical Medium teachings. If they do talk about metals, where's the rest of the information to fill in the blanks? It's here.

Health experts will sing the praises of "healthy fats" and "fish oil" and "high protein" for the brain. Meanwhile, following that advice oxidizes toxic heavy metals in the brain more. That means that however advanced a source sounds, it's providing you with the opposite of healing guidance, such as what foods and supplements really support our brain and neuron health. The world is oblivious to this toxic heavy metal battle in our brains. That's why here, now, it's time for *you* to become the expert.

RISE ABOVE THE MACHINE

We're taught that the medical powers that be—meaning the medical establishment, the pharmaceutical industry, and the health care industry in general—are all looking out for us. We learn from the start, as children, that medicine has our best interest in mind. There are a lot of great reasons to think so. The nurse at school puts a bandage on your scraped knee. You twist an ankle, and your pediatrician puts you in a boot and hands you a crutch. As we grow up, we hear about family members and elders going through hard times and getting care in the hospital, including surgeries that could be life-saving. We hear about a distant friend who got into a car crash and survived due to life-saving ER care. We're told about the great technological advancements in

medicine and see the headlines splattered across newspapers and other media. And so we believe that the whole of medicine is in our best interest, and we get a sense of safety in that.

We're taught in universities that science is ruler or king, that science is even God, that science has all the answers. Even with the plague we're faced with today, we're being taught every day that science has it under control and has sensible, reasonable answers—and then we learn every day this is not true. There are thousands of examples where the teachings that medical professionals are handed by medical research and science in medical school are actually cover stories—cover stories that are then repeated and told to the rest of the population. One example is the saying that the shingles virus and chicken pox virus are essentially one and the same. This is incorrect. They are two separate, different viruses.

When you scratch the surface, you can't get a straight answer or reasonable fact out of medical research and science. Yet every day when we're growing up, we're taught that everything science has to offer is concrete, indisputable, and legitimate. It's easy to believe this when you break your leg and you have a great orthopedic doctor and you leave the hospital in a cast. That kind of visible assistance is part of the smoke and mirrors of the medical industry. It's the deception of the medical machine. Have one thing right and a hundred things wrong. And still we're taught to believe that medical science and research, and the medical health care system, are sanctuaries, safety blankets, and can do no wrong. We're taught that they're looking out for our children, our babies, and pregnant women.

In a perfect world, the publicly known medical industry would be advanced enough to understand the full severity and complexity of toxic heavy metals inside our brains. Instead, alternative medicine has to learn about it from the publications of a prophet. Even as we quickly see "toxic heavy metals in the brain" become adopted as law in the alternative medical community, scientific studies aren't the original source. These Medical Medium publications are the original source of the knowledge of what symptoms and conditions are caused by metals.

The medical machine runs and runs and runs, an unstoppable bureaucracy of medicine. Billions of dollars go into scientific studies that are not applicable to children with chronic brain inflammation causing neurological fatigue and weakness of the limbs, not applicable to people on feeding tubes due to gastrointestinal disorders stemming from the brain, not applicable to individuals living through the daily realities of brain fog or bipolar disorder or autism. Medical research and science are sopping up all the billions of dollars going into medicine and using it for medical bureaucracy. Meanwhile, no dollars are being directed to investigate hundreds of examples of chronic symptoms and conditions. The medical machine completely ignores what should be some of the most obvious and profound discoveries in chronic illness—such as toxic heavy metals inside our brains.

Why is it that they don't know about this? How can it even be possible? Is it that they do know and they're avoiding it altogether? Is it because they simply haven't discovered it or stumbled across it? Is it due to a lack of funding, direction, or purpose in the industry? You make your judgment call. Here's my call: the classified medical industry does know, to a certain extent, that metals can reside in the brain and cause problems, and they're avoiding it. The publicly known medical industry is unaware, aside from the individual health professionals who are starting to have their suspicions now due to 35 years of Medical Medium teachings about the buildup of trace amounts of various toxic heavy metals inside the brain and organs causing dozens of chronic symptoms and conditions. Bits and pieces about toxic heavy metals are starting to enter the conversation, yet the whole story isn't there. The hows, whys, whats, and wheres are missing.

One reason the classified medical industry wants to avoid this information getting out is that a big part of why we have toxic heavy metals in our brains in the first place is from the medical industry itself. It's been one of the major sources of mercury, aluminum, and toxic copper inside us. So of course the topic is going to be avoided. It may very well continue to be avoided many, many years after this book has been in people's hands to read. Another reason why it's avoided is that in order to rectify the situation with toxic heavy metals in our brains, we would need to take initiative, and that would ultimately lead us to extremely alternative means, since the medical industry doesn't have a solution.

Even if the medical machine decided to put toxic heavy metals at the top of its list so billions of people would have a chance to heal, it would be stuck because there is no pharmaceutical treatment that would remove the subtle yet life-damaging levels of toxic heavy metals from inside our brains. Pharmaceutical and medical treatments actually *contain* toxic heavy metals. This conundrum would force the machine to go natural, because it's only a completely natural approach that's effective here. And once the medical industry went natural—if it even got the natural approach right—the house of cards would fall down because they wouldn't consider it science anymore. You can put all the science you want into alternative therapies, and while it may be respected among certain natural authorities, it will still seem like 100 percent quackery to the conventional model. Not to mention that if the medical industry discovered and owned up to the truth, who would be held responsible for toxic heavy metals and the damage and injury they have caused within babies, children, and adults, even causing miscarriages in pregnant women? How would they provide restitution?

All of this means the medical industry will find it nearly impossible to acknowledge all of the toxic heavy metals in our brains and the conditions they cause that you'll read about throughout this book. Instead, it will all be passed off as genetics, or they'll find other scapegoats. Billions of dollars go into genetic science, not to provide us with

answers about why we're sick and to help us heal but to learn how to clone or destroy our genes—even if the individuals working within this industry aren't aware this is the real endgame. There's great darkness in the genetic world of medicine. If there weren't, those billions would go into looking at the toxic heavy metals inside our brains, how we can work to heal or reverse conditions, and how to remove metals from pharmaceuticals and pharmaceutical treatments.

So yes, we learn as children that the medical industry works in our best interest. As a society we're taught to believe that there's always a medical solution to a problem, which is accurate in some areas of life. The truth is that the medical industry works in its own best interest. Many individual doctors compassionately work for our best interest while their hands are tied. The industry leaves doctors in the dark about what's wrong with their patients, so we're not offered the solutions to our problems. And when a doctor steps out of the box and finds the problems and the medical industry doesn't like what the doctor is discovering, the doctor gets in trouble—sometimes tragically so, in ways that threaten their livelihood and the well-being of their own family.

That's why it's critical for you to know that now, finally, the solutions are in your hands. In this book, you'll find critical information about the precise role of toxic heavy metals in a wide variety of mental, emotional, and physical health issues, how these metals enter our brains in the first place, and what you can do about them.

If you're someone who wakes up in the morning and shakes your head wondering why there's a lack of answers out there for the chronically suffering, now you understand why. *You're* learning the answers. You're learning the truth so you can do something about your health and your family's health.

By knowing what that critical truth is—that, for one, toxic heavy metals are saturating our brains and we can remove them to enjoy better quality of life—we supersede the machine. We rise above the so-called authority of our well-being so that well-being is in our own hands. We rise above the machine.

"Toxic heavy metals are the shadow we can't see until they create disease—although even then, we still can't see them; we can only see the disease. In other words, we can't see the metals when they create a symptom. We can only see the symptom or the symptom's effects. Along the way, maybe we can sense a presence, because when we're not well, we can often sense there's something wrong. If we get a name for our symptom or condition, we may still doubt ourselves and our intuition about what's really causing it. If we don't get a name for it, we can doubt ourselves even more."

— Anthony William, Medical Medium

CHAPTER 4

Your Viral Brain

When someone is struggling with chronic, recurring, invisible, mysterious, intermittent, or life-interrupting symptoms, enough visits to enough doctors, specialists, and experts in the field of medicine—including even psychiatry—will usually result in at least one diagnosis, if not multiple diagnoses. They may land upon a diagnosis of "You're just living with anxiety." They may land upon a diagnosis of "merely headaches." They may land upon a diagnosis of "autoimmune" without a specific condition name. They could diagnose fibromyalgia without an answer about what really causes it or how to find lasting relief from its true root cause.

Today in medical research and science there are so many different symptom and condition labels to choose from that relate to the seen and unseen. And yet for a world that prides itself on medical advancements, achievements, intelligence, expertise, and ingenuity, there couldn't be a greater disconnect when it comes to the brain—understanding even the smallest symptoms and being able to connect the dots correctly to the central nervous system.

ANSWERS IN INFLAMMATION

So many of us walk around with inflammation. We're not just talking about soreness in the elbow, knee, back, or big toe. We're talking about inflammation that is always undetected—undiscovered by the publicly known medical industry and purposely ignored by the classified medical industry. We're talking about brain inflammation.

If you're a medical professional or even a layperson, when you hear "brain inflammation," you may immediately think of someone falling off a bike and banging their head on cement or someone getting a concussion playing college football. Maybe "brain inflammation" brings to mind a vehicular accident and CT scans and MRIs, and yes, all of this describes one type of brain inflammation. These are obvious injuries that doctors understand can create inflammation and pressure inside the head. There's also the undiscovered, localized brain inflammation you read about in the previous chapter, "Your Alloy Brain," which is caused by toxic heavy metals.

There's another type of brain inflammation that occurs without toxic heavy metals *or* obvious injury (although it can also occur at the same time as either or both of these other types of inflammation). We're talking about brain inflammation that is never seen on scans, so it can be very deceiving, very mysterious, and very troubling for so many. Experiencing mystery symptoms that confound doctors can be maddening for anyone to live through. Experiencing a symptom that a doctor puts under the auto-immune umbrella—which makes it seem like the doctor's not confounded when really, they're still confounded—can be just as maddening. People are pushed into psychiatrists' offices by the thousands upon thousands. By the millions, people struggle with their minds, thinking their bodies are playing tricks and failing them, or that they're manifesting their illness with their thoughts or creating their illness because they're bad people or deserve karmic payback. Even our best experts in the field of medicine aren't able to determine accurately what's going on with these patients, from subtle to more extreme conditions that involve symptoms of the body and mind.

There is a greater truth underneath it all. There are answers to why people feel the way they do. What's behind this type of brain inflammation? Viruses.

Brain inflammation is one part of understanding a viral brain. Now, please don't confuse viral brain inflammation with having a virus inside your brain. Some people do contract viruses that find their way to the brain, make a home there, and wreak havoc. Yet for the majority of people, the viruses are in other parts of the body, sometimes close to the brain and sometimes causing brain inflammation from afar. Still, inflammation is only a *piece* of an answer. It's only one part of what's really going on inside the brain and body.

Envision this: publicly known medicine (both alternative and conventional) standing in perpetual quicksand. If it attempts to find or expose the truth to help you, it only sinks deeper, because exposing the truth would mean exposing all the reasons why the classified medical industry has kept us from the truth. And so publicly known medicine is stuck: little do those working in publicly known medicine realize that the medical industry would lose all credibility by revealing the truth, and it would have to let go of all the ground it has gained. All the billions of dollars of research and all the classified medical industry cover-up would be unveiled by bringing us the truth. Just as you read about regarding toxic heavy metals in the previous chapter, the medical establishment doesn't remain a hero by bringing us the real answers when it comes to viruses either. That would mean undermining itself at the same time. The only way the medical establishment stays a hero is by continuing to bring us the non-truth in the form of misleading stats, studies, numbers, percentages, reasons, and excuses.

Because the publicly known medical industry is not there yet, *we* need to be. Kindhearted, committed practitioners can escape the quicksand trap and help their patients if they learn the truth. So can the individuals they're trying to treat who are struggling with symptoms and conditions. We all deserve to know that subtle, undetected brain inflammation is behind so many people's struggles. That's the one piece. What's the other important piece? *Why* they're experiencing that inflammation.

When publicly known medical experts (both alternative and conventional) try to explain inflammation, the best explanation they have is the theory that grains, gluten, lectins, nightshades, processed foods, dairy, environmental pollution, stress, the sun, sugar, and carbs are inherently inflammatory. (Funny thing is, it's taboo for alcohol, cannabis, and caffeine to be thrown into that list.) When they reach past the theory that these factors are directly, inherently inflammatory, they theorize that these factors are forcing or triggering the body to attack itself and become inflamed. When they reach past *that*, they theorize that pathogens are triggers for the immune system to turn on the brain and body and attack itself. Unless they're learning the true answers about precisely how pathogens are involved with brain inflammation (which is Medical Medium information), and unless they're citing this as the source so people can discover how to heal, publicly known medical experts' theories only put the industry right back where it started: a whole bunch of fragmented, confused, trendy,

misunderstood pieces of the puzzle without the details that matter.

HOW VIRAL BRAIN INFLAMMATION REALLY WORKS

Let's fill in how viral brain inflammation happens. If you're familiar with my work, then you know how often viruses take up residence in the liver. From there the viruses will often release poisons that find their way to the brain; that alone can cause hundreds of symptoms and conditions, from anxiety to body pain to burning skin to brain fog to confusion to fatigue and much more. There's a group of viruses that most often cause these problems: the herpetic family of viruses (*Herpesviridae*).

Publicly known medical research and science have identified roughly nine types of these herpetic viral varieties out of hundreds that the classified medical industry has put out for them in a large-scale Easter egg hunt. Every now and then over the past five or six decades, a virologist who has dedicated countless hours to their field of medicine has miraculously discovered one of these "Easter eggs" and placed a name on the herpetic virus they've identified. The most common herpetic viruses are Epstein-Barr (EBV), shingles, herpes simplex 1, herpes simplex 2, HHV-6, and cytomegalovirus (CMV). (In Chapter 18, "Viruses and Viral Waste Matter," you'll find a fuller list of herpetic viruses, along with critical insights about how we're exposed to them and how to shield ourselves from future exposure.) As

I've written about throughout the Medical Medium series, these very common viruses are a major reason for our modern-day epidemic of chronic illness.

Of the herpetic viruses we can have breeding inside us, some viruses expel a lot more toxic waste in the form of *neurotoxins*. These viral neurotoxins then float around in the bloodstream and can find their way to the brain and even sift through the blood-brain barrier to the cerebrospinal fluid. In this way, viral neurotoxins create subtle levels of inflammation in the brain. This is a critical understanding of brain inflammation, one we'll explore in more depth soon. Viral neurotoxins are how a virus living anywhere in the body can create brain inflammation from near or far.

Living, Hungry Viruses

For the record, viruses *are* living. In the publicly known arena of science, there is a battle about whether viruses are dead or alive. No one can agree, and neither side has proven facts. Here is a pillar of truth: Viruses are alive. Viruses are cells. Viruses eat.

For a virus to live long enough inside the human body to create a chronic symptom or condition, it has to be able to find food to sustain itself. A virus does not have a mouth, as if it's an animal or human eating. Instead, a virus absorbs fuel through its viral cell membrane. To eat, a viral cell creates a vacuum effect, temporarily drawing in water within the blood that's filled with viral fuel through any area of the viral cell membrane and then immediately excreting

that fluid through any other part of the cell membrane. If a virus is highly active, it will need to feed on viral fuel on an hourly basis. If the virus is inactive or even dormant, it will need to feed on viral fuel on a weekly to monthly basis. The virus has an ability to expel almost all fluid out of its cell structure so it can then be refilled with new fluid that harbors viral fuel. When the virus is active and feeding regularly, its viral cells are continually excreting all of their contents through their cell membranes, making someone who has the viral infection experience heightened symptoms.

The publicly known medical industry is completely unaware that viruses eat. The classified medical industry knows, because the classified medical industry feeds viruses, breeds them, keeps them alive in labs, and uses viruses' foods of choice: preferably raw egg, iron, and mercury. Other foods the classified medical industry feeds viruses to keep them alive are gluten, dairy, and GMO medical-grade corn.

One of the problems of the publicly known medical industry when it comes to viruses is that it's so underfunded in this area. No one can find the truth even if they want to—so they hash out theories that are all on paper because they're not allowed to study viruses adequately, never mind take a virus of choice and look at it under a microscope. Very few doctors or scientists get authorization, and the outcomes are always vague, obscure, and inconclusive. So the publicly known medical industry stays stuck in its war with itself over whether viruses are just a dead strand of RNA and protein or they're alive. Many medical professionals believe viruses are only alive if they're an influenza (flu virus) strain, and even then, it remains questionable because of this ongoing internal war.

The publicly known medical industry has to work with theories kind of like astronomers do. As an astronomer, you go to bed at night dreaming about what you might discover behind the stars with your telescope. As a virologist in the publicly known medical industry, you go to bed at night dreaming that someday you may get funded and truly discover what a virus does. Or if a virus is even a virus. In the meantime, you keep yourself busy in your career attending meetings and medical conventions, and reading other colleagues' theoretical papers, and you listen to that lucky devil who was funded briefly, who's up on the stage at a convention talking about their theory of what they think they discovered. That's the grim reality of the publicly known medical industry.

The classified medical industry is a whole other game. They know that viruses eat. They feed the viruses. They grow viruses, proliferate viruses, and alter viruses, and every now and then, one escapes the lab. This is what the classified medical industry has been doing for over 100 years now, since the Spanish flu was released in 1918. The classified medical industry knows more about viruses—much more—than the publicly known medical industry.

Remember this: viruses are alive, viruses eat, and viruses are single cell. (That is, viruses are single-cell living microorganisms.

While it's always possible, through a mutative change, for them to become multi-cell living microorganisms, we'll talk here about single cells.) The most appropriate term for these single-cell microorganisms is *viral cell*. As we get into the details of how viruses inflame the central nervous system and cause life-altering symptoms and conditions in the process, the reality that viruses are hungry, living microorganisms will be foundational knowledge.

Polluted Brains

Brain cells are highly vulnerable. They're highly sensitive. They have to be pure and clean. Unlike the liver, which is meant to be a filter for the body, the brain is never meant to be a physical filter; it should only ever be a filter in the sense of processing information—receiving communications from another source or human being. The brain houses a complex spiritual network. It also houses a complex physical network, which requires absolute purity to the highest degree. It can't be that expired piece of fish at the market with a fog glazing over its eyes and an odor coming off it because the fish had become a filter for a polluted ocean loaded with dioxins, mercury, nuclear waste, petrochemicals, and sewage filled with pharmaceuticals.

We can't look at our brain and know if our brain is going bad from cologne, perfume, scented candles, air fresheners, and toxic heavy metals. When our brain starts to develop problems, we don't see a symptom or experience a condition quite yet. We can't open our skull like an egg, take a look inside, and take a sniff to find out if it's going rotten—we can't use visual clues or our sense of smell, like we can with that egg or a piece of fish, to determine if our brain is getting toxic and dirty. Only when we start to develop symptoms from a brain that's been suffering for weeks or months or years do we start to get a clue about what's going on inside.

As you know from the previous chapters, the electricity of your brain is meant to be clean. The fluid of your brain (cerebrospinal fluid) is meant to be clean. The blood in your brain is meant to be clean. And so your liver, your brain's best friend, is working overtime to keep poisons out of your brain so your brain doesn't have to become the filter. And yet life here on Planet Earth doesn't work so ideally. Because our livers get so overloaded, our brains get saturated with poisons from all areas and angles, including prescription pharmaceuticals that are supposedly for the brain, toxic heavy metals, preservatives, chemicals, caffeine, and more that you'll read about in Part III, "Brain Betrayers."

The brain is meant to be a sponge for knowledge. Instead it becomes a sponge for waste. As blood is pumped to the brain, it is blood that's filled with many different toxins. The publicly known medical field doesn't want any part in knowing this, because the last thing it needs is to learn about the poisons that enter our brains. That would expose the crimes, neglect, and agendas of the classified medical industry, and maybe even the wizard that puppeteers it all.

Notably, some of the poisons that get through to the brain are viral toxins, including viral neurotoxins. The viruses giving off these toxins usually come from elsewhere in the body; they may reside in the liver, lymphatic system, spleen, intestinal tract, reproductive system, nervous system, even skeletal system. Viruses can even nest inside bone marrow, where many toxic heavy metals such as mercury reside and settle. This is one of the foundations of blood cell and bone marrow disease. Mainly, the viruses reside in the liver.

As I mentioned earlier, these herpetic viruses range from Epstein-Barr virus and its over 60 varieties to shingles and its over 30 varieties to cytomegalovirus (CMV) and its many varieties to multiple varieties of human herpesvirus 6 (HHV-6) to well over a dozen varieties of herpes simplex and the hundreds of other HHV varieties and mutations, most of which are undiscovered by publicly known medical research and science. Classified medical research and science let the viruses out of the running gate. Publicly known medical research and science stumble across certain varieties of the viruses by chance.

Neurotoxins 101

The most common neurotoxin culprits come from your garden-variety EBV and shingles. Everyone at this point in time has at least one form of both EBV and shingles living inside their body. These viruses can produce large quantities of neurotoxins—chemical substances poisonous to our brain and nervous system. As we feed the viruses that live inside us, they get what they need to strengthen and grow in numbers, taking us closer to our first set of symptoms.

Eggs, dairy products, corn, and soy are just a few of the foods we consume that draw the viruses out of their dormancy into a feeding frenzy. Other exposures also become food to viruses, especially if they contain toxic heavy metals—exposures such as perfume, cologne, scented candles, fragrances, air fresheners, city or town tap water, and tattoo ink. All of these viral-feeding foods we eat and toxins we're exposed to build up in and overload the liver, where viral cells are already residing. With viral cells and viral fuel together in the liver, the virus can feed on what it loves, replicate, grow in numbers, and reach maturity—at which point the virus can produce and release lots of poisons.

Your liver stores pockets of these neurotoxins to keep them from reaching your brain. Yet because the liver gets too overloaded to filter and contain all of the viral waste, neurotoxins and other viral poisons get into the bloodstream. As the rest of your body tries to keep these neurotoxins from reaching your brain, neurotoxins start gathering and building up in your spleen, inside musculoskeletal tissue, and more. Neurotoxin buildup in the body creates its own symptomology that can come and go. The bladder, for example, can start to become sensitive and overactive from neurotoxins building up inside the kidneys and bladder and/or on the pudendal nerve. As another example, neurotoxin buildup in the

liver and lymphatic system can cause fluid retention (lymphedema).

Our organs and tissues aren't meant to serve as filters to catch neurotoxins, and so they reach overload. Eventually, viral neurotoxins can travel along the current of the bloodstream to the heart and finally get delivered to the brain. Some viruses, depending on where they're located in the body, can release neurotoxins that reach the brain before they even pass through the liver. Whatever path they travel to reach the brain, when neurotoxins get there, they start to build up and saturate brain tissue. This also creates a situation where neurotoxins are able to cling and bind onto major nerve channels, such as the vagus nerves. (You'll often hear these nerves referred to in the singular, as in "the vagus nerve." Our cranial nerves occur in pairs, which is why I refer to them in the plural here. Read more in Chapter 6, "Your Inflamed Cranial Nerves.")

The more aggressive the virus and the more food the virus has to fuel itself with, the more potent the neurotoxin it releases and the more this neurotoxin builds up in different areas of the brain, which means the more fatigued and brain fogged we get. In addition to brain fog and all-body neurological fatigue, neurotoxic buildup in the brain can cause confusion, anxiety, depression, tingles, numbness, twitches, spasms, tightness in the chest, dizziness, blurry vision, eye floaters, and much more.

As we continue in this chapter, you'll read the details of how viral neurotoxins and the resulting brain inflammation can cause or play a role in numerous other symptoms and conditions, including headaches, migraines, mood changes, weakness in the limbs, lupus, multiple sclerosis (MS), neurological Lyme disease, restless legs syndrome, POTS (postural orthostatic tachycardia syndrome), transient ischemic attacks (TIAs), strokes, and dysautonomia. In Chapter 6, "Your Inflamed Cranial Nerves," you'll also read about how viral neurotoxins can inflame cranial nerves such as the vagus, trigeminal, and facial nerves, causing and contributing to even more symptoms and conditions, from Bell's palsy to TMJ (temporomandibular joint dysfunction) to neuralgia. For more symptom and condition specifics, be sure to read Part IV, "Brain Invasion," and Part V, "Your Pain and Suffering Enlightened."

How Neurotoxins Hold Us Back

Once they reach the brain, how do neurotoxins inflame neurons, swell the brain, and cause all these problems? They can do so in different ways. First, it's important to understand that neurons and nerve cells have a sensitivity level. It's a sensitivity level that allows you to experience life: pain, pleasant sensations, your sense of hearing, smelling, seeing, touching, tasting. Neurons and nerve cells are supposed to be hypersensitive so they can receive messages easily from electrical signals that harbor information from your brain and travel down nerves throughout your body. This sensitive nerve messaging is what allows us to use our bodily functions, and what allows us to benefit from functions beyond our immediate control, such as peristaltic action and sleep.

In the same way that our skin is sensitive and can react to substances that damage skin tissue, our neurons and nerve cells are sensitive to neurotoxins, because neurotoxins can harm, injure, or damage neurons and nerve cells. That's what a neurotoxin is: a toxic substance to which nerve cells are allergic. Viral neurotoxins are pollutants that are extremely acidic. Viruses are also highly acidic.

A neurotoxin excreted by a virus was never meant to be in a human body where it could touch nerve cells. Prior to the 1900s, viruses did not excrete neurotoxins capable of causing enough harm to create serious neurological symptoms and conditions. Instead, neurological symptoms and conditions were only the result of direct exposure of neurons and nerve cells to large amounts of toxic heavy metals. The viral neurotoxin component wasn't a factor until the turn of the 20th century. Before that, viruses had not adapted to consume and use these toxic heavy metals as fuel.

Another reason why viral neurotoxins are damaging to neurons is that neurons harbor information. Neurons are part of information highways. When a neurotoxin saturates a neuron, it is coating the neuron with information that conflicts with the information the neuron is receiving and transmitting. Viral neurotoxins hold information ranging from where the virus was before you contracted it to the virus's mission to what the neurotoxin is made up of. When an electrical impulse traveling with its own information hits a neurotoxin-coated neuron, conflicting information that the virus embedded into the neurotoxin causes an overheating of the neuron. Information traveling from neuron to neuron is supposed to be pure, untampered with, and unadulterated. A virus's neurotoxic waste matter that harbors information about that virus is not supposed to be interjected into the information traveling through neurons and electrical impulses. The overheating that occurs as a result is the neuron deciphering what's legitimate information versus foreign invader information. Neurons can become inflamed through this process of overexertion.

THE UPS AND DOWNS OF BRAIN INFLAMMATION

Everyone experiences the spectrum of viral brain inflammation differently. Some people have a lot going for them—a lot of love, support, resources; a better diet earlier in life; less exposure to toxic heavy metals and pathogens; and less stress—and this brain swelling from neurotoxins doesn't create a lot of symptoms for them. Maybe they have a lower viral load, more electrolytes in the diet, stronger mineral salts inside the brain, stronger neurotransmitters due to fewer stressful periods of life, a more complete glycogen "storage bin" inside the brain, less insulin resistance (meaning that glucose can enter the brain more easily), and fewer toxic heavy metals inside the brain and body, in part due to limited exposure earlier in life.

Sometimes brain inflammation is chronic, lasting years. Sometimes it's temporary, causing balance issues often misdiagnosed as Ménière's disease. Sometimes the inflammation causes mild vertigo that's there all the time. Some people experience focus and concentration issues that last for years on and off. Some people feel perfectly clear one month, and then the next they're back to the drawing board with focus and concentration problems and brain fog all over again. Sometimes the symptoms are intermittent. Sometimes someone goes through a time of high stress, struggle, or hardship that breaks down the immune system and causes many fight-or-flight adrenaline bursts that create prime opportunities for viruses to expand, proliferate, and grow, leading to bouts of brain inflammation that go along with these difficult times. As we continue in this chapter, and in Part II, "Brainwashed," and Part III, "Brain Betrayers," you'll read more about the viral fuel, triggers, and exposures that contribute to these ups and downs in our experiences of brain inflammation.

Brain inflammation is rampant in our society today. Patients who've been filing into doctors' offices and clinics year after year, decade after decade—now more than ever before in history, and even more so in the coming days and years—should be leaving with not only a brain inflammation diagnosis; they should leave with a viral diagnosis. For all the reasons we've already explored, this won't happen the way it should. If it did happen, and it was acknowledged that people have brain inflammation, it would be spun in a direction that did not support the patient and instead supported the pharmaceutical industry. We're not supposed to know that viruses are causing our symptoms, unless it's a virus with tremendous propaganda behind it. The herpetic viruses that are causing the epidemic of chronic pain and chronic illness are the original viruses that classified medical research and science released into our environment over the last hundred years in a top-secret manner. Even though some of these viruses have been discovered by publicly known medical research and science, the viruses are not seen as a problem or a cause of neurological symptoms and brain inflammation. They're not recognized in this way—the viruses are not seen for what they are: biological warfare.

That's why we need to know, so we can heal ourselves: because getting help out there is not easy. The best that will happen now is leaving the doctor's office with a long-haul COVID or neurological Lyme diagnosis, whether that's backed up by a blood test or not. (Those of you familiar with the truth about Lyme disease are aware of what I mean here. For anyone new to the truth about Lyme, you'll read more about Lyme in Part V of this book, "Your Pain and Suffering Enlightened," and you may also want to check out the updated edition of *Medical Medium*.) Some functional specialty MDs who have picked up on Medical Medium information are starting to get one thing right: that COVID is reactivating the Epstein-Barr virus someone already has. They're still confused, giving a diagnosis of

reactivated EBV *with* long-haul COVID—when the problem is reactivated EBV itself, which can later inflame the vagus nerves, causing vagus nerve–related symptoms. And these well-meaning practitioners are not necessarily following through and providing the right protocols. The COVID virus itself does not injure the vagus nerves. Instead, the COVID virus weakens a person's immune system, allowing EBV to affect the vagus nerves. (More about long-haul COVID in a moment.)

Untangling the Epidemic of Neurological Fatigue

One reason people are filing into doctor's offices is that they're struggling with *neurological fatigue*. When someone's immune system is compromised and they develop a low-grade or high-grade herpetic viral load, a large amount of neurotoxins can be produced by that viral load, eventually saturating the brain and leading to a fatigue that seems to be everlasting, a fatigue that doesn't remedy itself with ample sleep.

No one is going to know this fatigue is caused by neurotoxins. Neither conventional nor alternative medicine will even know that it's neurological fatigue. They'll think it's simply fatigue from a thyroid disorder, neurological Lyme, long-haul COVID, or an adrenal condition, or they may call it ME/CFS (myalgic encephalomyelitis/chronic fatigue syndrome), without understanding what's really behind it. If a medical professional lines up the fatigue with EBV, that diagnosis is due to information gleaned from Medical Medium publications and teachings that reactivated EBV or other low-grade viral infections (detected or undetected) cause fatigue and even inflame or injure the vagus nerves.

This viral neurological fatigue is in a different class from everyday fatigue. Neurological fatigue is the result of brain tissue saturated with viral neurotoxins that elevate inflammation, resulting in swelling inside brain cells—swelling of glial cells, neurons, and glands in the brain—and/or swelling of nerves leaving the brain or swelling of tiny nerves on the outside of the brain, close to the skull. Neurotoxins can also land on nerves throughout the body, including the optic, vagus, phrenic, trigeminal, pudendal, hypoglossal, facial, and sciatic nerves, creating what starts as mild swelling that can create symptoms that make us feel uncomfortable and can then progress and worsen.

As nerve cells in the brain and body become saturated with viral neurotoxins and neurological fatigue sets in, you may feel like your legs weigh a thousand pounds. Your body can ache. Your feet may feel like sandbags are attached to them. It can be hard to hold yourself up; sometimes even sitting up is too hard. You may need to sleep a lot, spend a lot of time on your mattress island, and your thoughts may not be easy to process. Words may not be easy to formulate and express. Talking can be too difficult, take too much energy. Even a shower can be a difficult task, using up your energy reserves for the day. These are the more serious versions of neurological fatigue. There are also milder versions.

Again, we're not talking about a virus inside the brain inflaming the nerves or brain cells; it's neurotoxic viral waste matter that has made its way to the brain through the ocean of our blood. (In some cases, there can be a virus present in the brain itself causing more inflammation. Read more under "Direct Viral Brain Inflammation" later in this chapter.)

Part of what's so distressing about neurological fatigue is the mystery of it. When you're going through this debilitating fatigue and not able to find answers for it, you can reach a point of distrusting yourself. The world tells us that if we're fatigued, it means we need to exercise more or change our mindset or optimize our sleep or try the next trendy diet or health product. The world may even send us the message that we're lazy, or that we've created our fatigue. You gain power and set yourself on the path of healing the moment you understand this neurological fatigue for what it is: viral neurotoxins saturating brain and nerve cells.

With this knowledge, you also gain insight into one aspect of neurological fatigue (among many) that baffles the best of doctors: the intermittent nature it can exhibit. For some people, neurological fatigue is not so bad at times and then very difficult at times. This is because neurotoxins are floating around in the bloodstream, moving around, and landing on nerves at different times. Our body is in a constant state of rejuvenation; it has the tendency to fight off a problem and heal itself whenever it can. So as a nerve gets inflamed by a small amount of neurotoxins, the healing process kicks in to try to remedy that inflammation and rid those neurotoxins, and the neurological fatigue symptoms can start to lift on their own—until another batch of neurotoxins come and the symptoms get worse again.

If a greater quantity of neurotoxins is present in the bloodstream, and those neurotoxins are being produced by more aggressive viruses, then the battle becomes more difficult. This is when severe chronic fatigue that becomes deep neurological fatigue that doesn't seem to let up occurs. Neurotoxins are continually coating nerves, and the brain's and body's ability to remedy and restore the area can't keep up with the onslaught of neurotoxins.

Long-Haul Flu and Long-Haul COVID

Publicly known medical research and science have never had long-haul flu on their radar as a concern. By "long-haul flu" I mean when someone contracts an influenza virus, gets a high fever, becomes ill, and then doesn't seem to come out of it so easily. Rather than recovering quickly, they're now sick, fatigued, and dysfunctional for months and sometimes even years after having the flu. Medical research and science don't have a long-haul flu treatment. Long-haul flu has been around for decades, and it's gone unrecognized by publicly known medical research and science for all this time.

Long-haul flu is caused when an underlying non-flu virus or two that were already inside a person get triggered out of the running gate because a flu virus pushes that person's already-weakened immune system

to its limits. For example, a lowered immune system from the flu could allow EBV already in that person's body to reactivate. Millions of people around the world have experienced this type of post-flu-related sickness.

Publicly known medical research and science (both alternative and conventional) are unaware of the connection to the flu as a *trigger* for a different, underlying virus that causes lasting symptoms once a flu infection has cleared up. They don't realize either part—the presence of the underlying herpetic virus (such as EBV or shingles) or the flu as a trigger for that underlying virus to create chronic post-flu symptoms. Because medical communities don't understand long-haul flu, what commonly happens is that someone who's struggling after having the flu ends up with an autoimmune diagnosis. Or if they already had an autoimmune diagnosis prior to the flu, then after the flu, they can develop more symptoms, or more severe symptoms, and end up with additional autoimmune diagnoses.

Some flu treatments have been an ongoing trigger for decades, meaning a trigger for viruses such as EBV to reactivate, in turn leading to neurological symptoms and conditions that occur or recur. They have left a wake of people struggling with neurological symptoms because their viruses have been reactivated, resulting in brain and nervous system inflammation. This has been ignored completely by both conventional and alternative medical communities. Publicly known medical research and science don't have post–flu treatment symptoms and conditions on their radar.

What has gained recognition is the term *long-haul COVID* (also called *long COVID*). We are embarking into an era when a considerable percentage of the population is going to be suffering, both from long-haul COVID and from post-COVID medical treatments that will trigger chronic brain inflammation and lower the immune system. Just like some yearly flu treatments, some yearly COVID treatments will reactivate internal viruses in individuals that will create symptoms very similar to the diagnosis of long-haul COVID itself.

That is, some individuals will experience getting sick with COVID, and then not properly recover due to the internal viral inflammation from another, underlying virus such as EBV that was *triggered* by COVID lowering their immune system, allowing the EBV to reactivate. That will get labeled as long-haul COVID, or sometimes long-haul COVID *with* reactivated EBV—when really, the reactivated EBV or other herpetic virus should be the main focus because that EBV or other herpetic virus is the reason for the lasting symptoms that are labeled "long-haul COVID." Some COVID treatments will do something similar, lowering the immune system by keeping the immune system distracted, thinning out and overburdening the immune system so it's not able to watch out for other threats inside the body. As a result, the immune system will completely ignore the true, greater threats inside the human body, such as the herpetic viruses present that create brain inflammation.

For more about long-haul flu and long-haul COVID, see Part V, "Your Pain and Suffering Enlightened."

What Viruses Love to Eat

We gain ultimate power over the symptoms of brain inflammation when we understand where many of these ups and downs come from: viral fuel. The more of its favorite foods a virus has to feed on, the more it thrives and the worse our symptoms get. By removing foods and toxins that viruses love to eat from our brains and bodies, we start to starve the viruses that have been wreaking so much havoc with our health.

Now, there are different levels of viral brain inflammation. As I've mentioned, a factor that influences that level of inflammation is how aggressive the virus or viral strain is. The more aggressive the virus, the more potent the neurotoxin it excretes. The stage of the virus matters too. If it's in a dormant or early stage of infection, a virus will cause less inflammation than a virus in a more advanced stage that has built up a greater number of active viral cells in the body over time. The more viral cells, the greater quantity of neurotoxins they can excrete.

And then there's viral fuel: what level of brain inflammation someone experiences is largely determined by what the virus (whether it's an aggressive viral strain or a more moderate to mild viral strain) is finding inside the body to feed on and fuel itself. Here's a look at some of the most common virus-feeding foods and how they cause a virus—and its symptoms—to progress.

(For even more examples of viral fuel, see Part III, "Brain Betrayers.")

Gluten

Gluten is a favorite food of viruses. When a virus feeds on gluten, the virus can proliferate—grow and spawn and create more viral cells. Yet gluten itself is not a toxic substance. That's why a person can eat gluten and not experience any symptoms or conditions; the viruses they have may not have left dormancy and begun to feed on gluten yet. Gluten doesn't become toxic until it's consumed and excreted by a virus. So when a virus feeds on gluten, even though the virus is growing in number because it's eating a favorite food, the waste excreted from the virus will not be as toxic as the waste a virus excretes after consuming forms of viral fuel that are inherently toxic (such as mercury and copper).

Gluten is still problematic because it feeds viruses, so gluten increases numbers of viral cells, which creates more viral byproduct and waste matter, which creates inflammation throughout the body, even if it's sometimes very subtle inflammation with very subtle symptoms. The neurotoxins that a virus excretes when it feeds on gluten are still neurotoxic, so this variety of neurotoxin does cause brain and nerve inflammation, though on a smaller scale in comparison to some other forms of viral fuel. Sometimes when gluten leads to only very subtle inflammation and symptoms, it's because the virus is at an earlier stage, and as the virus advances, the inflammation and

symptoms that occur when eating gluten will worsen over time.

A stagnant and sluggish liver fills up with viral waste as a result of the virus replicating abundantly as it feeds on gluten. This can lead to symptoms such as mild fatigue, brain fog, and weight gain.

Eggs

Eggs are the perfect food for viruses. Viruses love eggs much more than gluten. While eggs themselves are a nontoxic food, they're certainly not the best food for the human body; hence all the heart attack warnings throughout the years. Eggs also stimulate and perpetuate viral growth and replication on a fierce level. This is because these viruses were originally raised inside chicken eggs in classified labs. More viral cells mean more potential for the virus to then find and feed on substances in the body that *are* very toxic (such as the chemicals in fragrances), which can in turn allow the virus to release upgraded, more noxious forms of neurotoxins that increase inflammation of the brain and nerves. Neurotoxins from a virus feeding on eggs aren't the most toxic or damaging of neurotoxins. They're a little bit more inflammatory than the neurotoxins excreted by a virus feeding on gluten, because as the virus consumes natural hormones and undeveloped proteins from the baby chicken, what was already foreign to the body (hormones and proteins) has now become *toxically* foreign to the body after being excreted from the virus.

Viral neurotoxins from eggs also cause the liver to become stagnant and sluggish, which means the lymphatic system is going to become stagnant and sluggish because the lymphatic system is only as clean as the liver is. Unlike gluten, eggs are high in fat. Higher fat means thicker blood, which means more stagnant blood and less oxygen in the blood, allowing viruses to thrive. Oxygen keeps viruses more docile. Fats are also extremely acidic, creating an acidic bloodstream, and an acidic environment allows viruses to thrive because the blood becomes thicker and more toxic as acid increases. Having more viral cells means more possibility of those viruses finding toxic heavy metals such as mercury and other substances to feed on.

When someone says, "My grandmother is ninety years old and eating eggs, and she's fine," that's not the reality. If you talk to that grandmother, she'll likely tell you she's on multiple medications, dealing with fibromyalgia, arthritis (maybe even rheumatoid arthritis), brain fog, memory loss, and weight gain, and has had these or other symptoms for a long time. Yes, maybe she ate eggs early in life without a problem to start with. Yet as eggs were feeding on viruses in her body over time, symptoms developed too.

People can go for years eating eggs without many symptoms. Then when symptoms do start to develop, they don't connect the symptoms to the eggs. Behind the scenes, viruses have been slowly growing inside these people's bodies from the eggs they consume, and it's these viruses that are creating their symptoms. Someone may say, "Well, I can eat eggs, and I'm fine." Meanwhile, they're getting diagnosed with polycystic ovary syndrome (PCOS) or prostate cancer or breast cancer or endometriosis or having miscarriages or reproductive problems and never making the connection with the eggs. Not to mention that they're also suffering with some degree of brain and nerve inflammation from the neurotoxins that viruses expel as they thrive on eggs. As viral cells steadily grow in number from the eggs they consume, there's a greater chance those viral cells will find more-toxic forms of viral fuel in the body—and that can have dire consequences for the central nervous system.

Toxic Heavy Metals and Everyday Toxins

Everyone has certain levels of mercury in their organs, including in their brain. Having more viral cells mean more opportunities to run across a small pocket of mercury inside the liver, spleen, pancreas, reproductive system, intestinal tract, heart, or brain. If someone is very low in mercury toxicity, it doesn't mean they won't get a dose of mercury exposure at some point that can feed a viral colony present in their body that's been supported by eggs. Once that viral colony consumes mercury, the viral cells are now excreting a powerful neurotoxin versus the milder neurotoxins they once had when the virus was feeding on gluten and eggs.

This powerful neurotoxin from a virus feeding on mercury is unlike other neurotoxins—because mercury itself is neurotoxic. Once it's processed inside a viral cell, the structure of mercury is changed. It's transformed into a methylmercury, meaning it's now composed of smaller mercury particles that have the ability to enter every part of the human body with ease and cross the blood-brain barrier with ease. This type of neurotoxin can saturate the brain, causing inflammation in different areas of the brain and resulting in a variety of symptoms. This is worse inflammation than the viral neurotoxins from gluten and eggs, which means that the symptoms someone experiences from mercury viral neurotoxins are worse too.

Viruses like mercury because it was originally used by labs to preserve viruses. While being studied and raised in classified labs, viruses would be kept alive and suspended in their present state in a mercury-based preservative solution. Viruses learned to adapt to mercury, using it as food.

Mercury is not the only toxic substance that allows viral neurotoxins to become problematic. Any toxic heavy metal can suffice. Any solvent or chemical created for industrial use can create potent viral neurotoxins too, including plug-in air fresheners, hair spray, other hair products, colognes, perfumes, scented candles, conventional household cleaning supplies, conventional detergents, fabric softeners, dryer dust (meaning the brew of laundry chemicals, air fresheners, perfumes, and colognes that spews out of dryer vents), fragrances, cosmetics, new toxic chemicals on fabrics, fungicides on new clothing and furniture, pesticides, herbicides, and gasoline fumes. All of these can provide fuel for viruses to create very toxic neurotoxins that create brain inflammation.

It's worth noting that more viral waste in the body means a more lowered immune system, which means more possibilities for the virus to reach the brain through the bloodstream to search for viral food in the brain. More viral waste and the resulting lowered immune system also mean more opportunities for the virus to cross into the spinal fluid to head to the brain on an alternative path, although most viruses, if they reach the brain, travel there through the bloodstream and not the spinal fluid. You could have debilitating neurological symptoms, such as what someone with neurological Lyme or multiple sclerosis experiences, and still not have the virus enter your brain itself. That's because the virus could be releasing neurotoxins from elsewhere in the body that are so potent that when the neurotoxins reach and enter the brain, neuron inflammation occurs, leading debilitating symptoms to develop.

It's also worth noting that someone could have a larger amount of mercury in their brain and body and a smaller amount of viruses or viral cells because they're not eating a lot of eggs, gluten, or other brain betrayers such as dairy and corn that would cause the virus(es) to grow in number. Therefore, the virus(es) remain smaller in numbers, less apt to find the mercury deposits. Even so, you can still experience symptoms from mercury deposits themselves, as you read about in Chapter 3, "Your Alloy Brain."

A Perfect Storm of Viral Fuel

As you've seen, there are nuances to how viruses, viral fuel, and neurotoxins add up to someone's individual experience. While mercury is a viral fuel, it's not a virus's food of choice, so it doesn't cause a virus to proliferate in large numbers. Yet if a virus is proliferating because it has other fuel present such as eggs, gluten, dairy, and corn, the viral cells can strengthen in number enough to go find mercury and other toxic substances to further fuel itself. A larger number of viral cells means more travel bandwidth for the virus as it looks for more sources of food, so more viral cells tend to travel deeper throughout the body. It's that combination of (1) growing the virus in number from eating foods such as eggs and (2) having enough mercury and/or other everyday toxins in your system for the virus to then feed on that leads to an abundance of potent neurotoxins, which makes for the more serious symptoms and conditions.

VIRAL REPLICATION

To get a complete picture of a viral brain, it helps to understand how viruses replicate in our bodies when we don't take antiviral action with the tools in this book and *Brain Saver Protocols, Cleanses & Recipes.*

Viruses will do anything to stay alive. They will adapt and realign and change their replication methods for survival. The viruses of today are all engineered and new in our modern-day history. This started in the first 20 years of the 20th century. Prior to the early 1900s, viruses were docile and untampered with by man. They may not have appeared docile because of the

severe deficiencies and lack of fresh water in many areas. A docile virus is not so docile when someone's diet consists of a single type of grain for two straight years, with no access to fresh fruit or vegetables or fresh, clean water for drinking and bathing. Plus, remedies such as vitamin C were a rarity. That's how viruses could take hold in areas impoverished in nutrients, food supplies, and fresh water. It's critical to understand this context for viruses prior to the 1900s.

When it comes to how viruses replicate, there are a lot of different theories. Experts often use terms like "DNA," "RNA," and "proteins" to make viruses seem like they're all about genetics. They purposely try to take viruses in the direction of being gene-related because that's where funding is going. They try to convince us that viruses are pieces of gene material, and that our genes are involved with the virus genes, and that these viruses aren't alive. They need us to believe viruses aren't the real problems, that it's our "weak" genes that are the problem and viruses are just the trigger. One of the theories out there is that viruses are attached to, and live within, our genes, and that when you trigger the gene, you can awaken the virus. No matter the popular theory of any given day, they're going to keep focusing on genetics when it comes to viruses.

Viruses have nothing to do with genes. Viruses are separate entities that we get exposed to, and then the viruses try to live the duration of their lives within our bodies. Viruses are actual living bugs that live within us.

Viruses are also replicators. Once inside us, viral cells grow in number, creating replicas of themselves. There are different varieties of viruses that cause brain inflammation, and the different viruses replicate differently. Here are some examples of how viruses replicate:

- **Viral Replication Method 1:**
  In this method a virus enters a human cell and then replicates inside the human cell. Then the human cell explodes, and from that explosion the virus replicas spread.

- **Viral Replication Method 2:**
  Many viruses replicate by viral cells coming into contact with one another. The viral cells need to touch each other, which sets off a stimulating hormone within each viral cell involved. That stimulating hormone starts off the process for each viral cell to create multiple replicas of itself within its viral cell membrane. Each membrane expands, stretches, and then snaps, and out come multiple new viral cells. (Each viral cell that snapped open now becomes a dead, toxic viral corpse. These viral corpses can form a sticky, jelly buildup in the organs that can make someone sick.) Once released from the old viral cells, the new viral replicas instantly go on the search for

food. This type of virus feeds on human cells that have already expired and died and whatever contaminants are in those dead human cells. When a viral cell has fed enough to mature, it seeks out another mature viral cell as a partner to start the multiplication process all over again.

- **Viral Replication Method 3:**
  Certain viruses don't have the ability to enter a human cell or to replicate on their own. To replicate, these viruses need fertilization, a type that occurs from another viral cell. While viruses are not male or female, with this type of virus, viral cells do fertilize each other. To do so, the viral cells will communicate between each other, and they will eventually find each other inside the body and join together for a fertilization process. One viral cell fertilizes the other, and then the fertilized viral cell releases eggs into the bloodstream or organs. This is one way the mutation process happens. If two viral cells of the same virus yet different mutations join together, their offspring after the fertilization process will be different from what the parent viruses were. While

the offspring viral cells will resemble the parent cells, there will be a slight mutation.

- **Viral Replication Method 4:** For this type of replication, no fertilization or stimulating hormone is required. Certain varieties of viruses attach to human cell tissue, with individual viral cells releasing viral eggs. It happens when a viral cell matures and nears the end of its life cycle, at which point the viral cell produces eggs within itself and tries to find a human host cell into which it can inject those eggs. These viruses can pierce and inject anywhere from a half dozen to over 50 eggs into a human cell, expanding that cell as the viral eggs hatch, exploding the human cell and releasing the hatched viral cells.

- **Viral Replication Method 5:** When a virus of this type is aging out and reaching its shelf life, it can replicate a newer version of itself as its old carcass and viral cell casing shed away. This is a transformational virus that replicates through cell transformation.

- **Viral Replication Method 6:** In this method, when a viral cell

reaches the end of maturity and will be dying soon, it releases a signal, through chemical compounds it excretes, that it's at the end of its life cycle. A number of other viral cells answering the call cluster around the mature viral cell to be fertilized. Once the viral cells are fertilized, the cluster breaks up and the fertilized viral cells search for human host cells. Each fertilized viral cell injects one egg inside one human host cell, and then each egg hatches inside each human host cell. This is a slow-replicating type of virus.

This is not an exhaustive list of how viruses can replicate. It's a look at some of the common examples. And keep in mind, most anything to do with viral replication remains undiscovered by publicly known medical research and science. They're still debating theories among themselves about the basic nature of viruses.

For the methods of viral replication that require viral cells to come into contact or fertilize each other, one single viral cell can live inside you without another viral cell, waiting for your exposure to another viral cell of the same virus. For example, if someone gets exposed to one single Epstein-Barr virus cell, that viral cell could stay dormant for two to three years until that person gets exposed to another EBV cell, at which point the virus can start replicating and creating symptoms. That said, when someone gets exposed to a virus, they're usually not exposed to only one viral cell. They're exposed to multiple virus cells, from dozens to hundreds at one time.

No matter what method a virus uses to grow its number of viral cells, the only way a virus can replicate is if viral food is present in the human body. Baby viruses need fuel sources inside human cells in order to grow—which is why it's so important to keep coming back to the information from the previous section, "What Viruses Love to Eat," and reminding ourselves that we can starve viruses if we want to stop viral replication in its tracks.

Viruses also need weakened human cells to enter—cells that are lacking in supplies. If a human cell is dehydrated due to caffeine, vinegar, and salt, and if it doesn't have enough vitamin C, zinc, and other trace minerals inside it, then it's a susceptible, vulnerable cell that viruses can break into. On the other hand, if a human cell is strong enough, hydrated enough, and abundant enough in phytochemical compounds, antioxidants such as vitamin C, melatonin, minerals, trace minerals such as zinc, and multiple antiviral compounds from fruits, herbs, leafy greens, wild foods, and vegetables, it's much more difficult for a virus to invade that human cell. When a virus tries to break into a healthy human cell, the virus could give up and look for a weaker cell. Because the process of trying to break into a healthy cell can take too long and require too much energy from the virus, it can even

ring alarms in the process that awaken the immune system to sniff out the criminal trying to enter the human cell.

DIRECT VIRAL BRAIN INFLAMMATION

Here in "Your Viral Brain," we've been focused on the most common form of brain inflammation. We've been talking about a brain *indirectly* inflamed by a virus that's living elsewhere in the body. Millions and millions of people globally are walking around with this type of undiscovered viral brain inflammation, and they are leading diminished lives because of it.

As I mentioned, there is also such a thing as a virus getting into someone's brain. Here's a little background on these more rare and extreme cases of viral brain inflammation, where a virus directly inflames the brain:

Sometimes a virus can stay dormant in the brain, not causing too many problems, although even a dormant virus in the brain can still cause mild neurological symptoms because it will release some pollutants as it's taking up residence. When a dormant virus in the brain becomes activated, or when an active virus enters the brain and causes an acute infection, that's when an explosive, acute condition such as Guillain-Barré or a condition that resembles a stroke can occur. That explosive, acute condition can occur from a combination of viral cells directly injuring brain cells while also releasing viral neurotoxins directly into the brain.

When a virus does enter the brain, or when a dormant virus in the brain becomes activated, it can create direct inflammation in a particular area of the brain, causing neuron damage and myelin nerve sheath damage that, if the damage becomes visible on brain imaging, could be diagnosed as demyelination or encephalitis. Although keep in mind that a diagnosis of myelin nerve sheath damage from brain imaging is not definitive. In many cases what medical professionals identify as brain lesions are actually oxidizing deposits of mercury and aluminum that have stained the nerve sheath, brain tissue, or nervous system tissue. And most of the time, they can't see anything in the brain.

Normally viral infections of the brain itself are acute and severe, leaving people in the hospital for weeks, diagnosed with meningitis even if the cause of the meningitis is unknown. *Meningitis*, by the way, is just a term for brain inflammation from a current infection, even if no one knows precisely whether it's bacterial or viral. Even after performing a spinal tap, they may not know; diagnosis comes down to theory and a doctor's opinion.

Spinal taps are almost always unnecessary and rarely offer any clues or insights into a medical problem when it comes to chronic sickness, or acute sickness that becomes chronic. Spinal taps were adopted by the medical industry when the industry realized it *could* administer a spinal tap. It's almost always a formality, versus an avenue that actually provides answers. Spinal taps can cause unnecessary damage to the spinal cord. Spinal taps are antiquated. The analysis of the spinal fluid is not advanced. The medical industry should stop performing spinal taps unless they learn to start testing for pertinent or relevant contaminants and viral byproduct inside the spinal fluid, which they do not.

As a result of the extreme inflammation of an active viral infection in the brain, patients can experience fever and severe neurological weakness, continual migraine, pressure in the head, or burning pain in the head. Symptoms can vary depending on where the viral infection is in the brain. And it's not easy to distinguish the difference between neurological symptoms from a virus inside the brain versus symptoms from neurotoxins traveling to the brain from a virus somewhere else in the body. For example, sometimes a person can experience what feels like a fever, where they have the sensation of their head burning hot even when a thermometer reading shows they don't have a fever. This is a case of nerves burning from the inside. It can be experienced without a virus in the brain and instead from a large degree of neurotoxins that have gone to the brain and inflamed brain tissue, or the feverish-without-a-fever symptom can occur from a virus in the brain directly injuring nerves. Chills without fever are a symptom of neurotoxins' effect on brain tissue. The feeling that the head is extremely heavy, that the head is swollen, or that it's hard to hold up the head on the body can be symptomatic of a virus in the brain latching onto nerves there, or they can be symptoms of viral neurotoxins.

OUR OVERBURDENED IMMUNE SYSTEM

Our immune system is looking out for us. I've always said that the body reacts to vitamin B_{12} shots as an enemy. When B_{12} is injected into the arm or leg, for example, and not delivered intravenously or taken orally, any kind of calamity can ensue, resulting in brain inflammation. Our body has a safety mechanism. Anything that breaks the skin is seen as an enemy if any kind of foreign substance is left behind. Our body will build an antibody to that foreign substance. The body does not consider it foreign if it's delivered intravenously: that is, by IV. That's why IV nutritional therapy is different from B_{12} shots. When B_{12} or any other type of nutrient or even medication enters in through the vein, the body will not consider it an enemy unless it's an outright poison.

If a B_{12} injection breaks the derma, travels into the muscle, and is then released into the muscle, leaving behind B_{12} or any preservatives, the deeper the injection injury is, the more chance your body has of retaliating and building an antibody or allergy to it. Retaliation can mean anything from a mild sensitivity to B_{12}; to a total breakdown of the body's ability to create, process, or convert B_{12}; to seeing B_{12} as an enemy, allowing for an inflammatory occurrence to happen, including inflammation of the brain. Also, B_{12} injections lower the immune system, allowing pathogens to take advantage and increase viral neurotoxin inflammation. Someone who has had B_{12} injections should switch to oral B_{12} in the form of adenosylcobalamin with methylcobalamin. (Steer clear of cyanocobalamin.) Intravenous (IV) B_{12} is okay, although B_{12} administered orally is best anyway.

The same applies to antibiotics delivered via injection and to allergy shots. If the needle goes deeper than the derma and enters into the muscle, there's a greater chance for the body to see the antibiotic or allergy shot serum as an enemy and to build an antibody, resistance, or allergy against that antibiotic or allergy shot. (Yes, allergy shots create more allergies.)

The same could happen with cosmetic injections. While cosmetic injections are usually just underneath the derma, cosmetic injection injuries do occur, where the needle accidentally goes a little farther and ends up directly in connective facial tissue, main nerves, or deeper in blood vessels and the bloodstream. When this happens, the body sees the cosmetic injection substance as the enemy and can build an antibody, resistance, or allergy to its components, such as to the botulinum toxin that is commonly used. The original trend was for women in their 40s and 50s to get cosmetic injections. Now younger generations in their teens and 20s are getting cosmetic injections, giving them an additional 20 to 30 years of exposure. That means 20 to 30 extra years to build up antibodies and allergies to the injections and cosmetic fillers, placing an additional load on the immune system, which weakens and lowers the immune system, allowing common, everyday viruses such as EBV to cause brain inflammation that much earlier in life.

Steroid injections often go deep into the muscle and connective tissue, which is why many people become sensitive to steroid injections. The body can eventually tag the steroid as a threat because it's not entering intravenously through a vein and is instead entering through a needle into muscle and connective tissue.

Anything that enters the body through this avenue has the potential to create sensitivities and conflict with other problems someone is struggling with, such as viruses. Our immune system is already burdened with viruses—many of the symptoms you'll read about in this book are caused by viruses creating inflammation, and the immune system is struggling to keep these viruses under control. Treatments that require an injection from outside the body that are not administered intravenously create a complication where the body's immune system pays attention to these distractions. Your immune system is now trying to decipher the poison, the toxin, or the foreign invader as friend or foe, and then making a decision about whether the body needs to create an antibody or chemical compound for resistance purposes, to protect the brain and other organs. This strain on the immune system can be a trigger for viruses to take advantage. Previously, the immune system might have had EBV, cytomegalovirus, HHV-6, HHV-7, herpes simplex 1, herpes simplex 2, or shingles under control. With the immune system's eye off the ball, these viruses can become reactivated.

A FUTURE OF BRAIN INFLAMMATION

Medical communities are starting to catch on to brain inflammation, acting as though it's a full and complete answer. The groundbreaking truth about viral-caused inflammation in the first Medical Medium book prompted great interest from the field of medicine. Doctors who are public figures and are aware of Medical Medium–published information are now talking about brain inflammation and its possible causes. Medical research and science have not yet discovered underlying, subtle pathogen inflammation, yet public-figure doctors are pretending the information exists in studies—which it does not. They've taken Medical Medium–published information on pathogen-caused inflammation and not cited its origin, yet spoken on behalf of the information as if they're all-knowledgeable. Some doctors who hold great integrity have cited Medical Medium publications as the source. Others who are public figures in the public eye pretend the information is fair use, and they use it for their own devices without citing it. At the same time they use the Medical Medium information about brain inflammation, they leave out critical parts of it, or twist it to suit their own agenda.

This is important for you to know so you can protect yourself from the misinformation out there as these figures manipulate Medical Medium information. When a public-figure doctor or even a healthy hobbyist takes information from Medical Medium publications about brain inflammation without citing this as the source, they make it look like it's been discovered. In reality medical research and science and medical schools are really not aware of this subtle type of viral brain inflammation. The public figures create the illusion that they're standing on the platform of medical research and science by finding one study, or more often just a theoretical research paper, that doesn't match the information they've learned here. They cite that one paper or study anyway, using it as a decoy. The real source they're using is Medical Medium–published information.

Accepting that there's underlying subtle brain inflammation in millions of people would be a colossal breakthrough in the field of medicine. It would also discredit decades of brain studies and literature. I know medical research and science, and I know the field of medicine, both alternative and conventional, and if they detected this subtle brain inflammation, they'd have to blame it on genetics or the autoimmune theory. That's what some public figures are already doing: saying that brain inflammation (that they've really learned about through Medical Medium) is the body attacking itself because of various triggers (which is not the real reason for brain inflammation). They say that the body is creating the brain inflammation from the body's own immune system attacking the brain. That's what I mean about twisting the information here. And that's as far as the field of medicine is able to go, because medicine is trapped.

We're heading to a place where chronic sickness is going to be redefined because more than half of the world's population is going to be greatly ill with neurological conditions, most of the time with brain inflammation present. In the coming years, there is also going to be an increase in human immunodeficiency virus (HIV). More people are going to be struggling with a lowered immune system, allowing other viruses such as EBV, shingles, HHV-6, and herpes simplex to create more chronic cases of brain inflammation and autoimmune disease. Medical research and science, both publicly known and classified, when steered correctly and monitored properly, can work in favor of humanity. When abused and not geared for public safety and instead geared for greed and sinister reasons, they can be the downfall of the human population, and most likely will be.

We've already witnessed what happened in the world over the last 100 years when engineered, manufactured viruses have left a lab and entered the population. We are learning that certain aspects of medical research and science are not working for the safety of the people.

With the knowledge about why you've experienced the health challenges that have held you back in life, you gain the healing tools and insights to *change* your experience and start living your life without the limitations of a viral brain, no matter what battles are waged in the medical arena.

CHAPTER 5

Your Emotional Brain

If someone told you they never get emotional, one of four things could be happening:

They don't realize what they're saying.

They're not telling the truth.

They handle their emotional state by convincing themselves that they never become emotional.

They spend time around people who express their emotions in a much more pronounced way, so in comparison, they think they don't get emotional.

Even when a person experiences depersonalization and says they're numb and they don't feel anything, the people around them would call that state of not feeling or expressing an emotional state in itself—an emotional state of being "checked out."

Emotions are a natural state of being for us all. Many people are trying to keep their emotions in. They don't want to be so emotional. They worry that emotions are a weakness, or they worry that their emotional reactions will get out of control and they'll melt down in front of others. Or people worry that if they say one thing wrong,

or express their viewpoint, the rest of the world will emotionally react. The world has gotten very emotional. Everyone is under so much pressure from so many directions. Our emotions are getting invaded and manipulated like never before from factors you'll read about in this chapter, factors that are clouding and disrupting and unsteadying and toying with what our emotions are meant to communicate.

So many people are misunderstood. Their actions, their words, their intentions, their emotional state—they're misunderstood by the people around them who know them, barely know them, or don't know them at all. This chapter is not going to be about hitting at a person's weaknesses, ripping a person down to then rebuild them from the ground up, fashioned in the way that others want them to be. This isn't about ripping yourself down to rebuild yourself the way you'd like others to see you, or to turn yourself into the person others want you to be. When we do that, we could be ripping the fabric of our good, important, even critical qualities and emotional strengths without knowing their value. Understanding our emotions should not be about judgment. It should always be the opposite. We should not be tearing each other down; we should be supporting each other. This chapter is about understanding why we get emotional—what happens inside us when we get emotional—because that knowledge can inevitably protect us from emotional damage.

EMOTIONAL CREATURES

Trying to change people by telling them about their egos, pointing out their emotional shortcomings and weaknesses, and convincing them that their thoughts are creating their illness—those aren't the answers to mental health, spiritual health, physical health, or emotional health. Supporting and strengthening an individual's emotional state, soul state, and spirit while providing tools for emotional recovery is far different from subliminally trying to teach them that they're a bad person, or that all their faults make them a bad person, or that something needs to be improved upon because they're not good enough.

We all become emotional on a minute-by-minute basis. We're emotional creatures. Some of us are more intense; for reasons publicly known medical research and science don't have a handle on, some people deal with more pronounced emotional responses and express them in a more pronounced manner. Every soul is unique, and everyone has their own emotional wellspring. We all have our emotional injuries and differences in how we process what we're experiencing, feeling, seeing, or hearing. Does emotional counseling help people through their wounds and processing? It can. Not that it's always the right fit or can help in every way, shape, and form. Because of the differences among us all, sometimes someone seeks support from a psychologist, psychiatrist, psychoanalyst, therapist, spiritual adviser, life coach, or counselor and has to switch out one professional they're using for another. Different professionals understand and respond to people's emotions differently. That affects the experience of the person who's going through and trying to process the emotions, which in turn determines whether that person is getting the coping mechanisms and management tools and as much help as possible from the professional.

As I said, emotional experiences can change by the moment, with some emotions being somewhat subtle and gentle and others being extreme. People handle them in a variety of ways—whether the reaction is to go running, scream out loud, throw things, break down and cry, blame someone, blame themselves, distance themselves from others, need to be around others, shut out the world, or act like nothing's wrong. This isn't about how to fix emotional problems by being a better person or how to fix the way you handle, deal with, or process your emotions. The truth is that no matter how cool or calm you are, something could happen that rocks your emotional state. Besides, if you say you need to "fix" the person you are, that's coming from a place of judgment.

So many others want to blame you for being emotional. They want to manage or control your emotional responses, whether through a drug, psychoactive plant medicine, catchy techniques, or trendy words on the neuroscience or spiritual scenes.

Speaking of neuroscience, there's a perception that it has advanced exponentially in the last 30 to 40 years. That is an illusion. Neuroscience is all still based on theorizing—when you hear advanced claims, what you're hearing is "We're theorizing that this is what happens with brain patterns." Calling a claim "neuroscience" makes people feel like there's a secret they don't know about yet. It makes us think, *Whoa, they've mastered something I'm not smart enough to understand yet.*

Neuroscience is fun. It's not the answer that gets people out of bed when they're sick and suffering and they've been everywhere and tried everything. Even with the most advanced approaches to emotional and mental health—including neurologists and alternative neuroscience modalities—the true workings of the brain with regard to chronic illness and chronic emotional struggles such as bipolar disorder, nervousness, depression, PTSD, and anxiety go undiscovered. Everything that's really happening in the brain goes overlooked because brain scan technology is not advanced enough to pick up on it. You can get an MRI or CT scan that gives you the green light and doesn't show any problems in your brain, and that sends you off on a search for neuroscience modalities to find relief. You think the problem must be your mind, your wiring, and that

you have to find a way to fix your thoughts to get better. What should be the true goal of any brain science—the understanding of what needs to be done to protect your brain—is missed. Neuroscience never even approaches the goal line.

And we can't forget the fraught history of how medical research and science have approached mental health in the past and the fraught legacy that leaves behind. Chronic illness and chronic emotional struggles have long confounded medical research and science, and the mystery of mental health has led to drastic measures in the name of "advanced science": for example, lobotomies to try to cure young women's anxiety. With this technique, the goal was to surgically slice through nerve connections and sometimes even remove brain material from the prefrontal cortex and other frontal-lobe tissue that was theorized to process and harbor emotions. After the surgical procedure was complete, the patient was not meant to "overreact" anymore with any kind of high anxiety, emotional outbursts, neurosis, or psychosis. The lobotomy was also meant to stop a patient from being up and down (what we call bipolar disorder now), or "all over the map" emotionally. Young women of the 1940s, 1950s, and even 1960s and 1970s were eligible for the procedure if they acted "out of the ordinary." Most of them were forced into the procedure. Many thousands of young women on record, and many more thousands off record, had small portions of their brain removed or surgically altered to basically quiet them down. It was a common practice. And again, this was "advanced" medical research and science—and just one prime example of some of the epic disasters involved with the medical industry and medical universities.

This was not 500 years ago. This happened within the lifetime of many reading this. This process is still happening today, behind the scenes in classified medical research and science, and even in publicly known medical research and science. Today, too, if your behavior is deemed out of control, family members can still have you admitted into a clinic and forced to be on heavy medications, with strict rules about not removing those medications, whether you, the patient, actually need them or not. It highlights how important it is that we apply critical thinking to any "answers" we're offered about the brain.

You may be at a point in your life where you're emotionally sound, thinking you're under control. And then . . . life doesn't always work that way. Events are going to come where you have to put on the brakes or you get some turbulence or you're under fire. Whether that's stress from daily turmoil or it's only once every 10 years, the most important part is protecting your brain so that when it's up against the worst or even the not-so-worst, it's getting what it needs. What people need now are answers. Answers to what actually causes brain problems, neurological problems, chronic pain problems, emotional problems, mental health problems—and answers about how to protect the brain. Because you want to protect your brain just like you want to protect anything else in your life.

THE TRUTH ABOUT EMOTIONAL TOOLS AND TECHNIQUES

Sure, we can do our breath work, yoga, alternative therapies, meditations, affirmations, and positive thinking. Do we know why we're still in pain, sick, struggling, and having brain problems? No, we don't.

You may be reading this from a standpoint of "I'm not sick and struggling." If mental, emotional, or physical symptoms haven't interrupted your quality of life yet, it may seem like these techniques should give us all we need, whether to keep our mental health steady in life or to emotionally handle the physical challenges of chronic illness. Know this: people who are sick now once stood in your shoes. They can tell you, "It wasn't until I started suffering that I understood there really aren't answers out there. Those techniques were just keeping me busy, and in some cases helping me manage and keeping me strong through my reactions, outbursts, and anger issues."

The real reasons why people get sick or struggle with mental or emotional health in the first place, and the real answers about how to heal, are very different from all the techniques and belief systems of the past and present. It can seem like certain techniques and belief systems are new and could therefore be the answers we've been seeking. In reality, the techniques and belief systems of the present are repackaged techniques and belief systems of the past. Not much has changed.

What has changed is how it's all repackaged with social media now. A younger generation that hasn't been sick yet uses their appearance and swagger and glossy lifestyle and seeming authenticity to showcase techniques of manifestation, meditations, morning routines, journaling, positive thinking, and breath work—as though these techniques are the reason for their privilege of health. Meanwhile, it's anything but authentic. The reason these individuals are able to project this shiny, successful image is that they were given resources and born with specific body types and looks. What you don't see is that they're an emotional mess behind it all. Far from balanced, they're self-absorbed, with anxiety through the roof. They may not have any health problems—yet. They still don't have it all figured out. Quite the contrary. They're painting a glossy picture to sell a package, while on the side of their lives not on social media, they're on antianxiety medications and having relationship issues left and right.

When a younger generation promotes positive thinking with a glossy image and sends the message "This is how I got here," they're not really selling anything new. What they're selling is old. Anyone who's been there and done that can tell you. It used to be that when someone repackaged or recycled an old technique and put it out into the world, they did so because they'd had an experience in their life that prompted them to seek out healing. If someone went on a stage with these techniques, they did it from a place of authenticity, hoping it would help others. Now there's a wave of repackaging that's not about authenticity. It's about flash, marketing, and promotion. It's

about "I'm going to package these goodies together. Here, this is why I am this way."

That social media persona may appeal to someone who buys into it, someone who may like an influencer's vibe, personality, body type, youth, and confidence. Someone who's suffering may come along and think, whether consciously or subconsciously, *I want that body type, I want that confidence, I want that swagger. I want to be that person. They're in their 20s, can fit into any clothing they want, and they've got the greatest lifestyle. Wow, did they get that body type and that life because of the meditations and tools they're promoting? I'll buy what they're selling.* Many who buy into it don't even know they're doing it. Some know they're falling for it hook, line, and sinker—and they still bite, because the flash and sparkle are that mesmerizing.

This doesn't mean we negate therapies and techniques for spiritual and thought-minded health. It doesn't mean you shouldn't implement or apply yourself to them if you like them. Many of these techniques are helpful and have some benefits. And yet, when you're suffering, you need the inner core of how to heal, not peripheral busywork. Especially when it comes to your brain, you need the inner core of knowledge and tools to bring yourself back to health—and then to *keep* yourself healthy, safe, and well. Once you've applied that inner core of knowledge and tools, that's when you can partake in a program or technique that's meaningful to you and truly enjoy yourself.

These tools can be really hard to apply when you're sick. How do you take action with breath work when your vagus nerves and phrenic nerves are inflamed and you're living with tightness of the chest, high anxiety, and panic attacks? How do you do workout routines and exercise programs when your body's inflamed? How do you accomplish thought building when you're so fatigued and severely brain fogged? How do you focus on positive thoughts when depression is taking over? We have to be respectful of the people who are really struggling, because these tools are not applicable at their stage of chronic suffering.

Thought-minded and emotional techniques do go too far when they teach us that our emotions are creating our physical symptoms and making us sick. It's the other way around: there are physical reasons for our mental and emotional suffering. If we address those physical needs of our brains and nervous systems, we find relief on all levels.

HOT HEADS

Imagine flying in a plane at night, about to land in a big city, and looking down at the entire electrically active urban grid below. Picture the twinkling lights laid out in a complex system spread out over miles and miles. That's basic compared to what's happening in your brain electrically. As you read in Chapter 2, "Your Static Brain," when we talk about the brain, we're really talking about an extensive and intricate network of neurons.

Because of that electricity in your brain, there's always heat occurring inside your brain. You started to gain insight into brain heat in Chapter 3, "Your Alloy Brain." Let's build on that knowledge. With every thought you have, every task you perform, every conversation you enter with anyone, that's instant heat in the brain. The minute anything jolts you on any level, good or bad, that voltage goes up. Instead of being 120, it's now 220. Instead of being 220, imagine it going up to 420. This voltage is not on the same scale as our power lines. It is a voltage scale that exists internally in the brain, unknown to medical research and science.

How a person copes with this brain heat depends on what kinds of reserves are in the brain. Are their neurotransmitter chemicals strong, or diminished and weak? Do they have good levels of melatonin? Enough glucose? Most of us have ample oxygen in the brain, even people who aren't exercising. Hydration is another matter. Are they hydrated enough? Do they have enough trace mineral salts—not the road salt that's on fast food, *mineral* salts.

And what else is inside the brain? Is somebody dealing with an alloy brain—are they dealing with various toxic heavy metals causing heat all on their own on the electrical grid? Is someone dealing with other types of toxic chemicals and brain betrayers? With pharmaceuticals that might even have been prescribed for emotion-related conditions in the first place? How much ecstasy, ayahuasca, marijuana, psychedelic mushrooms, or acid (all of which are high in toxic heavy metals) has someone done?

Is someone wounded emotionally, so that heat is always burning strong? Is the brain inflamed due to viruses inside the body? All these factors play a role in bringing brain heat to a higher temperature, and no one is in the safe zone unless they truly give their brain what it needs—what it *really* needs. Emotional healing is not just a mental state of being. It's the physical state of the physical brain.

Unfortunately, that information is missing from all the experts' talk about popular brain topics. The experts certainly *try* to offer tools. All sorts of theories abound about brain optimization. Yet without a foundation in what's happening to our brains, tools and theories can't offer true, lasting relief or protection.

The Heat of the Moment

As we go through life, we come across difficult situations—betrayal, loss, heartbreak, loneliness, confrontation. All of us experience these one way or another, somehow or someway. We get emotionally hurt. And the physical aspect of this goes wholly ignored. We need to address the physical core strength of your brain. So that no matter what we're experiencing emotionally or what we're thinking, that inner, core strength of our brain can survive emotional injuries.

When we have a loss or betrayal, our physical brain can become injured—especially if our brain doesn't have what it needs. Part of what injures the brain is not the broken trust itself; it's the fire that occurs when an event like this happens. That fire

is the heating up of the brain, an intense electrical heat. Someone had something right 200 years ago when they noticed that a friend needed to "blow off steam." Someone had something right 300 years ago when they called another person "hotheaded."

Not that someone needs to *seem* angry or irate on the surface for the brain to heat up. Sometimes when not showing emotion, the fire within the brain burns hotter than ever. You could be lying in bed hurt by betrayal, not expressing a word, and someone who saw you wouldn't even know you were upset—while the fire burned bright inside your brain and overheating occurred. (More on the electrical patterns behind this experience soon.)

Because publicly known medical research and science know only a tiny, tiny fraction about the brain, this brain heating can't be measured. If by some miraculous chance the earth is still alive a thousand years from now, and not a dead rock floating along, we still won't know everything about the human brain, no matter how advanced science gets, because there's a soul aspect of the brain intertwined with the rest of it, and science will never have those answers.

Even though the overheating of our physical brains can't be weighed or measured, it is just as real as the burn you'd get from touching a hot stove. It's as real as spilling hot coffee in your lap. It's as real as walking barefoot across a scalding parking lot to get to the beach. This heating of the brain occurs instantly when we experience an emotional challenge of any kind; it could happen in any minute of someone's life.

It even happens when people are merely frustrated with whatever situation is before them. The fire can burn at different heat levels; no matter the level, it burns.

If you've ever heard of the phenomenon of spontaneous self-combustion, it's actually related to this electrical heat. When there's a very specific recipe inside someone's body creating elevated ammonia levels in the bloodstream, a spark off the brain's electrical grid can cause combustion. Keep in mind, you need a lot going wrong for spontaneous self-combustion to occur. To begin with, the stage is set from (1) putrefied proteins rotting inside the intestinal tract and other sources of fermentation in the blood from weak digestion and foods fermenting inside the gut, all of which adds to the ammonia in the bloodstream; (2) chronic dehydration, meaning never enough water in the bloodstream; and (3) high blood fat levels from a high-fat diet. Then, if there's also continual overheating of the brain from a maxed-out electrical grid (due to brain betrayer toxins and a lack of electrolytes, trace minerals, and glucose), the grid can spark and catch the ammonia. Alcohol consumption increases someone's chances of self-combustion, as does smoking anything.

Brain heat can also be an aspect of someone feeling like madness is taking over. So many people doubt themselves when they're going through an emotional experience. They ask, "Am I going crazy?" They're not going crazy. They're experiencing intense heating of brain tissue in an emotional center of the brain, eventually reaching all areas of the brain at some point. This is often heightened by toxic heavy metals and other chemical poisons present in the brain's emotional centers.

Stress, loss, trauma, and betrayal burn hot as well. And we're not just talking about one angry spell of the year. We're talking about everyday frustrations too. For example, driving to work in traffic when you're late, slowed down, or stuck at lights causes the brain to heat up. Having a difficult conversation can cause the brain to heat up. Participating in a virtual meeting can cause the brain to heat up, because video calls often involve an additional form of stress, whether from spotty Internet connections that cause delays, participants talking over one another, or because we tend to raise our voice, increase facial expressions, or emphasize body language when we feel the format isn't allowing us to project our message.

The brain heat of life's challenges is harder on the chronically ill, because they're often stuck in bed. They're too fatigued to walk it off, go exercise, distract themselves, shake it off. A lot of people run from their stress. They burn off the adrenaline (also called epinephrine) created by mild stress and anxiety by keeping busy with the activities they like, wearing themselves out so that the thoughts don't keep cycling. People who are chronically ill don't have that option. When you're stuck on your mattress island, you can get caught up in your headspace with the brain fire burning hotter. It's like adding insult to injury because you're already dealing with the physical challenges that have isolated you in bed.

Brain heat can even burn on a different level, with a different kind of heat, when everything is good and happy. That's because when we're having fun, the brain still runs hot. The difference is that the brain's cooling mechanisms—which we'll explore later—are usually enough to temper that type of heat. That said, it's the reason why people with chronic illness can find that experiencing a little happiness is hard on them. It's why those who are very ill in the hospital can't have too many visitors wishing them well on a birthday; it generates way too much heat in the brain.

Even when we're not ill, the brain heat that happiness generates can be exhausting. I've known people who say they love every part of putting together a dinner party and have an amazing time talking all night, and then feel completely wiped out and exhausted the next day. If you asked them if they wanted to do it all over again the next day, they would feel reluctant. That's because the brain ran hot from all the fun—you can get burnt out from too much fun. There are people in the world who have the means to play all they want, and they end up needing vacations from their vacations, or "chill time" for days afterward, a chance to do nothing and increase self-care to recover from all the excitement they had on a fabulous trip (which was intended to be self-care in the first place). No matter who you are and how lucky in life you are, you still have to protect your brain and take care of it.

The solution here isn't to stop yourself from having emotions. We don't have total control over that anyway. We can make what

feels to be a lot of progress emotionally with conquering demons—we can move mountains in our emotional state—and that does not mean we will stop having emotions. Life is not a definitive, mapped-out journey. We know that our life is not somebody else's life. Yet if you look at the lives of others, they can seem to have a good run of it for a little while, and we can think they have life figured out, showing their best life moments in public. Behind the scenes, they're running into emotional quicksand more than we know. They're in another bad relationship, experiencing another friend betrayal, another career downer. They feel like they're drowning again, stuck at a bad Halloween party again, falling off the horse again, emotionally poisoned again. We just don't know it.

Some people do go for a little while without being challenged, without too much turmoil, sometimes many years before a big divorce or big life upset—before they get trapped in emotional quicksand again. Others have shorter stints of what feels like emotional freedom and progress. Either way, eventually adversity comes. And adversity becomes our greatest adversary if we don't know what's happening inside our emotional brains. In any moment of time, if we don't have our brain protected, the heating that can occur can set us back. These setbacks can feel very confusing when we believe we were taking the right steps for our emotional and physical health. Little did we know these steps might not have been the appropriate way of strengthening our brain's ability to sustain itself during an emotional storm. No matter how many meditations someone has done or what they've conquered emotionally, if they're not taking brain heat into account, they're not protecting their brain.

We can get worn down by the little ups and downs and challenges thrown our way. We can get worn down by the larger challenges that come along every so many years. Whatever life brings, whenever it brings them, our brains burn hot. Being prepared *ahead of time* is the ultimate defense and protection for our brain. It allows us to persevere through any kind of emotional hit or pain or even overwhelming joy we experience. When it comes down to it, being aware of our emotional brains is not about avoiding life's ups and downs; it's about learning to cool the brain and keep it from becoming scorched.

Toxic Fire

How and why does the brain even heat up? And what does the heat do, bad or good?

Well, the bad is that the heat kills brain cells—and we all know that we don't want to lose brain cells at a rapid pace. The cleaner the brain cell is, the greater ability for that brain cell to stay alive under heat; it takes hotter and more sustained heat levels to destroy a brain cell when the brain cell is clean. When a brain cell is dirty, filled with everyday toxins and toxic heavy metals, the brain cell heats up more quickly and stays hot longer. More toxins make the brain cell more conductive of heat, plus toxins coat the brain cell's inner cell membrane, not allowing heat to escape. If a brain cell doesn't die, the heat can render the dirty

brain cell out of service until the brain cell is restored. A clean brain cell can release heat more easily through its cell wall. That said, extended heating over a period of time can still render a clean brain cell temporarily disabled, forcing it into slumber and dormancy until the heating stops or shifts because the person switches gears with their thoughts or their project, taking a break and having some downtime or going to sleep. Dormancy of overheated brain cells is due to a shutoff mechanism that brain cells possess to stop large amounts of brain cells from dying at once. In this dormant state, brain cells wait for the opportunity to rejuvenate, replenish, and become restored so they can be of service and useful again.

Many times when someone is under extreme stress or emotional distress, that opportunity for brain cells to restore doesn't come. It's why someone who's going through a difficult relationship with constant fighting or emotional abuse may reach out to an old friend for help, saying it feels like what they're going through is killing them, that they feel like they're dying. These messages aren't just about the soul injury someone is experiencing from the cycle of abuse or the roller coaster ride of painful ups and downs in a difficult relationship. This person is experiencing brain cells themselves shutting down, going into dormancy, with some brain cells even dying.

Brain cell dormancy and death aren't all that happens when the brain heats up. There's also a diminishing of beneficial brain chemicals—including the hundreds of thousands of important brain-functioning chemicals that surge through our brain and remain undiscovered and undocumented by medical research and science. While some of these chemicals are inside the brain to combat heat, even they have their limitations. These chemicals get utilized. They get burned up. Then there are some brain chemicals that are there for other reasons of your well-being, and when the brain gets hot, these special types of chemicals make it hotter. For example, the chemical compounds in the brain involved with passion and creativity. These are invaluable brain chemicals that help us create and get inspired and express ourselves. The electrical grid of our brain should not be controlled when it comes to creativity, so these chemicals run hotter and our brain ignites, lights up, and explores for the benefit of our growth. This knowledge also explains what's behind creative blocks. When we have a lot of brain betrayers, these creative chemical compounds can be compromised, creating blocks in our creativity.

Have you ever heard of an explosion at a chemical plant, where there's a fire burning for a few days or weeks and the fire department is letting it burn rather than trying to die it out? That's because it's burning at too high a heat level because of the toxic substances feeding the flames. At the same time, that fire is releasing toxic substances that not even the best respirators can protect firefighters from. The mysterious chemicals inside our brain are a combination of natural chemicals from natural sources, good chemicals our body produces, and toxic chemicals from outside exposure that saturate the brain. When an emotional fire is lit in our brain, you don't get a combustion like a fire at an electrical plant. You get an internal combustion from the electrical heat of an emotional experience interacting with thousands of brain chemicals, both good and bad.

Offering relief is more than just trying to offer someone emotional comfort, if someone even has that privilege or opportunity to receive solace. Many people don't have someone reaching out and offering comfort. They feel they're in it alone. And even if someone does reach out a hand and tell them everything is going to be okay, it doesn't mean they're going to feel the comfort. When we're in the fire of hurt, betrayal, anger, or distress, our brain may be so physically compromised by the heat of emotional fire that we're not able to see through it with our own eyes.

You're Not a Bad Person

If we break robot status and express emotion such as anger, frustration, or pain, we can feel that we come across as weak. The self-help out there tends to lean on the side of "Let's change you as a person. Maybe you have some faults that are allowing these emotions to happen. We can make you a better person." This type of self-help tends to point out your flaws and imply you're a bad person. Even if it doesn't imply you're a bad person, it's an approach that's about learning not to react, learning to think logically, learning to meditate to control your emotions because you can't control the outside world and you can only control yourself—this still doesn't address what's physically wrong with your brain that's prompting this search for self-improvement.

Any approach that says, "You're the problem" can knock a person down, slightly injure them on top of what they're going through with their hard time. It can make them feel like they can't handle their emotions. It can even make them feel like they're creating their emotional reactions. What's never part of this self-help equation is telling people that there are toxic substances in their brain on a physical level that are allowing emotional fire to perpetuate and get out of control. This should be the main headline.

Especially if someone has dedicated time to practicing self-help techniques and hacks and then they blow their cork again, lose it, pop, they can feel like a failure and give up. What they never realize is that even if these life improvement hacks are helpful, they're still not enough to fix the core issues. The person's not a failure. The hacks they tried were only ever going to be temporary patches. When the patches fell off, it made perfect sense that their emotions heated up again, because they didn't die out the underlying fire—they didn't douse the flames, they didn't take away the fuel, they didn't repair the burns; the patches just tamped down the flames and kept it smoldering for a little while. People are blamed for "projection." They're told they're projecting their pain and anger at others. They're told, "Stop projecting." So they try self-care hacks and trends for betterment,

try to become better people, and then the minute they pop, they're blamed for projecting their pain onto others. What they're really doing is showing that their brain's physical needs aren't being met.

When an individual is suffering emotionally, they know something else is happening to explain why they're handling their hurt the way they are. They just can't put their finger on it. Sometimes anger and frustration come without an emotional trigger, and this makes it feel even worse, like they must not be a good person. If the person receives a diagnosis such as bipolar disorder, it still doesn't explain what's going on inside to make it happen. That person knows that what's happening in their brain is more than what they're getting from their therapist, doctor, or spiritual guru. The truth is there is always something more.

Emotional relief is not about fixing a person or their emotional state; it's not about making someone a better person. It's not about trying to shape or change someone and who they are. It's about removing the toxic chemicals inside the brain that are the fuel for the fire to burn hotter, and it's about restoring the good chemicals and supplies inside the brain that suppress fires and allow the brain to function at its optimum. That can give someone more of a fighting chance, so that when a self-help hack is applied, they may benefit. To experience better progress with these techniques—if we want them to "stick"—we have to address our brains' physical needs.

FIREFIGHTING SUPPLIES

There's something we all try to bring to our brain every day that's very important to it: oxygen. Without oxygen, we can't exist. The brain is extremely electrical, with electrical impulses moving and flowing around oxygen. Electrical impulses are actually fed by that oxygen. Because these electrical sparks need oxygen to occur inside the brain, it's critical that an ample amount of oxygen enters the brain. Oxygen is also highly flammable. You can't put a flame next to an oxygen tank, for example. And a campfire's flame burns hotter and brighter when it's designed to allow more air to flow in. These basic principles apply inside the brain too.

Because oxygen is flammable, other brain supplies must be present at the same time to prevent electricity from overheating and getting out of control. Traveling alongside oxygen, the water in our bloodstream circulates through much of the brain and is partly responsible for suppressing the heat of the brain's fire and keeping the brain engine cool enough. We also rely on ample glucose (sugar) in our blood because glucose helps cool brain cells and tissue. That's just the beginning of how our brain keeps electrical heat under control.

A Delicate Balance

To support your brain's electrical grid, your bloodstream is meant to carry a delicate balance of oxygen, glucose, water, electrolytes (made up of macro minerals, trace minerals, and trace mineral salts), amino acids, neurotransmitter chemicals, vitamin B_{12}, and healthy levels of adrenaline blends for everyday living. Oxygen, electrolytes, and trace mineral salts keep the electricity circulating around the grid alive. Water and glucose cool down the sparks that create the heat on the electrical grid while nourishing every brain cell. Amino acids also nourish brain cells, keeping the brain cells strong so they can handle the electrical currents. Vitamin B_{12} helps with brain cell repair. And neurotransmitter chemicals rely on electrolytes and trace mineral salts to keep them strong.

So ask yourself: Would hydration matter to lowering the amount of heat inside the brain? Would being chronically dehydrated play a negative role? Would getting ample glucose in our diet matter? Again, these brain supplies are meant to occur in a delicate balance. You have to have the right proportion of glucose, water, and oxygen. People are always breathing, so they're getting enough oxygen, yet if they're withholding glucose and water, the balance is off. When people exercise or do breath work at the same time they're doing intermittent fasting—meaning they don't have proper glucose, plus they're probably dehydrating themselves (losing water) with caffeine, yet they're increasing their oxygen levels—they're skewing the proper glucose, water, and oxygen proportions even more extremely. The electrical spark ignites hotter, then doesn't cool down enough.

We can throw off the balance of these three foundational supplies in other ways too. For example, it's possible to excessively drink water. If you try to drink gallons of water at once, you can effectively drown yourself. That said, our tendency is to override the glucose-water-oxygen balance of our bloodstream with too little glucose and water rather than too much, making the proportion of oxygen too high.

At the same time, we need the right balance of other electrical brain supplies, including electrolytes, amino acids, neurotransmitter chemicals, and healthy adrenaline. This is critical to stay emotionally balanced and strong.

Yet when we become emotional because we've been hurt, or we receive bad news, or we're shocked, the last thing we think about is, *How can I take care of myself, my bloodstream, my cerebrospinal fluid, my brain? How do I keep that balance of glucose and water so oxygen levels remain stable and don't cook my electrical grid?* The last thing we think is, *I should look for a food with glucose, electrolytes, or trace minerals in it.* And we certainly don't think ahead of time, *How do I prepare in case a shock comes? How do I get my brain up to par?*

Instead, when we're struggling in the moment with news about something that impacts our life, the first thing we do is go into mild shock. Don't eat anything, don't drink anything. Then our brain heats up as we think, *What if this? What if that? What did he say? What did she say? What did I say? I can't believe what I heard. Did I really see that? This can't be real.* At this nervous, scared pace, our breathing speeds up. We may scream, cry, go numb. Or we may exercise to try to control the anxiety. We end up

taking in a lot of air, a lot of oxygen, without giving our bloodstream what it needs to balance that oxygen intake. We go for more caffeine. All of this means more adrenaline too. We lose our glucose, hydration, and electrolytes in our bloodstream, and our electrical grid runs hotter than it should, making our situation much more difficult as we try to keep up a balancing act while already going through too much.

The adrenaline released in this type of situation goes beyond the healthy levels of gentle everyday adrenaline blends. Whenever there's a problem and the brain is being threatened, adrenaline is used as backup, emergency fuel. More aggressive blends of adrenaline are called for in these situations, whether they are related to fight-or-flight stress or induced by stimulants such as caffeine. Adrenaline can take over and override oxygen loss to try to keep a person alive. For example, if someone is drowning and they're losing their oxygen to the brain, adrenaline will be released and saturate the brain in hopes that it can keep the person alive enough for the moment to get them out of harm's way. As you'll read later in this chapter, these adrenaline surges are fuel on the brain's electrical fire and add to the brain's heat.

By the way, even though electrolytes are part of what keeps the brain's electricity going, a lack of electrolytes can cause emotional confusion and instability, which can elevate the heat of the brain. So when someone's electrolytes are low, they can get into an emotional funk, hit a little bit of gridlock. If this frustrates or scares the person, then they'll get an adrenaline surge, and that quick flame from adrenaline hits the electrical grid to take the place of missing electrolytes, trace minerals, macro minerals, and vitamin B$_{12}$. Ultimately, low electrolytes lead the brain to burn hotter.

Here's what an imbalance of electrical brain supplies in the bloodstream looks like in practice: If someone already has crippling anxiety and they're not eating even close to the balance of foods and liquids they need to keep their glucose and water levels high in the bloodstream, and then they go through some type of emotional turmoil, their adrenaline will be elevated, their glucose and water will be reduced, and their breathing will be increased, driving in more oxygen to the brain. Heightened oxygen and heightened adrenaline creating elevated heat on the brain's electrical grid without glucose and water to suppress the heat can even lead to hyperventilation in some situations. The electrical sparks on the grid run hotter and more sporadically, and can even go rogue, with brain electricity becoming reckless. The electrical grid becomes extra hot and travels to places it's not supposed to travel in the brain for what is occurring in the person's life. This can take a person to the level of being completely overwhelmed, push them into a panic attack, or shut them down so they're less responsive, lying curled up in bed feeling wrecked.

Taking Care with Breath Work

We're often taught to use breath work to help regulate emotions. Deep breathing

and breath work—certain types of it—do have their value. At the same time, breath work is not what people think it is. What people don't realize is that there is such a thing as too much oxygen. Even though we're in a world lacking oxygen, we're also in a world where people are lacking what they need in their diet. If you're not keeping a balance with other brain supplies such as glucose, trace mineral salts, and water, then driving up oxygen to your brain heats up your electrical grid, and that can be traumatizing to the brain and body. On top of which, people are often doing breath work while also consuming caffeine (which drives up adrenaline), putting their brain and bloodstream further out of balance.

Like many trends in health, breath work is a tool for the not-so-sick. If symptoms haven't sidelined you in life, you can bring breath work in and have fun with it. If you're really sick or struggling, breath work isn't going to fix you. Breath work is really difficult for people with anxiety and even worsens it for most anxiety sufferers, especially those with sensitive vagus nerves, causing neurological symptoms such as tightness of the chest. Breath work is not going to make lupus, neurological Lyme, eczema, fibromyalgia, Parkinson's, or MS go away. You can bring in simple, gentle breathing techniques—if they feel supportive and you're also staying hydrated and getting enough glucose, electrolytes, trace minerals, and macro minerals such as magnesium and trying to stay off caffeine.

Fanning the Flames with Fat

Another factor that throws off your bloodstream's delicate balance of electrical brain supplies is fat. If someone is eating a large amount of fat in their food, they're losing oxygen in their bloodstream at the same time they're losing glucose's ability to enter cells, because they're now dealing with insulin resistance. You don't have to be a diabetic to have insulin resistance. Everyone experiences insulin resistance when they eat a large amount of fat.

You would think diminished oxygen means the brain's electrical grid would diminish, and it starts to—until an emergency message gets sent autonomically to your adrenals to release a large burst of emergency adrenaline to thin out the fat flowing through your brain's bloodstream in order to save your brain. This surge of fight-or-flight adrenaline accelerates heart rate, which in turn forces someone to breathe more heavily, drawing more oxygen into the bloodstream. With adrenaline also acting as a blood thinner and a burst of oxygen arriving from the lungs, oxygen is able to get into the brain.

Someone may not feel this surge of adrenaline, because it's subtle. It may not give somebody a sensation. Someone else may feel this adrenaline surge from eating fat as a lift, a type of high.

Either way, now we're burning hot, hotter than ever. Before, we had a lack of oxygen and higher levels of blood fat with lower levels of glucose. The emergency flare this sent off brought in adrenaline to try to correct the imbalance, and for a quick moment, we ended up with a larger amount of oxygen and a large amount of adrenaline at once. This caused the brain to burn hotter. Now, as the adrenaline surge de-escalates and your system calms down, which could be hours later, blood fat fills up again in the bloodstream and oxygen levels reduce again. The heat from the extra adrenaline and oxygen that entered the brain is kept in, in part because we're still dealing with insulin resistance, which means that glucose can't enter brain cells to the degree it needs to in order to keep the brain consistently cool. We also have a scenario now where blood fat is insulating the brain, holding heat in the brain longer than it should be there. Now we have a longer-sustaining heat in the brain.

This fat-adrenaline heat cycle can occur multiple times a day, multiple times a night. People don't realize that with too much fat in the diet, they're chasing a high. The life-protecting adrenaline surges they get from eating radical fats can confuse someone, make them think they're making the right food choices, make them think their cravings are justified. In reality, the "feel-good" moments they get from eating high-fat foods are from an adrenaline surge that leaves them lost and far from intuitive about what they need. They don't really know what they need because they don't know about the delicate balance of oxygen-glucose-water-electrolytes necessary in the brain's bloodstream for true support. The "feel-good" moments come with a price; the brain ups and downs someone experiences from high-fat foods can make them feel emotionally imbalanced, whether oversensitive or noncaring or noncompassionate or irritable or combative or sad. Basically, someone can be all over the road map when this imbalance is occurring in the brain. And the constant frustrations this brings can make the fire inside the brain burn at that much greater intensity, allowing for the possibility of a future stroke. (More about strokes a bit later in this chapter.)

We're supposed to be able to handle emotional blows and recover more easily than this internal crisis allows us to do. Our brains are designed to bounce back. It's all the hidden physical problems we develop inside the brain that make it harder to have that resilience.

EMOTIONAL INJURY

When we say we've had emotional wounds and scars in life, this description is more accurate than we know. When we say, "I've been burned before," we really mean it. That's because when we go through upsetting or traumatizing experiences, we can experience physical injuries in the emotional centers of the brain from the intense heat generated (whether we're showing our emotions on the outside or not). These brain wounds can then influence how we think, feel, and behave.

Scorched Brain Tissue

For example, when you're lying in bed fixated on something hurtful someone said,

or some misjustice that occurred that was out of your control, or a hurt you experienced from betrayal in a relationship, and the hurt feels impossible to resolve, so it takes over your mind and dominates your thoughts, the electrical patterns in your brain don't just swirl around your entire brain and circulate. Part of your brain's electrical patterns can actually lose circulation, because the hurt that occurred has become such a singular focus that it has driven and pinpointed electricity into the specific area of an emotional center of your brain where the thought of that experience began to root itself and fester. It can feel impossible to keep your mind distracted with other thoughts in this situation—to simply change your brain's electrical patterns back to normal circulation—because the emotional injury that occurred was so shocking and hurtful that most of the electrical pattern of your brain is now dedicated to one thought pattern, in one direction, to one area, creating an obsession. That hurtful experience can become an obsessive cycle that can replay over and over and over again in your mind. A cauterization occurs from the intense heat generated in one area.

It may take a week for someone to be able to shift the brain pattern. Even if they try to get out of bed, take a walk, go for a run if they're physically capable, or keep themselves busy by being productive, the electrical pattern will keep shifting to that same wounded area, meaning the person will keep thinking about the betrayal or other form of emotional injury as they keep playing it back, trying to figure out how, where, or why it all went wrong to try to fix or resolve it. It becomes a battle of changing the brain's electrical grid, and that's hard to do.

Say the emotional injury had to do with a relationship. For the next few days, you try to go about your life. You get up, take a shower, try to make something to eat—yet everything you do that you shared with the other person becomes a reminder of the hurt, so the electrical pattern in your brain keeps heading into the direction of the hurt brain tissue. It becomes a fight and a struggle to heal emotionally. How serious the betrayal or other injury was, how many brain betrayers (such as toxic heavy metals) were present to fan the flame, how prepared your brain was with supplies to physically withstand the heat generated, and how many supplies you're continuing to give your brain to support it through healing—all these determine the size of the wound that's left over, what recovery looks like, and how fast healing can occur.

When we're emotionally healing, we have to remember this. We have to remember that physical tissue of the brain could have been injured, calloused, cauterized by the intensity of the electrical patterns driving into a specific area of an emotional center of our brain, and that brain tissue is in great need of healing.

Brain tissue is meant to be saturated with glycogen (stored glucose), meant to stay supple and soft, meant to have a form of elasticity and bounce-back sponginess. Brain tissue is not supposed to be hard. It is more difficult for electricity to run through

hardened brain tissue and hit the intended neurons. Brain tissue hardens when it gets scorched and cauterized from the overheating of an emotional injury—overheated brain electricity forms calluses and scar tissue in brain tissue that cause specific areas of brain tissue to lose their spongy, bounce-back quality. Neurons can even get trapped in this hardened, calloused brain tissue.

Hardening of brain tissue is most likely to occur when brain tissue is filled with toxins and poisons (including toxic heavy metals, petrochemicals, fragrances, MSG, and caffeine) and is constantly being overheated from emotional injury and high fats in the bloodstream. Toxic substances saturating the brain, without electricity even hitting them, lessen the elastic, supple nature of brain tissue. Plus, when the brain's electrical grid hits them, the everyday toxins and poisons in our brain can elevate brain heat, especially when glucose or glycogen is lacking to protect brain tissue. Electricity transforms toxins, making them more damaging to brain tissue. This means these toxins and poisons can create the beginning stages of some hardened brain tissue, although it won't be in the form of calloused tissue until an emotional injury occurs. When an intense emotional experience elevates the heat of a specific electrical pathway in the brain, now we have the perfect storm. That overheated pathway pinpoints electrical heat to a specific area of the brain, and if toxins and poisons are in that same specific area, there's a higher likelihood of hardening—of brain tissue getting cauterized and calloused and scarred—with the possibility of trapping neurons.

It's worth giving toxic heavy metals special attention when it comes to emotional injury. As you discovered in Chapter 3, "Your Alloy Brain," toxic heavy metals play a major role in brain heat and electrical patterns. Because metal conducts electricity and heat, when toxic heavy metals are present in brain tissue, your brain can heat up even more, which heightens the physical injury that can occur to brain tissue. This means we need to be that much more patient and proactive with the healing process, bringing back what the brain physically needs by following the healing guidance in Part VI of this book, "Bringing Back Your Brain," and, if desired, bringing in additional support from this book's companion, *Brain Saver Protocols, Cleanses & Recipes.*

Soul Protection

There can also be a soul aspect to emotional events. When something terrible happens, your soul—which normally resides in your brain—gets projected out of your body to protect you from a certain amount of soul injury. Some people can feel this out-of-body experience, watching themselves from afar or even above. This is a safety mechanism. This way, your soul doesn't have to experience the full amount of pain from betrayal or loss.

You may have heard of the supernatural occurrence of Mike the Headless Chicken. Mike was a chicken in the 1940s who survived long after his head was cut off. There are a lot of theories out there about how this happened. After hearing this story at the time, hundreds of farmers worldwide started chopping their chickens' heads off in experimental ways. It became an obsession, chopping the heads off in various places, because people were in such disbelief. Farmers would sever the heads higher up, preserving even more of a chicken's neck and brain stem than Mike's, trying to see if their chickens would live too. Over a hundred thousand chickens were beheaded in this process, and they never survived. Here's what no one knows about how Mike stayed alive, and why it's relevant here: a chicken has a soul, which normally resides in its brain, just like ours. At the traumatic time of having its head chopped off, this chicken's soul left the chicken's brain. Instead of floating away into the ether as the chicken's body died, the chicken's soul entered into the chicken's body, giving the physical body's will extra strength to survive, along with intelligence the soul had gathered from the chicken's brain. That is, Mike stayed alive because by entering his body, his soul gave strength of will and brain intelligence to his body.

Roller Coaster Relationships

When emotional injuries are repeated, an area of the brain can basically get electrocuted by intense electrical stimulation.

Relationships are a powerful example of how this happens. As we covered, when someone goes through a breakup, a tremendous amount of heat is generated in emotional centers of the brain. What if the couple gets back together, the relationship is mended, things get better . . . and then a breakup occurs again? Neurons in the same emotional centers of the brain that were just starting to mend will get shocked again—it's like an electrical shock treatment to that central nervous system tissue. If the relationship continues on this roller coaster of making up followed by turmoil again, emotional wounds will keep hitting in the same emotional centers. During the most traumatic moments on that roller coaster, the soul is outside of the body watching and waiting for things to subside so it can come back.

When a pattern like this develops, neurotransmitter hormones in the emotional centers of the brain start to gather information that another shock could be coming. This can make a person hypersensitive, even allergic, to the coming of the next breakup, fight, or cheat, causing additional emotional responses and additional emotional pain. That allergic response varies in severity depending on how much the brain is lacking in its nutritional needs and what the soul and physical brain both remember from past trust issues and other breakups, fights, and cheats. These old wounds are a big part of how allergic you get in the present. Because again, when we talk about emotional wounds, we're talking about physical wounds to brain tissue. These old wounds can physically tear open again and become fresh with a new emotional injury.

This isn't someone being "overly emotional." This is a person experiencing a physical brain response to repeated emotional and physical brain injury. Injured neurons in the emotional centers of the brain are receiving messages from neurotransmitter hormone chemicals as they try to send forewarning in hopes of stopping the situation. That's when a person learns their tolerance. An allergic reaction escalates and peaks to a point where you feel if you don't change your course in that moment, some serious damage is going to occur, or something's going to go terribly wrong. You're at your limit. You become so allergic that you feel if you stay in the game, you're going to get hurt past the point of no return. When this happens someone may leave the relationship for good, if they even have that option, before too much damage has been done in the emotional centers of the brain by calloused and cauterized tissue, and before too much soul injury has occurred.

Emotional Strokes

When you're lacking the brain supplies you need, it's easier to experience a stroke. If our brain environment isn't up to speed, we're more vulnerable. People who are most eligible for a stroke have elevated low-grade viral infections; combined with an imbalance of nutrients, food, and hydration; combined with toxic heavy metals and chemical poisons in the brain; combined with emotional shock or stress. We're not just talking about a classic stroke, the kind in which blood flow to part of the brain is interrupted in a readily diagnosable way. This combination of factors could also set somebody up for an emotional stroke that can't be diagnosed, where physical injury that's undetectable by any MRI or brain scan occurs inside an emotional center of the brain.

With an emotional stroke, a doctor will see no sign of physical stroke present in the brain (even though it is a physical brain occurrence), so they may classify your emotional stroke symptoms as an anxiety disorder or virtually any type of mental disorder, depending on the doctor and your symptoms. What *are* the symptoms of having suffered an emotional stroke? Examples include the inability to think clearly, panic attacks when someone is talking to you, feeling numb throughout your body, fear of communicating with anyone, inability to make decisions, losing sense of time, obsessing that something is wrong that you can't pinpoint, fear of starting anything new, fear of leaving the house, and allergic reactions to stressful situations, where something inside makes you feel you can't handle the stress.

Some people can have the mildest of emotional strokes, and some people can have more severe ones. You could be allergic to stress for a short time and then get past it because your brain is naturally healing; you're bouncing back. There's a resilience because you're getting what you need, or you already have what you need, inside your brain. On the other hand, you may not bounce back so easily. Your symptoms could be pronounced or prolonged; your allergy to any kind of stressful situation could stay around because the emotional injury was more severe and/or your brain is in greater need of the supplies to protect itself and heal.

What's going on in the brain with an emotional stroke? Tiny blood vessels in an emotional center of the brain get temporarily damaged. Brain tissue that bore the brunt of the brain's electrical heat from the betrayal, hardship, loss, or other trauma can also become calloused, making neurons oversensitized. Don't let this be cause for despair. When you give your brain what it needs, it can come back.

ADRENALIZED EMOTIONS

Adrenaline heightens everything going on in the brain electrically. When we get emotionally challenged on any level, whether good or bad, whether in a brand-new relationship with a partner, a new boss, or in a friendship with a coworker; whether with the excitement of going on vacation or taking time off to do something we love; whether deciding to go skiing one day or riding a motorcycle—anything we do, adrenaline plays a role.

Adrenaline Fuel on the Fire

When we have a good experience, adrenaline is released from the adrenal glands. When that adrenaline touches electricity, it's flammable. Healthy adrenaline helps fuel the electrical grid. It's undiscovered by medical research and science that adrenaline is filled with receptor compounds. These receptor compounds are designed for the electrical grid in the brain. When the compounds hit the electricity of the brain, they light up and ignite like fireflies, or like bugs hitting a bug zapper. Adrenaline is a necessity, in small healthy amounts. We require it in all of our everyday living and functioning.

Adrenaline behaves differently from oxygen. While adrenaline burns like oxygen inside the body, it does so with a more rapid, aggressive, intense heat. Adrenaline's fire doesn't squelch easily with water and glucose—although water (hydration) and glucose are still critical to address the brain heat from adrenaline. Imagine you're experiencing something good: skiing down a slope, your adrenals pumping because you're about to hit a tricky little spot that everyone forewarned you about, where if you don't handle it right, you'll wipe out. For the excitement of that challenge alone, it's worth it to you to go down the slope. Euphoria and clarity come when adrenaline is hitting the electrical grid during a good experience. It puts you in the feeling of being "in the zone." As your adrenals start filling your blood with adrenaline, all that adrenaline "gasoline" reaches your brain and ignites its electrical grid. It's more adrenaline, and a more intense blend of adrenaline, than the gentle, mild levels of adrenaline hitting your electrical grid when you're showering, brushing your teeth, or going to the bathroom.

What about an unhappy moment, a bad experience? What about betrayal? What about getting a message from your best friend that reveals she doesn't understand you after all these years? Everything you've poured out to this friend, all your vulnerabilities, weaknesses, and soul secrets, it's as if she never heard any of it, and she

delivers a blow you never thought possible. The adrenals release their chemicals, and an intense adrenaline blend geared to power you through the moment of betrayal rushes to your brain, hits the electrical grid, and catches fire. The reason you get this adrenaline fire is to provide clarity, faster thinking, and the strength to override any mental blocks or smaller injuries already in the brain—so you can be quick on your feet during this challenging emotional experience. The adrenaline fire is there to help set you on a new path, power you to a safer land and new experiences.

This adrenaline fire is also why, when somebody goes through an emotional experience, they can feel so drained and worn out afterward that it's difficult to function for months. When the adrenaline subsides from the electrical grid, feelings of sadness, depression, or brain exhaustion can be elevated. It's why bouncing back can take so long, and why some don't even bounce back. If the brain is up against acidity, deficiencies, poisons, and toxins, it's all the harder to recover from the intense adrenaline surge of an emotional blow.

The Bounce-Back Ability of Youth

When someone is young and goes through a hard time, elders will often say, "Get back on the horse and try again," or "Don't worry, somebody else is coming," or "It's okay you didn't get into that school; you'll go to a better one," or "It's okay you didn't get asked to prom. Better luck next year." We do tend to bounce back better when we're younger—because we tend to have fewer toxins in the brain and because the adrenal glands aren't fully developed yet, so they only release a limited amount of adrenaline for emotional experiences.

This doesn't mean you can't feel big emotions or be hurt emotionally when you're younger. Your brain electricity is still active and adrenaline is still being released, so you still feel and hurt. A teenager's first love going wrong, for example, can be devastating. Here's what's key: adrenaline won't fuel the fire and increase brain heat to the extent it does in adults. That's because children and adolescents have the control mechanism of underdeveloped adrenal glands. Underdeveloped adrenals release less adrenaline than fully developed adrenals do, and that protects a younger person's brain—it shields it from getting too hot because a younger person's brain is not fully developed yet. Even though emotions can be heightened in young people, and children often take things harder in the moment than adults, less adrenaline leading to less brain heat also means they can often bounce back more easily. This limited release of adrenaline also helps keep addictions from occurring in children.

You can still get an emotional wound early in life that you'll have to carry into adulthood and that can surface later. These wounds normally start to show themselves around age 30 or after, by which point the adult brain is fully developed. It's why so many unknowingly fear their 30th birthday. When your brain develops fully, you start soul-searching, and wounds start to surface.

And yet when you're younger, your adrenals won't flood your bloodstream the way they do for an adult. When you're still young, this protective measure gives you a dust-yourself-off, start-again ability. It gives you the power to recover fast, allowing your brain to enter a mode of "I'll look back at this and not even care about that one night Mom or Dad didn't want me to go out to the party." It takes a lot more adrenaline to power a fully developed brain and body, especially a brain and body that have accumulated decades of everyday toxins and other brain betrayers.

Given that we often see big emotional reactions in young people, this may still seem unexpected. In truth, for a child who's upset and reacts emotionally to a situation, adrenaline fire in the brain doesn't even touch the levels inside an adult who's staying outwardly calm and not reacting on the surface. When we see kids show extreme emotional reactions, it's often because of higher levels of toxic heavy metals in the brain and blood sugar crashes from insulin resistance.

As we get older, when we're lacking very important chemicals that are diminishing in our brains as we age—including glucose and glycogen storage banks—and our brains are becoming thick with toxins, toxic heavy metals, and fat because we don't know how to combat any of this, we can't recover the way we need to recover. Not only do we often have more problems as we get older; we have more adrenaline to scorch the brain than when we were younger and could still recoup easily. As adults our adrenal glands are fully developed; we no longer have the protective control mechanism of underdeveloped adrenals. When adrenaline releases, floods the body, enters the brain, and ignites the electrical grid, it causes an intense heat to burn.

TOXIN-CLOUDED EMOTIONS

Everyday toxins and poisons inside the brain are a large part of the brain limitations we experience, including emotional limitations. If an area of the brain is clouded with an abundant level of poisons and toxins—ranging from toxic heavy metals to solvents to plastics and other petrochemicals to pharmaceuticals to air fresheners, fragrances, scented candles, and beyond—that area of the brain that's clouded with brain betrayers can almost go into a sleep mode. This doesn't mean we'll be sleeping. It means an area of our brain is not functioning optimally, so we'll rely more on other parts of our brain that are less clouded and clogged up with toxins. It also means we'll be limited in brain function.

When emotional centers of the brain become filled up and clouded with toxins and poisons, we become more reliant on other parts of our brain. As a result, we can become limited in our emotional understanding of others. We can become limited in getting in touch with our own emotional state. We can become limited in feeling and expressing emotions, limited in harnessing emotions. Toxins and poisons clogging the emotional centers of our brain can also mean that we become extremely emotional without understanding why.

Dreams can become very intense, extremely emotionally challenging, where constant dream after dream after dream evokes emotions because the body is trying to heal the emotional centers of the brain. We do a lot of emotional healing through our dreams. People who have more toxins in the emotional centers of the brain tend to dream about drowning, being in water, playing in water, or being trapped in water—whether ocean, pool, lake, or river—because their emotional state is, in a way, underwater with toxins. They can also have dreams of running from people, not being able to get away when someone's trying to kill or harm them. While these dreams can have other meanings, many times they occur because of toxins in the emotional centers of the brain.

MAKING PEACE WITH OUR HEALING TIMELINE

When we get sick, we start to track the timeline. We count the days we've been sick, maybe even the hours. We count the weeks, the months, and eventually, if it lasts that long, we count the years. Something happens to us emotionally when we remember the month we got sick, the time of year. Many of us remember the people we were around when we first got sick, the job we were doing, the commitments we had on our plate. Time plays a large role in our emotional brain. It's as if our emotional brain is directly connected to time. Sure, we worry about time on a daily basis even when we're not sick or struggling. Our responsibilities and plans are based around time. Yet something changes when we're sick. We see time differently. We start saying, "It's time to get better," or "It's about time I'm feeling better," or we hear, "In due time, you'll get better."

Time is such a large aspect of illness because if we're sick, we feel like we're losing out. Time is passing us by. At the start it doesn't feel as threatening emotionally: "Yeah, I've been sick for a week, two weeks." The hands of time start to feel heavy when it goes on too long. You're not quite better, you're even getting worse, and now time becomes doctor appointments and your care schedule. Time is about how much energy you have, how much space you have around your illness to do what you need to do. Life can change when we're sick, causing restrictions, making us feel everything is so difficult. We have to slow down.

Our emotional brain puts due dates—and past due dates—on our recovery: "I have to heal before this date." And then: "I was supposed to be better already." We can feel trapped in a time war. Our emotional brain wants us to be healed by a certain time, and our physical body is not ready to heal because it's not getting exactly what it needs to heal. What's wrong with our physical body has not been identified yet, even with the best of specialists and best of diagnoses.

When we put ourselves on a timetable to heal, we get let down when we haven't healed yet. Then we register it as a failure: "I

failed to heal before the second semester of college." "I failed to heal before junior year." "I failed to heal before I was supposed to go back to work." "I failed to heal before my wedding." "I failed to heal before my child's first birthday." Failure syndrome sets in. "Why am I not healing? How is it possible that I didn't heal yet?" It feels like we're not getting better in time to live our lives. And then, when we're sick for too long, time seems to blur into itself. At a certain point, we're not keeping track anymore, only noting the landmarks along the way. Trying to get better has become too long, drawn-out, and time-consuming a process.

Having faith and trust in your body healing is a big part of not letting the time stamp of every moment spent being sick let you down. We have an emotional attachment to time when we become sick, some of it healthy, some of it unproductive. Part of this is the conditioning we've all experienced. Institutions have conditioned us to live on timetables that are industrialized. We're made to feel like we're wasting time, no matter what we're doing. We're made to feel like we have to be "on time" for everything. When we get sick, this conditioning is still at work, and the gears need to be shifted. The emotional centers of the brain need to get new messages. We can't be trapped by the everyday industrialized timetable we've been taught to live by. We can't apply that timetable to our healing. We have to learn to separate the two: the industrialized timetable and our natural healing timeline.

EVERYBODY WANTS TO HEAL

Everybody wants to heal. Nobody *doesn't* want to heal. No one wants to be sick or suffer emotionally. No one is afraid of healing; no one has a fear of healing that's secretly holding them back from getting better. As human beings, we want to heal. We want to live forever. We want to live at our healthiest for as long as we can.

There's also a trusting wire within us that's been taken advantage of by industries. This has created a brainwashing within us, a mechanism inside us that wants permission to do harmful things to ourselves. The desire for health is so strong inside us that we'll try to look for answers about why anything that's harmful could be good for us—we want validation that hurting ourselves is actually good for us. This can make it seem as if self-sabotage is part of our innate emotional nature, as if we want to harm ourselves, when we really don't.

We don't self-sabotage because we want to make ourselves sick. We self-sabotage because we're taught to self-sabotage, we're conditioned to self-sabotage, we're practically bred to self-sabotage. Alternative medicine cults, as well as top feeders and bottom feeders of the health industry, are always catering to this self-sabotage brainwashing, often using their credentials to manipulate our trust. They create their social media channels and give their five tips in 15 minutes. In those five tips, you'll almost always find at least one recommendation that provides validation and reassurance for self-sabotage.

A big part of the self-sabotage brainwashing is that we become programmed to seek validation that doing a harmful thing "in moderation" is perfectly fine. (You'll read more about this in Chapter 10, "The Moderation Trap.") For the not-so-sick, these self-sabotage measures are often a daily part of everyone's life. Coffee, vinegar, wine, pizza, fried and greasy food— if we hear these are not good for us, we look for someone else to say, "It is good for you in moderation." We don't want to face the reality of what we're really doing. We don't want to pay the consequences of osteopenia coming from vinegar, liver conditions coming from alcohol, adrenal problems coming from caffeine, so we'll never accept that these are true causes of these conditions. It's as if industry conditioning has placed a robot inside us that wants validation to slowly destroy ourselves, even though that's the last thing we really want.

We want to be healthy and strong and live forever . . . under certain conditions. Some of these conditions are "I'm going to have my dark chocolate and coffee and vinegar and wine and champagne and salt. You can't stop me. You can't tell me I can't. Because I'll go and find someone who's a health authority who says it's fine and even good for me to eat all that *plus* raw, aged cheese and grass-fed butter and green tea and matcha and kombucha and eggs, and I'll run with that. That will give me the comfy, warm, fuzzy feeling inside that I'm being validated for doing things that are actually helping destroy my body. I'll even convince myself that my body loves it, and my body's fine with it, and my body needs it." This brainwashing and conditioning becomes woven into the emotional centers of our brain. It also gets directed mostly to womankind, on purpose.

Yet the emotional centers of our brain can only be pushed so far. When you're sick or suffering enough physically, mentally, or emotionally, a survival mechanism kicks in, a survival mechanism in your brain's emotional centers that has been inside us since the beginning of time. That survival mechanism says, "No. I hear it's not good for me. I'm going to align my physical body to that understanding. I'm in too much pain—I'm too unwell to mess around now. I can't play games anymore." Something clicks in, where once you learn it's not good for you, you know it's time to stay away from that caffeine and that vinegar and that salt and that chocolate. You know it's time. Something rewires in the emotional centers of your brain that says, "I can't destroy myself anymore. I can't search for validation to support something that's harming me. I've been pushed around too much. I've been toyed with too much. I'm not in the business of destroying myself anymore because I want to live. I want to

heal. I'm not afraid to heal, I've never been afraid to heal, and it's time."

This enough-is-enough strength is inside everyone. It's the moment when you put your foot down. It's the moment when you truly find yourself, when you're working with and aligned with your body. Not even the snakiest salesman on social media videos or the snakiest chiropractor, doctor, or nutritionist on infomercials can give you the validation anymore to go into that robotic mode of "I'm going to destroy myself with a smile on my face, and be happy thinking about it, because my body deserves and needs what I'm putting in it." That old brainwashing that manipulated your trusting wire and sent a message to your brain's emotional centers to override common sense and sensibility about what your body really needs—that brainwashing won't work anymore. Even if everyone around you has been brainwashed, and they challenge you as you start trying to eat healthy, get healthy, get better, you'll know how to stand firm.

When that time comes, that's when you're reborn. It's the rebirth of finally moving out of mental and emotional pain, moving out of that in-between, and turning your life around.

CHAPTER 6

Your Inflamed Cranial Nerves

Inflammation of the cranial nerves plays a large role in chronic mystery illness. As I always say, "mystery illness" is a much broader category than anyone realizes. We think that if a condition has a name—such as anxiety, fatigue, POTS, vertigo, Bell's palsy, neuropathy, or ocular migraines—then it must not be a mystery to medical research and science. Anyone who has struggled with any chronic health issue knows this isn't how it works. Being handed a label for your set of symptoms isn't the same as receiving answers about why those symptoms are interrupting your life in the first place. Whether you're living with a diagnosis, a misdiagnosis, or a nondiagnosis, there are answers to be found in getting to know your brain stem and your cranial nerves.

CRANIAL NERVE ANSWERS

Your cranial nerves include your vagus nerves, your trigeminal nerves, and your facial nerves, among many others. Your cranial nerves extend out of your brain stem, and many symptoms of chronic illness derive from these cranial nerves. If a cranial nerve is inflamed in any way—because of viral neurotoxins, chemical poisons and toxins such as toxic heavy metals, or even physical injury—then symptoms can occur. Your cranial nerves are also affected by what's going on with your neurons. Symptoms can occur from compromised, contaminated, or inflamed neurons in the brain sending skewed, altered, or twisted messages to the brain stem and cranial nerves.

Viral Nerve and Brain Stem Inflammation

Most people with chronic illness don't have physical injuries directly to their cranial nerves. They have chronic cranial nerve inflammation. Chronic viral infections such as Epstein-Barr virus, shingles, herpes simplex 1, herpes simplex 2, HHV-6, or HHV-7 can cause cranial nerve inflammation. As you'll read in more detail soon, this viral inflammation can occur in the brain stem (where the cranial nerves originate), or the inflammation can occur anywhere along the cranial nerves themselves.

When someone's cranial nerves have been temporarily injured—for example, when someone sustains a head injury of any kind—those cranial nerves won't heal so easily if the person has a chronic viral infection at the same time. Injury to a cranial nerve causes tiny, fibrous root hairs to fray on the area of the nerve that was injured. If a low-grade viral infection such as EBV, shingles, or herpes simplex is occurring, the virus can attach itself to the cranial nerve's frayed root hairs, resulting in longer-term cranial nerve inflammation, sometimes long past the time of injury. The virus can station itself in the injured part of the nerve and live there, like lice in someone's hair. Some varieties of viruses will try to dig a little deeper into the nerve to settle in, leading to increased inflammation because the neurotoxins excreted from the virus are deeper in the nerve.

Contaminated or Inflamed Neurons

You can also have problems with cranial nerves where the cranial nerves themselves are not inflamed. In these cases, the problem is that the cranial nerves are receiving messaging from other areas of the brain that *are* inflamed or contaminated.

For example, your vagus nerves don't have to be inflamed to cause electrical heart palpitations, ectopic heartbeats, arrhythmias, and atrial fibrillations (AFib). When a doctor cannot find anything wrong with your heart, yet you're suffering from these heart symptoms, it can be caused by electrical

issues. The electricity running through your vagus nerves is filled with jumbled information from an upper echelon of the brain, where a group of neurons is contaminated with any number of brain betrayers, whether toxic heavy metals, fragrances filled with toxic heavy metals, chemicals from carpets or clothing, pesticides, or viral neurotoxins from a viral infection somewhere in the body. The result of this jumbled information being delivered to vagus nerves can be irregularities in heart rhythm.

This is the type of neuron compromise you read about in Chapter 2, "Your Static Brain." If groups of nerve cells acting as receptors in the brain stem receive distorted information from neurons in the brain, distorted information can then be transferred to cranial nerves, interfering with certain motor function.

UNTANGLING THE MYSTERIES

One reason why cranial nerve symptoms are so mysterious and misleading to medical research and science is that someone can have a little bit of everything. A person could have contamination and/or inflammation in a group of neurons in the brain from a source such as toxic heavy metals, viral neurotoxins, MSG, scented candles, fragrances, air freshener, carpet and clothing chemicals, tattoos (a source of toxic heavy metal contamination), or caffeine injuries. At the same time, they could have inflammation in the lower, middle, or upper brain stem caused by viral neurotoxins (or, more rarely, direct viral infection) and/or toxic heavy metal contamination in the brain stem. And then they could also have chronic inflammation anywhere along the cranial nerves due to viruses and viral neurotoxins. A person can have a little bit of it all—inflammation of the brain, brain stem, and cranial nerves—or more of one and less of another.

There is so much variation:

For example, a vagus nerve could be inflamed at the bottom (in the abdomen) and in the middle (in the chest), and yet not be inflamed higher up (in the brain stem).

Or someone's brain stem could be more inflamed in a particular area, inflaming certain cranial nerves where they originate.

Or someone could have more inflammation in a particular region of the brain that's skewing neuron messages to the brain stem and nerves. For example, someone could have more inflammation in the left hemisphere of their brain or the right hemisphere, or in the frontal lobe or occipital lobe or temporal lobe or thalamus or cerebellum. If inflammation is in an endocrine gland (hypothalamus, pineal gland, or pituitary gland), that can put pressure on adjacent brain tissue, squeezing the neurons in that neighboring brain tissue and affecting the messages the neurons send to the brain stem and nerves.

The precise location(s) of inflammation varies from person to person and can even vary for one person over time. The majority of the time, it's inflammation that you can't detect in a medical test.

Symptoms of Cranial Nerve Inflammation

The location where inflammation is occurring along specific cranial nerves determines the type of symptom someone experiences (such as tingles and numbness, aches and pains, stiffness, or burning sensations); where in the body those symptoms occur (such as the tongue, gums, jaw, temples, back of the neck, between the eyes, back of the head, top of the head, chest, or stomach); and what body functions they affect (such as swallowing or peristaltic action of the intestinal tract).

Mysterious cranial nerve symptoms also include blurred vision, trouble focusing the eyes, unusual movement of the eyeballs (including difficulty with the muscles around the eyes), visual disturbances, jaw pain, burning tongue, neck pain, head pain, migraines, face vibrating, head vibrating, ear popping, body buzzing and humming, pulsating sensations in the head, burning hot feeling with no fever, balance issues, dizziness, feelings of electrical shock to the head, loss of the ability to swallow, slurred speech, loss of hearing, drooping face, loss of movement of the face, pain in various areas of the face, feeling of a crooked jaw, pulling sensation in the face (such as nose, eyes, or forehead), twitching that's erratic and shifts all around the head and face, nausea, teeth grinding, tooth pain, gum pain, difficulty chewing, loss of smell, loss of taste, and mystery itches without rashes that don't go away with scratching. These and other symptoms of cranial nerve inflammation can either be caused by inflammation somewhere along the cranial nerve or by inflammation in the brain stem, where cranial nerves are attached.

Inflammation is really the secondary cause of these symptoms. The true cause is what's creating the inflammation: a low-grade or high-grade viral infection and/or toxic heavy metals and other chemical warfare. (Industries have been taking chemicals to a new level by adding toxic heavy metals to their chemical brews.) Most of the time, the inflammation is a combination of viruses and toxic heavy metals, especially because toxic heavy metals and other everyday toxins provide fuel to viruses to create more-toxic neurotoxins that further inflame the nerves and worsen symptoms.

The source of inflammation could affect multiple cranial nerves in multiple places. For example, two different cranial nerves could be inflamed separately, causing multiple symptoms. Or the inflammation could be in the brain stem and so pronounced that it's affecting two to three cranial nerves at once. For instance, inflammation of the brain stem could put pressure on the trigeminal nerves and vagus nerves at the same time, so someone could get a droop in their face, jaw pain, and grinding teeth while at the same time having vertigo, dizziness, and tightness of the chest.

Phrenic nerves are not cranial nerves; they branch out from the spine. Yet they receive signals from the brain stem similar to what cranial nerves receive. When cranial nerves are inflamed, often phrenic nerves can exhibit spasms and twitches. When phrenic nerves are inflamed, a feeling of anxiety or tension in the chest can occur, or pain in the upper back, tingles and numbness in the arms and shoulders, or a feeling of itchiness deep below the skin of the upper body that can't be relieved or soothed easily.

The Tree Branch Effect

The cranial nerves where inflammation can be the most common are the trigeminal nerves, facial nerves, vagus nerves, vestibulocochlear nerves, optic nerves, olfactory nerves, and hypoglossal nerves.

As I mentioned earlier, our cranial nerves occur in pairs, which is why I refer to them in the plural here. You'll often hear these nerves referred to in the singular—that is, "the vagus nerve," as though it is one single rope of a nerve running through your body. I say "vagus nerves" because there is a *pair* of vagus nerve branches stemming from your brain stem, just as there is a pair of trigeminal nerves and so on. This wording reminds us that there is more complexity at work than we realize.

Cranial nerves are like tree branches, which can make symptoms complicated—and which also spares us from even greater pain or debilitation. The human body is designed specifically so that if one nerve or one branch of a nerve is damaged, whether through viral inflammation, toxic heavy metals or chemicals, or injury, there's a hopeful chance that another branch of that nerve will be less injured or not injured at all, allowing somebody the chance to function, operate, recover, and heal. The tree branch system allows pain to not always occur everywhere around the head, face, neck, and torso. Instead, areas of pain will be localized in specific areas, versus broadcasting everywhere. Even though specific points of nerve inflammation can be painful, even devastatingly painful, this localization can make a condition more bearable, allowing for opportunities to function and live your life to some degree, and even to heal.

For example, one facial nerve can be inflamed, causing a facial droop due to temporary paralysis of that facial nerve. Yet the other facial nerve could be functioning, not having sustained paralysis, limiting the facial droop to only one side. This is the tree branch effect of the cranial nerves.

A similar experience can occur with trigeminal neuralgia. Someone could have pain in their jaw and cheek and not their eye, temple, or top of their forehead because only two areas of the trigeminal tree branch are inflamed.

Or someone could get a pain deep inside or outside one ear, where it's so painful you can't even touch it, while the other ear doesn't have any pain. Only one aspect of the facial nerve or vestibulocochlear nerve tree branch that's behind the pain is inflamed.

If both branches of a cranial nerve are inflamed because the brain stem has an aggressive viral infection, then instead of being localized, pain can oscillate throughout all regions of the head, face, neck, and torso. Sometimes this will give a person flashing pains, where pain will change locations after a few seconds, and then the spots where they're feeling pain will change again moments later, oscillating all around until the viral infection reduces and the brain stem becomes less inflamed.

VAGUS NERVE INSIGHTS

What you'll hear called "the vagus nerve" is not just one thick nerve that runs from one end to the other in a perfect line. The vagus nerves are a larger pair of nerves that leave the head region and travel down to the torso. The vagus nerves' size and reach make them more complex than shorter cranial nerves, which is why they deserve special attention here.

The Vagus Nerve Grapevine

We can think of the vagus nerve structure as a grapevine. Like the other cranial nerves, the vagus nerve grapevine is split in two as it leaves the brain stem, with those two main vines branching off on their own pathways. One vagus nerve vine branch could be inflamed while the other vagus nerve vine branch is not inflamed. This is a critical part of the human design that protects us. It means that if one of the vagus nerves is completely inflamed or damaged, there may still be a chance of survival while the other vagus nerve shares its functions.

Medical research and science haven't yet discovered all aspects of the vagus nerves. There are still new discoveries to be had. One future discovery is vagus nerve regeneration (VNR): that is, certain parts of the vagus nerves can regenerate and regrow themselves if the conditions are right. Medical research and science will also discover that the anatomy of the vagus nerves is not definitive. The vagus nerves are not designed the same way in every person. For example, the vagus nerve branches don't completely connect in the torso for everybody. In some people, the two vine branches merely cross over and touch each other, not actually connecting. The vagus nerves also vary in length in each person. This discovery is going to be forced upon the medical industry due to robotic surgeries, where robots programmed to perform surgery end up injuring patients' vagus nerves because the calculations are so unpredictable from person to person. Medical communities are going to start finding out that the vagus nerves' length, growth, size, and directions of travel are not as cookie-cutter as previously assumed.

The vagus nerves are made up of tiny strands and strings of nerve cells that run the length of the nerves. A vagus nerve is not just one solid nerve. It's a complex weave of nerve cells. (This is similar to how the other cranial nerves work, although not identical.) This complexity works in our favor. When vagus nerve inflammation occurs, it may affect multiple strings within a vagus nerve yet not every single string of the nerve. This means inflammation does not take over an entire vagus nerve. It also means symptoms can move and shift if nerve strand inflammation moves and shifts. If the cause of inflammation is aggressive, inflammation can breach onto other nerve strands. Or inflammation can go up and down, slightly pressuring

and pushing different strands of nerve cells within an area of a vagus nerve, leading to milder, phantom-like symptoms that come and go. This makes a lot of people feel crazy as they're explaining their symptoms to their doctor. Still, these phantom symptoms, and a person's main, more definable symptoms, are less severe than they would be if inflammation were taking over the entire nerve and creating more severe symptoms that would complicate someone's suffering further.

Because of the vagus nerves' size and reach, when inflammation occurs in the brain stem that affects the vagus nerve grapevine, the vagus nerves can exhibit a wider range of symptoms on the whole than other cranial nerves. These vagus nerve symptoms that result from an inflamed brain stem could include tightness of the chest, tightness of throat, mild dizziness, an imbalanced feeling, a sense of not digesting well, anxiety, pressure in the chest, difficulty swallowing (even if mild), a hard time taking a deep breath, pain in the throat, nausea, and sometimes erratic heartbeat. When vagus nerve inflammation is stemming from higher up like this—from the brain stem itself—it could be a little bit of everything. One possible experience is neurological asthma, a form of asthma where the airways are not impeded by visible inflammation. Instead, neurological asthma is the sensation of air restriction created by inflamed vagus nerves and/or other cranial nerves.

As inflammation ebbs and flows in the brain stem, from mild to more severe, some of the inflammation will lessen or intensify on the vagus nerve grapevine. Inflammation can come and go based on whether someone is getting more sleep or is lacking sleep, because when you sleep, your body is trying to heal inflamed nerves and your immune system is going after viruses. Other factors that affect inflammation include whether someone is less stressed or more stressed, whether someone is eating better than normal or a little out of control with their foods, and whether someone is exercising more or less. These changes matter.

On a day with lower inflammation, you may still have the tightness of the chest yet less pressure or pain in the abdomen region, less anxiety, and a better day with no vertigo, balance issues, or dizziness. If the brain stem inflammation becomes more pronounced, it can feel more drastic, with all of the symptoms combined at an advanced level. Viral inflammation combined with toxic heavy metals and everyday toxic chemicals that are inside the brain stem (located close to the vagus nerves there) can create most every vagus nerve symptom, with different variables and to different degrees, at the same time.

In many cases of brain stem and cranial nerve inflammation, the infection is not in the brain stem or nerves themselves. The viral infection (such as EBV or shingles, herpes simplex 1, or herpes simplex 2) is inside the liver or even the spleen. Wherever a viral infection is in the body, if it's releasing viral neurotoxins, those neurotoxins can travel through the bloodstream and land on areas of the brain stem and vagus nerve grapevine, creating additional inflammation and additional symptoms.

Wherever neurotoxins inflame a vagus nerve, they create an inflammation hot spot. That hot spot may lead to vertigo or dizziness, or that hot spot could result in tightness of the chest. Viruses themselves can also cling to parts of the vagus nerve grapevine, releasing viral neurotoxins while also creating hot spots where the viral cells have attached themselves to the nerve. If a virus attaches itself to a higher section of a vagus nerve, someone could experience a severe bout of vertigo where they feel stuck, sick, unable to walk, like they're falling when they walk, like they're on a boat, or they could get the spins when they lie down in bed. They could even end up vomiting.

The vagus nerves are channels for information delivery to the lungs, heart, stomach, and intestinal tract. When our brain's neurons get contaminated with toxic heavy metals, caffeine, MSG, petrochemicals, chemical fragrances, viral neurotoxins, or other brain betrayers, they can disrupt this flow of information. That is, contaminants interfere with the signals that neurons send down to the brain stem, which in turn affects the signals that cranial nerves such as the vagus are meant to deliver. (On rare occasions, brain tissue becomes inflamed from direct viral infection, and this can interfere with neuron messaging too.) When contaminated messaging travels from the neurons down the vagus nerves to the organs, such as the heart and intestinal tract, it's a skewed, erratic electrical signal with skewed information—all because the neurons from which the information originated were contaminated. This is how someone can have an electrical heartbeat issue without anything impeding or obstructing a heart valve or having any other heart problem. Another way an electrical heartbeat issue can occur is if the brain stem is inflamed where the vagus nerves exit. Messaging from neurons in the brain gets momentarily blocked in the brain stem, builds up, and then exits with high intensity, sending signals down the vagus nerves that hit the heart, which can cause heart palpitations and spasms in other places.

This is also how someone could experience gut pains, spasms, or peristaltic issues, often causing a gastroparesis diagnosis, without a physical problem in the gastrointestinal tract. Contaminated neurons in the brain—whether saturated with caffeine, MSG, toxic heavy metals, petrochemicals, chemical fragrances, air fresheners, carpet chemicals, new toxic chemicals on clothing (such as fungicides), or other contaminants—are sending distorted signals to the brain stem that then travel along the vagus nerve grapevine, all the way down to where the vagus grapevine connects with the small intestinal tract or colon. All of this can happen simply from neuron contamination, without vagus nerves even being inflamed. Or many times, the vagus nerves *are* inflamed near the colon, small intestinal tract, or stomach; the nerves inflame from viral neurotoxins from low-grade viral infection, or even from solvent or toxic heavy metal contamination on a section of vagus nerve itself. Both can also happen at once— neuron contamination affecting messaging

to the vagus nerves *at the same time* that vagus nerves are inflamed—making gut problems worse.

Vagus Nerve Healing

To heal vagus nerve problems of any kind, you want to address the different possibilities of why you're experiencing that symptom or condition by:

- Reducing and eliminating your exposures to toxic heavy metals, air fresheners, fragrances, scented candles, colognes, perfumes, scented detergents, fabric softeners, MSG, and other brain betrayers you'll learn more about in Part III;

- Lowering viral infection with support from Part VI of this book, "Bringing Back Your Brain";

- Going on a supplement protocol for your symptom or condition from this book's companion, *Brain Saver Protocols, Cleanses & Recipes* (if you don't find a supplement protocol for your specific symptom or condition, use the Cranial Nerve Inflammation and/or Vagus Nerve Problems supplement lists);

- And knowing how to restore the nerves themselves.

Let's fill in that last piece: how to restore our nerves. It's critical to know how the vagus nerves work and how they can feed themselves to get stronger or even heal. What do the vagus nerves need for nutrients, and how best can the vagus nerves receive these nutrients? The vagus nerves are made up of nerve cells. Nerve cells are the hungriest cells of all when it comes to sugar; nerve cells demand glucose.

When you're trying to heal a vagus nerve condition, it's critical that you don't have insulin resistance. Removing or lowering fat-based foods in the diet is a way to eliminate insulin resistance so that the glucose from critical clean carbohydrates can enter into nerve cells easily, without a lot of fight. Every single nutrient—every vitamin, mineral, trace mineral, electrolyte, amino acid, phytochemical compound, antiviral and antibacterial compound, antioxidant, and anthocyanin—can only enter into a nerve cell if it's attached to glucose. Nerve cells open up to be fed as glucose arrives, so that nutrient being attached to glucose is the only way a nerve cell can receive nutrients. It's the only way someone can receive, for example, vitamin B_{12}: if it arrives with glucose. If someone is on a high-fat diet, which causes insulin resistance, this means that glucose cannot easily enter into nerve cells.

Meanwhile, practitioners and doctors are taught to demonize glucose-rich foods such as fruit and potatoes, creating a fear of nightshades and "too much sugar" in fruit. Due to this lack of knowledge, medical communities unintentionally hold back a person's healing opportunity. As a result

of not enough bioavailable glucose in the diet and too much fat, whatever vitamin B_{12} and other nutrients that person is consuming are going to have a much more difficult time entering into nerve cells for restoration. For a chronically ill person, this matters greatly. There is no time to waste in the healing process.

What You Need to Know about Vagus Nerve Exercises

Because publicly known medical research and science don't have answers about why millions of people in the world are ailing from symptoms and conditions such as anxiety, depression, chronic pain, loss of motor skills, brain fog, confusion, and many other symptoms, this has resulted in a search for answers outside what publicly known medical research and science offer. In other words, it has resulted in creative ways to distract people in hopes that these distractions can be remedies. This is how vagus nerve hacks and techniques became a trend. While some techniques can be helpful as temporary measures for some people, the techniques are instigative and irritating on the nerves for most others.

Medical Medium information throughout the decades has made the connection between anxiety and the vagus nerves, and this has struck a chord in the health world. That information has stated that inflammation of the vagus nerves can bring about many symptoms that are involved in anxiety. As this information has been passed on from individual to individual, details that matter were left out—for example, the details that viral neurotoxins, toxic heavy metals, and brain betrayer chemicals are what can inflame the vagus nerves and bring about anxiety symptoms such as tightness of the chest, unexplained pressure on the throat, difficulty breathing even when the lungs are in good shape, unexplained nausea, anxiety, even the feeling that your stomach is flipping, and tingles and numbness running down the arms, shoulders, and abdomen. As someone runs off with the Medical Medium concept that the vagus nerves are connected to anxiety, the important details about *how* the vagus nerves become and stay inflamed fall to the wayside. As a result, we feel like we have to fix the vagus nerve with physical exercises.

The most common of the self-help trends are breathing techniques and exercises along with particular body movements intended to support the vagus nerves with the intention of fixing someone's anxiety. This is a noble intention. When we can't find answers, we don't want to just sit around not having any kind of direction at all. These techniques keep many people occupied and proactive in trying to get some relief.

What about the person who's never had to do a vagus nerve exercise? They're 80 years old, they've never had debilitating anxiety or other symptoms related to the vagus nerves—and they never had to do any special vagus nerve exercises to keep it that way. They haven't escaped health issues altogether: maybe they have osteoporosis, they had their gallbladder out 20 years ago, they've had cancer and survived it, and

they've had back surgery. And yet they've never had vagus nerve symptoms. The truth is that they didn't suffer anxiety and other neurological symptoms because they didn't have viral inflammation of the vagus nerves, or toxic heavy metals inside certain areas of the brain, or what people so commonly experience: the combination of the "right" blend of toxic heavy metals inside the "right" area of the brain *plus* viral-inflamed nerves such as the vagus nerves.

Temporary, quick-fix remedies such as exercises and movements in hopes of altering someone's anxiety by shifting, tightening, or toning the vagus nerves is not getting to the root problem, the cause of why someone is struggling with anxiety or other symptoms and conditions that Medical Medium information connects to the vagus nerves. I'm not opposed to creative ways to shift someone's being, or attempts to gently shift inflamed vagus nerves in hopes this will alter anxiety. Yet we have to be cautious. Most people who involve themselves with these practices end up worsening their condition because they injure their vagus nerves by poking or trying to manipulate the nerves when they're already dealing with vagus nerve inflammation for other reasons, such as shingles, EBV, or herpes simplex viruses. Their nerves have already become hypersensitive.

Gentle exercises aimed to calm or ease anxiety that have a label saying they're for the vagus nerves are unpredictable. Some people will get away with it, and some people will not. We have to remember to err on the side of caution and be careful with any vagus nerve exercises. Many people are really struggling with brain inflammation, brain stem inflammation, and cranial nerve inflammation—all due to viruses and/or toxic heavy metals or other brain betrayers such as pesticides, insecticides, and fungicides—and their nerves don't bounce back easily after they've been played with or manipulated in any way, even when using a technique that may be okay for someone who only has very mild anxiety and doesn't have a lot of inflammation yet.

The next time you come across a trendy post or video saying that vagus nerve exercises are the answer, remember what you read here. It's worth repeating: Vagus nerve issues can be hypersensitive. They're touchy areas. You need to handle the vagus nerve grapevine with finesse, treat it right, give it what it needs, and get rid of what's causing it to ail. Many people who are sick with chronic symptoms and conditions due to brain inflammation or cranial nerve inflammation don't have room for mishaps. Their reserves are low, their nerves are chronically inflamed for real reasons, and their anxiety is impeding their life for real reasons. The not-so-sick—those people who haven't had their lives upended by symptoms yet—can play around with exercises in hopes that it keeps a little anxiety at bay, and you can call these "vagus nerve exercises" if you want.

For the sick—those people who have to shape their lives around their symptoms—there's no room to play around. It's in these cases that many of these approaches either don't work at all, even temporarily, or they outright worsen the situation.

When the vagus nerves are inflamed, either at the brain stem or along the nerves themselves, there's a good chance we may injure an inflamed area more easily when engaging in exercises and hacks. There's a lack of understanding and knowledge about the vagus nerves because medical research and science don't have information on why our vagus nerves get inflamed, nor do they even realize we're living with inflammation of the vagus and/or other cranial nerves, and that can get us into trouble. A sensitive vagus nerve that is inflamed from viral neurotoxins can worsen when we experiment with ways to stimulate or move it.

For your well-being, it's best to learn how nerves such as the vagus, trigeminal, and facial nerves become inflamed, to address them at the core of their inflammation to heal from the inside out—and to be cautious about trying temporary patches that are applied from the outside in. The goal is to address the real cause of the vagus nerve issue, the real cause of the inflammation, with the resources in this book and *Brain Saver Protocols, Cleanses & Recipes*.

CHAPTER 7

Your Burnt Out, Deficient Brain

Picture a swimming pool with the water draining out. At the same time, fresh water is flowing in from a hose. You want to take a swim in that pool—you're burning hot, you're sweaty, you're desperate to cool off. Yet the water is draining out of the pool faster than it's filling up.

That's how it works when supplies can't reach our brain faster than our brain is using them up. If nutrients, phytochemical compounds, antiviral compounds, antibacterial compounds, macro minerals, trace minerals, trace mineral salts, vitamins, glucose, electrolytes, coenzymes, alkaloids, antioxidants, anthocyanins, polyphenols, and neurotransmitter chemicals leave the brain faster than we put them back into the brain, how can our brain function optimally? This is the foundation of burnout. Supply and demand. Deficiencies and burnout have more to do with each other than anyone knows.

THE BURNOUT SCAPEGOAT

The conventional medical industry loves to avoid real problems, the true issues that are causing people's chronic illness. They would love to pass the burnout concept along, identifying anything and everything that comes in as burnout. And yet at a certain point in time, people just don't want to hear the cause of their problems is burnout anymore—in the same way it gets old hearing that your health struggles are because of your genes. People want real explanations. Since medical research and science don't yet have real explanations for chronic illness, burnout serves as a good scapegoat, a free pass.

Burnout is very much real. What it truly is and how it works—that's what's missing from the medical explanation. Alternative medicine still believes that autoimmune disease is the body attacking itself, a concept it adopted from conventional medicine that was, and still is, a theory. Both alternative and conventional medicine believe, in essence, that autoimmune is your fault.

"Burnout" is another term for it being your fault. The implication is that you're just weak, you can't handle the heat, you need to take a vacation, you're inferior. We see that in how others treat us too: "You're burnt out. Let's get someone else in to do the job. They're not affected by burnout. They're stronger than you."

Here's what the journey of a burnout diagnosis can look like: *Why am I sick? What's wrong with me? Where do I need to go? Oh phew, it's all in my gut. But I'm not better yet. So what's wrong with me? I tried all your gut stuff. I did the brain scans, I did the MRIs, I'm on my fifth doctor, this probiotic and this parasite cleanse are not helping. So what's really wrong with me? Oh, it's burnout. Okay, I finally I got an answer.*

It's an "answer" that makes sense for about 10 seconds, an hour, or a day or two. After that, a burnout diagnosis doesn't feel so satisfying. *Why am I burnt out?* you'll find yourself asking. *How come I can't handle what someone else can handle?* If you're fortunate enough to have the resources to take a sabbatical or a week or two of vacation, you find that even with time off, you're still not better. You start to realize that "burnout" puts the attention on the surface, versus what's really happening deeper inside you.

Burnout should not be a sole diagnosis. We should be diagnosed with the deeper issues at hand: viral inflammation, toxic heavy metals, other poisons and solvents, MSG deposits, lack of glucose, lack of mineral salts, neuron injury, neurotransmitter deficiencies, adrenal complications, and vices that were brought upon us by drug pushers such as the caffeine industry machine. Burnout should be seen as a complex interplay of factors leading us to run low on what our brains physically need to sustain us and keep us strong.

SUPPLY AND DEMAND

The brain is a complex electrical grid, as you know well by now. Everything doesn't need to be perfect on that electrical grid. We have room to play—if we have the supplies we need. With the proper reserves, we have room to make mistakes. It's when those supplies are low, and they're low for too long, that restoring the brain with what it needs for its expert functions doesn't happen in a day or week. That's because burnout doesn't develop over just a day or week. Burnout happens before we see the signs.

Once we see the signs, we're already deep in it. For some, you could have a deficit for multiple years before you see the sign of burnout. Burnout happens even when we're not up against trials, stress, hardship, elevated workloads, or elevated demands—because it has so much to do with deficiencies, and we can experience deficiencies even when life is peaceful, if we don't have the proper knowledge and tools to fuel and support ourselves.

Burnout is all about whether we can get it in faster than it leaves. Can we get more of these packages of goodness into the brain at a higher rate than packages of goodness are used in the brain to meet need and demand?

When our brain doesn't have the supplies it needs, we suffer. Yet avoiding a deficient brain is not a clear-cut matter. It's not as simple as making sure we're feeding our brain what it *really* needs, rather than a trendy theory or idea about brain nutrition. Although lacking the proper, bioavailable nutrients in our diets is a critical part of the equation (and a topic we'll cover soon), it's not the entire formula for how we come to experience the brain deficiencies that lead to burnout and put our health in peril. Are we supplying our brains and bodies with *enough* of the right components to balance out the demands of stressors? Whether these stressors are daily or sporadic, whether minor or intense, whether emotional events, physical output, deadlines, or even the flu, is our brain getting enough support to power through, recover, and replenish its reserves? As your bloodstream is trying to deliver critically needed building blocks to your brain, many diminish before they can even get that far. In part that's because other organs and glands are desperate for attention as well. If they are in deficit, they're going to draw from the precious cargo that's heading up to the brain. Keeping your brain healthy and strong depends upon these important key components reaching your brain in time to support its vital functioning.

And then we must consider our body on a systemic level. Sometimes it's not even about nutrients themselves, or nutritional building blocks of brain hormones. Without realizing it, could we be fostering an environment within our body that undermines our best intentions for a well-fueled brain? In Chapter 9, "Your Acid Brain," you'll read about one way that can happen: through acidity. There's also hydration to consider—are we hydrated enough for our blood to properly carry supplies to our brain? You read briefly about the perils of chronic dehydration in Chapter 5, "Your Emotional Brain," and we'll get into more detail soon. There's also oxygen to consider—how oxygenated is our blood?

And, vitally, is the rest of our body functioning well enough to support our brain? Is our liver sluggish and stagnant from a high-fat diet, a viral load, and/or the numerous toxins we encounter in this world? If so, as we'll explore more in this chapter, the liver's ability to store and convert nutrients into bioavailable forms for the brain is diminished. On top of which, excess fat in the bloodstream from everybody's high-fat diets creates a form of insulin resistance, preventing cells from receiving precious glucose. Sugar brings nutrients into brain cells. Fat does not bring nutrients into brain cells.

One foundational truth is that you can get a blood test to measure your nutrient levels, receive results showing everything in the healthy range, and your brain (and other organs) could still be deficient. Just because nutrients are found in your bloodstream doesn't mean they go to the right places in your brain and body. Nutrients can be suspended around blood fat, trapped in your bloodstream and losing their efficacy, and eventually be urinated out of the body.

We also need to think about what else we may be doing to counteract the benefits of the good we try to bring into ourselves. For example, sodium bicarbonate (baking soda), charcoal, and clay treatments taken internally, intended to treat *Candida* with the theory that this will help the brain receive nutrients, actually do just the opposite. They suffocate the intestinal lining, blocking it from absorbing nutrients that would otherwise be delivered to the brain to support its functioning. (Read more about supplements that undermine our healing in Chapter 29, "Brain Betrayer Supplements.")

WHAT OUR BRAINS ARE MISSING

The top three nutritional components that your brain relies upon are glucose, trace mineral salts, and vitamin B_{12}. Your brain also relies upon supplies of critical brain hormones, proper hydration, specific amino acids, antioxidants, macro minerals such as magnesium and potassium, phytochemical compounds, coenzymes, alkaloids, anthocyanins, antiviral and antibacterial compounds, and polyphenols. Deficiencies in these essentials of brain function are rampant in our world today and lay the foundation for burnout, addiction, memory loss, brain fog, confusion, phobias, OCD, depression, and focus and concentration issues.

We'll focus here on glucose, trace mineral salts, vitamin B_{12}, brain hormones, and hydration. Without these components, the deeper problems such as toxic heavy metals and other brain betrayer toxins and pathogens do more damage.

Glucose Deficiency

Glucose (a form of sugar) is not exactly a nutrient. While we can call it a nutrient, it's different from the vitamins, minerals, trace minerals, and other nutritional components that support our brain and body's health. What makes glucose different? Glucose is an actual food source for your brain. Your brain runs on glucose. You'll read more about its crucial role in Chapter 39, "What Your Brain Is Made Of."

Glucose cools brain cells and brain tissue. Our brains are meant to be well stocked with glycogen storage (stored glucose) as backup for when we go without ample fresh supplies of glucose for too long. All too often, our glycogen storage gets eaten away and depleted. A prime example is intermittent fasting done the wrong way, with lots of caffeine and no available glucose for hours while someone runs on adrenaline.

With our glucose and trace mineral salt reserves low, our brain fire burns high because adrenaline takes over and becomes the fuel for our electrical grid. A lack of glucose reserves makes us more susceptible to emotional shock—on both big issues that come our way and smaller shock waves, bad news, and mild betrayal. As you saw in Chapter 5, "Your Emotional Brain," if we don't have enough glucose to cool down the brain when we're up against emotional struggle, our brain tissue can get scorched, leading to calluses and scar tissue. It's a pretty literal experience of burnout. Fortunately, that brain tissue can heal and recover and return. It takes the right tools. It takes time. And it takes an appreciation for how our brain really works.

Trace Mineral Salt Deficiency

Electrical conductors are another important part of brain function. Electrolytes serve as these conductors in your brain, and trace mineral salts are the building blocks of those electrolytes. Trace mineral salts, then, are part of the great foundation of your brain. Trace minerals in the brain are more critical than essential fatty acids. Electricity can't run through brain tissue without trace mineral salts. (These trace mineral salts are not to be confused with adding salt to food. More soon.)

Not all electrolytes are the same. Come-and-go electrolytes quickly get used up, dissipate, and disappear, traveling out of the brain or getting vaporized by electrical currents. These come-and-go electrolytes are made up of macro minerals such as potassium, magnesium, and sodium. Then there are foundational electrolytes: that is, longer-sustaining electrolytes that stick around. Trace mineral salts are the building blocks of these foundational electrolytes, which cling to neurotransmitters and help prevent them from dehydrating. These electrolytes don't cause extreme and explosive heating. They help the neurotransmitter reflect heat like a shield. These electrolytes made up of trace mineral salts also don't

get used up within a second. They can stay active for a longer duration of time.

Electrical impulses in the brain can only run with continuity if there's a steady stream of electrolytes and trace mineral salts. If there's an area of the brain where electrolytes and trace mineral salts are completely missing, then the electrical charge will diminish greatly in that area of the brain. As a result, someone could experience going blank and losing their thought. They had the thought, and now it feels like it's in the back of their mind and they're trying to retrieve it.

Brain cells are different from any other cells in the body. Brain nerve cells are different from any other nerve cells in the body. They require ample amounts of trace minerals to do their job. Other nerve cells in the body don't require as many trace minerals.

Keep in mind that salt is not the same as trace mineral salts that are bioavailable and have other minerals bonded to them. Consuming plain salt is similar to consuming processed sugar. Processed sugar is not the right kind of sugar the brain needs; it's missing most of its mineral content and becomes something different inside the body. Processed salt is the same. It doesn't have the trace mineral structure around the sodium, so what occurs when it enters the body is dehydration, versus providing the brain with what it needs.

Rock salt and sea salt do not remedy the trace mineral deficiency problem. If someone is going to eat salt, these are better salt choices than regular table salt. Still, these salts' composition is changed because they've been isolated and separated from their natural environment. These salts are too concentrated. Ocean salt (sea salt), for example, is changed because it was removed from its water solution. While ocean salt has more minerals than stripped, standard table salt, it still does not have an adequate amount of minerals due to its removal from the ocean. Plus sea salt's concentration, like rock salt's, causes salt shock when entering the body. Salt shock alerts the body that there's a problem, making the trace minerals in rock salt and sea salt less bioavailable. We get the best, most bioavailable trace mineral salts from healing sources such as lemons and celery juice.

Neurotransmitter hormones need trace minerals in order to be complete. They work side by side. Deficiencies of trace minerals inside the brain lead to temporary relapses of any type of symptom and condition as electrical activity drives through patchy spots of brain tissue in areas where trace minerals are deficient. Those patchy spots become the part of the electrical highway of the brain where electricity dims down. This creates inconsistency, causing someone to struggle, whether in receiving information or expressing themselves, delivering information vocally or writing it. Toxic heavy metals and viral neurotoxins in the brain worsen the effects of this deficiency.

The fewer trace minerals in the brain, the hotter brain tissue becomes—because again, trace minerals protect brain tissue. Trace minerals control the heat of the brain, while glucose cools down the brain. If someone is very deficient, void of many trace mineral salts and therefore electrolytes, it can almost

feel like it hurts when they think too hard. That's because brain cells near the electrical current pathway heat up excessively from the transmission of information, because trace minerals are not present in those certain areas to moderate brain heat. This electrical pathway overheating leads some people to try to remedy the situation by not thinking so hard, by shutting down. Then the brain tissue cools more than it should, because when there's a deficiency in trace mineral salts, the brain can't regulate heat well either way. Brain tissue goes from excess heating to excess cooling, even if thoughts are still highly active or intense as someone tries to shut down. Brain heat fluctuations can give somebody fluctuations between clarity and no clarity, or between feeling like they have to think too hard and then, as a result of trying not to think at all, feeling "out of it." Excessive heating and cooling take energy away from the electrical grid, essentially taking energy away from the brain.

This process is different when someone has ample trace minerals in their brain and they choose to quiet their mind. Because trace mineral salts are there to regulate heat in the brain, that person won't get a drastic fluctuation leading to excessive cooling. They'll be able to regulate their thoughts with greater ease.

Vitamin B$_{12}$ Deficiency

Vitamin B$_{12}$ is a necessity for the brain. A top reason is because B$_{12}$ strengthens brain tissue so that tissue can survive electricity. Every cell in the brain requires B$_{12}$ for that cell's survival. It's a required nutrient for brain cells to live longer. B_{12} is meant to be embedded into brain cell walls, allowing for quick cell repair when brain cells become intoxicated or damaged.

As we've well established by now, your brain gets hot from electricity. That may be from an emotional challenge or the brain storm of an emotional conflict. That brain heat may be from problem-solving or pressures in life, work, or school. Brain heat may come from exercising, when your brain is highly alert to every single movement you're making, sending signals to every single muscle throughout your body. Your brain tissue is an engine that's being used. How much B_{12} is readily available in each cell of your brain determines your brain's recovery from anything that challenges it.

For ideal recovery, every single brain cell has to be at 60 percent or more of its B_{12} capacity, and that B_{12} has to be bioavailable. B_{12} is brain cell soluble. The two organs that receive B_{12} the most, and the most easily, are the liver and brain. If a brain cell is under 60 percent of its B_{12} capacity, small damages occur to that brain cell. If a brain cell is under 30 percent of its B_{12} capacity, larger damages occur to it. And if a brain cell is under 5 percent of its B_{12} capacity, extreme damage occurs to that brain cell, and the brain cell walls may not be repairable.

Passing negative thoughts can't deplete your brain cells of B_{12}. Positive thoughts can't refill your brain cells with B_{12}. Yet negative experiences (betrayal, broken trust, losses, relationships, world tragedies) can deplete your brain cells of B_{12}, and even

positive experiences can deplete your brain cells of B_{12}. Happiness, joy, fun, play—for example, ski trips and other active vacations, new relationships, new opportunities, new babies, new jobs—all take B_{12}. If you lose your B_{12} from your brain cells, you can become played out, burnt out from too much play, and not recover easily. You can become drained from too much fun and need a vacation from your vacation. A difficult emotional struggle can do the same; it can burn you out if you're lacking B_{12} in your brain cells. Recovery is very difficult without that ample amount of B_{12}.

Very little B_{12} actually comes from our food. B_{12} deficiencies are as rampant as zinc deficiencies. And the B_{12} you get from eating a piece of meat or egg or cheese or other animal product is not the B_{12} that enters into your brain cells and allows those brain cells to work at their best capacity. That B_{12} from animals was designed for the animal's brain only. It's a different coenzyme altogether and is created for the sole purpose of that animal's brain and not for a human brain. A blood test doesn't tell you this. You could have a blood test showing you're high or level in B_{12}, yet it's the wrong B_{12}, not to mention that a blood test only measures what's in your blood. There is no test to determine how much B_{12} is in a brain cell, what kind of B_{12} is in a brain cell (if it's usable B_{12} or not usable), or how much B_{12} a brain cell is utilizing.

The B_{12} you're existing on inside your brain is still being created from that one piece of parsley you picked out of your garden 10 years ago. That's thanks to *elevated biotics*. Elevated biotics sit on the foods we grow or buy at the farmers market. When we eat these foods, the elevated biotics go to live in our ileum (a section of our small intestine), where they help produce B_{12}. Once B_{12} is produced in our body, our liver is there to be a storage bin for it. In most food and supplement forms, B_{12} has to be converted by the liver to allow methylation to occur. The B_{12} that our body produces in the ileum from elevated biotics doesn't have to be converted, only stored in the liver. If our liver isn't functioning well—meaning we don't store B_{12} and convert B_{12} from outside sources to make it more soluble and usable to brain cells—we become B_{12} deficient as a result of our stagnant, sluggish liver.

When we step on the gas in our car and hit it hard, we're relying on the strength of the nuts and bolts to hold that car together so it doesn't start falling apart. When we're using our brain, B_{12} is one of those nuts and bolts holding it together. Some people blow through their B_{12} supplies faster due to the different experiences and exposures using up their reserves. To some extent, everybody is depleted in B_{12}. Every nerve cell has to have a certain amount of B_{12}, and yet we walk around with nerve cells deficient in B_{12}. Many of us walk around with nerve cells at under 30 percent of their B_{12} capacity, and we suffer from that. One way we can suffer is burnout.

B_{12} deficiency also plays a role in how fast chronic illness that's neurological in nature hinders us and how long certain symptoms last—even after the core root of that chronic illness, such as the Epstein-Barr

virus, is destroyed. When you're in recovery, nerve recovery can take even longer due to a lack of B_{12}.

Brain Hormone Deficiency

Many of the hormones in the brain that are involved in communication and feelings of peace and happiness are originally derived from the adrenal glands. Medical research and science haven't yet scratched the surface when it comes to the role the adrenals play in our brains. In addition to producing reproductive hormones, our adrenal glands also produce some varieties of neurotransmitter hormones and hormone chemicals for brain functioning. Burnt out, weak adrenals can create a brain hormone chemical deficiency.

Our liver also has an ability, when functioning optimally enough, to produce some brain chemical hormones. As you'll read soon, most people aren't living with livers that are functioning optimally, so a stagnant, sluggish liver contributes to brain hormone deficiencies in its own way.

And there are neurotransmitter chemical hormones that are meant to be produced inside the brain and can be reproduced over and over again, developed to match specific neurons. That is, when a neuron cell develops, a matching neurotransmitter chemical develops with it. If we're missing the building blocks required for certain neurotransmitter chemical hormones to develop to match certain neurons, we can become deficient in these chemical hormones. Enough of them won't develop. (The brain actually has a miraculous ability to develop neurons themselves even when faced with severe deficiencies.)

Theories of neurotransmitter chemicals being created in the intestinal tract are misguided. In some cases, certain *foods* that we eat provide neurotransmitter hormones or substantial neurotransmitter building blocks via our gut. Melatonin, for example, is one of the antioxidant brain hormones contained in some foods, such as cherries. That doesn't mean that melatonin comes from our gut. Neurotransmitter chemicals can be *delivered through* our gut, not *produced by* our gut. While the food we eat can become building blocks to support the development of a neurotransmitter chemical compound, the intestinal tract itself does not create the neurotransmitter. Our brain, liver, and endocrine system (including the adrenals, hypothalamus, and pineal gland) contribute to neurotransmitter production, not our gut.

We've come to a place of oversimplification. We like to point to our gut for everything. People don't know why they're sick, yet they think the gut is responsible, because alternative medicine is in the process of brainwashing every individual that their problems all stem from their gut, that their small intestinal tract and colon are responsible for everything happening inside their body. They're brainwashing people because they're brainwashed themselves. At the same time, alternative medicine has people trained to consume lots of coffee, other forms of caffeine, wine, and CBD oil. Everyone is sharing bodily fluids in relationships. Then we have exposures to the dangerous chemicals in scented candles and perfumes that people select thinking they're tools for self-care. And yet none of that is considered the problem. Instead, your gut is the problem. Meanwhile, coffee, of its own merit, is like battery acid and destroys every beneficial living microorganism in your gut, despite any paid-for studies that say otherwise, so if your gut even did produce a neurotransmitter chemical, fat chance it would survive. Not to mention that when caffeine and alcohol enter the brain, they damage neurotransmitters in the brain. This oversimplification of "the gut is everything" plus brainwashing that nothing else we're doing is the problem is a new low in alternative medicine. It shows how much medical communities are struggling as they try to make sense of wave after wave of people seeking help for their burnout and other chronic symptoms and conditions.

Chronic Dehydration

Your brain needs to receive water, and it receives that water via your bloodstream. If your blood is lacking water, your brain will know. Water in the bloodstream is part of the brain's cooling mechanism, along with glucose. And you need water in your blood to carry that glucose. Water helps thin out your blood so glucose can be carried to your brain in a timely fashion, so your brain doesn't go hungry. Without a proper water level in the bloodstream, glucose won't arrive in the brain at a proper level either, even if you're consuming glucose-rich foods. It goes both ways because you need glucose for that water to do its job: the cooling effect of water on the brain only works when there's enough glucose to carry along with it. You also need both water and glucose in your blood to carry electrolytes and trace mineral salts, the regulators that allow the brain to function without overheating or becoming overactive or underactive.

When it comes to chronic dehydration, it's not just about whether we're drinking water that contains electrolytes or not. This is about the need for water, period. Drinking water without electrolytes and trace mineral salts doesn't mean the water running through your bloodstream to your brain is void of electrolytes and trace minerals. The water in your bloodstream can pick up electrolytes and trace minerals that have been provided to your bloodstream from food sources.

More relevant to chronic dehydration is the question "How thick is your blood?" If your blood is too thick, and there's not enough water in your bloodstream— regardless of how many electrolytes or trace mineral salts that water is carrying—the lack of water reaching your brain is a foundation for this type of chronic dehydration. Almost everyone is already on a high-fat diet, whether they realize it or not, so their blood is already thick, which makes it hard for glucose and water to travel to the brain at the levels the brain requires for maximum efficiency. Your blood can also get thick when you're not getting enough hydration in the first place, when your blood is filled with adrenaline from caffeine or fight-or-flight, and when your liver is stagnant and sluggish

(meaning that your liver is filled with poisons, toxins, toxic heavy metals, and pathogenic byproduct). Caffeine and adrenaline are dehydrating on their own, so these make it difficult to get ahead of chronic dehydration. Thick and gooey blood will not support the proper levels of glucose, trace mineral salts, electrolytes, and oxygen, meaning that brain cells become deficient easily when we're chronically dehydrated, setting us up for burnout.

YOUR LIVER IS YOUR BRAIN'S BEST FRIEND

When we go through a relationship breakup, we hurt. Our heart hurts. The same is true when we experience some type of broken trust or betrayal, when we go through an event that is traumatizing in some way. To get you through it, a large spurt of reserves is used up in your brain, due to an electrical storm that's occurring because of the traumatizing event or difficult situation you're up against. As your brain undergoes the stress of these challenges, neurotransmitters get dehydrated and many even get eaten up and destroyed. Neuropathway chemicals get overutilized while chemical compounds, amino acids, and enzymes get burned up. Glucose, glycogen, electrolytes, and trace minerals get eaten up quickly. On top of this, we don't know how to support our brain when we go through this trauma. We don't work on restoring our brain's reserves. Instead, we unknowingly strain our brain further by temporarily starving ourselves, or by bingeing on caffeine, chocolate, ice cream, pizza, chips, soda, sushi, desserts, and food deliveries, prompting adrenaline surges.

Our livers are meant to store bins of nutrients—backup glucose reserves, backup mineral salts, backup electrolytes, backup phytochemical compounds, backup brain hormones, and more—for times of crisis. When the brain runs through its supplies, the liver is called upon to release a well of stored-up nutrients into the bloodstream to get to the brain. Here's the trouble: most everyone has stagnant, sluggish livers. Those backups aren't there.

Keep in mind, even if liver backups are there, precious brain resources still burn away more quickly than your liver can refill them when you're going through a breakup, betrayal, or other trauma. Even in the best of circumstances, brain reserves take time to restore. So we don't want to slow down recovery even more by having maxed-out, depleted livers. Part of getting our brain back is getting our liver back. Part of our brain strength is strengthening our liver, getting it out of stagnancy and restoring its reserves so every time there's a crisis, our liver can exercise a quick response and replenish at least some of the loss to our brain.

We walk around in perpetual deficit. *Humankind* is perpetually in a deficit. We're raised on foods we were never supposed to eat to begin with, and then through adulthood taught to eat foods that we as humans were never supposed to eat. In both childhood and adulthood, we're trained to turn to high-fat comfort foods and stimulants

that we were never meant to eat or drink—comfort foods and stimulants we end up relying upon when we're faced with burnout. The first thing many do when they start to feel something is amiss—a struggle, a brain fog, a difficult emotion or thought, fatigue behind the eyes, neurological fatigue in the brain—is hit the stimulants. And the minute they feel an adrenaline high, with electrical fire at maximum, whether from that stimulant (for example, a daily psychoactive drug addiction such as caffeine) or from drama that's occurring in life, they reach out to high-fat "comfort" food that humans weren't even supposed to learn to consume in the first place.

Why aren't these foods as innocent as they seem? Because they aren't supportive of burnout or what's behind burnout in the first place. More than not supportive, these foods are *unproductive* for anyone dealing with burnout, hindering both the liver and the brain. And yet they're the foods we're taught to reach for to soothe ourselves, numb out, or power through. In Chapter 30, "Brain Betrayer Foods," and Chapter 28, "Brain Betrayer Food and Supplement Chemicals," you'll uncover much more about how foods and food chemicals can hinder us.

Our liver is meant to be our library of nutrients—a library of phytochemical compounds, antiviral and antibacterial compounds, trace minerals, macro minerals, enzymes, hormones, glucose, and more. When our liver gets stagnant and sluggish because of a high-fat diet, whether from poor or high-quality fats, our liver loses the ability to catalog, convert, process, and methylate the critical nutrients our brains need. That is to say, a high-fat diet is one of the bases of our deficiencies. As we obsess about getting our omegas, we deplete ourselves of every other nutrient, creating an acidic environment that atrophies the brain and draws critical trace minerals and phytochemical compounds out of our brain and even out of our skull. Let's be clear: no one is deficient in omega fatty acids. Omegas from sources such as fish, cheese, nuts, seeds, nut butters, seed butters, avocados, and oil do not make up for what you lose when you put them front and center in your diet.

LOSING PRECIOUS RESERVES TO FIGHT-OR-FLIGHT

Even when critical building blocks do reach the brain and storage is refilled, meaning that the brain has readily available assets of critically needed stabilizers like nutrients and phytochemical compounds, there's still fight-or-flight to consider. When we're up against a barrage of adrenaline, that has a significant effect on our stores of brain supplies. Floods of adrenaline can scorch brain tissue, and it's your reserves of nutrients and phytochemical compounds that help protect you and minimize damage from excess adrenaline's injurious, corrosive nature.

It's hard to keep a full storage bin of precious commodities inside the brain when, on top of using brain reserves for daily thinking,

emotions, talking, playing, doing our tasks, taking care of our responsibilities, living our lives, and trying to create our dreams, we're also drawing on these precious reserves to do battle in moments of fight-or-flight. Hard times of struggle, difficulty, challenge: whenever these occur, our adrenal glands release spurts of adrenaline (also called epinephrine, as I mentioned earlier), which go to the brain quickly. Adrenaline is there to burn fast, and it interacts with the electricity in the brain like gasoline to a flame.

Your brain's fire keeps you alive. It helps you navigate the difficult moments, make decisions quickly, defend yourself. Yet if you are consistently in compromising positions and this goes on for too long, all the supplies that are entering the brain are being used up—before they can even become reserves. What's coming in is not entering fast enough to make up for what's being lost.

It's okay to encounter fight-or-flight. Life is hard. We're up against a lot. It's okay, as long as we know how to restore and replenish our brain's reserves. We tend to do the opposite. When life is relatively smooth and we have more time on our hands, we don't tend to build up our brain's reserves. We latch on to vices: caffeine addictions, intermittent fasting, extreme heat activities (such as hot yoga and excessively long hot saunas), extreme body cooling treatments, alcohol, antidepressants. We indulge in foods and activities that are not always helpful or supportive for our brains. Caffeine beverages alone are very destructive to our brain's reserves. Caffeine puts us in a false state of crisis, creating fight-or-flight on a daily basis, even if everything is actually going okay around us. This slowly robs our brain's nutritional reserves.

COMPLICATING FACTORS

Many people are desperate to bring their health back. Yet if someone takes a normal natural-health direction, which relies on elementary measures such as removing processed foods, they all too easily run into the trend traps. Stuck in a world where their health results only get them so far, they're forced to test out trendy theory after trendy theory, acting as guinea pigs for misguided hypotheses. When that's the case, it's going to be a long time before that brain gets restored—if it ever does.

As you've seen throughout this chapter, brain burnout is complicated. Many people dealing with health issues have viral inflammation; neurological fatigue; deposits of toxic heavy metals, other poisons and solvents, air fresheners, fragrances, scented candles, perfumes, colognes, fabric softeners, scented detergents, clothing chemicals, and MSG inside brain tissue; not to mention long-term caffeine addictions and alcohol dependencies.

When someone experiences burnout for too long, they can get some depression with it. They can get some anxiety with it. They can get some depersonalization or brain fog. It's especially true if that person has underlying factors such as toxic heavy metals in the brain, which everyone does. The levels of toxic heavy metals in the brain,

what combinations they're in, and where they're located in the brain determine what kind of added "bonus" someone is going to have with their burnout—for example, depression with a little bit of anxiety.

And then there's viral brain inflammation. The person with small amounts of viral brain inflammation is going to burn out faster than the person without viral brain inflammation. Burnout is hard enough for someone without viral brain inflammation. The person with brain inflammation from low-grade viral infections such as EBV, shingles, herpes simplex, HHV-6, HHV-7, or cytomegalovirus is going to be even more susceptible to brain burnout. That's because when patches of brain tissue are slightly inflamed from viral neurotoxins, this already puts a damper and stress upon neurons, neurotransmitter chemicals, cranial nerves, and brain endocrine glands. Depending on where in the brain inflammation is more dominant, symptoms and conditions vary. This can affect the type of burnout one person is experiencing versus another.

When someone's brain is inflamed as a result of viral infection, more supplies are needed than for someone who does not have viral neurotoxins inflaming their brain, because neurotoxins swell neurons. A swelling neuron demands more supplies because the neuron is in a constant process of trying to repair itself. Someone with viral inflammation in the brain needs twice the glucose.

If someone with viral brain inflammation is not advised properly about diet, it makes it even more difficult. If a person is told to eat a high-fat diet, this minimizes oxygen to the brain, and oxygen is helpful both in repelling viral infection and in restoring brain tissue and creating new brain cells. A high-fat diet also inhibits glucose from getting into brain cells.

Just because someone is dealing with viral inflammation and toxic heavy metals in the brain, that doesn't mean we can't reverse brain burnout. We can still reverse brain burnout, at the same time heading in the direction of reversing viral inflammation and reducing toxic heavy metals. What's important to keep in mind is that someone dealing with extra complications will need more time and more help.

RESTORING OUR TRUE SELVES

We tend to think that managing our thoughts is the answer to burnout. Controlling our brain waves, our neurological pathways, with positive thoughts and meditation is believed to be a key to solving burnout. And yes, that can be helpful. Yet if pieces are missing in the brain's physical function, it's harder to succeed in meditation, creative thinking, positive thoughts, productive thoughts, happy thoughts, and even achieving goals and dreams. Many people who are burnt out and confused about why, who haven't found a way to fix their burnout and other symptoms yet, seek out these mental practices in hopes of ridding themselves of all their physical and mental discomfort. Mental practices only get us so far on their own. Lasting relief comes from addressing supply-and-demand

deficiencies in the brain and the factors that are draining our brains faster than we can replenish them.

The critical root causes of the physical burnout problem have to be fixed: our neurotransmitters are weakened and dehydrated, our neurons are atrophied, our electrical impulses are diminishing, our brains are bathing in acids, and our glucose reserves are disappearing. It makes the struggle of trying to balance the mind through self-care, love, positive thinking, creative thoughts, and realignment of our thought patterns, and learning how to minimize our triggers, much more difficult jobs—because there's always a physical component behind our struggles.

The best meditations we will ever experience occur inside a brain that has ample electrolytes, trace mineral salts, glucose, B_{12} reserves, neurotransmitter conductivity, neuron size and strength, and electrical impulse fire—and fewer toxic heavy metals, fragrances, MSG, caffeine, and alcohol. *Then* rewiring thought patterns and triggers, and rewiring for a present-moment existence, can take hold. Only with the proper brain supplies can thought productivity stick.

Someone living with brain burnout who is missing these key pieces of our brain health puzzle will find it's hard to correct an unhealthy thought pattern. It doesn't stick. It doesn't take hold. Which is why people with signs of burnout have a much more difficult time meditating, focusing, or even believing in themselves.

That's right—key trace minerals in the brain help support us in believing in ourselves. As you discovered in Chapter 5,

"Your Emotional Brain," a strong physical brain helps defend us from emotional injury. And a strong brain helps defend us from emotional triggers. When someone is cranky and irritable and tired, not feeling well or not at their best because they're struggling and exhausted, and then you trigger them, it's going to affect the person. It's much easier for that person to navigate a trigger if they're feeling more themselves, not tired, not irritable, feeling vital and thinking clearly because their brain has what it needs, and they're not addicted to adrenaline, caffeine, or other vices. When someone is able to process thoughts well and a trigger comes along, there's a good chance it will blow right over, or they'll pat you on the back and say, "No worries, I completely understand."

Brain burnout can bring something out of us that isn't us. It can make us unrecognizable. You're not even who you are. Brain burnout can bring us to our knees. Make us doubt who we are. Make us doubt if we're a good person or not, make us doubt what we're doing and where we're going in life, doubt our purpose, even doubt our existence. This doesn't make you a weak person. You didn't manifest burnout through your thoughts. It's physical.

Patterns can take over with brain burnout where we get heated up too quickly; we can become hotheaded, have tantrums, fall apart, experience meltdowns or even increased OCD flare-ups. Our brain engine burns hot quickly. It doesn't take much to spark a fire. Information coming in from an outside source processes and registers differently when you're in a weakened condition, when reserves in your brain are low. It doesn't take much to rev up that fire really fast. Your reactions could be intense even if you're not physically showing a reaction because that's not who you are. Internally there's still a reaction happening inside your brain. Smoldering fire is taking hold. When this occurs over and over again, when everything seems to be in your way, it develops into a pattern, a pattern caused by burnout—a deficiency of brain supplies—not a pattern caused by you. Someone says, "Boo," and you jump. Your brain jumps. The pattern can turn into an overheating, and reserves burn away quickly.

Medical Medium tools, such as those you'll find in Part VI, "Bringing Back Your Brain," and the Burnout protocol in *Brain Saver Protocols, Cleanses & Recipes*, are designed to heal your brain and keep your brain strong. They're designed to restore brain supplies faster than your brain uses them up and designed to remove the biohazards that aren't supposed to be in there. That's key to preventing and addressing deficiencies and burnout, and it's why the tools you'll find in the Medical Medium series are the most effective to find relief and restore your true self.

CHAPTER 8

Your Addicted Brain

When we think about addiction, we bring to mind the opioid epidemic and street drugs and alcohol, hotlines and rehab, programs to get dry and recover. We envision someone financially exhausted from their addiction. We see the turmoil that addiction can cause in their own lives and for the people who love them. There are plenty of theories: hardships at a young age, mistakes made, peer pressure, bad influences. Genes are now entering the picture too, the idea being that the person suffering was somehow born with an addictive gene.

Whenever you see gene blame like this, it's wise to employ some healthy skepticism. Genetic theories, usually papered with poor studies, are an easy out that make it seem like the very fiber of someone's being is at fault. They're a way of saying, "We don't have the real answers." Genetic theories can make it feel like addiction is inevitable, or unfixable, and like fighting to free yourself is a losing battle because your struggle is written into your DNA. Here's what's critical to know: genetic addiction remains an unproven theory. It's not the breakthrough or hard science it seems to be. (More on genetics soon.)

Addiction is deeper than all this, and also more widespread. It's more vast than fentanyl, heroin, cocaine, alcohol, pills, and cigarettes alone. We all have an addictive nature deep inside us. If you think you're completely immune to addictive behavior on any level, you could be in denial. I'm not talking solely about alcohol and drugs here. Addiction runs through all avenues of life and lifestyle. Have you ever heard someone say, "We all have our vices"? That's truer than we know.

Addiction could be as basic as being habitually fixated on a favorite food or meal. It could be an addiction to acting like someone you're not in a way that isn't good for you. You could be addicted to devices. You could be addicted to TV. You could be addicted to driving or confrontation or expressing toxic opinions on the Internet. Exercise addiction is real. So is addiction to shopping or adrenaline play such as zip-lining, hang gliding, or bungee jumping.

You could be addicted to looking outside your front door all the time, checking up on your neighbors perhaps more frequently than you should. You could be addicted to staying up late or staying up all night, using the excuse "The world is quiet then, so I can get a lot done." You could be addicted to collecting—pets, antiques, anything—because you feel like your collection is never complete. You could be addicted to hoarding, not wanting to throw anything out. You could be addicted to organizing, where the addiction runs so deep that everything has to be perfectly organized, and it pains you to have one little thing out of place.

Or you could have a more serious addiction: caffeine addiction. On top of the caffeine you'll find in coffee, black tea, and kombucha tea, there's caffeine in chocolate, cacao, matcha tea, and green tea. There are people for whom caffeine controls their existence, whether they realize it or not. It's common to get "the shakes" in the middle of the day as your morning caffeine wears off, prompting you to reach for that afternoon dose. Caffeine is an accepted, normal addiction that no one's ever supposed to question, even though it can create serious struggle. We often talk about caffeine addiction jokingly. "My family knows not to get between me and my morning cup of coffee." What we don't often hear is the reality that caffeine is a psychoactive drug.

Other serious addictions include sex addiction or gambling or driving too fast. Addiction to scented candles, air fresheners, perfumes, and colognes are serious too. These types of synthetic fragrances are injurious to health. They are actually engineered by chemical companies to have an addictive quality so that we won't be able to break the urge to keep buying them and keep contaminating our personal world and the world around us.

Not all addictions are negative. There are positive ones too. You could be addicted to getting a full night's sleep. You could be addicted to healthy hobbies. You could be addicted to being outdoors. As we'll cover at the end of this chapter, our addictive nature can help us in this way.

What about if our addiction doesn't help us? Our addictive nature can quickly turn unhealthy if we don't know what really causes serious, dangerous, or even destructive addictions.

THE STORY OF ADDICTION

It used to be that addiction was considered a person's problem with a substance itself. Illegal substances were most recognized as sources of addiction. After that, overuse of legal prescriptions such as opioid painkillers was recognized as a type of addiction. In many cases, people ended up in this position because they were in pain and the medical industry, which doesn't understand chronic illness, dealt out their opioids. It wasn't these people's fault, even though they were often blamed.

It took a long time in human history for us to identify alcohol as an addiction. We still don't even want to go there. If you're a drinker, it doesn't mean someone is going to consider it an addiction. It often takes a person getting numerous DUIs, waking up on a street bench practically vomiting to death, or ending up in the emergency room multiple times before someone else will start to say, "Hey, maybe you have an addiction to alcohol." Alcohol is so coveted in our world today that it's almost immune to blame, until that connecting line becomes very obvious. It usually takes someone destroying their life or someone else's life with alcohol to end up in a 12-step program. We reserve the "addict" and "alcoholic" labels for these extreme situations.

Everyone else tries to get away with masking their addiction by saying they only drink socially, or only with friends, or only on weekends, or only one glass a night. Meanwhile, it's all addiction when it comes to alcohol, because of the nature of how alcohol interacts with our system. (Read more about alcohol in Chapter 12, "Alcohol.") Alcohol is a prime example of how less-obvious addictions become protected by the covenants of societal norms.

We've always wanted to separate ourselves from the idea of addiction. Historically blame usually fell on the person struggling with addiction for lack of willpower or for some form of weak-mindedness, mental flaw, or lack of inner strength. Compassion was conspicuously absent from the conversation.

Willpower is still very much part of the conversation. People look at someone struggling with drug abuse, alcohol abuse, gambling, or shopping addiction and think, *Well, how are we going to reshape and change this person? There's obviously a weakness here.* Those who struggle with addiction are often considered insensible or out of touch with reality. Sometimes addiction is even blamed on stupidity. It's simply not true that people who get caught up in addiction are weak or stupid. Intelligent people get caught up in addiction. Besides which, everyone is intelligent.

Lately addiction has been called a disease—and that gets closer to the truth, which is that something is happening inside the brain that explains why bringing a substance into the body or engaging in a certain activity sets off a dependence. That brain reaction explains why someone is reaching for that caffeine or other addictive substance or activity in the first place.

Nobody knows the full truth of what's going on in the brain to create addiction. Naming it a disease does not mean it's understood. It's only gotten that status because of its recurring nature: the observation of a person's desire to go back to the same destructive addiction. If an addiction is destructive enough on an obvious level, and it's an addiction that most of the world does not partake in at that level, then we deem it a disease. This is why alcohol is borderline: because such a vast proportion of the population partakes in it. Again, it takes a person destroying their life with alcohol to consider calling it the disease of addiction, calling it alcoholism, because everyone is drinking.

Not everyone is doing cocaine, heroin, acid, or other street drugs. Not everyone is on psychedelic mushrooms. With addictive substances like these, a smaller percentage of people are engaging with them, so we can more clearly observe someone getting into that addiction cycle. We see the desire to go back to the drugs, even after surviving withdrawal and sobering up. That's when we determine that it must be a disease. With some substances, there isn't that gray area, with someone just doing a little bit of heroin each weekend. There isn't a socially accepted ritual of a glass of heroin every night, the way you may see someone drink a glass of wine each night. A drug such as heroin can quickly spiral into that destructive place that makes it clear addiction is at work.

While alcohol is milder, it can still be abused, and that abuse can become severe. There is also a gray area before that point. You can have a glass of wine every night and not call that a disease—because alcohol is socially accepted and protected in this way. Almost all the population drinks, and we don't want to think that's a problem. Only when someone is on their tenth DUI (or has injured someone while driving under the influence, or has been revealed to be abusive toward family members when drinking, or has lost family and friends due to their alcoholism) and then finally goes into rehab, gets dry, gets their life back in order, and then ends up on a park bench again with a bottle of wine in a brown paper bag—only in this small percentage of the population are we ready to deem it a disease. It's taken a lot of attention to even get here, where we will call that a disease rather than a lack of willpower or a moral failure. In cases like this where it is pronounced, we observe enough

repetition of patterns, enough struggle, that we've come to accept it as addiction and brain-related, even though we still don't understand the rest of the equation.

WHAT REALLY CAUSES ADDICTION

The truth is that four main types of causes can create a susceptibility to addiction:

1. Toxic heavy metals and other contributing brain betrayers

2. Deficiencies in the brain, particularly in glucose, glycogen, and/or trace mineral salts

3. Emotional injury, whether early in life or later

4. Early caffeine exposure (whether in the womb or as a baby, toddler, or child)

A person can experience only one of these causes or any combination of them. Toxic heavy metals in the brain, for example, can create an addiction all on their own, even for someone who grew up in a nurturing home with every resource. Or someone could be dealing with toxic heavy metals in the brain at the same time they're dealing with other brain betrayers or nutrient deficiencies or emotional injury, creating that person's unique experience of addiction. Toxic heavy metals play a very large role in substance abuse and other risky addictions.

It's worth noting that the four causes listed above are the *main* causes of addiction—that is, the causes responsible for the majority of people's addictions. Early drug exposure and early alcohol exposure can also lead to addictions. Even minimal alcohol consumption during pregnancy and breastfeeding can set the stage for addictions. Still, because there is awareness around the risks of drug and alcohol use while pregnant and breastfeeding, it's a less common cause of addiction. Caffeine use in the form of chocolate, green tea, and even coffee is a common, everyday occurrence among those who are pregnant or breastfeeding. We also give kids chocolate on a regular basis. That's why early caffeine exposure gets the attention in this chapter, along with the other three main causes of addiction, which are also common and everyday.

A common thread connects these various causes of addiction: toxic heavy metals and other brain betrayers, deficiencies, emotional injury, early caffeine exposure, and even early drug and/or alcohol exposure. It's a thread that everyone shares, no matter the particular combination of causes that led to their addiction, no matter the type of addiction, no matter the scale of it. That common thread is adrenaline.

THE ADRENALINE OF ADDICTION

The role of adrenaline is central to understanding addiction. When we're addicted to a substance or activity, we are essentially addicted to the adrenaline it triggers.

Let's take a look at how that works, starting with the first type of addiction cause: toxic heavy metals and other brain betrayers.

Adrenaline + Toxic Heavy Metals and Other Brain Betrayers

Nearly everyone walking around on Planet Earth has an underlying toxic heavy metal load in the brain. Some people's toxic heavy metal load is mild, and some people's load is more extreme. When adrenaline saturates brain tissue, it's almost like an antidote to these underlying levels of toxic heavy metals because (1) the adrenaline is like a temporary patch, allowing electrical signals to travel in and around the metals more easily, and (2) adrenaline acts as a temporary anti-inflammatory for any areas of brain tissue where toxic heavy metals are causing mild inflammation. So when a substance or activity triggers an adrenaline surge, that gives us a feeling of relief from the toxic heavy metals hidden in our brain, and then we want to keep reaching back for that relief in the form of whatever substance or activity triggered the adrenaline.

Let's not forget: toxic heavy metals aren't the only toxins in our brain. Someone's brain can be really toxic with brain betrayers. On top of toxic heavy metals, there could be multiple chemical poisons and acids, plastics, radiation, and/or other brain betrayers circulating in the brain and inhabiting brain tissue. And MSG deposits, toxic calcium deposits, and salt deposits create crystallizations in the brain that act as obstructions to electrical pathways in the brain. Adrenaline can feel like sweet relief from any kind of toxic overload in the brain. Just as with toxic heavy metals, adrenaline offers that antidote effect by patching over electrical impediments and temporarily reducing the mild brain inflammation that results from toxic overload. In this way, toxic overload creates a susceptibility to addiction. The fewer toxins in the brain, the less susceptible someone is to addiction.

There are more obvious addiction sources that trigger adrenaline surges, and there are less-obvious sources. Some people fall into substance abuse, for example, whereas others develop an addiction to heated arguments and confrontations that put them within arm's length of danger and therefore pumped up with adrenaline.

Many people, without knowing it, use exercise to treat mild brain inflammation or mild anxiety or depression caused by toxic heavy metals. The adrenaline produced by the exercise provides a temporary feeling of relief. This is how exercise addictions can develop.

Some people have severe health conditions that prevent them from exercising much, so they can't use exercise adrenaline surges to manage the effects of toxic heavy metals on their brain. Even those people who are physically capable of exercise find that it's self-limiting. We can't exercise every minute of the day and night to hold back anxiety and depression. People often resort to the drug caffeine as an adrenaline-producing treatment, whether they realize it or not, sometimes even consuming caffeine before their workouts.

No matter what substance or activity someone uses, what no one realizes is that they're using the substance or activity as a tool to trigger adrenaline highs for momentary relief from toxic heavy metals and everyday toxins in the brain. An individual's degree of toxic heavy metal burden especially is part of what determines how extreme an addiction can get and how heavily someone leans on adrenaline as a quick fix.

Adrenaline + Deficiencies

Meanwhile, when our brain is deficient in critical supplies, we have another reason to seek relief from adrenaline: to help us power through our deficiencies. Shortages of critical supplies in the brain are the norm with our exposures and diets today. Living day in, day out with deficiencies of glucose, glycogen (stored glucose), and trace mineral salts in the brain—not to mention amino acid deficiency and brain hormone deficiency—takes a toll. We're not taught to maintain our glucose levels and store up glycogen. We're not taught to feed our neurotransmitters with trace mineral salts from sources such as celery juice and leafy greens. Instead, we're so often presented with a high-fat, high-protein diet as the norm—and that means we unknowingly look for adrenaline to fill in for the lack of desperately needed brain supplies. Hence, brain deficiencies can create a susceptibility to addictive impulses as we reach for substances and activities to provide those power-through adrenaline surges.

By the way, a high-fat diet is an addiction itself. Every time we consume fat, our adrenal glands release an adrenaline blend to give our heart strength to tackle thick blood from the fat. Adrenaline is also a blood thinner. This adrenaline release is why eating fat gives us a quick, feel-good moment. The moment never lasts. Once the feel-good moment passes, we're back to eating fats again as we chase that high. Fats are really addictive, and they are the real cause of unproductive sugar addiction, which we'll cover later in this chapter.

Adrenaline + Emotional Injury

When someone experiences emotional trauma, whether in their upbringing or later in life, it can lead to obstructions in the emotional centers of the brain in the form of scar tissue, blood vessel stagnation, inflamed blood vessels, hardened tissue, or even mild cases of missing tissue, where brain tissue starts to recede from the inside out in small pockets. Any of these impediments and obstacles can lead to a continual need for adrenaline to bring relief as a temporary patch over the impediments and obstacles.

Other factors can heighten our craving for adrenaline. For example, someone could have high electrical output in the brain from constant emotional demands and stress, leading to extreme electrical grid heat, coupled with a combination of brain tissue saturated with acid, an acid bloodstream, and acidic spinal fluid. Someone could have

a little bit of brain inflammation in an area of an emotional center of the brain. Any of these factors can make symptoms even more intense and make the need for adrenaline feel all the more pressing.

Adrenaline sometimes also has a soothing effect. It can be an anti-inflammatory. If the emotional centers of our brain are calloused from the intense electrical heat of emotional challenges or constant ups and downs, adrenaline is called in as a quick treatment and we feel temporary relief. We become addicted to that adrenaline because it's soothing our calloused brain tissue, basically treating our inflammation in the brain. In turn, we can become addicted to the sources that trigger that adrenaline—sources such as caffeine, alcohol, chocolate, sex, confrontation, and fats.

Adrenaline + Early Caffeine Exposure

Early exposure to caffeine is another hidden cause of addiction that can occur with or without the other causes. We train little ones to eat chocolate, a form of caffeine. And if someone who is pregnant or breastfeeding is consuming chocolate, coffee, coffee drinks, green tea, black tea, cacao, or kombucha tea, that creates caffeine exposure for the baby. When babies, toddlers, and children become caffeine-addicted from these sources of early exposure, it can set the stage for all other addictions later in life.

Caffeine addiction is adrenaline addiction—when we get hooked on caffeine, we're hooked on the adrenaline release it triggers. (The same is true for addictions to other forms of drugs, as well as alcohol addiction: they're adrenaline addictions.) The caffeine industry wants children addicted at a young age, even before birth. That's why chocolate is so accepted. Pregnant women are now drinking green tea because they're told it has health benefits. Meanwhile, the baby goes through withdrawal every day in the womb, and this sets the stage for a lifetime of addictions. Once the baby is born, if the mom is breastfeeding, caffeine in the breast milk can create a situation where the baby doesn't sleep well at night.

If a pregnant woman is under serious stress like a loss, that creates adrenaline surges too. The baby in the womb will be saturated in adrenaline and then have to go through withdrawal from the adrenaline as the surge subsides. This is another form of early addictive exposure, when a baby goes through a roller coaster ride of adrenaline saturation during pregnancy. Like the adrenaline roller coaster ride of caffeine exposure, this experience of a pregnant mom going through a period of enormous stress can possibly set the stage for addiction later. The same is true when a child is up against a traumatic situation in early life. Abuse, for example, triggers intense adrenaline surges. At this early, formative time of brain development, this can set a child up for susceptibility to more adrenaline-seeking in the form of addiction.

It's good to keep this information in mind so that if your baby or child has experienced these early exposures, you can focus on improving nutrition and keeping away as many brain betrayers as you can.

A Sustainable Solution

Adrenaline can take its toll over time. While it can be a temporary soother, it is corrosive in its own way—especially when we're relying on frequent surges of intense adrenaline blends. An adrenaline surge to help us patch over brain betrayers, power through brain deficiencies, and/or soothe impeded and inflamed brain tissue is an emergency system meant to keep us alive in crisis situations. Yet repeated surges of adrenaline in the brain, not to mention in the rest of the body, are not sustainable. The wear and tear will show through weight gain, emotional instability, fatigue, aging, and hair loss in women.

Rather than rely on this emergency adrenaline system day after day, we serve ourselves best by directly addressing the underlying needs and issues that we've just seen addictions reveal: toxic heavy metals and other contaminants in the brain (including MSG, salt, and calcium deposits); deficiencies in critical resources such as glucose, glycogen, and trace mineral salts; brain tissue obstructions such as calloused tissue in the emotional centers of the brain; and caffeine exposure early in life. Addressing your brain's needs is what this book and *Brain Saver Protocols, Cleanses & Recipes* (which includes an Addiction protocol) are here to help you do.

SUGAR ADDICTION: NOT WHAT IT SEEMS

What we call sugar addiction is not technically an addiction. It falls into a different category from other addictive substances. Unlike substances such as nicotine, MSG, and caffeine, which our brains and bodies don't need, sugar (glucose) is essential. Our brains and bodies require sugar. While processed sugar is not the ideal, we don't turn to processed sugar for adrenaline the way we turn to other addictive experiences and substances for the adrenaline they trigger. We turn to sugar to get glucose directly to the brain. What prevents that glucose from getting to the brain is insulin resistance from fats being in the bloodstream at the same time. So even though we've eaten the sugar, we want more because our brain cells aren't receiving most of it. That's why it can be so difficult to engage in "moderation" around processed sugar and refined carbohydrates such as white bread.

There are many more nuances to this that you'll read about in Chapter 33, "Eating Disorders." What's important to know here is that processed sugar addiction or fixation can perpetuate addiction of any other kind, whether in the form of other food addictions or prescription medication dependency (most often for depression, anxiety, ADHD, or bipolar disorder). Why? We often find ourselves with a sugar addiction in part because we're trying to treat ourselves—not in the sense of giving ourselves a treat, but in the sense of treatment. We're subconsciously trying to self-treat on a medical

level because of the lack of glucose and glycogen storage in our brain. If we want to find true relief from impulsivity around processed sugar, we can actively address our brain's glucose and glycogen deficit by lowering the fats in our diet, bringing in foods that are rich in bioavailable glucose (such as fruit) to replace the fats, and supporting our brain with the other Medical Medium healing practices and protocols in this book and its companion.

THE TRUTH ABOUT GENES AND ADDICTION

It's easy to convince us that addiction is genetic. We look at long family lines of addiction running through the generations, and it seems to make sense that addiction is in the genes. Even if addiction doesn't follow a linear path through a family, we're still told it's genetic. If Grandpa had a drinking problem, for example, and any family member develops an addiction, we'll hear, "You inherited that gene from Grandpa." Someone may ask, "If it's genetic, how come Mom doesn't struggle with addiction and I do?" They'll be told, "Oh, it skips a generation." Because we're not aware of the true causes of addiction, inheriting an addiction can seem this simple.

Addiction isn't this simple because addiction isn't genetic. We're told it's genetic because that's easy to swallow. Genes aren't answers to addiction.

The reason addiction *seems* to be genetic is that addiction can indeed show up in generation after generation—because those family members (1) experienced the same nutritional deficiencies and emotional upheavals due to common circumstances, (2) were exposed to the same toxic heavy metals and other brain betrayers due to common circumstances, (3) followed the same patterns of early caffeine exposure, and/or (4) because the same toxic heavy metals and other contaminants were passed down through their bloodline.

Yet none of this is common knowledge, so when we see a headline trending about addiction and genes, it seems to make logical sense. We can't see the toxic heavy metals and other obstructions in each other's brains. What we can see are the effects of addiction—the actions of someone struggling with addiction and the reactions of the people in their lives and how these may repeat themselves in a family. We can also see the physical traits of someone struggling with addiction, and how maybe they have the same facial features as an ancestor who struggled with addiction. We're led to draw conclusions. "You got the same nose and ears. Addiction must be in the genes too."

Genetics is in the same realm as neuroscience. Both genetics and neuroscience seem like such lofty, high-minded fields of medicine that their inner workings must be beyond our comprehension and grasp, and we should therefore bow down and accept either label as divine decree. Especially if genetics and neuroscience are put together, as with addiction—if you hear that genetics and even epigenetics and gene expression are determining our neurochemistry and

neurobiology—it's essentially "game over" for any questioning of what's really going on with addiction. That sort of terminology must mean theorists know what they're talking about. Right?

Blaming addiction on genes is a great mistake. For one, when you blame a condition like addiction on someone's genes, it sends the subliminal message that it's unfixable. If you believe your genes are the reason for your addiction, it can feel like that much bigger a fight to free yourself. It can even feel like there's no sense in trying, because in the back of your mind, it may feel like an unwinnable fight. If we follow the theory that genes are responsible for addiction, then what does that theory have to say about how you fix your genes and get rid of your addiction problem? That you don't. This is one of the greatest shortcomings of blaming addiction on genes. How do you beat your genes? Checkmate. Your genes win.

Another limitation of blaming addiction on genetics is that it can be an excuse to keep an addiction, to surrender and give in to it. *I'm going to keep smoking or drinking because the doctor says it's in my genes,* someone may think. It's used as a reason not to fight to get to the other side.

Not to mention that when we blame addiction on genes, we invalidate someone's emotional injuries, abuse, struggles, and hardships. "That's not why you have an addiction problem," is the message we send. "It's not because you have emotional wounds from difficult experiences in your life." When you're told it's all in your genes, it can make you doubt yourself, doubt the validity of the trauma you suffered and how that could have led to your addiction.

When we hear terms like *genetic switches*, it can sound like definitive science. Keep in mind that turning genes on and off is still a theory. There's no proven science to date that shows this happening and causing an issue. It's not like scientists have a window into a person's genes and can watch genes being switched on and causing an addiction. Science hasn't even proven that there's a possibility for genes to simply be switched into gear, or for gene changes to match the circumstances that are occurring. It's an interesting theory—what if genes could just be activated or turned on?—yet it's only that: theory.

When it comes to genes and addiction, no matter what terminology is applied, it's all theory. And we have to be careful about theories that travel through the ether with no substantiation, no legitimate studies behind them. Often what occurs with genetic studies is that once there's a study on a gene, theories evolve that have nothing to do with the study itself. The study gets cited even though it's completely unrelated to the theory that someone else is proposing, other than the mere fact that both have to do with genes.

Billions of dollars go into genetic research in the belief that the purpose of the study of genetics is to fix our problems and try to help people with their diseases. It's quite the opposite. Classified medical science is purposely using the study of genes to find ways to worsen our lives and health conditions so the industry can profit. Even if the individuals studying genes within the publicly known medical industry have the purest intentions, their work is being used against them. Genetic research isn't about helping others, unlocking our genes, and bettering our lives. Although the classified medical industry hasn't accomplished it yet, genetic research is ultimately about a thirst to use genes to find ways to control human nature and humankind.

So remember, keep your wits about you when you hear assumptions and theories, even seemingly scientific ones, that addiction is all in the genes. If addiction is blamed on genes, then the very fiber of someone's being can be blamed as the source of the problem—and the publicly known medical industry doesn't have to look further for answers and risk exposing what the classified medical industry doesn't wish to expose.

EVERYDAY ADDICTION

What's behind our addictive nature? It's not because we're flawed or wired wrong. As we noted at the beginning of this chapter, not all addictions are unhealthy. Living life to its fullest potential, having dreams and aspirations and visions of what we're searching for in our lives, having loves and joy and happiness—these can all be addictive. Even the simplicities of basic living—watching the sunrise, watching the sunset, taking walks—can be addictive. We can become addicted to extremely healthy practices.

Positive addictions, like other addictions, come down to adrenaline. Unknown to medical research and science, our adrenal glands produce 56 different blends of adrenaline in response to different circumstances and emotions. More than half of these adrenaline blends are for everyday situations (including walking briskly, conversing with strangers, bathing/swimming, and dreaming). The release of these adrenaline blends can provide pleasant sensations that we want to feel again, which is how a beneficial addiction to a good night's sleep, a healthy hobby, or being in the outdoors can take shape. These everyday adrenaline blends are milder than the harsh adrenaline blends for crisis, plus they're triggered at gentler levels—and milder adrenaline blends at gentler levels translate to a more nurturing and sustainable experience for our brain and body.

We need adrenaline for healthy addictions and healthy practices. So if we use our adrenaline and burn out our adrenaline reserves with unhealthy practices, we're not going to get the best out of the healthy addictions and practices. We're not going to have the best sensations, experiences, feelings, or even have the best energy for them if we're trapped in unhealthy practices that are requiring adrenaline for the wrong reasons. Chances are that someone's unhealthy addictions are outweighing and even diminishing the benefits of their healthy ones.

It's also possible to become addicted to unhealthy practices that are *said* to be healthy practices. We can be fooled by unhealthy practices because of their addictive nature and the feelings we get from their adrenaline highs. Just because many addictions are life-supportive, life-friendly, life-healthy, and life-lengthening doesn't mean that everything we hear is healthy actually is.

Everything in moderation is a popular term that we use as permission to try anything. To understand why moderation is misled, and to understand the addictive nature of these practices that makes stopping at "moderation" unrealistic for so many, you'll find entire chapters on the subject in the next section of the book. There in Part II, "Brainwashed," you'll dive into three prime examples of how addictive substances—psychedelics, alcohol, and caffeine—truly interact with the brain, even in microdoses.

Whether you find yourself in an addictive cycle with caffeine, drugs, alcohol, nicotine, MSG, sex, pills, gambling, confrontation, shopping, electronic devices, TV, staying up all night, scented candles and other fragrances, unproductive foods, hoarding, organizing, work, exercise, acting like someone you're not, or any other substance or activity, it is not a fault with who you are as a human being. If you've never been that person who could have just one drink, or smoke just one cigarette, or take just the prescribed opioid dose, it isn't because you are weak. You are strong to have gotten this far. You are strong to have lived so long with a brain so in need of support. It was never about "knowing better." You were always smart. With your new knowledge about how our addicted brains really work, you can use that intelligence to give your brain the helping hand it's been asking for all along.

CHAPTER 9

Your Acid Brain

Alternative and conventional medicine understand very few aspects of chronic illness. Traditionally, alternative medicine has had just a few placeholders to explain chronic symptoms and conditions: (1) acidity causes disease, (2) something can go wrong in your gut and become a problem, (3) you can have a complication with your immune system, and (4) you can have a deficiency. These are the golden rules of the alternative medicine model and even the conventional-alternative hybridized model of medicine now. They package up these "rules" into one big box of charms, in hopes that you get lucky in your healing.

That's not a responsible way for a medical model to go about its days—because publicly known alternative and conventional medical communities still don't see what's responsible for chronic illness, unless they previously learned Medical Medium information or took Medical Medium information without citing it. Alternative medicine and its hybrid models hang their hat on that first placeholder, that acidity causes disease. Here's the issue: saying that the body

is acidic, and that this is tied to disease, is only the pig's ear and not the whole pig.

Who's to say anyone knows what makes us acidic? Because on almost all accounts, alternative and conventional medicine have called the shots wrong when it comes to chronic illness. Here, too, they misunderstand. They misunderstand where acidity fits into the big picture of our health, and they misunderstand what to do about it. That's in part because they misunderstand what even makes us acid and alkaline. Diets, cleanses, supplements, and protocols deemed alkaline actually make us acidic. In their pursuit of the "acidity causes disease" golden rule, they are working against exactly what they're trying to solve.

FATS ARE ACIDS

The alternative medical theory is that processed food, processed sugar, fast food, and fried food are responsible for making someone acidic and solely responsible for disease. These same sources claim that the answer to acidity is to eat healthy whole foods and lots of healthy fats. You would think that's a great solution. Yet people drowning in their chronic illness, who are really sick, don't recover by simply switching to a seemingly healthy diet. One of the reasons they don't recover is that no one knows why they're sick to begin with, even if they're offered suggestions like *Candida*, small intestinal bacterial overgrowth (SIBO), gut flora problems, microbiome issues, parasites, not enough fiber, not enough pure water, protein deficiency, oxalates, lectin issues, too much sugar, goitrogens, fructose intolerance, and food sensitivities. These still aren't answers about why they're sick, so people who are drowning in their chronic illness end up drowning in healthy fats and healthy proteins (which are high in fat). This is true regardless of whether someone is eating a vegan, plant-based, or animal-based diet. Peanut butter is high fat, high protein. Chicken and fish are high fat, high protein. Nuts and seeds are high fat, high protein. Cheese, milk, and eggs are high fat, high protein. The truth is that fats, including healthy fats, are highly acidic.

So one of the "answers" of alternative medicine for the last 10 years—to increase intake of healthy fats—has worked directly against its theory that acidity is the origin of disease. It's amazing how 10 years could be thrown away like that, with hundreds of thousands of sick individuals led the wrong way. Yes, some people may have improved by getting rid of processed foods and exercising more or starting to exercise for the first time, especially if they were never really chronically ill to begin with. If their only complaint before making changes was that they were overweight and sluggish, with mild fatigue and some headaches, then exercising and cutting out processed foods could have made enough of a difference to get them by until more limiting symptoms surfaced or a heart attack or stroke occurred. Most everyone who was chronically ill and tried this approach still stayed sick and lost 10 years of good time. The goal of the alternative and conventional medicine systems and all their indoctrinees and dogma-based practitioners is to eat lots of fats, basically fatting everyone to death without realizing it.

High-fat diets and moderate-fat diets incorporate generous amounts of overt fats—what I call *radical fats*. These include nuts, seeds, nut butters, tahini, other seed butters, nut milk, soy milk, oat milk, coconut oil, olive oil, sesame oil, other oils (whether healthy or unhealthy), avocado, raw cheese, pasteurized cheese, milk, butter, other dairy, chicken, beef, pork, and fish. Whether plant-based or animal-based, fats are all acid producers. The fats within these foods are acid-producing for six reasons:

1. **Fats are acids.** Fats' consistency grants the illusion that they're not acidic. Even though they don't burn your tongue—fats feel smooth and silky on your tongue—fats are very acidic and should be seen as straight acid. Fats contain acidic compounds, and fats' pH lowers when they enter the body. Fats contain phosphorus, which is

acidic inside the body. And think about the term *fatty acid*: their composition makes them a form of acid. Triglycerides in fats are extremely acidic and don't need to be high as measured on a blood test to cause problems such as acidosis.

2. **Fats don't allow toxins to leave our body easily.** Toxins get absorbed into fat, making fat even more acidic than its original state.

3. **Fats push and squeeze water out of the bloodstream, supporting chronic dehydration.** Water loss in the bloodstream makes it less possible to flush out acids. Fats hold on to acids in the bloodstream, and dehydration means less water to bind onto acids and draw them out.

4. **Fats thicken the blood.** This causes your adrenals to flood your bloodstream with adrenaline purposely, to thin out the fat so your heart doesn't have to strain greatly pumping your blood, and so oxygen can still get to your brain (because fats thin out the oxygen inside the bloodstream). That flood of adrenaline is extremely acidic and corrosive. It takes the adrenal glands' most acidic adrenaline blend to thin out fat because the adrenaline has to play a role similar to bile, only in the bloodstream.

5. **Fats trigger insulin surges.** When you're eating radical fats, large amounts of insulin are produced to try to gather any sugar in the bloodstream and deliver it into cells—because fat gets in the way and doesn't allow sugar to enter cells easily. Insulin's job is to get sugar, not fat, into cells. Without this response—if insulin weren't released by your pancreas in large amounts—there's a good chance glucose would not get to your brain so easily and your brain would start to starve. Insulin has to maneuver around the fat that you're eating. Insulin is another substance that's highly acidic. When larger amounts of insulin are produced, larger amounts of acids accrue because fat keeps insulin in the bloodstream longer than insulin should be there. Insulin is supposed to release quickly from the pancreas, attach to sugar, and drive it into cells. It's not supposed to be stagnant in the bloodstream, trapped in fat. Insulin has a

shelf life in our bloodstream. Like other hormones (including adrenaline, sex hormones, and thyroid hormones), if insulin sticks around too long in the bloodstream, it starts to expire, creating more acid.

6. **Fats trigger bile surges.** In response to radical fats in the diet, your liver has to produce large amounts of bile to break down and disperse the fat in your bloodstream, so some of the fat can be utilized. What can't be utilized either has to be stored or discarded. It's not supposed to be like this. We're only supposed to eat as much fat as our body can use. Instead, because people are eating an overabundance of fat, it's a calamity. Some of the fat gets stored and stuck in the liver and other parts of the body, and some of the fat gets discarded by the digestive tract. Bile's job is to remove as much of the fat you've consumed as it can, and to get it out of your intestinal tract and into the toilet on a daily basis. It takes a large amount of bile to do that, and bile is highly acidic.

This is all to say that fats in the diet, even healthy fats—the very recommendation of the same communities diagnosing acidity—are the leading *reason* for acidity. Fats themselves are acidic, plus fats prevent other acids and acidifiers from leaving the body, plus fats trigger the release of acidic adrenaline, insulin, and bile—natural substances that work for our survival that we're nevertheless not meant to flood ourselves with multiple times a day, every day. Consuming moderate to high amounts of dietary fat is the natural way we acidify ourselves here on earth.

EXTREME ACIDIFIERS

On top of this, we bring in more acid bombs—that is, extreme acidifiers such as vinegar. Almost everyone consumes vinegar regularly, whether they know it or not. Vinegar is in most restaurant dishes, in home-cooked food, in "healthy" prepared food from natural food stores, and in processed food, salsa, hot sauce, dressings, mustard, ketchup, bone broth, pickles, barbecue sauce, sushi, and many soups. Plus vinegar is in alternative therapies such as those based on apple cider vinegar (ACV). Vinegar's acetic acid acts as a barrage of acidic corruption to the body all on its own, never mind the natural, normal way we acidify ourselves with fat.

Then there's caffeine. Caffeine is highly acidic itself, plus it prompts the adrenals to produce excess adrenaline, which is itself acidic. This means that coffee, black tea, green tea, matcha tea, chocolate, kombucha tea, and caffeine pills and products bring on a whole other round of acidity.

These are only the basics. Pharmaceuticals, contaminants, pollution, alcohol, perfume, air fresheners, scented candles, dryer sheets, other fabric softeners, scented laundry detergents, incense, cologne, fragrances, and other exposures are also acidifiers, contributing to acidity in their own way.

Toxic heavy metals are also extremely acidic. As I mentioned earlier in the book, they're not like the trace minerals from foods. Toxic heavy metals are industrialized. Their composition has been damaged. This increases their acidity. Toxic heavy metals both contribute to an acid environment simply by being present in our brain and body and also serve as food for the pathogens that cause more acidic body systems. When toxic heavy metals oxidize, leach, outgas, and rust, killing additional brain cells and other cells in the body, the dead cells create acid as well.

You'll read more about toxic exposures in Part III, "Brain Betrayers."

HOW ACIDITY AFFECTS US

That's the truth of how we become acidic. What about how acidity affects us on a disease level?

Peeing Out Our Bones and Atrophying Our Brains

Acidity causes reactions to occur where our body must release precious minerals to buffer the acid. This goes beyond the toxic calcium in dairy products causing osteoporosis. Multiple acidic actions upon the body from all of the acidifying sources you've just

read about begin to remove minerals from bones and teeth, which aren't supposed to be releasing minerals. An acidic environment in the body causes us to urinate out our calcium. Put less delicately, when we're acidic, we pee out our bones and teeth. If proper calcium isn't entering the body from bioavailable sources such as lemons, then we're never going to neutralize the acids in our bloodstream enough to stop the leaching of calcium, magnesium, potassium, manganese, chromium, silica, selenium, molybdenum, and other precious minerals and trace minerals from our bones and teeth. (Another tool to battle acidity is the Nerve-Gut Acid Stabilizer recipe in Chapter 42, "Medical Medium Brain Shot Therapy.")

The reason why you'll hear a story of someone over 40 slipping on ice and cracking their skull in three places so easily at the same time they break their hip is a lifetime of acidity. Compare that to someone who's 20 years old who slips and hits the ground at the same force and doesn't come away with a single fracture. Bones thin out as each year goes by.

What does this have to do with the brain? If we're acidic, we essentially excrete calcium every morning as we pee, and our skull thins out. As our skull thins out, a gap widens between our brain and skull. At the same time, a lifetime of a high-fat diet starves the brain of glycogen, aging the brain faster, causing it to shrink more. Acids and deficiencies contribute to brain atrophy as well, so that with each passing year, our brain shrinks a little as it bathes in acid and loses critical trace minerals and phytochemical compounds. This makes the gap wider. Acids are the great divider of the brain and skull. With more space between the brain and skull, the skull can fracture much more easily due to this hollow quality, not to mention that the acids have thinned the bone of the skull itself.

It's not the acidic environment so much that creates chronic illness. If someone is too acidic, yes, they'll lose their bone mass and atrophy organs such as the brain. Yet even in these circumstances, they can still live a relatively disease-free life. A true cause of chronic illness is pathogenic activity—that is, viruses and bacteria.

Allowing Pathogens to Thrive

Viruses thrive in an acidic environment. They thrive in a lowered immune system environment. And here's what happens: acids deplete the brain and body of precious trace minerals (which are neutral to alkaline in nature). Trace minerals are supposed to be there to keep the immune system strong. Immune cells feed on trace minerals. Trace minerals are part of what makes up an immune cell's composition. Acids lower our immune system because our immune system gets weakened and scorched and breaks down from toxic acid.

Many of us lose immune cells just from being in chronic acidic states. With lower levels of trace minerals in our brain and body due to an acidic environment, pathogens can take advantage. Plus, as you read in Chapter 4, "Your Viral Brain," an acidic environment allows viruses to thrive because

the blood becomes more thick and toxic as acid increases. Pathogens sustain their existence in a toxic, acidic environment, especially when fats are contributing to the acid. Further, Medical Medium information has always stated that the viral neurotoxins, viral casings, and other byproduct released from these pathogens create more acid.

Pathogens such as viruses and bacteria also thrive on eating foods such as eggs, dairy products, and gluten. Eggs, dairy, and gluten already create acidity in the body on their own. At the same time, these foods feed the pathogens that inflame nerves and create chronic illness and chronic neurological inflammation. Pathogens thrive in a high-fat environment. The fattier the foods we eat, regardless of whether they're healthy fats or not, the less oxygen is in the bloodstream. The natural amount of oxygen in our bloodstream is a viral suppressor—a pathogen suppressor. The less oxygen present in the bloodstream, the more viruses and bacteria thrive.

Losing Our Good Acids

The reason why the gut looks like the cause of everyone's issues is that when we lose our hydrochloric acid—our good acid—the resulting environment in the gut allows unproductive yeast, mold, fungus, and bacteria to overgrow, creating toxic acid. Hydrochloric acid is an alkaline acid. Its chemical composition starts out acidic as it's squeezed out of the stomach glands, then changes in composition to alkaline as it leaves the stomach and drops into the duodenum and small intestinal tract.

(By the way, there's also such a thing as good acid when it comes to food sources. Healing foods such as lemons and other citrus contain fruit acid that is highly alkaline as it enters the body, due to its composition derived from alkaline minerals such as beneficial calcium, potassium, and trace mineral salts.)

The hydrochloric acid produced by our stomach glands destroys pathogens in the gut. Yet we destroy our stomach glands through high-fat diets, caffeine, vinegar, and alcohol. So we essentially lose out on producing hydrochloric acid, which in turn allows more unproductive fungus, yeast, mold, bacteria, and viruses to thrive in our intestinal tract, creating more bad acid to contribute to the problem.

Then we add even more bad acid to the gut with high-fat diets. Again: fats, even healthy fats, are acid producers and therefore deficiency creators. Everybody's so brainwashed to get their essential fatty acids from healthy fats that they're unknowingly making themselves deficient in every other vitamin, mineral, and other nutrient. Nutrients can only enter cells when bonded to glucose (sugar) and then driven in by insulin. Nutrients cannot enter cells using fat. Fat blocks nutrients from entering cells and even blocks nutrient absorption in the intestinal tract. The trend of eating fats with your leafy greens to absorb the greens' nutrients does the opposite of what is claimed.

(Read why in Chapter 39, "What Your Brain Is Made Of.")

FAULTY TESTING

Alternative medicine uses pH testing to help determine if a patient is acidic. What they don't realize is that they're misguided in how they interpret the results:

When they see an alkaline reading on a pH strip, they think that means a person is alkaline. They don't realize the alkaline reading could be because the person's body is so acidic that they're losing all their alkaline minerals.

Or say you *are* acidic. You could finally start to become alkaline, and pH testing will show acidity—because you're expelling acids as part of your healing.

We can't simply say that every pH test should be interpreted opposite from the reading, because another scenario is you're so chronically acidic that you have no alkaline minerals left in your body. In that case, your pH test reading could be acidic when you are indeed acidic.

No one trying to interpret a pH test can know which scenario is which. Do the results match someone's body environment, or are they the opposite? On top of which, no one knows what the best time in someone's schedule is to get a pH reading, or how what a person is eating and drinking is affecting a test. There is no proper time of day to find an answer. All of this means that pH tests are not really readable. Relying on pH tests is like chasing ghosts.

ACIDIC GAMES

We can play acidic games all day long. The simple truth is that acidity on its own doesn't mean someone's going to be bed-ridden with chronic fatigue. Just because a person's skull has thinned, their brain is atrophying, and their hip has been replaced twice, it doesn't mean they're going to experience the wide range of symptoms and conditions that alternative medicine has tied to acidity. It's the pathogenic factor that's so important to consider—and how the immune system breaks down from acidifiers and deficiencies. Having an acid brain and body makes us more susceptible to viruses and viruses' effects on our health. That is, more susceptible to developing inflammation of the brain, inflammation of the brain stem, and/or inflammation of the cranial nerves—and all the life-limiting symptoms that can result. The acidity isn't the cause of the disease. The acidity makes the environment right for the pathogens that are the true cause of disease to thrive and create our symptoms.

Plus, as you read in Chapter 3, "Your Alloy Brain," an acid brain influences our brain's heat scale because acidic blood doesn't allow toxins to leave the body easily, which raises the brain's temperature. That has several effects. It makes us more susceptible to the toxic heavy metals in our brain, which can melt and move and form alloys from excess brain heat while oxidizing and corroding from the acid itself. The increased heat of an acid brain also intensifies emotional blows and makes it harder to recover from them. And by raising brain heat and contributing to our deficiencies, acidity makes us more susceptible to burnout.

To blame any of these health struggles on acidity itself is to misunderstand, ignore, and even be entirely unaware of the other factors involved. The alternative and conventional medical industry doesn't even understand acidity. We're made to feel like we're the problem for being acidic, like we just can't get it together enough to foster an alkaline environment inside ourselves, and that's the cause of our suffering. Meanwhile, the medical industry is pushing an agenda that's nowhere close to being alkaline. The very diets and protocols they propose to remedy the situation make us more acidic.

An acid brain and body set us up to be more vulnerable to a static brain, an alloy brain, a viral brain, an invaded emotional brain, inflamed cranial nerves, a burnt out, deficient brain, and an addicted brain. Yet acidity itself is not the cause. Nor are we learning how to truly make ourselves alkaline from any of the sources that use "acidity causes disease" as a golden rule. To find relief, we need to hold on to this knowledge. We need to bring the true alkalizers into our lives while removing the other factors—such as viruses, toxic heavy metals, acidifying foods and drinks, and other brain betrayers—that tell the bigger story about why we struggle with our brain.

"Your brain is electricity. The electricity created in your brain exists through a combination of two supernatural forces (one receiving power from the ether and the other receiving power from your soul) plus a physical component (your heart's and brain's programming to thrive since your inception of life). This is the foundational basis of your brain's life force and how it runs."

— Anthony William, Medical Medium

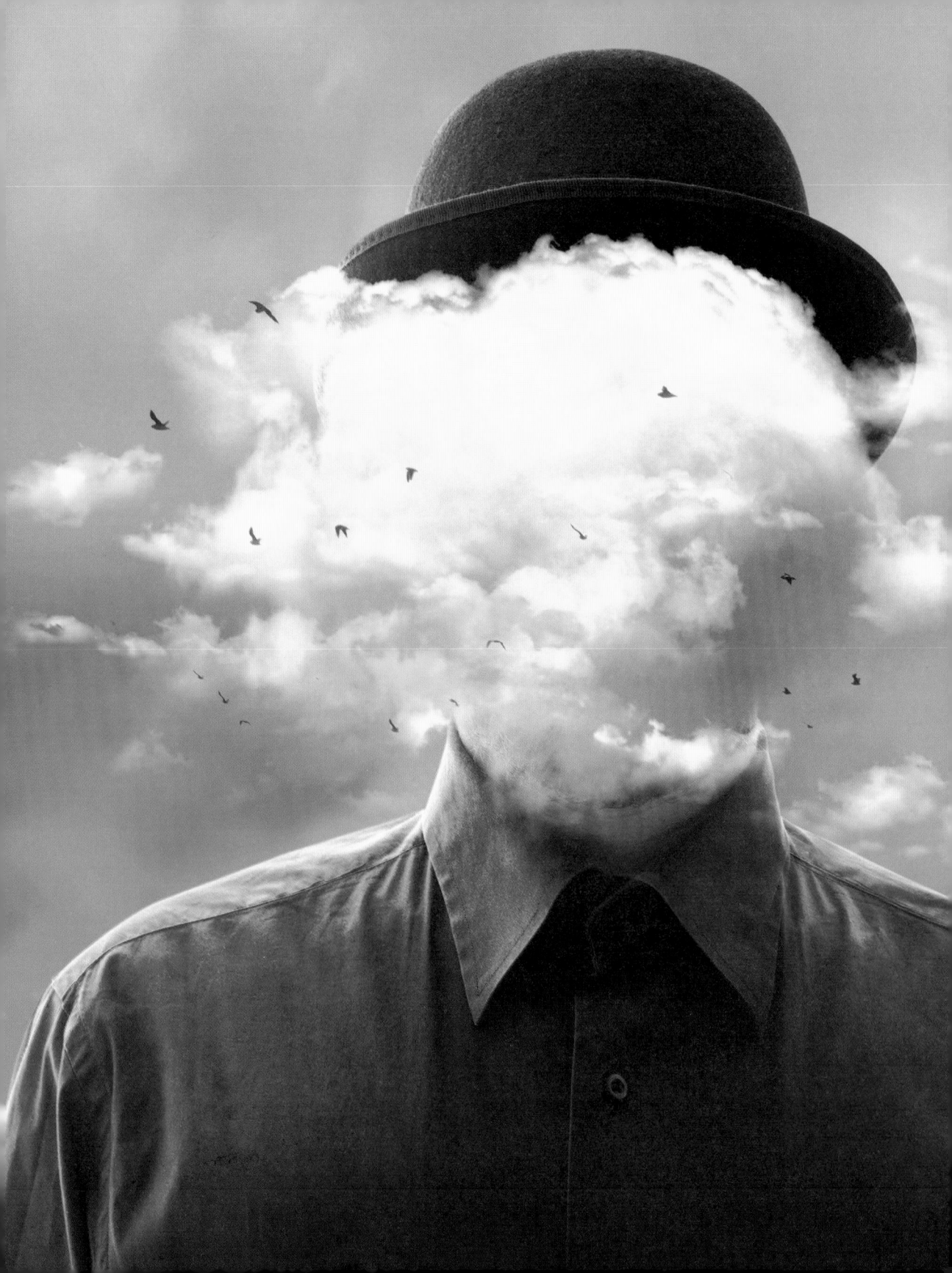

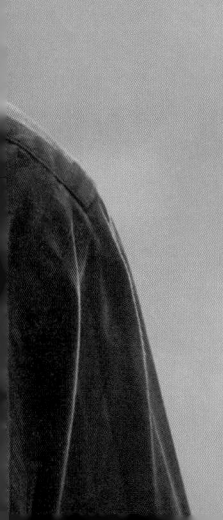

PART II

BRAINWASHED

"Not until you experience a neurological symptom, a mental or emotional health stumbling block, or another brain-related condition do you realize how very little is known about the brain. Only then do the misinformation, missteps, and smoke and mirrors become clear."

— Anthony William, Medical Medium

CHAPTER 10

The Moderation Trap

Moderation never works for anyone. It's permission to do things that aren't great for us. Our physical body does not like "moderation." Yet our body is governed by our subconsciousness and consciousness—our mind—which can be injured or persuaded to want something our physical body doesn't want. Our free will is part of how we step outside the box in life. It's how we embark on trying to heal when we aren't being given the true answers.

We can make two kinds of mistakes. In the first kind, we can have a test in front of us in school and get several true-or-false questions wrong; we can make a mistake crossing our t's and dotting our i's; we can make a mathematical mistake. In this type of mistake, there's no free will. Or rather, not your free will. The free will behind that test was the free will of an institution or the person who designed it. We only used our free will to decide to sit down, fill out the test, and try to answer the questions.

Then we can make mistakes that affect our soul: mistakes through decision processes using our conscious mind that aren't about exact calculations, formulations, or word choices. We can make mistakes that are outside the realm of punching numbers and answering questions that we've studied and prepared for and memorized. While making these other kinds of decisions, our soul can be impacted. These are the mistakes we make with our free will.

When we're sick, the diagnostic testing process is similar to being in school. Here's a physical test that the doctor prescribed, here's a drug that the doctor prescribed, here's another test, here's another drug. We use our free will only to try all these tests and these treatments, just like we use our free will only to sit down and take a test at school. We go through the MRIs, CT scans, blood panels, and more. We're still not better. That leaves us in the realm of not finding answers. We find ourselves sitting at home one night, telling ourselves we really need to heal. We have to find an answer.

Now we have to use our free will like never before to find answers for our physical body. It's not about black and white, we discover. It's not about taking a test in an institution on a memorized set of answers. It's not about being indoctrinated to place all our eggs in their basket. Instead, finding health answers becomes a journey, kind of like when we're looking for love. We're lonely, we want a partner to share our lives with, and there can almost be a desperation of our consciousness in some situations that brings the soul into a different realm. Just like in the search for love, when we reach this point in our search for healing, it's not about what looks perfect on paper anymore, or even what makes sense anymore. We end up taking risks. That's where the soul has no choice but to go along for the ride with whatever we're being pushed into and whatever our consciousness is pushing our soul into, even if it's not best for our soul and physical brain and body. This is where we can make mistakes if our consciousness is peer pressured, convinced, persuaded, or conditioned into using information or practices that don't align with healing, or that even interfere with healing.

CONDITIONED TO GO AGAINST OUR INSTINCTS

"Moderation" is one of those practices. "There's nothing wrong with having that," "You should have what you want," "You need to balance it." We're told that if we only engage in "reasonable" amounts, questionable foods and certain practices such as microdosing, caffeine, and even alcohol can benefit us. So we give them a try, and we end up set back even more in our healing, whether we know it or not. Because our conditioning is so strong, we blame ourselves for these practices not working out instead of blaming the substances themselves. We may even become so attached that we guard these practices with our lives, even though they're harming our lives. We've been pushed so often into finding fault with ourselves, with our brains and bodies, that self-blame becomes our default setting.

Moderation cannot be defined. Even though you'll see a definition of the word *moderation* if you look it up in the dictionary, we should see it as undefinable because "moderation" is not measurable. It's a ruleless definition because it's different for everyone. Each individual's limitations are different. One person's moderation can kill another person. That's true whether we're talking about alcohol, psychedelics, or even food. Someone who's allergic to nuts could die from someone else's level of nuts "in moderation."

We hear moderation talked about a lot with food. Choosing to eat a food in moderation is born out of knowing somewhere deep inside you that the food you're choosing may not be safe to eat a lot of, or to eat constantly. We use the term *moderation* to give ourselves permission to consume that food. Something inside us knows we're not supposed to be eating fried, greasy food every day. Or cakes, cookies, and doughnuts every single day. Or large amounts of these foods. We learn along the way that it's not the best choice and could lead to some kind of health complication. So we do it "in moderation." Moderation is permission to self-indulge or self-sabotage.

Drinking in moderation is also a term you'll often hear. Maybe you even use the term. As with any other substance, using the term *moderation* around alcohol gives us a fuzzy, safe, warm feeling inside. It's permission to drink in any capacity we feel is appropriate. That's a slippery slope. One person may drink every single day and still call this moderation. Another person may drink in the afternoons and feel that's moderation because they're not drinking in the morning. Everybody's moderation when it comes to alcohol is different. For some, it may be on weekends only. For others, it may be one glass of wine a night all week. And for yet others, "moderation" may be getting straight-out drunk once a month. We hide our alcohol addiction behind the word *moderation* as if it's a shield keeping us from harm. Meanwhile, we make those who recognize themselves as addicts feel different or faulty, when that's far from the case. (More on alcohol in Chapter 12.)

MODERATION ORIGINS

Even when we know better, when we know not to consume something that isn't the best for our health and well-being, someone around us or something we see in the media tells us we can do it in moderation. Sometimes it's stated explicitly, and sometimes the moderation message is subliminally out there. The suggestion is always in our face, wherever we turn.

Moderation is nothing new. It goes back hundreds and hundreds of years in human civilization—for as long as it's been human conditioning to eat ourselves sick. The concept of "everything in moderation" arose in ancient times, when people first started to have the type of access that allowed them to indulge in excessive consumption of all kinds. Hand in hand with this newfound instant gratification, the concept of moderation developed as a way to rein it all in. This moderation knowledge has now been in our consciousness for centuries: if we're not taught to be careful and put limitations on what, how, when, why, or how much we consume, we can kill ourselves in one capacity or another. Even before the word *moderation* emerged, the concept emerged as a way to protect ourselves.

Now moderation is being used to unprotect ourselves. We're using it as permission to poison ourselves. Whatever we want to indulge in or harm ourselves with, we can do so in good conscience by saying we're doing it in "moderation." We're meant to have the tools and knowledge and resources to not go down this road.

It's hard to break away from the status quo of moderation because it's so built into society. If you choose to fight the brainwashing of moderation, you get your wrists smacked. You get punished by others who don't want to break their own habits and lifestyle of using moderation to consume foods and substances that aren't benefiting them. Those who give themselves permission to indulge in what they know deep down isn't good for them find it unsettling and even threatening when you decide to go in your own direction. It makes them uncomfortable when you start to find empowerment and take control over your health and become aware that certain foods and substances, even "in moderation," aren't doing you justice. Instead of questioning their own practices, these moderation champions tend to point to you as out of balance. The more uncomfortable they feel, the higher and more insistently they start waving the moderation flag.

A CHANCE TO GROW FREE

We are smart. Our souls are wise. When we're finally given the knowledge, the correct knowledge, about how to heal, we have the potential to recognize it. If we have struggled enough with our health that the blindfold of health dogma has come off, we can see the information here for what it is: the truth. Then it's like recognizing a soul mate after years of relationships gone awry. Whether suddenly or slowly, we realize that those past relationships we contorted ourselves into in desperation didn't go wrong because of some flaw in who we are. Just

like a healthy relationship, the truth about healing may push us to grow. If we give ourselves that chance to grow, we give ourselves the chance to heal.

When, on the other hand, we take moderation and apply it to the world of poisons and toxins, we push it too far. Now we're taking the basic, problematic standard of moderation and exalting it to a place of recklessness. That's what you'll read about in the coming chapters. You've already discovered from Chapter 8, "Your Addicted Brain," why it's so easy to get hooked on certain substances and activities. In the next section of the book, Part III, "Brain Betrayers," you'll see how many of the items we're told are healthy aren't, even in small amounts.

And before we get there, we'll continue Part II, "Brainwashed," with a close look at three examples of how substances that we're told are beneficial in "moderation"— psychedelic microdosing, caffeine, and alcohol—actually interact with the brain and body. Afterward, we'll explore why fighting about food belief systems is a losing battle for everyone. With this knowledge, you can free your soul from conditioning and give yourself the chance to grow and heal.

CHAPTER 11

Microdosing

Psychedelics that are considered plant medicine have gained popularity recently with the theory that "everything is okay if you microdose it."

Now, we're very confused in the health world about what plant medicine is. It's a trend to take something toxic and put the term *plant medicine* in front of it, as if that makes it not toxic or even dangerous. The "plant medicine" label is like an excuse to use plants that have chemical compounds that hinder our body, hurt our body, or set our healing back. As long as we put it in that plant medicine category, a substance has immunity and is considered a safe, viable way to heal.

Really, the term *plant medicine* should be all about fruits, leafy greens, herbs, wild foods, and vegetables that are not mind-altering or adrenaline-surging sources of plant chemical compounds. Plant medicine should be about blackberries, wild blueberries, lemon balm, rosemary, ginger, thyme, celery, spinach, cilantro, and shiitake mushrooms, as just a few examples. Instead, "plant medicine" is being used to give benediction to psilocybin mushrooms (also known as magic mushrooms or shrooms), ayahuasca, or even cacao, matcha tea, and other green tea.

PLAYING WITH POISONS

The problem we have with both alternative and conventional medicine is the same problem we have with discerning what plant medicine really is: no one knows why anyone lives with chronic symptoms and conditions. No one knows why someone has anxiety, depression, bipolar disorder, or OCD. No one knows why anyone has brain fog, fatigue, or the myriad of neurological symptoms that we explore throughout this book. Medical communities may categorize a given struggle as "autoimmune." That's not the answer. "Autoimmune" still means we don't know why anybody has any of these symptoms, conditions, or health struggles.

It all falls into the same pot of guessing-game soup. The conventional doctor doesn't know why you have depression yet offers an antidepressant. The alternative doctor doesn't know why you have depression yet offers you a better diet, a regular exercise routine, the recommendation to get rid of processed foods, and the instruction to take some vitamin D, a multivitamin, and some fish oil. While not every doctor's visit will yield these exact recommendations, whatever the varying recommendations are, they still won't be based on knowing the true, underlying *why* of your suffering. Perhaps a doctor believes gut health is causing your depression—that *Candida* or SIBO or leaky gut or microbiome is to blame. Perhaps a doctor believes you have a chemical imbalance—a neurotransmitter issue such as a dopamine deficiency. Whatever the case, it's still a case of "We don't know why you're sick. We don't know *why* you have depression or any chronic symptom."

The same guessing-game technique has led to widespread interest in psychedelics and microdosing. Someone's search for anything to try, any answers, leads them to the door of the darker side of plant medicine. I've said for years that just because something falls under the umbrella of ancient doesn't mean it's safe or perfect. Over the years I've heard this hundreds of times: a family reaching out to me because their daughter or son was at an ayahuasca or other psychedelic ceremony and barely made it out alive and was still to this day suffering from the brain injury. Defenders of ayahuasca or other psychedelics will say the practitioner leading the ceremony was the

problem, and that you have to be careful who you choose to guide you.

This is not to disrespect anyone involved in ayahuasca ceremonies or any kind of indigenous technique of spiritual healing. Indigenous cultures have also grown bananas. Indigenous cultures have also grown spices such as vanilla bean, cinnamon, turmeric, and ginger. These are nontoxic and have healing properties. While some of these can be self-limiting, meaning that large quantities can be irritating, they are not dangerous. Our brain does not see them as an enemy, nor does our immune system or body. At the same time, whether we're an indigenous culture or not, we can all grow, eat, and play around with poisons. Many non-indigenous people become guides or practitioners who administer psychedelics.

What I mean to address here is the person who's looking for answers to chronic illness, the person who's desperate to try anything and gets further injured in that process, landing a life of much more suffering and hardship than they already had with their condition. People in their lives may pass it off as a bad trip, sweep it under the carpet, and call it their journey, saying, "It was supposed to happen, they had to learn something from it." Meanwhile, it was an injury and not a positive experience of any kind for anyone. Maybe no one even realizes that their brain health is declining from injury—whether a decline that continues over time after one trip or a steady decline with each psychedelic experience.

MICRODOSING: NEW MARKETING FOR PSYCHEDELICS

The landscape around psychedelics has changed in recent years. The mistakes of the past, consuming high dosages of psychedelics, are less common. Too many obvious injuries have occurred. Now there's the term *microdosing*. We talk it up as though if we microdose, we give ourselves permission to partake, as if it's now a controlled environment. The term *microdosing* makes us feel safe. To the human psyche, *microdosing* also implies that there's some scientific nature involved. We feel secure in the sense that there's some type of science advising it, that some type of study has occurred that proves efficacy. As you've learned about scientific studies, they're really just theories combined with never-ending games of trial and error.

Labeling drug use as "microdosing" provides a sense of safety to a wider variety of people. Now it's tempting to many more people who would never partake if they didn't feel it was scientifically evaluated and monitored. It's no longer just a niche crowd of people who go into the desert, sit around a campfire, and drink a whole bowl of psychedelics. Marketing has now made it seem like science has been applied to psychedelics, a tactic that pulls in a much bigger crowd.

The term *microdosing* acts as a safeguard. It makes someone believe that the person offering a therapy and using the term *microdosing* knows a lot, that they're very smart or well educated in the process they're offering. Maybe that's true to some degree, that the person offering a microdosing technique knows a lot about the *theory*. Yet even if you know a lot about a game, it's still a game. There's still a wake of people injured from psychedelics, people who went into microdosing therapy with migraines, for example, and ended up with migraines that were far worse, coupled with additional symptoms.

What psychedelics do is put the body in a crisis state. When we go through a crisis state and come out of it, we change in some ways as a person. It's like surviving a 10-car pileup on the freeway. Your car flips over two or three times, and you seem to walk out of it with a mild concussion while others around you died. There's something that happens inside us when we survive any kind of crisis, and that falls into spiritual change. And when we induce ourselves with a toxic chemical compound that throws our body into chaos, after it subsides we feel we spiritually grow.

ADDICTED TO SURVIVAL

There's an addiction process that occurs with any dose of psychedelics: the addiction to "How did we survive that? That was a heck of a ride!" and "My spiritual teacher told me how much I've grown by doing it" and "I think I'm ready to do it again." One of the addictive aspects of psychedelics is the adrenaline surge that occurs when the poison enters our bloodstream. When any kind of poison enters the bloodstream, our body has to release a steroid compound to soften the blow so the brain, heart, and lungs don't take the hit as hard. A dose, even a microdose, of psychedelics is no different. As our brain starts to get poisoned, it sends an emergency signal to the brain stem and then out to the adrenals, looking for the adrenals to save the brain. An intense adrenaline blend is released to stop strokes from occurring and blood clots from forming, in part by thinning the blood and in part by opening blood vessels back up with steroid compounds as the vessels are closing from the poison.

Why do we need that blood thinning effect? Because our immune system responds to any poison in the body as a foreign invader, trying to stop the invader before it gets to the most critical places in the body such as the brain, heart, and lungs. Our immune cells trying to devour the poison can develop into a blood clot. Our immune system is built with knowledge in it, information in it, to take risks to protect us. Our immune system knows that a kerosene-like, corrosive substance (adrenaline, also known as epinephrine) is coming its way in seconds to dissolve the clot, which will separate the immune cells and try to open blood vessel passageways so there's less constriction, and poisons can leave the brain and body.

Now, adrenaline isn't kerosene. It isn't paint thinner. Yet it has a similar property in that it can start to dissolve and break down a blood clot that's thickening. So as our immune system gathers around the poison—in this case, a psychedelic substance—and tries to eat it up and absorb it, a large number of white blood cells surround the drug's poison chemical compounds. The white blood cells start to group together and become a clump that can get caught in blood vessels. That's a blood clot. Then adrenaline enters the scene and starts to break down this clump.

This chaos is part of the addiction to psychedelics, even to microdoses of psychedelics, or any other poisonous substance. That adrenaline released into the bloodstream to thin the blood and protect the brain in that moment from the onslaught of chemical compounds also saturates the brain, creating extreme adrenaline highs. At the same time, these poisonous chemical compounds, such as the ones found in psychedelics, start hitting neurotransmitters and neurons, and a hallucinogenic effect occurs. The brain effects we associate with these substances—both the adrenaline high and the hallucinogenic effect—occur because what's being consumed is toxic.

The aftermath is that we're coming down off that adrenaline high. Our body is in the process of recovery as the poisonous chemical compound is dissipating, and we survived it. It's not exactly the same as recovering from a party where you got completely drunk and stoned and puked in the bathroom all night, and then spent the next day in the stupor of a hangover . . . yet there are similarities. Whichever substance sent your body into survival mode, they're parties you'll never forget, experiences that become etched in your consciousness. The parties we never forget aren't cures for depression, anxiety, brain fog, fatigue, or neurological symptoms. They only worsen them.

One of the saddest parts of psychedelics is knowing a 25-year-old or 28-year-old who doesn't have any idea why they're sick, has seen a number of doctors, tried a number of medications, can't find relief mentally or physically, and then stumbles into the world of "This can heal you physically and spiritually." It's one thing if you're not healing so you take some junky vitamins, try a range of animal-protein and plant-based diets, try a few different therapies and healing techniques, try conventional pharmaceuticals, and you're still stuck and you're still sick. That's a better place to be than getting caught up in the world of psychedelics, believing that maybe you have a spiritual block that's keeping you physically ill.

When we lose time and we're exhausted and we don't have answers that are working or helping, the next easy sell is "It has to be you. You're the problem. This is a spiritual issue, a mental and emotional problem. The psychedelics will shift something within you, bring you spiritual growth, take you on a spiritual journey where problems can be solved so the outcomes in how you feel physically and emotionally can improve or be healed."

If I didn't know the truth about health, and I went to five or six or more doctors and was still suffering emotionally, mentally, and physically, I could just as easily fall into the same trap as anyone else. It's no one's fault. I'm not blaming anyone for the decisions they're making during their process

and journey. I'm simply trying to let the person who's on the journey searching for answers know that the trendy terms *microdosing* and *psychedelics* are not a viable, productive direction in healing. Everyone who's physically ill, physically and mentally struggling with symptoms and conditions, only gets worse with psychedelics.

This takes us to the understanding of the sick and the not-so-sick, a concept you can read about at the end of this book. Someone who is not-so-sick, which is to say that they are able to live their lives without symptoms getting in the way, may try out psychedelics because they're insecure, lacking confidence, or feeling lost. Their chances of injury from the substances may be a lot less, depending on how much and how often they partake in the psychedelics, because they're not already living with limitations. If someone lives with more persistent symptoms such as insulin resistance, acne, mild depression or anxiety, or what their doctors deem "hormone imbalance," they're going to feel the effects of those psychedelics a lot more. Then there is the person who is outright sick, who's been diagnosed with multiple conditions, who experiences 30, 40, or 50 different symptoms. Someone in this position can get injured with psychedelics quickly, resulting in a setback that creates even more symptoms and worsens the symptoms they already have. These people who get injured are the canaries showing us that psychedelics are not helpful or fruitful.

EVERY ADDICTION STARTS WITH MICRODOSING

Which brings us back to the moderation teachings that have been ingrained in us. *Microdosing* is just a new term for moderation. Instead of ten cups of coffee in a day, someone decides to do one or two, calling that moderation. Instead of a full-blown psychedelic experience, someone decides to take a smaller dosage, calling that microdosing. Here's the wrinkle: Who's to say exactly what moderation is for anyone? One person's "psychedelics in moderation" is very different from another's. It varies for everyone.

When we take the term *moderation* and flip it to the trendy, hip term *microdosing*, it gives us a feeling inside. That feeling when we hear "microdosing" is *That sounds like exact science. That sounds like it's been vetted. It sounds right for me because I'm somebody who doesn't want to do a lot of something that could potentially be too intense, so I like the sound of that*, microdosing. *Sounds right for me.*

It's like someone's first tattoo. I've got nothing against tattoos besides the toxic heavy metals they contain. They can have an addictive quality, though, that draws a useful parallel here. We tend to start with something small—a butterfly tattoo or a few words, some scripture or a quote. Something we feel connected to that we want written on our bodies. Most don't start out with a full sleeve or body tattoo, planning to spend entire days at the tattoo studio. That comes later, once we're so addicted to our tattoos, so in love with them that we want to keep getting more. It's not the first tattoo. You go in saying, "Okay, I'm going to try this out. I'm going to get this little one." It's tattoo microdosing.

Every addiction starts out with microdosing to some extent. Our first experience of alcohol may start with just a few sips of beer. Maybe by the third time you're drinking beer, it's a whole six-pack. To begin with we started with a microdosing mentality. While some people are "all in or nothing," for the majority of people, there's something that sounds very sane about microdosing. No one wants to go to an ayahuasca party and drink a whole bowl of ayahuasca for their very first time—although many have, without realizing it, ingested a large dose of ayahuasca or mushrooms all at once.

THE ULTIMATE PRICE

Many of us want to feel we have control over what we're putting inside our bodies. Microdosing gives us this false sense of security that we're in control. Our consciousness and thought process can be very different from, even defiant to, what our body and soul really need or want. We might say, "No, microdosing is controlled. It's careful. I'm going to heal with this." Our physical brain and our metaphysical soul are not saying that. Our physical brain is saying, "Don't let that poison enter this temple. It doesn't matter if that psychedelic is trendy right now, in this time in history and in earlier times in history. Do not let it enter the temple."

The ghost that lives inside our brain—our soul—is saying, "Don't shorten my time here on earth and slow down your spiritual growth." It's our consciousness and subconsciousness that can be tricked. Our subconscious and conscious mind can be peer pressured, convinced, persuaded, or conditioned to partake in psychedelics or other substances and activities in which our body and soul don't want to partake.

So remember, when someone uses that fancy term *microdosing*, they're really using an old, misunderstood term: *moderation*. "Let's do smaller dosages more frequently" sounds so logical and reasonable. It sounds less rigorous and precise when you consider it within the context of the rocky road that led here: "We're going to do a smaller amount more often, instead of drinking a whole bowl of psychedelics in one night, screaming and vomiting, and then feeling lifeless and energy-less until the next one." Microdosing is an attempt to get the trip, the journey, without paying the price, when in truth you're paying the ultimate price: your health.

"Tips, tricks, and trends for the brain are really for the ones who haven't suffered with any brain-related complication, disease, or condition. When you have suffered, that becomes clear."

— Anthony William, Medical Medium

CHAPTER 12

Alcohol

Throughout the centuries, all the way up through today, we have associated someone who's had too much to drink with slurred speech, the inability to walk in a straight line, the inability to think or speak clearly. We call it being drunk. If it becomes more severe and that person is vomiting or incapacitated, we may call it alcohol poisoning. Do we really know what happens when our bloodstream is saturated with a high volume of alcohol? We don't, and we never did.

We assumed, because medical research and science assume, that more alcohol in the bloodstream leads directly to these actions and symptoms—that alcohol itself affects the brain to cause these experiences. Here's the truth: no one knows exactly what happens inside the brain with alcohol. Intoxication is not fully understood; it's only one aspect of what happens to the brain when someone drinks.

Alcohol's effects start out with what is called getting a little "tipsy." Some say alcohol helps them loosen up and speak their mind. Some say a couple of beers help them

relax. Some say wine helps numb them out. Yet *how* does alcohol seem to loosen them up, relax them, or numb them out?

BRAIN CHARADES

As we've discussed throughout this book, your brain survives on glucose. A lack of glucose to your brain can slowly starve it over time. And if glucose were eliminated from your bloodstream and never entered your brain, you could go into brain failure within moments. Alcohol is the all-time trick on your brain. That's because your brain believes alcohol is sugar, sugar it can use. It believes it's like the glucose that's created by the foods you eat that contain carbohydrates and sugar. Really, alcohol is *methyl*-sugar. It's a hybrid of what *was* sugar—more of a vaporized sugar versus a usable sugar. Alcohol's essence is sugar, yet it's not.

As a result of this charade played on your brain that leads it to identify alcohol as critically needed glucose, several things go wrong. The more alcohol in your bloodstream, the harder it is for your brain to use any real source of glucose in your bloodstream. And alcohol dominates over any glucose storage left in the brain.

Your liver is your main glucose storage bin. Its job is to release glucose congruently as your brain needs it. There are moments when we aren't getting sugar or glucose or fructose or any kind of carbohydrate in our diet, and we go into glucose deficits in the bloodstream. Your liver's job in that case is to release glucose so your brain doesn't completely starve. This includes circumstances where you aren't eating for a long period of time. Remember, without glucose, your brain can't survive. The liver fulfilling this role is why someone can do a water fast and their brain can survive the experience—because the liver is releasing ample glucose for the brain. Glycogen reserves in the brain and glucose reserves in the liver determine how long someone can withstand a water fast. Now, not everybody's liver functions that well. Many people's glucose storage bins can be minimal due to the liver being sluggish or stagnant, so drinking alcohol can affect these people more than alcohol affects people with strong livers. That's why some say, "I can't handle alcohol," or "He can't handle his liquor." Because their livers are weakened, especially as they age.

Regardless of someone's alcohol tolerance, when enough alcohol is consumed, the effects are all the same. As you're drinking alcohol, it starts to poison and numb the liver, and your liver is your defense mechanism to stop alcohol from getting to your brain. By the time you start getting tipsy—or whatever you personally call the beginning stages of feeling alcohol's effects, no matter how mild—your liver is already at its saturation level for protecting the brain. When we talk about "moderation" with alcohol, we miss this crucial point.

Alcohol is toxic in any amount, so the liver's job is to soak up every last drop it can. When your liver is being poisoned by alcohol, it can't release glucose anymore. Even if someone has a large storage bin of glucose, eventually the liver becomes paralyzed by the alcohol in this vitally important function—because the liver's job of releasing glucose is halted. Its job instead becomes soaking up alcohol.

At the same time, alcohol pushes aside any glucose that is in the bloodstream, so alcohol becomes the brain's number one choice for fuel, because alcohol seems like glucose, even though in the end, it isn't. Alcohol is a byproduct of glucose. It's a byproduct of sugar. It's a ghost of what sugar was. So the brain becomes a victim of the ghost effect of alcohol. As more alcohol enters the brain, a person exhibits more drunken (that is, inebriated) behavior. When someone gets to the point of drunken behavior—slurred speech, inability to function normally—that means the brain is already starting to starve to death. And here's a key understanding: most of the symptoms we associate with drunkenness and alcohol poisoning aren't only from alcohol itself. Most are symptoms of the brain starting to die.

The more alcohol you consume in an evening or day, the less glucose the brain absorbs and then fuels itself with. If we think of the optimum as 100 percent of glucose entering the brain and keeping it alive, then drinking alcohol brings that glucose percentage down to 5 to 10 percent, depending on how inebriated someone is. It's like taking a fish out of water, watching it gasp on the beach as it takes in oxygen instead of water, then putting it back in the water to revive it, and then taking it back out and repeating. The fish will stay alive, although it pays the price for being thrust into survival mode. This is what happens when someone drinks alcohol regularly. Just enough glucose is getting to the brain to keep the person alive, yet it's so little that the person loses the ability to function. You become a walking, talking example of a dying brain.

Alcohol dominates over glucose getting to the brain because not only is the liver intoxicated and paralyzed and cannot release enough glucose to get to the brain—but the brain chooses alcohol over glucose. This is not because the brain needs alcohol, or because alcohol is good for the brain. Again, it's because the brain is being tricked into thinking the alcohol is the most accessible, viable form of glucose.

THE INTOXICATION ELEMENT

The effect of alcohol on the brain isn't solely from this trick sugar effect, where the brain becomes starved of valuable glucose. Alcohol is indeed a poison, and as a poison it does have an effect that can be intoxicating and debilitating. Yet the slurred speech when someone is on their third drink is

because the brain is starting to starve from glucose and therefore losing the ability to function.

When inebriation becomes extreme and drastic and someone drinks so much that they collapse, conk out, and fall asleep, that drunken sleep is a game of Russian roulette. Because if the brain doesn't get any glucose at all due to the intensity of intoxication, the brain can actually starve and that person can die in their sleep. Or due to alcohol poisoning (one aspect of inebriation that's not about lack of glucose), they may need to vomit. As the brain is dying from a lack of glucose, the nerves are not functioning optimally. The vagus nerves can become paralyzed as the brain is losing deeper glucose reserves, meaning that as someone is vomiting in their sleep, it's easier to choke and die.

Eating enough glucose-rich foods and keeping your fats low is important before a drinking night so you have ample storage bins of glucose freshly available. This is why when someone says, "I'm drinking on an empty stomach. I haven't eaten today," you'll see them get buzzed faster, showing those first effects of drinking early. We think this buzz, this tipsiness, is because the brain becomes intoxicated with alcohol. Really an alcohol buzz is a brain starving of glucose. The liver is starting to mop up the alcohol, so it's not releasing glucose anymore, and because someone didn't eat, they also don't have freshly available glucose in the bloodstream. For someone who did eat that day, it takes longer for the alcohol to affect them as they start drinking because they at least have that fresh glucose for the brain.

It takes a larger volume of alcohol for intoxication to come into it—that is, for the poison aspect of alcohol to play a role in someone's symptoms. Even then, drunkenness is part intoxication by alcohol and part brain starving of glucose.

If drunkenness were only about intoxication of alcohol, the symptoms would be limited: someone would be nauseous, vomiting, feel sick in the head, feel dizzy, yet while greatly sick, they would still be coherent. It's the starvation of the brain happening at the same time that leads to loss of motor skill function, slurred speech and other difficulties speaking, not understanding what someone is saying, and at the same time, saying things you don't know you're saying. As the brain is getting very little glucose, on the edge of staying alive, certain parts of the brain start to shut down.

MISGUIDED HANGOVER CURES

A hangover, like drunkenness itself, is part from starvation of glucose, part from intoxication of alcohol. The worst approach for recovery is to drink again the next day. Even though that's the advice given to many people who drink, it's the worst option. It doesn't work. It doesn't shake a hangover—because once again, you're starving the brain of glucose.

The reason people tend to gorge on food the day after drinking is because their brain is asking for glucose. Depending on how much alcohol someone consumed, the brain narrowly missed starving to death from lack of glucose, so now the organ sends messaging throughout the body that it needs large amounts of glucose desperately and immediately. At the same time, someone could still be nauseous from the alcohol, feeling sick to the stomach and like they can't really hold down food yet. That queasy part of a hangover is from the toxic nature of alcohol.

Many people don't drink to the point of nausea and vomiting. They are still looking to scarf down food to sober up. The same night they drank, they're looking for a diner or drive-through at two or five o'clock in the morning, ordering a whole stack of pancakes with maple syrup, toast, eggs, bacon, waffles, hash browns, burgers, fries, tacos, or burritos. Or they're turning to ample food the next day. The common phrase is "sopping up the alcohol." It even happens when someone is actively drinking, out at a party or a bar when a companion says, "You've got to eat something to sop up that alcohol." What no one realizes is that eating food after drinking alcohol is actually about getting glucose to the brain so it can come out of its starving state and start to function again.

Because we misunderstand what's going on in the brain and body, we're still not getting what our brain really needs—because we're adding fat. Mistakenly, we reach for a combination of carbohydrates plus fat, and that fat inhibits the carbohydrates' glucose from getting to the brain. For example, frying hash browns in oil, butter, and grease inhibits the potato's glucose from easily getting to the brain. Now we're getting insulin resistance, and our body has to fight to divide the sugar and fat so the sugar can get to much-needed places in the brain and other parts of the body. It's not like we're trying to recover from a drunken stupor by consuming fruit such as bananas or papayas or mineral salts from sources such as spinach, other leafy greens, or celery juice. Instead we go for a plate of eggs, which is fat. Or we go for toast with avocado, or oatmeal with nut butter—and avocado and nut butter are both fats getting in the way of the glucose from the carbohydrates of the toast or oatmeal. Across the board, pizza (again, sugar plus fat) is often the most popular go-to after a night or even day of drinking.

ADRENALINE SURGE OF SURVIVAL

Why is starving the brain of glucose addictive—that is, why is alcohol addictive? Because there's an unexpected adrenaline high that comes with the brain losing its fuel source to stay alive. The more alcohol that gets to a brain, in turn starving the brain of glucose, the more adrenaline (epinephrine) is released. This adrenaline can affect each person differently. It can determine if someone is going to be an angry drunk, or if someone is going to be sitting down on the ground crying or outright bawling when they're drunk.

When we say alcohol is talking for someone, what we're really witnessing is adrenaline being used by a brain starving to death. Any time we're in danger on any level, our adrenals send out an adrenaline blend in hopes of changing the chemistry of our bloodstream to help in any way possible. Adrenaline becomes a backup fuel when the brain has no fuel. And remember, adrenaline in itself is an addiction. The more inebriated we get and the more our brain starves of fuel, the more adrenaline is released.

This adrenaline surge often affects people based on what experiences they've had in their life. We each feel different emotions when adrenaline is released. Life experiences and wounds tend to peek their heads up when someone drinks. That's one reason why each person has a different emotional experience when they drink. Some people call alcohol relaxing, some say it gives them a migraine, some say it makes them sad and depressed, some say it makes them happy, some say it gives them strength, energy, and courage. It's all about how someone's reacting to the adrenaline surge. Some people get pumped up when they start to drink—excited, screaming, and yelling with their first round of beers, whether cheering at a sports event or simply celebrating that happy hour moment.

They call it "happy hour" for a reason. The sensation that occurs when you're knocking back that first drink is this adrenaline surge of survival in the face of brain starvation. If we understood this, what we'd be shouting instead of "Cheers!" is "My brain is about to start starving to death! My adrenal glands are going to release a tremendous amount of epinephrine to keep my brain alive! At the same time, I'm going to feel the brain effects of intoxication from alcohol's poison! All in one, it's going to give me a great night!" Except it wouldn't feel like such a great night after all.

"The emotional centers of our brain can only be pushed so far. When you're sick or suffering enough physically, mentally, or emotionally, a survival mechanism kicks in, a survival mechanism in your brain's emotional centers that has been inside us since the beginning of time. This enough-is-enough strength is inside everyone. It's the moment when you put your foot down. It's the moment when you truly find yourself, when you're working with and aligned with your body. When that time comes, that's when you're reborn. It's the rebirth of finally moving out of mental and emotional pain, moving out of that in-between, and turning your life around."

— Anthony William, Medical Medium

CHAPTER 13

Caffeine

Caffeine has been around since long before the 20th century. Yet it was the 20th century when caffeine became popularized because people were losing their ability to function optimally.

The epidemic of chronic illness truly surged in the 1940s. Doctors' offices were overflowing with new cases of women experiencing neurological symptoms that doctors had never witnessed before. At the same time this was happening, caffeine was being advertised in various forms, more than ever before in our history. So as women and some men were living with depression, anxiety, chronic fatigue, aches and pains, neck pain, jaw pain, migraines, restless legs syndrome, vertigo, OCD, listlessness, malaise, loss of libido, heart palpitations, weight gain, hot flashes, and night sweats, the caffeine industry was investing large amounts of resources to take advantage of a population declining in health.

These symptoms were slowing people down. It was the start of mostly women, and some men, losing their ability to function on the level they could back in the 1920s and

'30s. To exploit this new wave of chronic illness, the caffeine industry was getting them addicted to a stimulant.

Simultaneously the pharmaceutical industry started putting caffeine in almost all pharmaceuticals as an ingredient. Most every pharmaceutical drug produced in the 1940s into the 1950s had caffeine in it, and that has continued ever since. So the caffeine industry wasn't just the beverage consumption world. It also became the pharmaceutical world.

Back in the 1940s, the pharmaceutical world had a wholesome appearance. You'd go into the pharmacy and you could sit down and have an ice cream soda and a chocolate brownie while waiting for your prescription to be filled. Usually pharmacies were small, run by one or two individuals that the whole town or village knew. At the same time, coffee products, tea products, and chocolate products also had a wholesome perception. Little did anybody know back then that these two seemingly small, wholesome industries—pharmaceuticals and caffeine—which had images of being rooted in small-town, family-run business, had actually exploded into gigantic industry monsters devouring countless people through their missions.

The numbers of people suffering with chronic illness never declined. Those numbers have only expanded as the years have moved forward. And with those increasing numbers of the chronically ill, the caffeine industry has expanded as well.

Part of chronic illness is the inability to think clearly—brain difficulties such as brain fog, confusion, ADHD, focus issues, and the inability to concentrate. As these symptoms were exploding in the 1940s and beyond, it was interfering with the working world. So the caffeine industry placed heavy emphasis on a campaign to make sure coffee and tea were in every factory, workplace, and corporation worldwide. Prior to the 1940s, most individuals didn't drink coffee or even black tea. Most individuals drank water out of the tap, a glass of orange juice, or milk in the morning. Tea was far less common as a morning drink, and coffee was even less common.

So most workers weren't addicted to caffeine at the outset. They only gravitated toward it due to the campaign of the caffeine industry that coincided with brain issues developing in the workplace. As more people developed neurological issues, more mistakes were happening. The 2 o'clock or 3 o'clock lull, with people falling asleep or getting tired or foggy-headed on the job and needing a mid-afternoon picker upper was a new phenomenon. Then came the 11 o'clock lull and the need for a

late-morning picker upper too. What no one realized was that this struggle in the 1940s and 1950s was due to the beginning stages of the epidemic of chronic illness that continues to plague our world. It was also the beginning stages of caffeine addiction that we still have today.

JUDGE FOR YOURSELF

The classified medical industry created the pathogens that cause chronic illness and exposed us to them. They also exposed us to toxic heavy metals, causing future decades—and what will turn into centuries—of sickness ahead of us, so that the medical industry has a future in making money. With all this the classified medical industry brokered a deal with the caffeine industry to keep our addiction strong. To buffer and hide our symptoms and add to our decline as we age. Caffeine slowly robs the youth and vitality of adults, teenagers, and even children and babies.

The caffeine industry is not what it seems. The caffeine industry is not a tiny mom-and-pop coffee shop with finely roasted, fair-trade, and sustainable coffee beans, just like the tobacco industry isn't a mom-and-pop cigar store with assorted cigars from around the world and a clerk wanting to light one for you so you can taste a fine smoke. The caffeine industry sometimes gives us this wholesome illusion, when really it's a systematically structured, weaponized industry that has think tanks of individuals hired to dictate and plan your every move. The caffeine industry relies on your future of consuming caffeine products and pharmaceuticals with caffeine inserted into them.

(Caffeine has even been used in prisoner-of-war torture experiments. They injected caffeine into people to see if it would work as a truth serum, and to see what it would take to push them to their breaking point. Often the prisoners would have heart attacks right in their seats or drop dead after being injected.)

Caffeine industry think tanks are people hired to ensure the longevity of the caffeine industry. Their number one goal is exposing newborn babies to caffeine because this guarantees the next generation of caffeine consumers. At the same time, the pharmaceutical industry has think tanks of individuals strategizing for future generations to be addicted to caffeine because the pharmaceutical industry uses caffeine to mask how bad the epidemic of chronic illness is.

Caffeine is ironclad, covenanted, and treated as holy. You can't break the caffeine monster. It's like an evil demon, a shapeshifter, a sea serpent, a machine. You get hooked on caffeine. Welcome to the machine.

TAKING ADVANTAGE OF MOMS

In order to expose newborns, the caffeine industry's tactic is to get pregnant and nursing mothers to continue their pre-pregnancy caffeine addictions. Almost all women consume chocolate during pregnancy, and this creates a caffeine addiction for the baby. The caffeine industry depends on this as part of its strategy. Pregnant women are also now being told to consume coffee, matcha tea, green tea, or even kombucha tea during pregnancy, with the direction that it's healthy for them. This is one of the directives from the caffeine industry passed down through various channels, so that even the alternative medical industry promotes green tea, cacao, kombucha tea, and matcha tea for pregnant women, leading alternative medicine to do the caffeine industry's bidding.

Maybe a pregnant woman holds off all caffeine until giving birth, and then consumes caffeine while still breastfeeding. If she consumes caffeinated beverages, chocolate, or cacao products while nursing, the breast milk is filled with caffeine, and that's exposure for the baby, creating caffeine addiction. If moms had any idea they were being used by the caffeine industry in this way, they would be appalled and motivated to make change.

It's not a mom's personal choice to consume coffee, matcha tea, kombucha tea, or green tea during pregnancy. It's a choice *conditioned* by the industry. It has taken decades of conditioning to get to this point, with the caffeine industry spending billions of dollars to learn how to think for moms and womankind and to be one step ahead of them.

CAFFEINE IN OUR LIVES

Womankind in the 21st century is suffering from brain conditions. Chronic illness is on the rise more than ever before, and neurological problems are number one. This means that the dependency upon caffeine is also greater than ever before in history. We're at a point now where womankind has a difficult time functioning without caffeine because of the internal struggles of central nervous system conditions. Men, too, are suffering from central nervous system conditions more than ever before in history, so their ability to function is also reliant upon caffeine.

Caffeine tends to put your body into fight-or-flight every single day when no outside crisis is happening, making you numb to real fight-or-flight situations. We tend to get so used to the caffeine fight-or-flight on a daily basis that when a real situation occurs where we're in danger, we tend to delay—even in the most critical situations. That delayed response can make or break our survival.

Caffeine also lowers the immune system throughout the body, allowing your brain to be more susceptible to attacks from invaders such as pathogens and toxins. This happens due to the continual adrenaline surges from continual fight-or-flight. The intense rushes of adrenaline challenge immune cells, making them less productive or even killing the immune cells.

All this fight-or-flight also means that caffeine weakens adrenal glands on a daily basis. Since many reproductive hormones are produced by the adrenal glands, as this weakening process adds up as the years go by, it causes hormone imbalances and loss of libido. And not only do you lose precious reproductive hormone production; you lose the specific hormone responsible for hair growth, leading to hair thinning for women. Many women in this situation who notice hair thinning or loss, or even get a diagnosis of alopecia, never realize that they've experienced this because of a specific hormone missing from their adrenals—and in many cases, caffeine consumption has contributed.

Meanwhile, an endless sea of money is used in caffeine studies—to try to prove the antioxidant levels in caffeine products, to try to prove the presence of any other type of nutrient. There are going to be many studies to come doing the same. The industry knows that if they deem anything positive from caffeine studies or they keep including caffeine in studies, it gives people more permission to consume caffeine products.

Difficult Childbirth

A strong childbirth depends on strong adrenals, and caffeine consumption weakens the adrenals, especially in women.

Adrenaline is how a pregnant woman finds the strength to push a baby out of the uterus and vaginal canal. That push takes large amounts of adrenaline to use muscles' core strength and keep nerves strong, with the adrenaline delivering messages to the brain so the brain can activate every single nerve within every single muscle to gain the strength to propel the baby out.

Oftentimes women are putting their adrenals in fight-or-flight every single day through caffeine use. If the adrenals aren't performing at their best or if one adrenal is weakened from continual caffeine use for years, it can create a much more difficult childbirth experience than it normally would in someone who has strong adrenals.

While there are women whose adrenals are still hanging in there, still staying relatively strong even with caffeine use, it's not like this for most people. Most women's adrenals are already challenged by the stressors, circumstances, and struggles of life, or by everyday life's ups and downs. Workloads, relationship challenges, underlying chronic illness, or symptoms and conditions such as anxiety—these can all wear down the adrenals if the glands aren't getting a chance to heal and recharge.

So someone's adrenals may already not be as strong as they would naturally be. Then someone uses caffeine for strength and energy to power through their day, energy that's coming from their adrenals. When we use caffeine, we're using it to trigger our own adrenaline, meaning we're using the precious reserves that the adrenals provide.

The adrenal weakness that regular caffeine use creates can, and normally does, lead to a situation where labor and delivery time can be doubled, tripled, or more—many times leading to C-sections. It's because the adrenals don't have the strength to release the quantity of adrenaline needed to set off the alarms in the proper channels of the brain that send signals to the nerves inside the muscles needed to gain strength to propel the baby. The duration and difficulty of

labor and delivery often depend on how strong the adrenals are, and caffeine undermines adrenal strength.

Dehydrating Brain Cells and Aging Us Faster

Caffeine itself is a diuretic. It's not just what the caffeine is in that's a diuretic. Whether caffeine is in matcha tea or other green tea, the caffeine is a diuretic. Whether caffeine is in fully caffeinated or decaf coffee, it's a diuretic. Whether caffeine is in kombucha tea or cacao, it's a diuretic. Whether caffeine is in soda or another soft drink, it's still a diuretic.

Caffeine's diuretic property is different from other diuretics. Some diuretics that are naturally in plants expel non-useful, unproductive fluid from areas such as the lymphatic system, the liver, kidneys, or even intestinal tract. Caffeine doesn't have any of that ability; it doesn't expel fluid that's not useful from the body. Caffeine dehydrates our cells, expelling their useful fluids and disrupting cells' important fluid composition.

Caffeine is especially dehydrating to the brain, where it expels fluid from brain cells. Caffeine is a psychoactive drug, one that enters brain cells such as glial cells, forcing the fluid composition in those glial cells to change. This does not detox a glial cell or a brain cell of any kind. Rather, it intoxicates the cell by removing fluid, while leaving an abundance of toxins behind inside a much more dehydrated cell. It's similar to the water distillation process: as you heat the water, vapors of the water leave while many of the toxins stay behind.

This brings us to caffeine and brain heat. The psychoactive drug aspect of caffeine creates a hotter brain cell—electrical fields burn hotter when caffeine is present. This contributes to the expulsion process, where the fluid is forced to leave the brain cell because the temperature changes within the brain cell. Caffeine tends to heat up and hold its heat. (We can see this in action: a cup of coffee will hold its heat longer than a cup of herbal tea that has no caffeine because caffeine retains heat.) As this psychoactive drug saturates brain cells, the brain's electrical grid burns hotter, heating the caffeine. The caffeine enters cells and changes the temperature inside them, which expels water from the cells while leaving some water behind, just like the distillation process. That's different from how normal diuretics work.

Caffeine's dehydrating effect ages a person faster, speeding up all brain diseases. It also fast-tracks people into more wrinkly skin and age spots (also called liver spots or sunspots), creating situations where people need more body lotions, body creams, ointments, moisturizers, moisturizing makeups, and moisturizing skin treatments. It also leads many people into early plastic surgery and early cosmetic injections—and they never realize it was because of chronic dehydration occurring from their coffee, matcha, cacao, kombucha, and green tea consumption.

Bathing Our Brains in Acid

Your body sees caffeine as a poison. As a result, caffeine doesn't simply leave the body. Your body forces caffeine out of your body every single day. That's part of what you feel during caffeine withdrawal.

Caffeine is not a detoxifier. It's an intoxicator. Therefore as it's pushed out of the body, it takes nutrients (such as trace minerals, macro minerals, electrolytes, antioxidants, amino acids, and enzymes) out with it. The body is forced to expel everything good as it's trying to force the caffeine out.

Caffeine contributes to the brain bathing in acid, creating an acidic environment in and around the brain. Caffeine is so acidic that it depletes the bones and teeth of calcium. Caffeine also contributes to the thinning of the skull, similar to vinegar. The more caffeine you consume, the more microdeposits of calcium you lose from your skull, which causes a thinning of the skull, so that as you age, you're more vulnerable to fracturing your skull in a car accident, ski accident, or basic fall. Caffeine forces calcium to leach from your bones to buffer its acidity. Your body therefore wants caffeine out of your body. Caffeine leaves with all the nutrients mentioned above—and you urinate out all these important nutrients.

(Caffeine, by the way, is one of the reasons why people go along in life and then their teeth just seem to start falling apart at the seams. Some people can go 5 years on caffeine and see this problem, some can go 20 years before they see this problem. It most certainly comes.)

Reverse Polarity

Many young women, and even some men, who never had a health problem end up dying as they're working out or going for a run, or dying in their sleep. There have been thousands of these stories over the years, and you often won't hear about them. These stories don't make the media, the news. And the diagnoses of these deaths normally remain unknown. No one is able to properly piece together what happened.

In many of these cases, the undiscovered cause of death is caffeine jumping the heart. That is, these are unexpected heart attacks caused by a reverse heartbeat due to an electrical surge. Why does that electrical surge occur? Because of a buildup of caffeine deposits in and around neurons of the brain.

This buildup often happens because someone is consuming caffeine before a workout and at the same time, not consuming enough food before the workout. Caffeine tends to saturate the neurons in the brain. And then as the person's working out, they're engaging their adrenals 100 percent. Because the adrenals are fully occupied responding to the exercise, the brain doesn't send a signal to the adrenals to release adrenaline specifically geared to enter the brain and disperse caffeine deposits away from neurons, as it would otherwise. The special fight-or-flight adrenaline can't be accessed because the adrenals are maxed out as someone goes for their run or other high-intensity workout.

As a result, all the neurons saturated with caffeine send a signal to the brain stem, which creates a small explosion through all the brain stem nerves in hopes of forewarning the heart that there's an accumulation of poison surrounding the organs. This emergency signal from the brain stem to the heart places such a shock upon the heart that it stops for a split second and the blood pressure that was surging to the heart as someone was exercising stops in its tracks. The blood propels backward for a split second, causing an undiscovered *reverse polarity syndrome*. This is a condition that has caused thousands to drop dead on their treadmills at young ages and older ages for no apparent reason. Many times it's classified as a heart attack in a seemingly perfectly healthy heart, with no health condition present.

By the way, many people who have died after struggles with drug addiction didn't die at the height of drug addiction. They died when they were coming down off drugs and jacked up on caffeine instead. They experienced this same type of reverse polarity.

If someone dilutes their caffeine and consumes enough glucose or food before a workout, the chances of this reverse polarity syndrome happening are far less. The accumulation of caffeine around neurons won't be as concentrated and therefore won't trigger or warrant this degree of emergency messaging.

THE OTHER ONE IN THE RELATIONSHIP

Often when a relationship is starting, both partners are consuming caffeine. It's rare that a relationship can prosper and blossom with one person on caffeine and the other not. This isn't because caffeine is an aphrodisiac. It's because if one person is not on caffeine, their awareness of their partner's caffeine dependence creates tension. You're constantly witness to the time caffeine dependence takes. "I can't do this, honey, until I have my coffee." "I can't go anywhere until I pick this coffee up." You see your partner going through withdrawal on a daily basis. You see their behavior on caffeine versus off caffeine. You see how they have to stop everything and drop everything until they have their caffeine, and you may feel frustration about what gets stopped and dropped. The partner on caffeine may not feel comfortable being seen through these eyes. That's why usually, partnerships blossom when both people are reliant on caffeine—or better yet, when neither partner consumes caffeine.

CAFFEINE WITHDRAWAL

A continual shock wave occurs throughout the brain from the everyday caffeine withdrawal process. Caffeine's psychoactive drug properties tend to rule the brain's electrical grid, forcing it to change patterns throughout withdrawal. This is very taxing on the brain as a whole.

There's also a brain hormone aspect to caffeine withdrawal. One of caffeine's dangers as a psychoactive drug is its ability to destroy brain hormones. Caffeine is an all-around brain hormone blocker. One brain hormone that gets disrupted and destroyed is dopamine. Dopamine production occurs both inside the liver and inside the brain, and caffeine blocks this production. Caffeine also stops dopamine and other brain hormones from delivering information to specific neurons. That is, caffeine renders dopamine and other brain hormones inactive to specific neurons that require these brain hormones. Unable to find the neurons that need them in time, recently produced dopamine and other brain hormones eventually get destroyed.

This is why caffeine withdrawal is so brutal and caffeine withdrawal can spiral somebody into a depression rather quickly. When someone is coming down from caffeine and they have moments where they're off caffeine completely, whether it's for multiple hours, half a day, or a day or more, what they're feeling is a recalibration of dopamine and other brain hormones starting to work again. You would think this feeling of dopamine becoming reactivated would give the feeling of joy and peace. That takes more than a day off caffeine. It could take weeks off caffeine before you feel the reactivation of dopamine's role in the brain. Short stints of being off caffeine instead tend to result in anxiety, depression, more depersonalization, unexplained sadness, or a feeling of being confused and lost. This effect with dopamine can be ongoing for years, and no one will realize it's happening. Again, caffeine doesn't just interfere with dopamine production or activation. It interferes with all brain hormones to some degree or another. You can support yourself through caffeine withdrawal with the supplement protocol in this book's companion, *Brain Saver Protocols, Cleanses & Recipes*.

Look, I realize that people rely on their caffeine to survive. They're not feeling well and their symptoms are not being addressed or understood, so they become dependent on caffeine. Some people rely on caffeine for driving, some for jobs, some to function.

I'm not shaming anyone at all for being on caffeine. If you're someone going through this, I completely understand why. The system set you up. Maybe now, with this new understanding of caffeine, you have a new relationship with it. Maybe you can start to replace caffeine, start to wean yourself off, try the Adrenal Fight or Flight Stabilizer Brain Shot from Chapter 42, use the "Caffeine Withdrawal" supplement protocol, heal your underlying condition using the tools in this book, its companion volume, and the rest of the Medical Medium series—and find healing on a whole new level.

"Many people who are burnt out and confused about why, who haven't found a way to fix their burnout and other symptoms yet, seek out mental practices in hopes of ridding themselves of all their physical and mental discomfort. Mental practices only get us so far on their own. Lasting relief comes from addressing supply-and-demand deficiencies in the brain and the factors that are draining our brains faster than we can replenish them."

— Anthony William, Medical Medium

CHAPTER 14

Food Wars

We hear "moderation" often as advice about food itself. We don't see a lot of moderation in how people debate about food. It's very common to see people go to extremes in defending their chosen food belief system, even if that belief is "everything in moderation." Meanwhile, regardless of their food belief system and the science they use to defend their argument, everybody gets sick and nobody knows why they're sick. As soon as vegans or people eating plant-based get sick, they tend to run back to animal foods. When people already on animal-based diets get sick, most of them tend to stay with animal foods and keep searching, searching, searching for other reasons they could be sick and suffering. There are not a lot of vegan or plant-based families where the children are born and bred vegan and stay that way. Nearly everybody is raised on an animal-protein diet, and that's why most people who become vegan or plant-based will run back to animal proteins once they're sick, or once the temporary benefits they first received dissipate. They're

scared into it by practitioners, doctors, and family members, or they scare themselves into it, thinking they're lacking something based on material they read or a video they watched somewhere.

Both sides—animal-based and plant-based—believe that protein is the answer for everything. They think the reason they're alive is protein. This partly comes from most people being raised on animal protein. Vegans and plant-based people won't adopt this way of eating unless someone convinces them in a confident manner that there's protein in a plant-based diet, which there is. Both animal-based and plant-based folks are brainwashed to think it's all about protein because "protein" sounds scientific. They have to feel that their diet belief system, no matter what kind of name it gets to fancy it up, is science-based.

Both sides are also brainwashed for confrontation. Before people who've gone plant-based eventually revert to eating animal products, first they fight back. Plant-based folks don't look at animal-based folks and say, "Look, we're all sick." Instead each side seeks out their weapons of choice in the form of studies and research papers. Both the committed animal-protein people and the committed plant-based and vegan people call themselves researchers now. They spend a lot of time on the Internet looking around for information. They throw articles at each other that they feel are based on science. They say, "Well, this keto study says—" when it isn't even a real study. It's a survey or an uninformed observation or a theoretical paper put together by health professionals with limited experience on the subject. And if they do reference an actual clinical study, how reputable was it? Who funded it? Was it based on a handful of paid participants from the same age and background monitored over a very short time span, leading to gross generalizations and misinformation?

Meanwhile, they're all still getting sick. If someone hasn't gotten sick yet, they think it's because they've found all the answers. The reality is that they've simply been fortunate for all the reasons we talk about in the Medical Medium book series—fortunate enough to dodge the poisons and pathogens in our midst due to luck, chance, or privilege.

BOTH SIDES ARE BRAINWASHED

The bottom line is that both sides are brainwashed. They're brainwashed that they can trust the science behind their diet. They're brainwashed that protein is everything. They're brainwashed to confront each other.

Both sides of the food wars are brainwashed that intermittent fasting is healthy.

Both sides are brainwashed that caffeine is good, that adding quality salt to food is good, that apple cider vinegar is good.

Both are brainwashed that you can fix all your problems through breathing techniques or through manifesting.

Both sides are brainwashed that chocolate is plant medicine that's good for you.

Both are brainwashed that they don't create any waste with their food decisions and diets.

Both are brainwashed that their diet belief systems are sustainable—and are all about sustainability.

Both sides are conditioned to run to the conventional doctor for antibiotics the moment they get sick.

Both sides are brainwashed to believe that autoimmune symptoms are a result of the body attacking itself.

Both sides are brainwashed to believe that their genes dictate why they're sick.

Both sides are brainwashed to be afraid of fruit, so much so that even if they do start believing it's okay to eat a little more fruit, all it could take is one whistle from a food brigade that sends them right back into fruit fear once again.

Both sides have B_{12}, iron, and calcium deficiencies—while both sides are brainwashed to believe that only plant-based and vegan people are at risk of these deficiencies.

Both sides are worried about vitamin D deficiency, both sides are vitamin D deficient, and both sides believe vitamin D megadoses are the answer.

Both sides believe in fermented foods.

Both sides believe that all your problems stem from your gut.

Both sides believe that the brain is made of fat and you need fat in your diet to survive.

Both sides believe their blood tests are all accurate.

Both sides unknowingly get too much blood drawn when they get a blood test.

Both sides believe that a diet of processed foods, bad eating habits, and fried and greasy foods was the sole cause of any symptoms before they changed their diet, when really there's much more to it.

Both sides believe their food choices now make them spiritually enlightened.

Both sides believe they're very much different from the other side, that they're opposites, when they're not.

They are the same side, the same belief system, they shop at the same markets to get their food, and the only difference is that one eats meat and one doesn't.

Still, they face off against each other. And both sides use flawed science, fake science, underdeveloped science, and broken science to back up their positions. Animal-product science doesn't believe in plant-based science. Plant-based science doesn't believe in animal-product science. These science entities are against each other. And the conventional mainstream medical science entity does not support any of the sciences that either plant-based or animal-based believers are projecting.

On top of all this, food war battlers go for the emotional. Vegan and plant-based believers tell animal-product believers they're killing animals, destroying rain forests, clueless that animals have souls, and making their children eat dead animals. Animal-product believers tell vegan and plant-based believers they're causing malnutrition in their babies and children, starving them of protein, not preparing them for "real life," and keeping them away from moderation.

No matter what food belief system someone belongs to, whether plant-based or animal-based or even everything-in-moderation, they use science to attack anyone who doesn't share their belief system. That any group can find science and data to back up their position—that science hands out the weapons to both sides of the battle—should make us question the very war.

Everybody's fighting, both sides are at war, and their eye isn't on the ball about what creates chronic illness.

LOST AND EXPOSED

When a person—or a person's child—gets sideswiped or blindsided by health challenges, and neither they nor their revered publicly known medical research and science can understand why, whatever belief system they've consumed themselves with starts to break apart. It doesn't matter what study or research paper they've tried to prove their beliefs with in the past. When neurological Lyme, MS, ME/CFS (myalgic encephalomyelitis/chronic fatigue syndrome), anxiety, depression, brain fog, digestive problems, vertigo, tingles and numbness, migraines, ADHD, OCD, auto-immune, or eating disorders start to inter-rupt life, any doubts someone has had in the back of their mind about a plant-based diet or veganism start to grow like weeds. The doubts usually take over fast, and once again that person goes into the land of the lost, as disoriented and searching as they were when they first made the decision to go vegan or plant-based. Some hold on to that plant-based or veganism belief and fight for a little while in that lost land while they're sick. They'll see their functional medicine doctor or their plant-based natu-ropath, and they'll fight for it until a family member or friend ignites that tiny doubt that was in their head, and the doubt grows into a monster. They defect. They change their diet belief system.

Unless someone has found Medical Medium information, they don't know why they're sick so they believe it's caused by their diet. It's not just a rookie thing in health to believe that diet is why you're sick. It's an entrenched belief system among long-term diet believers too. Again, people commit-ted to diet belief systems believe that their diets beforehand were the sole reason for any symptoms they experienced instead of understanding pathogens, heavy met-als, and chemical exposure as the source of their symptoms. This is part of the brain-washing mechanism. When symptoms come up once they're following a diet belief sys-tem, if it's plant-based they'll fall through

the trapdoor of believing they got sick from the lack of animal products. If they get sick on an animal-based diet, on the other hand, they won't blame their diet. They'll be more apt to blame factors like stress or unhappi-ness. They'll be more afraid of fruit than ever before. They'll feel like maybe there's a spiri-tual or genetic reason why they're sick.

Each side, plant-based and animal-based, has part of its underbelly exposed. Plant-based believers are most susceptible to get-ting slammed about deficiencies because they've long been fed doubt about whether a plant-based diet offers them all the nutri-tion they need. Both sides are susceptible to fear. Both sides get sick with the same types of symptoms and conditions. Once they become sick, both plant-based and animal-based believers start worrying about the microbiome, bacterial overgrowth in the gut, metabolism issues, nutrient deficien-cies, *Candida*, leaky gut, fructose intoler-ance, histamine problems, food allergies, oxalates, gene mutations, autoimmune, or whether they're exercising enough.

It's a constant revolving door of trying to get improvements from mixing and match-ing, flip-flopping, and guessing games. "Try this," "Try that," "Eat this differently, but yet eat that a little differently." It's a game that occupies you while your body's fighting for temporary results, temporary improve-ments, and temporary relief. Some prac-tices could be supportive, some not. You can't be sure which are which because you can't read the signs and symptoms that your body's providing you, because whether you believe in plant-based or animal-based, you don't know why you're really sick. The game could go on for so long. It could go on forever in a person's life, until they can finally find a way out.

A WAY OUT

Healing from a symptom, condition, or disease isn't about choosing sides. It isn't just about going plant-based or animal-based or everything-in-moderation. Recovery isn't going to be reliant upon a scientific study. We may have that illusion. In the end, healing is about understanding that we've been tricked along the way, duped. The wool has been pulled over our eyes; we've been bamboozled. Healing is about learning that all sides are continually fooled. Once you learn why you truly became ill, opportunity opens up. The light does appear at the end of the tunnel, and health freedom is possible.

"We can't open our skull like an egg, take a look inside, and take a sniff to find out if it's going rotten—we can't use visual clues or our sense of smell, like we can with that egg or a piece of fish, to determine if our brain is getting toxic and dirty. Only when we start to develop symptoms from a brain that's been suffering for weeks or months or years do we start to get a clue about what's going on inside."

— Anthony William, Medical Medium

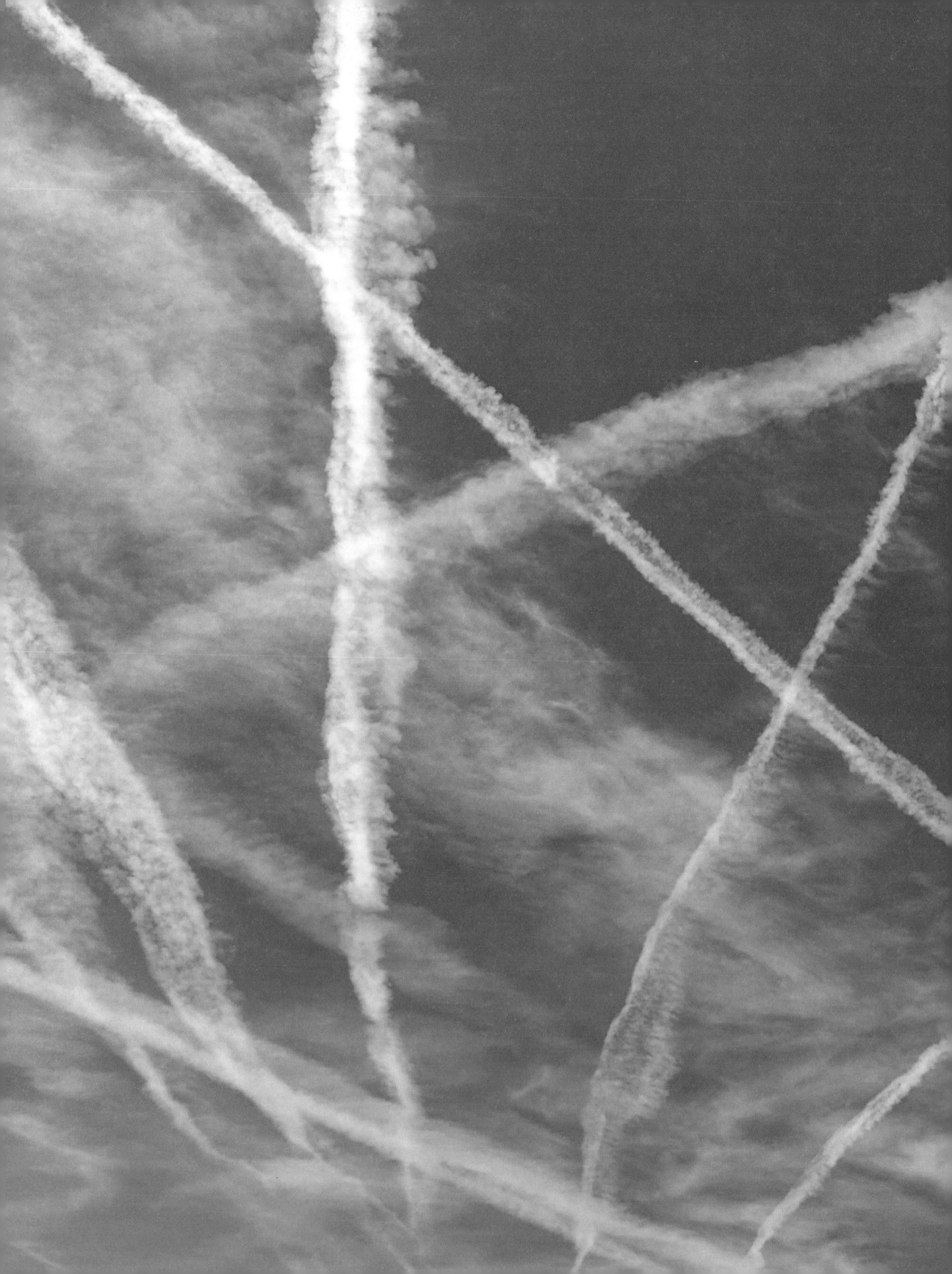

PART III

BRAIN BETRAYERS

"If you're someone who wakes up in the morning and shakes your head wondering why there's a lack of answers out there for the chronically suffering, now you understand why. You're learning the answers. You're learning the truth so you can do something about your health and your family's health. By knowing what that critical truth is—that, for one, toxic heavy metals are saturating our brains and we can remove them to enjoy better quality of life—we supersede the machine. We rise above the so-called authority of our well-being so that well-being is in our own hands. We rise above the machine."

— Anthony William, Medical Medium

CHAPTER 15

Evolving Backward

We think humans are evolving and advancing. What's really evolving are the toxic chemicals we're exposed to, the electromagnetic fields (EMF) we're up against, the pathogens we're exposed to, the brain betrayers designed by industries to supposedly make our lives better.

We confuse the long-standing theory that humankind is evolving with the advancements in technology that we see all around us. We see advancements in life-saving surgical medicine, advancements in how far we can reach into space with our telescopes. It gives us the misperception that humankind is getting ahead by leaps and bounds. In some ways that may be true, when it comes to technology.

What about our physical brains and bodies? What about the physical existence of humankind? Is that evolving? Life expectancy will decrease at a gradual pace during this decade, and then life expectancy will decrease at an unprecedentedly drastic pace over the next decade and beyond. Already, the new normal is to struggle with symptoms, whether you identify as "sick" or not.

EVOLVING EXPOSURES

Virtually every human being on the planet experiences at least one symptom at this point. We're at a place where chronic illness is growing at rates we've never seen before in our history. There are different levels, from very mild to devastatingly severe. There's the not-so-sick group, those who are experiencing symptoms and still functioning, working, being productive, even playing all day if they have that privilege. Then there's the sick group, those who are frightfully ill, those for whom each day is about surviving.

This increase in sickness like never before is only going to keep developing. So are we evolving in the right direction, or backward? Are our physical bodies any different than they were in ancient Rome 2,500 years ago? And if you believe that we have evolved since then, are we evolving faster than what's evolving around us now that's destroying us?

We need to be aware that we are going backward, not forward, with our physical health. In the next one to five years, we're going to see chronic illness rise to levels no one could ever imagine. And that's because instead of our bodies advancing, everything wrong about the world is evolving. Environmental pollution is evolving. The ocean is becoming more toxic. The Great Pacific Garbage Patch is becoming bigger. The chemical industry is evolving, creating new chemical soups by the hour around the world. The pharmaceutical industry is evolving, even overreaching and controlling the nutraceutical industry, and not always evolving in our best interests.

Pathogens are evolving—more and more new strains of pathogens that have been released from labs over the last hundred years and keep people sick with chronic illness are mutating and strengthening as we pass those pathogens around to each other, whether through our family line or any other means of exposure.

Genetically modified food is evolving, with more and more land bought to grow more and more varieties of GMO food. Dangerous chemicals in our world are evolving. The caffeine industry is evolving. Corruption is evolving, corruption on all levels.

Chemical fragrances—scented candles, air fresheners, fabric softeners, conventional cleaners and detergents, colognes, perfumes, and fungicides—are all evolving. The very air around us is evolving. We're getting to a place where you can't smell fresh air anymore, inside or outside. Twenty-five years ago, you could still smell the air at the beach, smell the wind, and not worry about what direction the breeze was coming from. You could walk through a busy area

with a crowd of people and not be choking on hundreds of different makes and models of chemical poisons. Now you can't take a walk, can't even go to a beach, without smelling fabric softener, perfume, cologne, aftershave, scented sunscreen, body spray, or scented candles wafting from someone or somewhere. People everywhere walk around emitting these toxic chemicals off their bodies. Plus fragrance is in public buildings, it's in offices, it's in hotels, it's in cars, it's in people's homes. Fresh air has been taken from us, courtesy of the chemical industry.

OUR IMMUNE SYSTEM'S FIGHT TO DEFEND US

There's no way humankind could physically evolve faster than any of these forces against us. Which brings us to the immune system, which is responsible for protecting the brain. Our immune systems were never made for what's evolving around us. They weren't designed to fight off engineered viruses that were manufactured in labs and released into our environment. Our immune systems weren't made to put up with the amount of chemicals—either the number of varieties or the outright quantity—that we're up against or the EMF evolving around us—the radio frequencies, the cell tower signaling, the radiation. Every time something foreign enters into our body, even if it's in the form of radiation, our immune cells have to gobble it up. Our immune system is the security system against any attackers that want to invade our brain. Our immune system has a big job in defending our brain.

How long a white blood cell lasts against a toxic invader depends on how toxic the substance is. Nano poisons from perfume and cologne have to be gobbled up by our white blood cells in order to protect us. Nanoparticles from air fresheners and scented candles have to be gobbled up. Pathogens such as the viruses that everyone lives with now (e.g., Epstein-Barr virus [EBV]) cause low-grade viral infections, and our immune system has to seek out these pathogens and gobble them up. Flu viruses and COVID have to be gobbled up by our white blood cells. Toxic heavy metals have to be gobbled up by our white blood cells.

Meanwhile, with the caffeine industry evolving around us, new caffeine abominations are created, and we're trained to become addicted, which lowers the immune system. On top of its already enormous job, our immune system has to defend us against caffeine products on the daily. White blood cells die when they're defending us. They're the soldiers we're completely unaware of who are fighting for our lives.

Here's how it works: As a white blood cell gobbles up nanoparticles of, say, air freshener fragrance or toxic heavy metal, it can get filled up. It's taking the hit for us, and that hit is like a stab. It means the white blood cell won't last long. It continues to gobble up the toxic nanoparticles until the white blood cell ceases to live because it either outright dies or it explodes. It's the same with fighting pathogens. When a white blood cell fights a pathogen, the pathogen explodes, and the white blood cell often explodes with it. In many situations, a white blood cell dies when it's killing a pathogen. White blood cells are not as easily replaced as we think they are. The more white blood cells that die quickly due to exposure, the bigger the gap before newly created ones arrive.

This battle is part of how we're evolving backward, not forward. If you believe in other planets that humankind may have existed on, can you imagine any of those planets getting to a point of destruction, where humankind was evolving in the wrong direction because everything harmful to humankind was evolving at that much greater magnitude?

Our immune system isn't evolving in the direction of strengthening. We're becoming more deficient, more intoxicated, and our immune systems are further weakened, our brains further threatened—unless we're proactive about our exposures, alongside restoring and rebuilding our immune system. We can adapt if we're knowledgeable about the brain betrayers all around us—and if we support our brain and body by giving our immune system what it needs to defend us.

CHAPTER 16

Blood-Brain Barrier

Our human body is not geared for the levels of exposure we experience on this planet. The blood-brain barrier never anticipated the Industrial Revolution and the Classified Medical Industry Pathogen Revolution. Convincing us that we're equipped to handle any toxins that come our way is like convincing us that our human body is equipped to handle nuclear waste; we create it on the planet, so we should be fine. Our blood-brain barrier should have no problem protecting us against nuclear waste or any other toxic material. Right?

No one is measuring the levels of toxins in our environment in relation to how our bodies handle and receive them. Medical industries don't want to admit there are toxic heavy metals in our brain. They don't even want to entertain the idea, never mind that we're living with inflammation from pathogens. Publicly known medical research and science are in the infancy stages of recognizing a chronic illness could be pathogen-related. If they're that early in the process of understanding chronic illness, how advanced can they be in

understanding our body's complex mechanisms, such as our blood-brain barrier?

Our blood-brain barrier was not made for any of this. We act like it's an impermeable structure that has no limitations. Nuclear waste? Industrial waste? Solvents? Toxic heavy metals? All someone has to do is use the term *blood-brain barrier* to make us feel like we're protected. And yet the reality is that all these and more inevitably cross our blood-brain barrier. Many pharmaceuticals are specifically engineered to cross our blood-brain barrier. Even the pharmaceuticals not designed with this in mind can cross our blood-brain barrier.

Our blood-brain barrier was designed to keep natural, mostly bodily toxins out of the brain. When someone has a little too much uric acid buildup because a kidney is weakened, for instance, that uric acid is not supposed to permeate the blood-brain barrier. If someone gets a cut that goes deep and leads to a skin infection, then that person could develop the beginning stages of sepsis, in which case the blood infection is not supposed to cross the blood-brain barrier. If someone ingests a toxic plant that's been on Planet Earth for 10,000 years and was never meant to be human food, the blood-brain barrier is there to hold back at least some of the toxins in an effort to prevent the brain from going into toxic shock.

Our blood–cerebrospinal fluid barrier is also overtaxed. Cerebrospinal fluid, which surrounds the brain and spinal cord, is supposed to be pure, with no contamination. That's the gold standard. In this time on Planet Earth, our cerebrospinal fluid is not pure. It's harboring chemical soups from industry, pathogenic byproducts, toxic heavy metals, and more. A thousand years ago, cerebrospinal fluid may simply have had some toxic heavy metal contamination, and that was only for people living in cities with lead in the drinking water. Cerebrospinal fluid had a whole different purity hundreds and thousands of years ago. Today, we walk around polluted.

OUR BRAIN: NOT LICENSED FOR INDUSTRY

The blood-brain barrier has limitations and vulnerabilities. It's only geared for the small stuff, not for anything industrially engineered. If an industry creates a battery, for example, and that battery corrodes, and battery acid appears on the battery and then is accidentally consumed, that battery acid is going to enter through the blood-brain barrier. Industrial toxins and mercury from that battery are going to enter the brain. The blood-brain barrier's

construction is porous. It acts as a type of thin filtering wall of tissue. The blood-brain barrier is only licensed by our human bodies to keep back certain contaminants that are natural, mostly bodily toxins.

There are many pharmaceuticals designed to pass through the blood-brain barrier. Morphine is one of them. It's one of the reasons why morphine can kill you: it can cross through blood vessels of the brain and spinal fluid vessels.

Remember, all pharmaceuticals have toxic heavy metals in them, so engineering pharmaceuticals to cross the blood-brain barrier means that toxic heavy metals from those pharmaceuticals also cross through the blood-brain barrier. Whether platinum, titanium, copper, mercury, or aluminum, we're exposed via pharmaceutical pills, creams, liquids, and more.

And when toxic heavy metals from any source oxidize in our body, the oxidation seeps past the blood-brain barrier.

PATHOGENIC INFILTRATION

Viral neurotoxins also pass through the blood-brain barrier. A virus itself is small, so imagine a neurotoxin coming from a virus—how small that is. One of the reasons why publicly known medical research and science don't even identify neurotoxins is because they're so small. Neurotoxins are excreted from virus cells as a liquid, and that neurotoxin liquid slips through the blood-brain barrier as if there is no blood-brain barrier. If classified medical research and science discovered viral neurotoxins, publicly known medical research and science would not be allowed to further research viruses and make this key discovery.

Certain varieties of EBV can themselves cross through the blood-brain barrier. As for the varieties that can't cross, their neurotoxins still can. That's what Guillain-Barré syndrome is: pathogens and pathogenic toxins crossing through the blood-brain barrier. The pathogens that can cross the blood-brain barrier do so by latching on to that barrier and inflaming their way through. They slowly do tissue damage to the barrier so the pathogens can enter and cross, eventually permeating it and leaving microscopic barrier scars. (Remember, only some varieties of pathogens do this, not all.)

Keep all of this in mind as you read about the brain betrayers to come. As easy as it is to convince us that our blood-brain barrier is an impermeable presence that makes us impenetrable to the dangers that industries release into our world, all we have to do is look around us at the suffering on this planet to be reminded that this doesn't add up. If we want to save ourselves, we can't take advantage of our body's protective mechanisms. We can't take our blood-brain barrier for granted. We have to protect our brain and body right back, and that starts with bringing awareness to the daily exposures in our midst.

"Our brains and bodies have not betrayed us. They've been betrayed by industrial chemicals and other contaminants in our everyday lives that have only accelerated in development in recent years."

— Anthony William, Medical Medium

CHAPTER 17

Your Protective Guide

Our brains and bodies have not betrayed us. They've been betrayed by industrial chemicals and other contaminants in our everyday lives that have only accelerated in development in recent years.

What we're going to explore in the chapters ahead are the brain betrayers we're up against every day, the ones that challenge and defy our immune systems, the ones that take up residence in our brain tissue, the ones that contaminate our neurons and neurotransmitters.

These brain betrayers can also defy our brains from afar, as is the case with viruses that take up residence in our liver and send viral toxins into the bloodstream that can eventually reach the brain.

We're talking about the brain betrayers that, whether from near or far, scatter our brains, fog our brains, inflame our brains, undermine our brains, disrupt our brains, fatigue our brains, pollute our brains, scramble our brains, distract our brains, burn out our brains, heat up our brains, rob our brains, scar our brains, drain our brains, addict our

brains, shrink our brains, age our brains, acidify our brains, and even rot our brains.

The chapters to come are not meant to make you fear life here on Planet Earth. We can't avoid everything that isn't great for our brains. We have to live in this world. These chapters also aren't here so you can accept everything listed and move on with life, ignoring these brain betrayers as if they don't exist.

We *can* make life in this world better. By learning to stay away from even a handful of brain betrayers—some of which you've been reading about throughout this book and some of which you'll discover here—you'll be doing yourself and your loved ones justice in a world that doesn't always do that for you.

Every little bit counts when it comes to avoiding or decreasing the saturation of your brain with these contaminants. You may be able to easily avoid the ones you never realized until now were the most detrimental. Or you may look at a category of brain betrayers—for example, the domestic invasion brain betrayers—and find ways to replace or cut them out. Sometimes we can't stop ourselves from being exposed to brain betrayers—viruses especially. We can still take steps to lessen exposure, and when we do get exposed, we can do plenty about it by strengthening our immune system, removing viral fuel from our body, and staying hydrated.

Rather than being here to scare you, the chapters ahead are your protective guide, not just for your brain or even your body; it's a guide to a better life. With a little knowledge about what we're exposed to on an occasional or constant basis and the role that plays in harming us—even if it's as simple as aspartame triggering a migraine—we're so much better equipped to live the lives we see for ourselves rather than get sidelined by symptoms or illness.

If this is your personal copy of the book, feel free to take out a pen or pencil and start marking up these pages with your thoughts about what you already do a good job of steering clear of and what you think you can watch out for next. Use it as a journal or checklist to mark your progress along the way: *How many items can I check off this list that I really don't need in my life?* See what makes sense for this moment in time.

Maybe, for instance, you're finally ready to remove the air fresheners and scented candles in your home, and you can switch to a natural, fragrance-free laundry detergent. Then in a few months, maybe you'll be able to check off a few more items. It's these simple yet powerful steps that can protect your friends, your family, your pets, your children, and your own future.

THE BRAIN BETRAYERS LIST

- Viruses and Viral Waste Matter
- Pharmaceuticals
- Toxic Heavy Metals
- Fragrances
- Bacteria and Other Microbes
- Chemical Industry Domestic Invaders
- Chemical Neuroantagonists
- Petrochemicals and Solvents
- Chem Trails and Rainfall Exposure
- Radiation and EMF
- Harmful Food and Supplement Chemicals
- Harmful Supplements
- Harmful Foods

BRAIN SATURATION

Any of these toxins and poisons in any amount can reach and saturate any aspect of the brain, some more commonly ending up in certain places in the brain than others.

For example, petrochemicals often end up in the cerebral cortex, an outer layer of the brain, although some petrochemicals can also end up deeper within the brain.

The amount of exposure has an influence. If it's a fair amount of exposure at once, or extended exposure (meaning for more than just a few minutes), you could get deeper saturation of petrochemicals or other brain betrayers entering the brain. When exposure is small, tiny, occasional, here and there, you may not react or experience symptoms if you are not sensitive.

Someone may be on a pharmaceutical for a month, or they may be on pharmaceuticals for 10 years. Someone may be exposed to fumes for a few minutes at a gasoline pump, or they may have some gasoline spilled on their skin as they're also breathing in the fumes. Everybody has different exposures, and that's why penetration of the brain varies. Smaller amounts build up over time. Larger amounts speed up the process of sensitivity.

When brain betrayers settle in the cerebral cortex, they may not affect critical brain functions right away, unless someone is already sensitive and living with brain betrayer complications—such as low-grade viral infections and symptoms. In that case, the smell of fresh paint could set them back for days or weeks.

On the other hand, someone who isn't on the verge of that tipping point—who hasn't been saturated with brain betrayer toxins, isn't dealing with low-grade viral activity, or doesn't have a diminished or challenged immune system—won't necessarily see immediate effects from exposure. They could be exposed to something like fresh paint every day and not see a decline in their health until they've accumulated more brain betrayer toxins or developed viral infections or a compromised immune system due to any and all exposures. If someone's life is painting and they're free and clear of most other exposures, they may only experience slowly weakening brain function from the paint exposure for the first 20 years, if the toxins stay in the outer banks of the brain or even saturate deeper into the brain. Then one day, exposure can cross a threshold, and they can decline much more quickly.

When it comes to brain betrayer exposures, it's death by a thousand cuts. Instead of cuts, it's contaminants building up in the brain. Just what those contaminants are, where they settle in the brain, and how early in a person's life they add up vary widely. That's why there's such variability in every individual's symptoms and experience. Even when some brain betrayers enter deep into the brain, they may not cause symptoms yet. Or brain betrayers don't have to enter deep layers of brain tissue in order to create a symptom or weakness or sensitivity.

Whether we feel their effects yet or not, these contaminants aren't helping out anybody's brain. One way that brain betrayers affect the brain is by slowly causing it to atrophy and shrink. Another is by serving as fuel for viruses. You'll read about many more effects of brain betrayers in the pages to come. With this information, you hold power.

Keep in mind that Part VI, "Bringing Back Your Brain," is also a resource for you. There, you'll find tools to cleanse, detox, repair, and protect your brain and nervous system—including Chapter 42, "Medical Medium Brain Shot Therapy," which has a special set of recipes to help you deal with brain betrayer exposures. You'll find even more support in this book's companion, *Brain Saver Protocols, Cleanses & Recipes*.

"For the record, viruses are living. In the publicly known arena of science, there is a battle about whether viruses are dead or alive. No one can agree, and neither side has proven facts. Here is a pillar of truth: Viruses are alive. Viruses are cells. Viruses eat."

— Anthony William, Medical Medium

CHAPTER 18

Viruses and Viral Waste Matter

Common Herpetic Family Viruses

- Over 60 varieties (most of them undiscovered) of Epstein-Barr virus (EBV)

- Over 30 varieties (all but one undiscovered) of shingles

- Multiple varieties of human herpesvirus (HHV)-6, HHV-7, HHV-8

- Multiple varieties of the undiscovered HHV-9, HHV-10, HHV-11, HHV-12, HHV-13, HHV-14, HHV-15, HHV-16

- Over 20 varieties (all but one undiscovered) of cytomegalovirus (CMV)

- Over 100 varieties of herpes simplex virus (HSV) 1 and 2

- Viral waste matter (byproduct, neurotoxins, dermatoxins, and viral corpses) from the above herpes-family viruses

Common Fever and Respiratory Viruses

- COVID

- Influenza (flu)

Viruses are in our lives much more than anyone realizes. It's not just the standard cold and flu symptoms that signal a virus, or the symptoms of flu and COVID we see on the news. So many people walk around with low-grade infections from the herpetic viruses listed in the bullet points above without knowing it—because much of the time, detecting them is beyond the capabilities of current medical testing. The medical world doesn't yet link the multitudes of autoimmune conditions and symptoms with chronic viral infections. Or someone can harbor a virus without exhibiting symptoms.

Herpetic family viruses want the host to remain alive. These viruses do not have an end goal of trying to extinguish a person. Viruses such as flu and COVID do have an end goal of trying to extinguish the person. They have been manufactured to do so. Of course, weak versions of the flu and COVID rarely succeed in this programming that was created through manufacturing.

Flu and COVID viruses do not stick around long inside the body after they've been conquered by the immune system. They either conquer you, or your immune system conquers them. Herpes-family viruses maneuver around the body, staying alive, eluding the immune system, creating a situation of having to live with these viruses for a lifetime, unless we learn how to put them in dormancy or eradicate them from our bodies.

When someone is in an active viral infection stage, they're contagious, and that means it's easy for us to pick up the virus too. Because herpetic viruses so often fly under the radar, we may not know if someone we're around has a virus, and since symptoms are (1) frequently delayed due to a viral incubation period and (2) often not identified as viral by the current medical model, we may not know we've contracted a virus.

With some herpetic viral varieties, we have to be exposed to infected blood to become infected ourselves. With some newer viral mutations, we can contract the viruses from exposure to saliva, tears, mucus, and other bodily fluids, or from touching certain viral pustules that present on the skin. It's even possible to get one of these herpetic viruses at conception from your parents and live with it unknowingly until the virus is given just the right triggers later in life to interfere with your health. In Chapter 4, "Your Viral Brain," and Chapter 6, "Your Inflamed Cranial Nerves," we explored just how these herpetic viruses such as EBV and shingles interfere with your brain and nervous system. You'll discover more details throughout Part IV, "Brain Invasion," and Part V, "Your Pain and Suffering Enlightened."

Any virus can interfere with the brain in its own specific way. For example, flu and COVID viruses affect the brain through fever and blood toxicity. Flu and COVID can damage the kidneys, causing backup of toxins in the blood that eventually enter the brain. These viruses can also prompt adrenal dysfunction and electrolyte depletion, causing the adrenals to react to a cytokine storm that the pathogen invader is creating by challenging your immune system, and this crisis can rupture the adrenal glands, spilling a tremendous amount of adrenaline into the bloodstream, harming the brain. These viruses can also fill the lungs with mucus, hindering the ability to take in optimum levels of oxygen, which could affect the brain. That's why it pays to protect yourself.

SEXUAL TRANSMISSION AND THE AUTOIMMUNE WAVE

The herpetic viruses that plague us with autoimmune disease are viruses that get transmitted through intimate contact such as kissing and basic fundamental sexual transmission, in addition to other methods of transmission you'll read about in this chapter. The viruses that create autoimmune conditions are passed around like this on the daily, all around the world.

We've lost consciousness about how to protect ourselves. For many years, the standard was "Do you have an STD?" To which a sexual partner might say, "I had chlamydia. The doctor prescribed an antibiotic, I took it, and my chlamydia's gone." That tends to be the extent of what people worry about with STDs. They know herpes simplex 2 (genital herpes) is a concern, yet they don't ask for test results from a partner, even though they should, because herpes simplex 2 can actually be discovered through a blood test in many cases. People are concerned about HIV, although nowadays it's uncool to even think about asking someone you're about to have sex with if they've been HIV-tested, especially if you're falling in love or trying to make something work with a brand-new partner.

We're in a sex-positive time. Is it done responsibly? We live in a world where people aren't entirely mindful—or informed. Nowhere is anybody being taught or educated that a virus such as herpes simplex 1 (oral herpes, aka the cold sore/fever blister virus) can cause a lifetime of misery for some people. Debilitating trigeminal neuralgia; painful scalp; gum, teeth, and jaw pain; and an inflamed brain stem and cranial nerves are all possible complications from simplex 1. It's not even simply contracting herpes simplex 1 that's the only concern. What if you're contracting simplex 1 over and over

again from different people, meaning that you're picking up different mutations of simplex 1? Some strains have been altered by the pharmaceutical antivirals those people took to suppress symptoms. Some of these herpes simplex 1 varieties and mutations have different intelligences and strengths, because they've been in different people with different immune systems taking different medications.

This isn't a campaign on whether someone should be sex positive, intimate with others, searching for the love of their life, or on the dating scene. This is about supporting someone, educating them, so they can protect themselves, and if they do get sick, have a way to heal it. Someone may have intimacy with many partners and be lucky only to contract a mild form of EBV or a mild form of herpes simplex 1. Another person may have intimacy with only one partner yet contract more than one variety of EBV, CMV, herpes simplex 1, HHV-6, and shingles, because maybe that partner has picked up multiple viruses from being intimate with many people.

This also isn't about living in a box, being fearful of the search for love. Say you've had a decade of relationships, gathered multiple viruses, and now want to heal with the right tools and information so you can recover, become strong, and then pursue a new relationship. Moving forward is about healing past viral infections, strengthening your immune system, protecting yourself and your brain, being mindful, and erring on the side of caution when you can. Starting fresh is about knowledge and wisdom on better ways to navigate through life. You don't have to feel pressure to quickly jump into something. Even if passion is taking over, you get to methodically think about things a little more with this new knowledge and wisdom in hand.

There's a herpes explosion right now among people coming out of long-term relationships. They've been part of a long-term couple that breaks up or divorces, and then they meet someone who's been on the dating scene for a really long time. The older that new partner is, the more partners they're likely to have had, which means the more bugs and strains they've likely picked up along the way—and the more you want to make sure they've been herpes tested or inquire if they are on medications for herpes or have a history of herpes.

We have two problems here: (1) it's uncool to even think that the person you're courting could have bugs; (2) it's uncool to ask them if they have bugs. It's understandable if it's hard to even ask someone if they have a symptom. It's still worth doing. How do they feel? What's their health history like? A lot of people are so sex positive they don't get to know a partner. Also, on the dating scene, there are people who are treating their herpes with medications to suppress it, and they're not telling anyone they're dating. Asking them takes it to a place where if they are on a medication like valacyclovir for herpes breakouts, they may be more inclined to tell you.

Testing is really hard with most other herpetic viruses. EBV, cytomegalovirus, shingles, and HHV-6 are hard to test for.

You could have EBV and it may not show up on certain tests. On the other hand, herpes simplex 1 and herpes simplex 2 are, in general, pretty detectable through testing when someone's had them for a while. Testing is still not dependable. You don't know when someone has had their last date, transmission, relationship, or exposure, on any level, to bodily fluids. It could take months or, for some varieties, even a few years before the virus surfaces and becomes detectable through testing.

Sexual transmission is not the only way to pick up herpetic viruses. Yet however someone gets infected—from family, from parents passed down to offspring, or from public places, which we'll discuss more soon—it's possible to pass the viruses along through intimate contact. It pays to be educated. That's what this comes down to. Being educated is a way to avoid a lot of autoimmune diagnoses that could be coming your way.

Feel free to question your potential partner. Ask them if they have a history of mono, frozen shoulder, cold sores, acne, or urinary tract infections (UTIs). With Medical Medium information, you can decode their symptoms and understand what types of viruses and bacteria they may have.

Whether you're 20 years old and you feel awkward asking about herpes or you just had a divorce and now you're on the dating scene, it's worth being mindful and talking about it. Everybody who has herpes says, "I wish I had known better." Meanwhile, nobody who's sick with autoimmune disease from EBV, CMV, shingles, or another herpetic virus they picked up through intimate contact even gets to say, "I wish I had known better," because they're still in the dark about why they're sick. They're living with symptoms, they don't know why, and they're out there on the dating scene, contracting more viruses and viral strains.

Not every stage of EBV, shingles, and cytomegalovirus is infectious, and it's the same with certain strains of the herpes simplex viruses. If you work on healing yourself, you're making yourself less infectious so you're not the person infecting anybody. You're still going to be around people who are full of bugs and aren't doing good things for themselves. When you find someone who really cares, you can help them clean up. Both of you can be on Medical Medium immune system protocols for EBV or other herpetic viruses. While herpes simplex 1 and 2 are different beasts, it's still the same approach. It's all about building yourself up, strengthening your immune system, putting any viruses into dormancy, and healing yourself so you can be in a much better place.

PUBLIC RESTROOMS

People have to realize there are bodily fluids left on toilet seats. Those bodily fluids can contain varieties of *Streptococcus* (strep, many strains of which are antibiotic-resistant), *E. coli*, *Staphylococcus* (staph), herpes simplex 1 and 2, EBV, shingles, HHV-6, cytomegalovirus, and human papillomavirus (HPV). That means these bugs can be on toilet seat surfaces and usually are.

Covering toilet seats is critical—flopping down straight onto a public toilet seat is not a wise practice.

Then there's the toilet water in the bowl. Even if the toilet was flushed, a toilet's never truly flushed. There's always invisible leftover material floating around in the toilet water, and as you go to the bathroom, splashes from the water can pop up back into you. It's very easy to get infected in restrooms because when you're going to the bathroom, you're exposed. For example, when someone is having a bowel movement, their rectum doesn't immediately close. As their fecal matter torpedoes into the water, it's very easy for that water to splash up and enter into the rectum as it's still closing. Before you poo, it's best to place a sheet or two of toilet paper on the surface of the water to mitigate splash. To protect yourself further, it's important to flush a public toilet before you even use it. (If it has a lid, put the lid down before flushing. Otherwise, try to turn away or back away while it's flushing. The mist can project outward with viruses or bacteria in it.)

Many people won't use enough toilet paper to wipe. They use a few tiny sheets, perhaps in the name of saving trees, or if they're in the habit of using less to save money, or they just miss the target. They end up with a handful of feces. That hand will then flush the toilet, if it's not automated. Then that hand will touch the soap dispenser and the sink handles, leaving behind more fecal particles, and then after they wash their hands, they'll touch the dirty handles again to shut off the sink. Even if their own hands are clean, they're touching handles that other people have touched. Those other people could have touched their eyes, blown their nose, or just touched their face while applying makeup in the bathroom mirror. Then as everyone exits the bathroom, they're touching the spot on the door everyone else has put their hands on.

Hand sanitizer does not stop all of these hand-body exposures. It's a noble idea, partially helpful sometimes, and yet hand sanitizer is random in its ability to kill pathogens. It's not good enough. We have to be careful about how we use public facilities and stay mindful that pathogen transmission is common in restrooms.

SHARING FOOD AND DRINK AND DINING OUT

Be mindful of sharing food and drink. You're also sharing saliva and sometimes even microscopic blood particles.

Sometimes we share food and drink knowingly, as when we eat off the same plate or drink out of the same bottle or glass. Sometimes we share with other people unknowingly:

Restaurants do not usually clean their glasses properly. There tends to be residue on all the glasses. Lipstick residue, for example, tends to hold on to pathogens on glasses—lipstick encapsulates pathogens, keeping the bugs sustained on glasses for days. Many men have extremely sticky saliva because men often go around chronically

dehydrated, eating protein-heavy diets, and proteins are extremely sticky foods. Higher-protein diets tend to make saliva very, very gluey. Men's saliva can sit on glasses for a week after multiple washings.

Forks in restaurants, just like forks at home, create small injuries in the mouth. The steel in forks is also porous. Metal forks stick into the person's gums, dislodging tiny bits of plaque and gum bacteria, compressing it into the pores of the fork. So the pores in silverware get clogged up with cells from the inside of people's mouths, including micro amounts of blood. Forks in restaurants can be biohazards. They're not sterilized as if you were at the dentist's office, where a sterilized tool goes in your mouth. Instead, eating with bar or restaurant silverware is like going to a dental office where they take all their dental tools and wash them by hand or throw them into a common dishwasher that may not even be high-heat (because most dishwashers do not get hot enough to kill pathogens) before putting them into the mouth of the next patient. That's why I say that utensils in restaurants can be biohazards, potentially spreading every pathogen and disease.

And for years I've said that busy chefs in busy restaurants often cut their hands and fingers daily, which is Russian roulette for transmitting any kind of pathogen.

Here are some tips if you have to eat out:

- Bring alcohol wipes, and wipe your forks and other utensils. Or ask for a mug of scalding hot water (like for tea) and place your utensils in that.

- Alternatively, bring your own utensils or order food that doesn't require utensils and eat with your hands, as long as your hands are clean.

- Ask for your food to come very hot. If the chef cut their finger while preparing your meal, the heat of the food and the plate is a great way to kill viruses that may be in that blood.

- Ask for beverages that come in bottles that haven't been opened to avoid drinking out of glasses. Wipe off the top and neck of the bottle with an alcohol wipe before drinking, as your lips may slip past the part of the bottle that had been under the cap and onto the area where the server was touching the bottle as they carried it. (If bottles aren't an option, ask for a can, in which case, try to wipe down the rim and pour area of the can before opening.)

- If you're forced to drink out of a glass, ask for a wrapped straw or bring your own straw. If you can, bring your own cup or glass.

DENTAL VISITS

The dentist's office is another place where pathogens are transferred. Often, dentists, hygienists, and assistants will put on their gloves and then start touching everything with their gloves. They're touching the handles of the lights, adjusting them, and also touching chairs, controls, computer keyboards. In the end, their latex or nitrile gloves are only protecting the practitioner, not protecting the patient. Yes, they put on a new pair of gloves between patients. Yet the surfaces they're touching with those new gloves may have saliva, blood, and mouth tissue cells on them, and those surfaces have often not been sterilized between patients. That's how pathogens can get transmitted.

To avoid this situation, bring your own disinfecting wipes to the dentist and ask them to wipe down high-touch spots such as controls, buttons, and handles that they think they're going to use during your procedure, and ask them to put on fresh gloves afterward. You can't be afraid to ask your dentist for better sanitary steps to be taken. If people learn to request this, it will become more common practice.

MORE VIRAL EXPOSURE TIPS

We've covered many of the basics of viral transmission, such as intimate contact and group restrooms, and tips for how to protect yourself. Another basic tip is to practice good hygiene like hand washing when you've been in a public space. And in Chapter 22, "Bacteria and Other Microbes," you'll read about why it's worth taking care with shopping cart handles.

It's also important to stay aware when handling objects we've just brought into our homes. Packages can be a huge source of transmission for flu, COVID, methicillin-resistant *Staphylococcus aureus* (MRSA), and strep, especially when you're setting down packages on your cutting board or kitchen counter; placing a new package in a crib or on a bed or couch; or rubbing your eyes, fixing eye makeup, or moving your hair constantly while in the middle of opening a package. Wash your hands after handling packages. Find a designated area for your packages that isn't a high-exposure spot in your home. If you are not in a rush to open a package, let it sit before opening—a practice I call decanting the package. Because packages can have people's mucus, saliva, traces of fecal matter, skin flakes, or any other bodily fluid contaminant, this is a worthwhile protection. If you give a package three to five days to decant in your designated area, there will be a lesser chance of being exposed.

Beyond all of this awareness about exposure sources, you can limit the damage a virus can do by making your body an inhospitable place for viruses. How? You can limit the other brain betrayers in your life. You can incorporate the healing foods and cleanses from later in this book to remove toxins that serve as viral fuel from your brain and body. (Every Medical Medium cleanse is antiviral.) You can even try the protocols in the "Supplement Gospel" section of *Brain Saver Protocols, Cleanses & Recipes* to provide your immune system with the best possible support for your health situation.

"There is a greater truth underneath it all. There are answers to why people feel the way they do."

— Anthony William, Medical Medium

CHAPTER 19

Pharmaceuticals

Common Pharmaceuticals

- Antibiotics

- Antidepressants

- Anti-inflammatories

- Sleeping pills

- Biologics

- Immunosuppressants

- Prescription amphetamines

- Opioids

- Statins

- Blood pressure medications

- Hormone medications

- Thyroid medications

- Steroids

- The Pill

- Pharmaceutical alcohol

- Recreational drugs

If you're on medication or you've received a medical treatment, you're aware of it. You may not be completely aware of what was in the medication. You at least know it was administered. What you might not know is what you were given in your early childhood or even babyhood that could still be in your system. It's very common to receive antibiotics early in life, pre-memory. Even if you've never taken medicine, pharmaceuticals could be in your brain and body systems.

WATER SUPPLY

More and more, pharmaceuticals are entering the water supply because people who are taking them then eliminate them when they go to the bathroom. This also means that medication-laced water can become a part of our food through reservoirs, irrigation, public water supplies, well water near septic tanks, and fish swimming in lakes, rivers, and oceans. There are other ways to get this pharmaceutical-laced water, such as brushing our teeth, cooking with tap water, and swimming in lakes and rivers, pools, or water parks. Restaurant water normally contains pharmaceutical runoff.

POOLS AND WATER PARKS

Swimming in a pool or water park doesn't only lead to pharmaceutical exposure via the water supply. There's also the runoff coming from people's bodies. When you're swimming in a hotel pool, for example, there's pharmaceutical runoff coming from people's skin and out of their armpits, their genitals, their mouth if they get water in their mouth, and even their urine or feces, if they urinate, defecate, or pass gas in the pool. (The pool water becomes a filter for what's in the gas.) It's a pharmaceutical bath.

Sure, they chlorinate the water to shock it for parasites, bacteria, and algae. That chlorine doesn't remove any of the pharmaceutical residue in the water supply or the runoff from people's skin. Those pharmaceuticals stay in the pool water unless the pool is fully drained. Pool water can stay in the pool for a very long time without ever getting a repair that calls for it to be drained. At a hotel, for example, you could have pharmaceutical-filled water for five straight years or more, where it concentrates year after year and doesn't dissipate. And pools never get tested for pharmaceutical levels, ever.

FOOD SUPPLY

Antibiotic-fed animals translate to our ingesting antibiotics when we eat their eggs, meat, fish, and dairy. Even if you take care to find the highest-quality, best-treated animal products for when you prepare food at home—which is a great protective measure if you eat animal products—you've likely been unable to avoid eating conventional animal products when dining out or eating at a friend's house, and that means antibiotic exposure. Even if you take great care to avoid eating animals fed antibiotics now, what about the first 10 years of your life, or the first 20 or even 30? Those antibiotics that you were exposed to during a previous chapter in your life store up over your lifetime.

Keep in mind, grass-fed animals—grass-fed beef; free-range, pastured chicken; organic-fed pigs—still occasionally get infections, get sick, and get treated with steroids and antibiotics. They're just not as saturated, for the most part, with antibiotics for chronic contagious infection as conventionally raised animals are. When chronic infections do occur with grass-fed animals raised free-range and pastured, some animals are out of commission for a while due to an ongoing infection that takes a month to treat. Once recovered, the animal is back in the running again. It's still listed as grass-fed beef and ready for market when time comes. We're shielded from this information, kept from the inside goings-on. We think it's inconceivable that the animals have ever had something wrong with them, any kind of infection or illness. I don't want you under the illusion that you're not going to get antibiotics from grass-fed meat, because it's not true.

MORE PHARMACEUTICAL EXPOSURE SOURCES

A lot of people get medication exposure from the flea or tick powder or cream they apply to their dogs and cats, or from flea and tick–repelling pet collars.

Intimacy is another form of pharmaceutical exposure—for example, kissing someone who's on medication.

Then there are medicated creams that have a powerful outgas. A large variety of medicated creams, from steroid creams to chemotherapy creams, outgas a very potent, pungent smell that the person using the cream is unaware of because they live in it. Breathing in this outgassing is exposure.

Basic contact with shopping cart handles is another surprising source of exposure because those handles are where a lot of pharmaceutical residue resides, often from pharmaceutical creams and sweat from individuals' palms, which contain pharmaceutical residue if they're on medication.

PHARMACEUTICALS AND OUR BRAIN

Pharmaceuticals are manufactured to affect the brain or body in specific ways, generally stimulating or suppressing certain neurological or bodily processes. So when you take a medication, it could very well be for the purpose of trying to enhance or subdue particular functions of the brain. At the same time, pharmaceuticals can affect the functions of the brain in ways that aren't always ideal. That is, there are side effects, sometimes debilitating and life-altering and even creating a dependency that outweighs the original problem for which the person took the medication.

Medications can be, in general, toxic to all areas of the brain. Here's how it works:

When a medication enters a person's body system, the liver absorbs some of it. Much of that medication enters the bloodstream directly, bypassing the liver at first—because some medications have an uncanny ability to absorb into your bloodstream through your mouth, throat, esophagus, stomach, and duodenum. When medications find their way as far as the small intestinal tract, that's when they find their way into the lining of the tract and eventually into the hepatic portal vein and up into the liver. Even medications that bypass the liver at first eventually find their way there through the bloodstream, when the liver absorbs the medications as part of its bloodstream cleanup. (The kidneys aren't the only part of the blood cleanup equation.)

When the medication is out of your bloodstream, it's living somewhere else—such as stored deep inside the liver, where the medication is then time-released back into the bloodstream over future years. Inevitably, a stagnant, sluggish liver with a storage bin of old pharmaceuticals has to pop a cork every so often, releasing residuals that find their way to the brain if someone's not cleansing. That is, the liver is up against a lot when we don't know how to care for it, so it can't hold on to every brain betrayer forever. As the liver gets oversaturated with various cocktails of medications you might have taken long term (including over-the-counter medications), it starts letting go of some, so they circulate through the blood-stream again and find their way back to the brain, no longer just affecting the receptors the medications were originally intended for. The longer the medications stay in the body, the more efficacy the medications lose for their intended purpose. Now the pharmaceutical brew can act as a toxic sub-stance to the brain overall.

Plus pharmaceuticals contain toxic heavy metals. Pharmaceuticals also contain caf-feine. These additives are part of how medi-cations affect the brain so potently.

Medications of any kind, whether intended for the brain or elsewhere, have the ability to get past the blood-brain barrier and enter every part of the brain because phar-maceuticals are tissue-soluble—there's no part of the brain that's immune or unexposed. Medication also gets stuck in the brain, in which case, it doesn't get time-released. It stays there indefinitely, raising toxicity lev-els within the brain tissue, slowly denaturing brain cells, and never leaving the brain until

someone learns how to actively and proac-tively work to clean it out of brain tissue.

(For information on how recreational drugs can affect our brains, see Chapter 11, "Microdosing.")

Some medications can be useful in crisis situations, such as injuries or severe infec-tions. There are times when they are truly necessary. What we need to be aware of is how long-term use of pharmaceuticals ends up saturating brain tissue and dampening the central nervous system's ability to per-form. When we're not given answers from the medical industry about how to heal chronic illness, our symptoms and condi-tions continue for far too long, and we may find ourselves on medications for extended periods, with the medications possibly mak-ing our conditions worse. Medical research and science don't even know what the cause of chronic illness is to begin with, so they also don't realize they could be making the condition worse from the medication. One thing to keep in mind is that sometimes multiple medications are prescribed by dif-ferent doctors, creating a stronger brew than anyone intended that can alter or hin-der the brain's ability to function optimally. If you're actively relying on medication, I respect that. You can still work on healing your brain and protecting it from the dozens of other brain betrayers here in Part III.

CHAPTER 20

Toxic Heavy Metals

It's unknown that toxic heavy metals are a leading cause of today's epidemic of brain dysfunction, deterioration, and disease—and that they are incredibly widespread, at our fingertips in daily life.

Common Toxic Heavy Metals

- Mercury
- Toxic copper
- Aluminum
- Lead
- Cadmium
- Barium
- Nickel
- Arsenic
- Toxic calcium
- Toxic chromium
- Strontium
- Uranium
- Toxic iron
- Toxic platinum
- Titanium
- Tin

(Please note: This is not an exhaustive list of toxic metals.)

Toxic heavy metals are also passed along through the bloodline via metal-contaminated sperm and egg, so generation after generation comes into this world with inherited toxic heavy metals such as mercury.

Toxic heavy metals are behind some of the most life-altering brain-related and mental health symptoms and conditions of our time, from depression to obsessive-compulsive disorder (OCD) to Parkinson's to Alzheimer's. Toxic heavy metals are also behind many of our daily challenges and frustrations, from anger issues to anxiousness to focus and concentration issues and brain fog.

Keep in mind that the Medical Medium definition of *toxic heavy metal* is any toxic metal—because any toxic metal does heavy damage upon the body. As we covered in Chapter 3, "Your Alloy Brain," keeping a metal out of the toxic heavy metal category because of its weight definition undermines our understanding of the metal's damaging effects upon the body, giving it a license to harm people without any concern or worry. Including lighter metals in the toxic heavy metal definition alerts us to their ability to harm us.

METALS IN OUR MIDST

"Your Alloy Brain" also covered how toxic heavy metals tend to accumulate in our brain: through the brain's electromagnetic field, which is meant to draw in beneficial trace minerals. It's standard to feel some skepticism about how toxic heavy metals even find their way into our bodies in the first place. Maybe we picture a ball of aluminum foil and think, *How could that possibly find its way inside me?*

Well, one source of toxic heavy metal exposure is touch. When we pick up an aluminum can or a battery, or wear copper-based jewelry, oils from our hands and skin extract and absorb minute levels of the metals, drawing them into our derma and then deeper into our system. Oil is extremely acidic, and that acidic nature reacts to metal specifically. This reaction means that oil corrodes and eats away at the metal, causing the metal to leach when oil touches a metal.

An acidic chemical interaction occurs, forcing the metal to release metal byproduct molecules.

We ingest toxic heavy metals too. Metal utensils scraping metal bowls and pans in the kitchen leads to metal shavings in our food that could be microscopic, nanoscopic, or even smaller. When your silverware and cookware get worn down, when your knives go dull, where do you think that metal goes? The metal particles are going into your food, into your body, into your system—and can slowly accumulate in your brain.

All pharmaceuticals have some level of toxic heavy metals in them. Some people have been taking pharmaceuticals for most of their life, and these metals build up inside the brain. Antianxiety, antidepression, and stimulant medications are among the pharmaceuticals that have toxic heavy metals within them. So the irony is that we're often using pharmaceuticals that contain toxic heavy metals to treat conditions caused by toxic heavy metals themselves.

Mercury, lead, aluminum, and copper especially are in our midst. Handling batteries, handling some varieties of light bulbs, getting or removing mercury amalgam fillings, and most all dental work involve toxic heavy metals. Every ceramic filling has metal to some degree (although less and in different forms than amalgam fillings), and fluoride is an aluminum byproduct. Eating fish, taking fish oil supplements (even the high-quality ones that claim to be mercury-free), and spending time swimming in lakes and other water sources are a few of the ways to encounter mercury.

When it comes to toxic heavy metals and our central nervous system, there are three concerns: (1) past exposure to toxic heavy metals that has led to toxic heavy metal buildup in our brain, (2) present exposure to toxic heavy metals that we can limit or avoid altogether with the awareness in this chapter, and (3) present exposure that we can't avoid—and therefore want to catch before the toxic metals reach our brain. Toxic heavy metals are very much a part of our everyday world. A key to safeguarding yourself and your loved ones is acknowledging this—because then you can minimize new exposure while putting Medical Medium protocols to work to clean up toxic heavy metals in your brain and body and repair the damage they've left behind.

EXAMPLES OF LEAD EXPOSURE

Lead can get into our system through old lead pipes or lead sealers on newer pipes, and we can also be exposed through lead paint. This can happen in surprising ways.

For example, lead paint chips can seep into soil, exposing us when we're gardening or growing food in contaminated soil. Many people grow gardens around their home, and lead paint chips can leach lead into soil for hundreds of years unless it's remediated.

Up until the early 1980s, lead was even in the paint on pencils, so you could get exposure from handling and biting pencils. Some people keep pencils around for

decades in a desk drawer for a grandchild to find one day and use or even chew.

Plus there are always traces of lead in the water supply, even water that's supposedly filtered in restaurants and coffee shops. There's even lead in fish, especially freshwater fish.

EXAMPLES OF ALUMINUM EXPOSURE

Speaking of which, many people bite the metal caps on pencils, which is aluminum exposure.

Aluminum is everywhere, especially in the kitchen. When we simply handle aluminum products, the oils from our skin extract and absorb toxic metal particles on a nanoscopic and even smaller scale. When we eat out, that food was often prepared with aluminum pots, pans, and utensils that were scraped and worn, sending particles into our meal, plus our leftovers are served up in aluminum takeout containers. Aluminum is also a common ingredient in cosmetics and sunblock and sneaks into tap water. When you drink off the top of an aluminum can, you're getting aluminum from that process. You also get aluminum exposure simply from holding cans.

People often think they're safe with aluminum cans because of the thin epoxy coating inside some cans. Once they're told, "Hey, these cans are lined, you're safe," all doubts about aluminum toxicity drift away. People think this lining means aluminum won't leach into the beverage. Yet all cans expand and contract. Placing aluminum cans in the refrigerator causes the metal to contract and weakens the liner inside the can. Then when you take the can out and handle it, the can starts to warm up—maybe you're even out in the sun—and that warming means the metal expands quickly, pulling apart the liner inside the can. This is why you hear countless stories of people tasting metal in their canned beverage even when there's said to be a liner present. Liners also disintegrate over time on the store shelf if not purchased soon enough after manufacturing. The liners get eaten away by the liquid within the cans.

EXAMPLES OF TOXIC COPPER EXPOSURE

Copper is often in pipes, meaning it ends up in our drinking and bathing water, plus it's showing up more and more in kitchenware. Copper mugs and thermoses and water containers are really big right now, purposely created to leach copper into the water, as if this were a positive thing.

The trend derived from a practice hundreds of years ago in certain parts of the world where water supplies were scarce. Storing water in copper vessels such as copper-lined barrels, copper canisters, or copper pots was a technique to keep certain (but not all) microbes from proliferating in still water. It was a survival technique. The upside was that water was less contaminated with parasites, because the parasites, specifically certain varieties of amoebas, were poisoned by copper. (Bacteria and viruses in today's world don't die from copper poisoning. They thrive on copper.) The downside of storing water in copper vessels was copper poisoning for the individual consuming the water on a regular basis. It was a trade-off of one evil for a lesser evil. This storage technique could keep somebody from being bent over vomiting and having diarrhea from dysentery from a parasite (even though that did still happen; killing off parasites with copper wasn't guaranteed). Instead of being sick to their stomach, that person could be functioning, consuming the water, living their life—and developing symptoms, conditions, and diseases because of the copper toxicity. It was the way to stay alive in certain parts of the world where water was scarce. The choice was to go completely without water for a long period of time or consume water that caused neurological disease while keeping you alive longer. We can't confuse this survival choice with a health-promoting practice.

Somehow we've upgraded this survival tactic to a trend. Like all trends, the details are missing. Little does anyone know that if the trend blows up any bigger, we're going to have more eczema, psoriasis, and psoriatic arthritis cases than ever. We're going to have even more unexplained neurological symptoms and diagnosed diseases. We're going to have worsening of emotional and psychological conditions. High levels of copper toxicity in the brain can cause madness, personality disorders, paranoia, and worsened OCD.

Promoters of copper containers for water storage believe that it's healthy because they believe that we're deficient in copper. This thinking deserves to be corrected for two reasons: (1) we're not deficient in copper, and (2) ironically, the copper thermoses, copper water containers, trendy copper kitchenware, and copper jewelry all meant to provide you with usable copper don't even provide the beneficial, healthy, usable form of copper. They're all made from toxic industrialized copper, just the same as copper pipes delivering your water.

And again, we're not lacking beneficial copper. Most every food we eat has copper, both toxic industrialized copper and the healthy trace mineral copper from our soil. Even food produced organically has traces of toxic copper. How does that happen? Most organic growing fields are refurbished conventional growing fields. Depending on the local certification rules, they can usually get the organic designation after seven years of not spraying conventional pesticides, herbicides, and fungicides. Meanwhile, copper from pesticides, herbicides, and fungicides stay in the ground for more than seven years—so both organic crops and conventional crops end up with industrialized toxic copper. There's also healthy copper in every food we eat. Some foods are abundant in it. Copper is a metal we have too much of, both in trace mineral form and toxic industrialized form. No one is void of trace mineral copper. A lack of copper is not why anybody is sick. The fear of deprivation of copper is misleadingly wrong.

HERBICIDES, PESTICIDES, AND FUNGICIDES

Herbicides, pesticides, and fungicides are common sources of many toxic heavy metals, from mercury to lead to copper, cadmium, barium, nickel, and arsenic. Keep in mind that even organic vapor sprays for organic produce have toxic heavy metals within them. Not to mention that organic sprays can contain MSG, caffeine, and especially nicotine. The purpose is to paralyze an insect nervous system. All three of these chemicals are problematic to the human brain, and it's easy to consume them if you don't wash your organic produce carefully.

Crops aren't the only place where fungicides, which are very high in copper and other toxic heavy metals, are sprayed. Industries are using fungicides on clothes, blankets, sheets, furniture, couches, chairs, rugs, and more—practically everything, especially items that end up close to our skin.

TATTOOS

Tattoos are a source of toxic heavy metal exposure. The ink from a tattoo is basically on a time-release, leaching metals slowly from the derma into the bloodstream over a lifetime. From the bloodstream, those toxic heavy metals find their way to the brain, where they end up residing in brain tissue.

As of today there are no sources of tattooing that are free of toxic heavy metals, not even tattoo inks that are vegan and cruelty-free. In order for tattoo ink to be seen clearly through the skin, there have to be metals inside the tattoo ink. As light hits your skin from the sun or any source of light, it reflects off the metal inside the tattoo ink under the skin. That reflection allows the tattoo to pop and be seen clearly. As the years go by and tattoos' toxic heavy metals are time-released deeper into your bloodstream, tattoos fade. The light reflecting off your body ink doesn't have as much to reflect off anymore—toxic heavy metals within the ink were what gave the tattoos their clarity.

If you already have tattoos, you don't have to remove them. Instead make sure you're following Medical Medium protocols to sop up and expel the metals as they're time-released into your bloodstream, so the metals don't build up in your brain. If you choose to remove a tattoo because you don't like your tattoo anymore, the procedure could release more metal into your bloodstream faster, so following the Heavy Metal Detox guidance from Chapters 44 and 45 would be wise then too.

MERCURY IN FISH AND SEAFOOD

Ocean saltwater contains an abundance of trace minerals, which clash with toxic heavy metals. The ocean is alive. It's composed of living energy from trace minerals floating in it. Ocean minerals are living minerals that are grounding. Toxic heavy metals disrupt this energy. Living minerals and toxic heavy metals don't mix well. They don't run on the same frequency or charge. Because toxic heavy metals such as mercury have been industrialized, they have changed and become

destructive. Industrialized toxic heavy metals such as mercury are on a rogue and radical separate charge that disrupts grounding. Acting as free radicals, these toxic heavy metals alter electrical frequencies and energy wherever they are—our air, our ocean, our body.

This conflict causes a mineral-metal separation within fish. That is, the trace minerals and toxic heavy metals within fish, which the fish harbor from living in the ocean, conflict with each other. The minerals and metals can't join together. They react and repel each other. This reaction causes most trace minerals that are inside the fish to end up in the muscle tissue of the fish, while the mercury and other toxic heavy metals absorb into the fat and oil of the fish. This is due to the difference in formation of toxic heavy metals versus minerals. Toxic heavy metals are oddly shaped and denatured through industrialization, so the metals are not in their natural form. Industrialized metal particles' odd shapes pierce oil, getting stuck and trapped in oil and fat more easily than muscle tissue. As a result, the majority of toxic heavy metals end up in the oil and fat, while the minority end up in muscle tissue.

Because the fat and oil in the fish tend to absorb the toxic heavy metals, and the presence of those toxic heavy metals repels trace mineral absorption in the fish's fat and oil, this leads the fish oil to become void of nutrients and trace minerals. Oil in fish is supposed to be high in trace minerals. Instead it's high in radical, damaging metals and extremely low in trace minerals. This is why, if you're going to eat fish, choosing less oily fish is your safest bet. (You may have heard out there in the health world to eat less oily fish. No one knows the real reason why less oily fish contains less mercury.) Leaner fish is not free of toxic heavy metals. Mercury and toxic heavy metals can still end up in other parts of the fish besides the fat and oil. They're simply most concentrated in the oil and fat of the fish.

Fish oil supplements are a common source of toxic heavy metals in part because mercury and other toxic heavy metals concentrate in the oil and in part because the extraction process used to produce fish oil supplements destabilizes the mercury in the fish. This destabilization creates a methylmercury that becomes that much easier for our brain to absorb and that much more potent because of its homeopathic dilution.

VAPORIZED HEAVY METALS

Metals fall out of the sky. Toxic heavy metals are in the jet stream. They're in the breeze we inhale. Chem trails expose us to a large amount of metals of all kinds. Petrochemicals coming out of jet planes vaporize metals in the atmosphere, and industries all around the world are releasing toxic heavy metals into the air as they make products for commerce. Wind can carry pesticide and herbicide drift for hundreds of miles. If the weather is just right, wind patterns can carry pesticide drift thousands of miles, from continent to continent. Fireworks leave us breathing in toxic heavy metals such as strontium.

We also live with toxic heavy metals in our indoor air. Industries have created ways to vaporize fragrances via plug-in air fresheners, scented candles, and scent diffusers so that when we breathe in these synthetic fragrances—which can contain toxic heavy metals, among other brain betrayers—the vapors penetrate the sinus cavities the way sniffing cocaine does, allowing those toxic heavy metals to get to the brain.

SPINAL TAPS

When spinal taps are performed, they don't even look for toxic heavy metals, yet toxic heavy metals are abundant in spinal fluid. Spinal taps are a standard practice that never yields enough information when someone is chronically ill. They're a formality that weakens and traumatizes patients further.

TONGUE DISCOLORATION

When someone gets dark gray or black discoloration on their tongue and they're sure food or tobacco didn't stain it, it's a sign of heavy metals deep in organs surfacing, especially mercury and metal-related viral toxins. If you're proactive in cleansing, metals and viral toxins surfacing is a positive sign. If you're not proactive on any level, your body is showing that you have an overload of mercury or metal-related viral toxins overflowing. Depending on where metals and viral toxins are positioned in your body, you may not experience a black tongue either way.

CHAPTER 21

Fragrances

Common Fragrance Exposures

- Plug-in air fresheners

- Scented candles

- Aerosol-can air fresheners

- Spray-bottle air fresheners and mists

- Cologne and aftershave

- Perfume

- Car air fresheners

- Incense

- Scent diffusers

- Scented body lotions, creams, sprays, washes, and deodorants

- Scented shampoos, conditioners, gels, and other hair products

- Scented laundry detergent, fabric softener, and dryer sheets

- Cosmetics and makeup

- Dryer dust (exhaust in outside air from dryers in homes using conventional laundry products, colognes, perfumes, scented candles, and air fresheners)

The fragrance sector of the chemical industry is far from innocent. The industry has a set of goals. One goal is to keep their chemicals in mass production. To do this, they want to keep people purchasing their chemicals—and to do that, they want to condition and train people to believe they need these synthetic fragrances and scents. Last but not least, they want to take away any future chance for someone to know what nature really smells like. Whether smelling ocean air at the beach, smelling the earth and fresh air of the forest, or smelling flowers and freshly mown grass as the wind rustles through trees in your backyard, they want to disrupt the authentic experience. We're coming to a time when we're not going to know what any of these natural surrounding smells are like. We're only going to be surrounded by contaminating fragrances.

Fragrances are unlike other toxic chemicals. Many toxic chemicals have a shelf life and dissipate over time. The rain can dilute certain outdoor toxic chemicals, for example, thin them out and make them less harmful. The rain cannot thin out a toxic chemical that's saturated with fragrance. Fragrances are being created to last for an extremely long time and not dissipate. In many cases, fragrance can be unstoppable. We're on the verge of never being able to smell what the ocean air is like when we're standing on the beach because we're just going to be smelling fragrances blowing off other people.

FRAGRANCE LABELING

Fragrances are unidentified chemicals, even more so than other domestic chemical industry invader products, which you'll read about in a few pages. One loophole in the chemical industry is this: fragrances don't have to list the multiple chemicals within them. When you see the word *fragrance* in a list of ingredients, you're looking at corruption. Because in that word are a host of different chemicals that will not be listed as ingredients in that product.

Using a product that lists *"natural fragrance"* is not a way out. There are still chemical industry fragrances in natural fragrances. The chemical industry is allowed to call a fragrance "natural" if there's one single essential oil added to the mix of industrial chemicals.

Whether scented products seem conventional or natural, what you'll find listed in them are *"fragrance"* or *"natural fragrance"* or *"perfume"* or *"parfum."* You will not see the list of chemicals in that fragrance or perfume, so you'll miss out on any understanding of how many industry-created chemicals go into making that scent. Even if it says "naturally derived," it still doesn't mean it gets a free pass.

Many people in the health scene are concerned about conventional products, so they're using clean makeup, clean hair care products, clean skin products. Meanwhile, these products all have either fragrances or natural fragrances or perfume in them, or any combination. If you were to sit inside a chemical factory watching people with hazmat suits walking around giant containers of swirling chemicals, and then you saw those chemicals being put into a fragrance and that fragrance sold to all the different companies that sell all these products, you would be shocked to say the least.

SABOTAGED SELF-CARE

We're adopting healthier lifestyles, we're eating healthier foods, we're concerned about our environment, and at the same time we're allowing perfumes, colognes, and fragrances to be inside everything. Many people are concerned about climate change, and at the same time, they're contaminating our climate with chemical industry soups that are highly toxic and even affect wildlife.

One reason we turn to fragrances is self-care. We're picking out perfumes and scented candles and scented lotions and scented everything because they're supposed to relax us and put us in the right frame of mind. We think we're promoting well-being by using fragrances. Another reason we use so much fragrance is that our bodies have smells, and fragrance is how we hide our smells. It means all these fragrance chemicals are inside our brain. We're allowing chemical giants to hurt our brain, age our skin and body, age our lungs and organs, speed up the disease process, and at the same time, age our pets.

Fragrances are in air fresheners; scented candles; makeup (including clean makeup); skin care, hair care, and body care products (whether clean or regular and conventional); and laundry products. The more organic or clean we go with our domestic products for body care and more, the more loopholes the chemical giants find to put their fragrances with unidentified toxic chemicals into these products. It's imperative we get wise to it and avoid fragrances, including perfumes.

FORCED EXPOSURE

We also need to get wise to the ways the chemical industry tries to expose us to these fragrances even when we don't personally use them. For example:

Scented candles and plug-in air fresheners saturate walls. Even if the person using them moves out, anyone who moves into the home or office afterward has to contend with this lingering scent.

Fragrances can become mold-harboring. A film begins to develop from burning scented candles or using plug-in air fresheners, and that film collects on every fabric and fixture inside the home, trapping particles of dust and debris that float in the air. Trapped in the film, this debris can harbor moisture, creating a perfect situation for mold to grow. Someone often uses fragrance in the first place to cover the smell of mold or mildew in a space. In a situation like this, where mold is already present, adding fragrance products such as air fresheners or scented candles can accelerate the mold.

Fulfillment centers and warehouses are shipping out products such as clothing that are saturated with air fresheners, contaminating the products that arrive at our homes and workplaces.

Dryer dust is extremely toxic when any fragrances are used in the home, which means that neighbors get exposed. This dryer exhaust is a combination of the air fresheners in the home plus perfumes, colognes, scented candles, cosmetics, and body products saturating all of the clothes being laundered combined with the fragrances of the laundry detergents and fabric softeners used, all blowing out with hot air and polluting the environment.

CHAPTER 22

Bacteria and Other Microbes

Common Bacteria and Other Microbes

- Over 50 groups of *Streptococcus* strains

- *H. pylori*

- *E. coli*

- *Salmonella*

- Foodborne toxins (Includes many uncataloged microorganisms. Even when killed off through cooking, the microbe bodies remain toxic and can build up in the system.)

- Methicillin-resistant *Staphylococcus aureus* (MRSA)

- *C. difficile*

- *Staphylococcus*

- Mold

- Parasites

Most of these microbes enter through the mouth—that is, through food, water, shared food and drink, contaminated dishware and cutlery, eating with unwashed hands, or intimate contact. It's also possible to pick up a bug such as strep or *H. pylori* from bathrooms and restaurants. Essentially, you can pick up bacteria in the same ways you can pick up viruses, as outlined in Chapter 18, "Viruses and Viral Waste Matter."

(Note that the bacteria associated with neurological Lyme disease are not in the above list of common brain-betraying bacteria. As you'll read in the entry for Lyme disease in Part V, "Your Pain and Suffering Enlightened," there's a reason for that.)

SHOPPING CART HANDLES

Shopping cart handles are a popular place for bacteria. Pre-COVID shopping cart handles were one of the mega transports of all transports for bacteria. And not bacteria that make us stronger, as some theorize. Bacteria that make our lives more difficult, even miserable. At the height of COVID sanitization efforts, when surfaces such as shopping cart handles were regularly disinfected, shopping carts had never been safer.

Strep, the leading bacteria type on shopping cart handles, can cause chronic sinusitis, chronic allergies, chronic lung infections (including pneumonia), chronic postnasal drip, chronic ear infections, chronic sties, conjunctivitis, strep throat, sore throats, itchy rectum, irritable bowel syndrome (IBS), chronic or intermittent diarrhea, bloating, cramping, gastritis, yeast infections, bacterial vaginosis, pelvic inflammatory disease (PID), overactive bladder (OAB), UTIs, acne, interstitial cystitis, sebaceous cysts, and boils. Strep can also contribute to pediatric autoimmune neuropsychiatric disorders (PANDAS), as a coinfection with a virus such as HHV-6 or EBV.

How do shopping cart handles become such a hotbed of microbial activity? People often grab a shopping cart with dirty hands—and that shopping cart handle is already saturated with bacteria from other people's hands. So they add their own strain(s) to the mix while picking up another variety, or multiple varieties, of Streptococcus or other bacteria. When shopping carts and hands were being sanitized regularly, strep transmission minimized greatly. Once COVID was misrepresented as "over," shopping carts were once again filled with strep bacteria, with very few people sanitizing or washing their hands regularly. So we're back to square one. People are even back to eating samples or other food while shopping.

STREP AS A STRESSOR

Most people carry more than one strain of Streptococcus bacteria throughout a lifetime. Out of all the bacteria that are harmful to us, strep is what people contract and live with the most. People pass different strains of strep to one another in all the ways mentioned in Chapter 18, "Viruses and Viral Waste Matter." Because strep can be antibiotic-resistant, it's becoming the new superbug. Some strains of strep can cause chronic conditions and not give in or let up, leading someone to live miserably. A person can end up collecting several varieties and strains of strep that eventually camp out in the liver, intestinal tract, and other organs. One way strep can stress out our brains is by causing chronic conditions such as severe cases of acne. Acne can be devastating to individuals suffering from it, causing excessive emotional injury. It's traumatic for many people who are getting severe breakouts of acne on their face and body.

Strep is also a threat to our brain because it's an immune system complicator, weakener, and overloader. By lowering our immune system, strep allows viruses to prosper and thrive. Strep and EBV in particular have an affiliation. They work with each other: as strep weakens the immune system, EBV can proliferate and create neurological conditions of the brain.

There are certain varieties of strep that cause high fever—high fever that can run for days and even weeks at a time. A severe case of strep throat that's not succumbing to antibiotics can give someone a fever of 100 to 103 degrees for as long as three months. This continual fever compromises the brain and weakens the central nervous system by burning up storage bins of glycogen, neurotransmitters, and key electrolytes.

Other bacteria and microbes can affect the brain by causing fevers too. Even though fevers are natural reactions of your body that serve a purpose, mild fevers that surpass a few days can tire the brain. That's why someone who's been sick with a fever for three or four days tends not to be too sparky when they come out of it. It's not just the body that's been affected; the brain has been affected too.

GOOD BACTERIA DON'T FIX BAD BACTERIA

Drowning our digestive system with helpful, beneficial microorganisms does not alter the level of bad bacteria in our intestinal tract in any way.

For example, if someone has small intestinal bacterial overgrowth (SIBO) or bloating or IBS, the strep residing in their intestinal tract does not get crowded out by good microorganisms. Alternative medicine, without understanding these gastrointestinal conditions, has placed a gut balance theory upon avid health-goers, claiming that all their problems will go away by increasing beneficial

microorganisms—whether through a trendy product or fermented foods—to create balance within the intestinal tract environment. The very basis of the theory is misguided. Good bacteria don't destroy bad bacteria, and it's not possible for alternative or conventional medicine to properly measure or understand what balance means inside the intestinal tract.

Let's say that again: good bacteria entering your intestinal tract will not destroy any strain or group of strep or any other unproductive bacteria such as *E. coli*. They don't compete. They don't conflict. They don't eat the same food. They don't go to war with each other. A beneficial microorganism does not attack a nonbeneficial microorganism, does not push it out of its environment, tell it to go somewhere, or destroy it. Instead we need specific Medical Medium protocols, both with food and supplementation, to do that job of breaking down and eliminating toxic bacteria such as strep, and we need to build our immune system in the process.

Here's another reason this "good bacteria fight bad bacteria" theory is misguided: fermented foods and many other recommended sources of "good" bacteria do not actually contain good bacteria; they contain unproductive bacteria that thrive on something dying, not something living. Probiotics and toxic drinks, powders, tablets, or anti-*Candida* protocols outside of Medical Medium information don't provide healing because they don't come from an understanding of the real, underlying problem. Alternative and conventional medicine do not even understand yet that strep is the leading bacteria in the intestinal tract environment causing problems such as SIBO. Even if they did know strep was the problem, they still wouldn't understand that fermented foods and probiotics do not kill or stop *Streptococcus*.

FOOD POISONING

Food poisoning is more detrimental than we know. Not only because of the fever it may prompt or the stomach upset, diarrhea, or vomiting—it's also because of the microbes' effects on the brain. When someone gets food poisoning, it's not uncommon to lose control of the mind and thoughts, to not know where they are, to develop double vision, and in some cases, to practically hallucinate. That's because the active, living bacteria, parasites, and other microbes behind food poisoning produce a poisonous excretion that's highly problematic and injurious to the brain; when these toxins reach the brain through the bloodstream, they have a hallucinogenic effect.

The toxins produced by these foodborne microbes such as parasites and bacteria are not neurotoxins, the way that viruses produce viral neurotoxins. These bacterial and parasitical toxins are not poisoning and injuring the brain in the same way that neurotoxins from a virus do. Foodborne pathogens have a different toxicity level that they release and excrete along with their dead bodies, in cooked or living form. This toxicity triggers an acute allergic reaction in the body and brain in the form of vomiting, diarrhea, and pain. The reason this eventually becomes neurological—the reason your brain can have an allergic reaction once your body starts to—is that your brain detects a threat occurring: the possibility of your organs shutting down. So your body and then your brain go into crisis.

Different microbes have different effects. For example, a dangerous *E. coli* can eat away at the intestinal linings very quickly, causing internal wounds. Meanwhile, a microbe never even recognized in the lab or studied before that's sitting on a piece of raw fish may not eat through the lining of your intestinal tract and may instead release a toxin that your intestinal tract fiercely tries to expel—the cells in your intestinal tract are reacting to the toxin because the cells are being poisoned, and this becomes an allergic reaction. If these toxins eventually reach the brain through the bloodstream or cross the blood-brain barrier, the brain can exhibit an allergic reaction, creating the hallucinations, seizures, and other symptoms that can occur with food poisoning.

Even if a piece of raw meat or chicken that was harboring live *Salmonella*, *E. coli*, or any of thousands of other microbes gets cooked thoroughly so that the bugs die, the microbes still have a toxic nature in corpse form. Most of the time, people don't feel the effects of these microorganisms. In some cases, though, the brain can become allergic to the toxic microbe corpses, prompting a violent reaction such as vomiting or losing the ability to function, in a near-paralysis state.

Any section of the brain is susceptible to microbes, microbe toxins, or microbe corpses. Some microbe toxins won't affect certain areas of the brain and will affect others. Some toxic microbes can affect all of the brain. Some parasites excrete toxic substances that can affect any part of the brain. It all varies. It all depends. It's the luck of the draw.

There are so many undiscovered, unresearched, unanalyzed microbes—we're talking thousands of microbes in our food and water that are not cataloged. Their harmful effects on the brain can range anywhere from fevers, seizures, and hallucinations to acute attacks of the shakes, blurred vision, loss of eyesight, glaring pain in the head and neck, tightness in the throat, trouble swallowing—a mix of brain and body effects. And very often, it's not the microbes themselves reaching the brain; it's their poisons. That said, these extreme reactions are more of a rare situation, not the everyday situation of people eating toxic microbes and not knowing why they have hives, feel utterly sick, and vomit. In this more common scenario, they'll often pass it off at the doctor's office as maybe just 24-hour flu. Meanwhile, they ate something somewhere that gave them a case of food poisoning.

Food poisoning from a parasite can weaken the immune system, becoming a trigger for viruses already living in a person's body to proliferate. As a result, viral symptoms can develop, creating chronic illness. It's easy to mistake these symptoms as coming from a parasite, since they developed after the food poisoning. Yet parasites can't live and breed inside someone in the long term. Lasting symptoms come from viruses that were triggered into activity.

Worms aren't parasites. Worms are worms. Almost all worms can live inside us and not create chronic illness.

"For the most part, *brain* is a mystery word. It keeps us far away from our problems within the brain itself. It keeps us from looking deeper inside."

— Anthony William, Medical Medium

CHAPTER 23

Chemical Industry Domestic Invaders

**Common Chemical Industry
Domestic Invaders**

- Fragrances

- Sunblock and suntan lotion

- Laundry detergent, fabric
softener, and dryer sheets

- Cleaning products

- Body lotions, body oil, body
wash, body scrubs, soaps, and
other body products

- Hair spray and other
hair products

- Makeup and cosmetics

- Dry cleaning chemicals

- Nail chemicals (such as polish,
remover, adhesive)

- Spray tan

- Hair dye

- Talcum powder

These domestic invaders are the ultimate Trojan horse for the chemical industry. By disguising their dangerous toxic chemicals inside a bottle or other appealing packaging, chemical companies find a way to put these brain betrayers into people's everyday lives—and even condition us to believe we can't live without these chemical-laden products.

Most of these products are scented—and as you read in Chapter 21, "Fragrances," that comes with its own toll on our health. It's no coincidence that chemical industry domestic invaders contain fragrances. Toxic chemicals that are manufactured by chemical companies throughout the entire chemical industry have an unpleasing smell. Chemical giants that produce chemicals for any industry cannot control the outcome of what that chemical will smell like. This, in large part, is why fragrances were created: to mask every chemical-made product for domestic use inside the home, office, car, and around the yard so people would not be turned off by the chemical smell. No one wants to use a chemical-made laundry detergent from a chemical company that makes you nauseated when you smell it. Although the chemically sensitive are attuned enough that they'll often be nauseated by (or experience other symptoms from) both the underlying chemicals and the synthetic fragrance.

Chemical industry domestic invaders are more threatening than the other petrochemicals we'll look at later because chemical industry domestic invaders are sneaky. Domestic invaders often seem friendly and necessary for our lives, which means that we tend to end up with more exposure to them than to straight petrochemicals that we know warrant caution. These products seem like they should naturally be around us. We're taught they should be a part of our life, that we can't live without them. We're taught they're safe, pleasing, helpful, and even supportive of our emotional and mental state. Domestic invaders are accepted—and that makes them all the more dangerous.

Normally, most people aren't going to question that we need to wash our clothes or clean our homes and workplaces, so when we're handed a laundry detergent or cleaning supply, no one's going to question the product. This gives these chemical industry domestic invaders immunity in our

lives. Many of these products are marketed based on our appearance and our hygiene and cleanliness. Some of these products are also considered important for our safety and important if we want to be around others. Some of these products hide our body smells. We are not supposed to believe they can harm us in any way. We are trusting of products created by the chemical industry because there is a façade that people are looking out for us, and these products must have been through scrupulous testing. The word *natural* is a safe word in our consciousness, so we especially tend not to question products that are marketed as natural as much as we should. We're trusting they will not harm us.

CONTINUAL EXPOSURE TO HABIT-FORMING PRODUCTS

Domestic invaders are everyday items all around us—including, as the name suggests, in our homes. We get into the habit of using them, sometimes even becoming dependent upon them. On top of which, domestic invaders are often in our environment beyond our control—for example, plug-in hot oil air freshener or cleaning products in a waiting room, or scented candles in a store, or fabric softener on the clothes of someone we're standing near, or somebody's hair products or body lotions, where our only recourse is to walk away. Unlike smoking, which has gone out of favor to a degree, and where you can at least ask people not to smoke around you, you can't ask someone in an elevator with you to go back in time and decide not to put on his overpowering aftershave.

With chemical industry domestic invaders, contamination through exposure is not a one-time deal. If we're using the products every day or every other day or once a week, that continual exposure has an accumulated effect inside our house, apartment, car, office, body—and inside our brain. These betrayers enter our brain and body systems all the time, and that accumulated volume makes them even more dangerous to our children, families, pets, and selves.

We have to remember these are toxic chemicals made in chemical factories. This isn't someone plucking soapwort out of the garden, rubbing it between their hands with a little bit of water, trying to create soap. Conventional detergents and soaps don't just wash off your skin. They wash through your skin. That is, there are chemical agents inside these products that absorb way past our skin's surface, enter our bloodstream, and have an easy time getting deep within our organs such as our liver and brain and then inhabiting our liver and brain, giving us a harder time trying to get them out. Our body isn't naturally designed to detox manmade chemicals from industrial chemical factories. These toxic chemicals become a part of us long term, which inevitably contributes to the disease that eventually plagues us, or even the disease that takes us down in the end.

UNMONITORED CHEMICAL AGENTS

When we speak of chemicals, we are speaking of any kind of chemical created by the chemical industry, whether we know that chemical exists inside a product or not. Chemical companies are exempted, for the most part, from full disclosure in labeling. They have free rein in the creation and use of their chemicals because they produce so many different chemicals for so many different industries. There's no proper regulatory system designed to monitor, safeguard, calculate, and keep track. It would take rebuilding the entire chemical industry and beyond.

Thousands of chemicals are churned out daily, so they get thrown into extremely large categories instead of individually tested for safety. You can have 10,000 chemicals in one category and have that category deemed safe by an authority. Meanwhile, out of those 10,000 chemicals, more than 5,000 of them are life-threatening in large dosages, while the other 4,000-plus chemicals may not cause immediate, obvious health effects within the first decade of use, yet with continual exposure will contribute to diseases, symptoms, and conditions as the years go by.

There's such a vast array of chemicals in production for these domestic invader products—thousands upon thousands of chemicals. Once these chemicals enter our body through the nose, mouth, lungs, or skin, they can saturate any aspect of the brain, whether deep in the inner core inside the brain stem, inside the hemispheres, or in the cerebral cortex. Some domestic invaders are petrochemical derived. When they settle into the brain, domestic invader products often end up deeper in the brain's grooves than other petrochemicals. Domestic invader chemicals are created to have radical absorption abilities, and the brain is vulnerable and easy to invade.

Different chemicals do different things. There's no wall up that stops certain chemicals from entering any part of the brain. They go past the blood-brain barrier.

This raises one of the foundational problems: these chemicals aren't brain-tested. It's not like the chemical industry knows what these chemicals can do inside the human brain or how they can penetrate the human brain. There's no authority overlooking this either. If the chemical doesn't burn the hair off your arm, then it goes to the next stage of testing for use. No one's monitoring any of these chemicals entering the brain. With current medical tools, it's not even possible to monitor the full scope of these chemicals' effects on the brain. We can't just cut open someone's brain, remove a portion, and look for these chemicals. So the industry's ultimate protection is that they're creating chemicals with effects that can't be measured or monitored.

Meanwhile, chemical industry domestic invaders can create immune system weaknesses that allow brain disease to take root, feed viruses, and fuel the creation of tumors. These domestic invaders also contain traces of toxic heavy metals—and you know by now what those can mean for your brain.

AN EXPERIMENT ON HUMANKIND

It's no secret that we encounter and use these products all the time. What's hidden is what their ingredients do to us. Humankind is one big chemical industry experiment.

How many dangerous chemicals can a person sop up in their lifetime before it becomes apparent that it's hindering their health and well-being and even injuring them? It's almost like a joke or a prank—how far can the chemical industry push the envelope before it's blatantly obvious? The key to chemical industry domestic warfare is to slip everyday items through the door and never have the finger pointed at whatever evil is slipping through that door. It's the ultimate con on humankind.

Families want to be safe, want to protect their children. A child means everything to a parent. The chemical industry takes advantage of families, driving their poisons into their homes by exposing them to seemingly safe products that are toxic.

Laundry detergent, fabric softener, and dryer sheets, for example, do the opposite of making us fresh and clean. The chemicals from their harsh scents and other additives get into our lungs and onto our skin and into our brain, increasing our internal toxic loads. Sure, detergents remove dirt. They also put something far worse than dirt inside your body. You look squeaky clean, you feel squeaky clean, yet now you're dirty and intoxicated with harmful chemicals. (Not to mention that many laundry chemicals are created from petrochemicals.) Makeup also contains harsh ingredients, including toxic heavy metals. Cleaning products—other items designed to make us think they're helping us—are potent cocktails of chemicals.

Whenever possible, opt for natural, unscented versions of the products you use every day. Watch out for ingredients such as *"parfum,"* *"perfume,"* and *"fragrance,"* and seek out labels that say "unscented" or "fragrance free." It's a good sign that your natural products could be safer.

If you work someplace where you have control, consider putting in place a scent-free policy to protect yourself, your coworkers, and your visitors from the surprising effects of chemical industry domestic invaders.

"One distinction between being not-so-sick and sick is the difference between being able to engage in self-care versus relying on desperate care.

The sick don't have energy or time to play games. Their hours aren't filled with lots of play time and self-care appointments that are fun. The chronically ill—the sick—need to use their time wisely, accomplish what they can where they can. Stringing them along, luring them to buy into something that isn't for their best benefit: this isn't productive, and yet it's happening, so stay mindful."

— Anthony William, Medical Medium

CHAPTER 24

Chemical Neuroantagonists

Common Chemical Neuroantagonists

- Chemical fertilizers

- Lawn treatments

- Insecticides (including ant killer, roach killer, spider killer, wasp killer, silverfish killer, tick killer, flea killer, mite killer, mosquito killer, termite killer, and gypsy moth killer)

- Nighttime aerial insecticide spray

- Larvicides

- Rodenticides

- Other pesticides

- Chem trails

- Herbicides

- DDT

- Fungicides

- Smoke exposure of any kind (including cigarettes, marijuana, and vaping)

- Fluoride

- Chlorine

Chemical neuroantagonists sounds like such a serious category that it must be difficult to come into contact with these chemical agents, right? Quite the contrary. We're up against these brain betrayers more than we know.

Walk through a park, golf course, campus green, or town common; eat conventionally grown produce, food made from a conventionally grown crop, or even organic food grown on former conventional fields; eat conventionally raised chicken, pork, beef, or fish; handle conventionally grown flowers; sit in your neighbor's chemically treated yard; walk down a sidewalk where someone has sprayed weed killer or is mowing the lawn, and you could come into contact with pesticides, herbicides, and chemical lawn fertilizers and treatments. People often spray the interiors and exteriors of schools, offices, apartment complexes, dorm rooms, hotels, houses, warehouses, storage facilities, and other buildings with roach killer, ant killer, termite killer, wasp killer, mosquito killer, tick killer, and more. So it's all too easy to breathe in or even touch chemical neuro-antagonist contamination.

ROGUE SPRAYING PRACTICES

Organic crops, while they aren't sprayed with conventional pesticides and herbicides, still come with exposures. For one, organic farming relies upon the same solvents, degreasers, and cleaning agents for their equipment, tractors, and trucks as conventional farming. Exhaust coming out of the tractors gets blown on all the crops. This exposure finds its way into produce.

Plus, dangerous mosquito sprays and other insecticides are dumped out of helicopters and planes all around the U.S. and in other places around the world. These high concentrations of mosquito spray from low-flying planes and low-flying helicopters douse organic crops, including fields where grass-fed cattle are grazing, just as they do any other farm or yard. The chemical companies providing the spray and flight patterns do not purposely avoid organic farms. This occurs every single year.

Whole cities and towns are sprayed by helicopter for bugs like mosquitos and gypsy moth caterpillars, so see if you can find out the local schedule and stay indoors

with windows closed at those times. Keep in mind that scheduling is never a definitive operation. Even if you have the local schedule in hand, it isn't guaranteed to be correct. Timing is never exact; it's always extremely loosey-goosey, and spraying is often done without forewarning. Trust your instincts if you see, hear, or smell something suspicious.

If you like going to a public park, find out its particular treatment schedule too, and see if you can wait for a good rain between when it's sprayed or fertilized and when you visit. When you do go, take along a blanket so you don't end up sitting on treated grass. Pregnant women should take special care with all of this; direct pesticide, herbicide, or fungicide exposure can be enough to cause pregnancy complications.

DDT ISN'T GONE

DDT is in a pesticide class all its own. This toxin that seems like a problem of the past is still very much with us today. It's in our oceans, lakes, streams, reservoirs and other water resources, agricultural fields, and more. Plus it's still in use in some parts of the world, and winds can even carry it from continent to continent. What's more, DDT passes along through bloodlines from generation to generation, so if one of your forebears was exposed in DDT's heyday, that same DDT from back then could now be in your body and brain.

In farming, a lot of fields are recycled. Almost all the farmland in use today is farmland from the 1930s, 1940s, 1950s, and

1960s that was heavily sprayed with DDT, so DDT is still in the dirt. That's true whether the farmland is used for conventional or organic farming today. Most organic farmland was converted to organic from conventional farming. The organic certification rules usually state that in the range of 5 to 7 to 10 years without conventional spray, land can be deemed suitable for organic farming. DDT lives many years past that in soil. DDT has a half-life of a good 100 to 200 years.

And that's just crops. Animals, whether raised conventionally or organically, graze in fields that were once fields conventionally sprayed with DDT.

UNREGULATED FUNGICIDE EXPOSURE

Fungicides are secretly everywhere too, coating more and more items you buy and encounter in daily life. No one's told, "This was sprayed with a fungicide." There's no warning on a package, no tag on clothing, no forewarning. It is a secret campaign that no one speaks about, no one knows about, other than big fungicide companies and manufacturing.

What happens is this: Any corporation that manufactures a product is sought out by suppliers. Chemical companies will send sales reps to meet with manufacturing companies and sell them on the fungicide chemicals that they want the corporations to spray on everything they manufacture. The manufacturers then take the fungicides, put them in spray jets, and spray these dangerous

chemicals on every single item and package. No one's monitoring this. There's no federal law. This is total rogue contamination. When you handle items sprayed with fungicides, nowhere does it say, "Patent number 1732284 applied." Nowhere does it show a skull and crossbones. Nowhere does it warn IMMUNE SYSTEM DIMINISHER with a list of side effects. And yet fungicides are in every country. Manufacturing plants throughout the world are sold this fungicide. You're not allowed to be informed of any of this.

Fungicides are sprayed on new clothing and manufactured goods; applied on crops, in hospitals, on new and used cars, and in airplanes; and even applied on garbage cans, garbage bags, and the exteriors of some water bottles. Cardboard boxes; packaged foods, including organic packaged foods; and beverages are sprayed with fungicides. Fungicides are on or in couches, appliances, tech products, lawn furniture, beds, blankets, sheets, dog shampoos, cat shampoos, other pet care products, medication boxes, cosmetic and self-care products, medical supplies, health care supplies, cleaning supplies, cleaning solutions, and much more. Basically, it's a trillion-dollar business for chemical companies to produce this much fungicide to sell to every manufacturer. They've made it a standard of industries to grandfather in fungicides against any ramifications from these dangerous chemicals.

Whenever you can, wash, wipe down, or air out new purchases. Fungicides have an odor that, once you know the smell, you'll never forget. If you have an odor-free-enough environment, stay on alert for their perfume-y scents that sizzle the nose, signaling you to these damaging fungicides' presence. On the other hand, if you live with other scents saturating your environment, chances are you won't smell the fungicides. If you're surrounded by perfumes, colognes, scented candles, and air fresheners, don't assume fungicides aren't on something because chances are, you can't detect them. You may have become smell-blind. Just the same, you're still exposed to the fungicides. There's a high likelihood that the outsides of the scented candles you buy are coated with fungicides.

SMOKE EXPOSURE

The smoke from any cigarettes, cigars, vaping, and marijuana is not the only smoke that's detrimental to our brain and neurological health. On top of the chemicals that smoking, vaping, and secondhand smoke draw into the lungs, bloodstream, and brain, there's chemical exposure from recreational fire sources such as fire pits burning treated lumber, treated logs in a fireplace, and charcoal grills. Fires on people's properties set to burn sticks, twigs, rotten logs, and leaves often have garbage, plastic, cardboard, and rubber thrown in, taking the smoke's toxicity to a whole other level. Burning pesticide-laden plastic row covers is also a common agricultural practice across the country, and without detecting or knowing it, we all breathe in this white smoke.

On top of all this, if someone's home is saturated in scented candles, air fresheners, detergents, fabric softeners, hair spray, cologne, and cleaning products, the air inside their home enters the fireplace, gets cooked by the heat of the flames, goes up the chimney chute, and contaminates the air outside with even more toxic renditions of the chemicals—because they've gone through the flame and become distorted, taking them to a new toxic high.

Smoke inhalation in any of these ways lowers the immune system, intoxicates the liver and lymphatic system, and compromises the nervous system.

FLUORIDE AND CHLORINE EXPOSURE

Fluoride and chlorine are very common in our lives, made all the more widespread because we think of them as being on our side. The obvious exposure to fluoride is in dental treatments. For chlorine, it's swimming pools, power washing, and cleaning products such as bleach in office buildings. These brain betrayers are also very commonly in tap water, including beverages and foods in restaurants. Even if you know to find fluoride-free toothpaste and ask your dentist for a fluoride-free cleaning and seek out swimming pools that use little or no chlorine, you may be ingesting and bathing in fluoride and chlorine at home if you don't use water filtration. Fluoride and chlorine are highly toxic to the immune system and central nervous system.

CHEMICAL NEUROANTAGONISTS AND OUR BRAIN

One of the reasons chemical neuroantagonists antagonize us is that they are potent viral fuel—in part because they often contain toxic heavy metals. However you're exposed to pesticides, they can find their way into your spinal fluid. By feeding viruses in our body or even brain, chemical neuroantagonists result in more-toxic viral waste such as neurotoxins, which heighten nervous system symptoms. Because of this, chemical neuroantagonists make a viral brain more viral and inflamed cranial nerves more inflamed. And because chemical neuroantagonists cross the blood-brain barrier very easily, they also make an alloy brain more alloy, an emotional brain more emotional, a burnt out brain more burnt out, an addicted brain more addicted, and an acid brain more acidic.

Chemical neuroantagonists tend to enter into the brain in four main ways:

- First is when we breathe them in and they enter our sinus cavity, from which they can seep into the brain. (Whether we're breathing in chemical neuroantagonists through our nose or mouth, it has the same effect.) Walking through a yard or park that's being sprayed with pesticides, for example, brings those toxic aerosolized particles into your sinus cavities, and that means fast delivery straight to your brain, similar to how cocaine or fentanyl

would be delivered. You'd think the bloodstream would derail the contaminants. In this case, it doesn't. In the sinuses, chemical neuroantagonists bypass blood currents, with a saturation rate unsurpassed by anything else—meaning chemical neuroantagonists can cross connective tissue and travel into the brain almost instantly upon breathing them in, saturating the frontal lobe.

- Breathing in chemical neuroantagonists also sends them to the lungs. From there they immediately enter the bloodstream and can travel throughout the brain via the blood, ending up anywhere inside the brain. Chemical neuroantagonists can even absorb into the spine and enter the spinal fluid, eventually reaching the brain that way.

- Pesticides, fungicides, and other neuroantagonists entering the mouth—whether you're breathing them in or eating them—can also mean that you end up swallowing and ingesting them. These chemical neuroantagonists absorb quickly into the stomach lining or intestinal tract lining, from there entering the bloodstream rapidly.

- Not every neuroantagonist enters the body through the air. The skin is the fourth main avenue for these brain betrayers to enter our bodies and eventually brains. Say you're pouring insecticide into a spray bottle. A few drops can easily splash onto your arm, hand, or leg. Then when you're spraying it, the spray can drift or splash onto your skin and even soak through your clothes. Absorption into the epidermis, derma, and beyond sends these chemical neuroantagonists into the bloodstream. From there they can reach the brain over time, sometimes even in a time-released vapor form.

"The brain is meant to be a sponge for knowledge.
Instead it becomes a sponge for waste."

— Anthony William, Medical Medium

CHAPTER 25

Petrochemicals and Solvents

Common Petrochemicals and Solvents

- Chemical solvents, solutions, and agents

- Lacquer

- Gasoline

- Diesel fuel

- Carpet chemicals

- Kerosene

- Propane

- Exhaust fumes

- Engine oil and grease

- Lighter fluid

- Gas grills, stoves, and ovens

- Dioxins

- Paint

- Paint thinner

- Plastics

Petrochemicals and solvents form another brain betrayer category that sounds like it's too serious for someone who works, say, in an office job to get regular exposure to it. Then again, take another look at that list. How everyday are some of those items?

We breathe in gas exhaust every day, whether when walking down the street, sitting in traffic, or walking behind our own car that we've just started in the driveway.

We often pump our own gas, starting as soon as we get a license. That means breathing in the fumes from our pump and the pumps around us, fumes absorbing into our skin from the air, plus the inevitable drips of gasoline on the skin. Gasoline, a solvent, can bypass the blood-brain barrier very easily and enter spinal fluid.

If you've ever eaten food cooked over a charcoal grill, fire pit, or a bonfire started with lighter fluid, you've eaten food with lighter fluid residue cooked into it. Not to mention that if you started the fire, the lighter fluid could have spilled onto your skin, plus you likely got a big inhale of its fumes. Or if you're someone who uses newspaper or cardboard to light a fire, the solvents on the newspaper or cardboard burned and became more toxic, and then you breathed them in. Plus the wood used in fire pits is often treated with solvents.

EXPOSURE ROUTES

Which brings us to just how petrochemical and solvent betrayers enter our bodies and make it to our brains: mostly through the same avenues as chemical neuroantagonists:

We breathe in petrochemicals and solvents through our nose and mouth, which guide them to our sinus cavities and in turn our brain, directly to the frontal lobe and other areas of the brain. Breathing in these brain betrayers also coats our mouth, which means they enter our saliva, which we then swallow, meaning the petrochemicals and solvents end up coating our stomach lining. At the same time, petrochemicals and solvents enter our lungs, from which they enter the bloodstream and become rogue contaminants that can reach almost any part of our brains.

Petrochemicals and solvents also absorb into our skin and, from there, enter our bloodstream. This happens, for example, when we check our car's oil and get oil on our hands or arms, when we handle cheap plastics day in and day out, or when we get paint or paint thinner on our hands.

On top of which, we sometimes eat petrochemicals and solvents—as in the case of grilled items becoming saturated from lighter fluid, treated charcoal, or gas grills—which brings them into our digestive systems and can mean they enter our bloodstream that way too. We also end up breathing the residue that's being cooked into our food, in addition to eventually consuming it.

DEMYSTIFYING CHEMICAL SENSITIVITIES

If your thought is *Well, I know my sister is sensitive to chemicals, but I never have been*, don't think that you're unaffected by petrochemical brain betrayers. Your sister (or mother or other family member or friend or coworker) is the canary in the coal mine. They became sensitive due to other contaminants such as toxic heavy metals, pathogens, or toxins that could have entered their life at one time or another. When someone has a reaction to a carpet that's just been shampooed, a newly painted room, or a freshly lacquered item from the woodshop, the instinct is to call out that person as the problem. Really, they're calling out the problem for the rest of us. All sensitive people have done is reach a certain saturation point with poisons and toxins over the course of life; those same petrochemicals (and other contaminants) are building up in your brain and body too, and simply haven't reached the same tipping point—yet.

Sometimes a pathogen is the behind-the-scenes reason for a reaction. When a person is chemically sensitive, it can be because they have a pathogen that's willing to feed on these brain betrayers, and the pathogenic activity stirs up symptoms. A person could also be loaded with toxins and poisons yet not have a virus present (or not have a virus that's out of dormancy or hungry enough to feed on those toxins and poisons). Someone's immune system could be lowered from these toxins and poisons, making the person more susceptible. Often people walk around like this, very toxic, with a high saturation level of neuroantagonists, petrochemicals, and other toxins, and then they contract a virus. That virus has found a treasure trove awaiting it, and a viral feeding frenzy begins that pushes someone over the edge into experiencing symptoms such as viral inflammation from exposure to industrial chemicals.

MORE ON PETROCHEMICAL EXPOSURE

Petrochemicals are pervasive. They're everywhere. Imagine, for example, a world coated with a dust too fine to see that's inhaled and eaten by every creature on the planet. Chem trails and dioxins are that "dust." (More on chem trails in a few pages.)

You already know how much we come in contact with cheap plastics; not only do we touch them all day long, but we ingest their particles from sources like plastic wrap, plastic food containers, plastic utensils and dishes, the water supply, pharmaceuticals (which are filled with plastics), and

packaged foods that were prepared using plastic assembly line parts. (Although note that plastics used in high-end food processors, blenders, and juicers are of good quality and less likely to leach, making them safe to use because these plastics are less porous or are non-porous. The very little plastic contamination you receive can be remedied easily with Medical Medium protocols.) Plastics saturate brain cells such as glial cells, making it harder for nutrients to pass through.

Even if an item such as kerosene seems out of favor now, it doesn't mean you weren't exposed from a space heater or camp stove back in the day. And propane is still around—for example with grills, hot water heaters, generators, ovens, and stoves.

Paint is still really toxic. Don't get so dazzled by "clean" paints that you think they're 100 percent safe. Many paints are partially less toxic than they were, and it's definitely worth seeking out low-VOC (volatile organic compounds) and no-VOC paints. Still, even if they smell better, it doesn't mean you're not breathing in toxins. They're not predictable. Also beware of paint thinner. Breathing it in or dripping it on your skin while fixing up your home is a common source of exposure.

Since we aren't taught how to properly cleanse and protect our bodies, all our everyday exposures from past and present could still be taking up valuable brain real estate. With their presence, these brain betrayers can slowly weaken brain function. Chemical solvents can build up in a painter's brain for 20 years, for example, and it might not have a discernible effect in that time. Instead an overall diminishing can occur as these brain betrayers build up, decreasing brain function bit by bit and setting that person up for brain disease later, especially if the petrochemical exposure is ongoing. Petrochemicals catch us later.

"The not-so-sick fall every day and become the sick. That's commonly when the realizations come. The fall they take brings them to a new awakening about how they've perceived the world."

— Anthony William, Medical Medium

CHAPTER 26

Chem Trails and Rainfall Exposure

Common Exposures

- Chem trails

- Precipitation contaminated with chem trails (not just contrails)

There are planes that fly over every city, town, and village in the world that are not planes filled with passengers, tourists, travelers, or cargo. These are airplanes that are empty of people except for a pilot and sometimes copilot. Inside, these planes are hollowed out, with large plastic tanks installed, tanks that can be filled with toxic chemicals. With the flick of a switch by the pilot, the contents of these tanks can be pumped out of the plane, creating a trail of dangerous toxic chemicals.

These planes are off the normal flight grid. They're exempt from following any flight pattern laws. And there are thousands upon thousands upon thousands of these planes flying all around the globe releasing what's called a *chem trail* day in and day out.

This can be a difficult topic for anyone who believes that all human beings on this planet would never sabotage other human beings. Thirty years ago, there were fewer than half of these planes in the skies, so it could be much more challenging to accept this frightening reality. Today, when you look up in the sky on Easter Sunday, Memorial Day, or any given weekend and you can count 5, 10, 20, or even 100 chem trails crisscrossing each other in all directions, it's a much easier awakening. As you read the following words, keep an open heart. The next time you see a blue sky streaked with white vapor turning into cloudy haze, you may have a whole new perspective.

CHEMICAL WASTE DISPOSAL

Project Chem Trails started in the 1960s as only a very small number of planes and only in small parts of the world. Now it has flourished into endless numbers of planes on rogue flight patterns all over the globe.

Chem trails are not governed by the governments or the militaries on the planet. Chem trails are separate from all of this. Governments are aware of chem trails, and they ignore them as if chem trails don't exist. Most chem trail planes are abandoned airline passenger planes from the 1950s, '60s, '70s, '80s, and '90s that have been refurbished. The purpose of these planes releasing toxic chemicals is to discard byproduct from the chemical industry in a discreet way.

There are hundreds of thousands of chemicals used in our industries every day. They're put in our food, they're put in our cleaning supplies, they're used in everything that's manufactured. Many of these chemicals are so toxic that if the human body were dipped into a vat of these chemicals, it would be a very quick death. On their storage containers, these chemicals carry the death warning, a skull and crossbones. And every single chemical that's manufactured for industrial use equals thousands upon thousands of gallons of waste. From the chemical's inception to the chemical's release in the marketplace, the amount of byproduct that results from perfecting that one chemical far surpasses anyone's imagination.

In the old days, industries just dumped chemical waste right into rivers, oceans, and land. The chemical industry cannot dump into our lakes and waterways and oceans to the same degree anymore. The chemical industry cannot leach into our land to the same degree anymore. With more chemicals being produced than ever before, where does all the chemical waste go? There's too much chemical byproduct and

no place to store it or release it. It can't be recycled. And so, since the chemical industry cannot dispose of their waste in the ways they once did, now chemicals are systematically dumped on us from the skies. Again, this happens all around the world. Planes filled with chemical industry byproduct release these toxic chemicals into the sky.

FALLING FROM THE SKY

Chem trails are composed of every toxin possible that the chemical industry creates. This includes toxic heavy metals such as mercury and copper. It also includes old, outdated, antiquated chemical storage bins that have been backlogged in storage for decades—chemical waste that has sat in tanks for 50, 60, 70, or even 80 or 100 years. It's a combination of chemicals, both old and new, being placed in planes and dumped out of the sky.

When the weather is nice around holidays such as Easter and the Fourth of July, when a lot of people will be outdoors, chem trails are usually increased substantially on purpose, to the point where the sky loses its blue color and the streaks in the sky spread out. It can look like a constant mild cloud cover along with streaks you see in every direction.

Chem trails are a stealth brain betrayer. When we get alerts about poor air quality, mostly that bad air is due to chem trails, without anyone's knowledge. Chem trails fall from the sky during the day and mostly during the nights. Overnight is when they start to settle in the lower atmosphere. Chem trails then becoming stagnant and clustering is the leading reasons for poor air quality alerts.

We live in a world where we're being taught to fear the future of our climate. At the same time, there's a terrifying reality that's being ignored, which is the unprecedented high level of dangerous chemical contamination and saturation being released, within our sight, onto our children. A debate about flying private jets, driving cars, and burning fossil fuels is occurring while humankind is being poisoned.

Did you ever hear about thousands of birds falling out of the sky? That's from a migration of birds running into a very thick patch of chem trails, being poisoned in the sky and falling to their death. It happens all over the planet.

Algae blooms and chemical clusters in oceans and lakes are from chem trail fallout as well, causing schools of choked fish and other sea life to wash up on shore.

Even with all the energy, time, and knowledge that have been invested into why our bees are dying, it's still a mystery. While theories float around about whether bees are disappearing due to bacteria, genetically modified organisms (GMO) food, or a mysterious bee disease, chem trails are the real main culprit. That's why we're losing our bees.

IGNORING THE TRAILS

No one is allowed to know chem trails are there or believe they're there. This is why everyone who's a public authority ignores chem trails and chem trail planes. This is why militaries and governments ignore chem trails and chem trail planes. This is why the air traffic control towers ignore chem trails and chem trail planes. This is why school institutions don't teach children about chem trails and chem trail planes. This is why universities and university professors don't utter a word about chem trails and chem trail planes. We just go about our lives.

You could be the most powerful public figure in the world having a cookout in your backyard, you could look up at the sky watching the chem trails, and you can't say a word because the people behind it are above all. They are above even the most powerful public figures and above the people who run every country in the world. Most public figures aren't even aware of chem trails. If they inquire, they're told they're just seeing contrails—normal exhaust coming out of a normal plane.

RAINFALL EXPOSURE

It probably isn't hard to remember a time when you got soaked in the rain— whether going for a run in the rain, taking a hike or boat trip without rain gear, or getting caught on the street without an umbrella. Rainfall contains whatever contaminants were suspended in the sky when the rain clouds formed, many of them rogue byproducts undocumented by any agency, that can fill the atmosphere by the hundreds of thousands.

Rain very often carries chemical neuro-antagonists and other brain betrayers such as radioactive particles, barium, jet fuel, vaporized material from chemical factories, and dust particles from agricultural land, both domestically and from other countries, that contain residue of pesticides, herbicides, and fungicides. Yet pollution spewing out of factories, exhaust, dioxins dusting around the atmosphere, and radiation fall-out only represent a fraction of what contaminates the atmosphere. Chem trails are our greatest threat when it comes to rainfall.

As beneficial as rain is, and as pleasant as it can feel to stand out in a warm summer rain, if you're dealing with any sort of chronic or neurological symptoms, it's good to be aware that rain is not as pure as it should be. The term *acid rain* doesn't even scratch the surface as far as what's actually in rain. Even if the rain isn't always really acidic, it still can be loaded with contaminants that are much more problematic and dangerous than the acid factor of rain. Not only does rain soak into our skin; we also breathe in its moisture—and its contaminants—at the same time.

PATHWAYS TO OUR BRAIN

Rain that falls on your head can saturate your scalp and enter your bloodstream quickly, eventually finding a pathway to your brain.

Some of the most dangerous chemicals dropped out of chem trail planes are so highly absorbable that they can absorb into

bone with ease. If you're in a certain part of the world where those most potent chemicals are being dropped in that moment, or where precipitation has gathered around a cluster of the chem trails that have this poison, this variety of chemical can even absorb through your skull. Your skull is living bone and material that's porous when it comes to solvents and nanotechnology chemicals, so in these cases, your skull is not a barrier to the chemical agents that toxic rainfall contains. And because these brain betrayers are so minuscule—basically diluted homeopathically when that condensation formed in the sky—these rainfall contaminants are much more absorbable and aggressive.

This isn't an everyday thing. Most rainfall chemicals absorb into the bloodstream through the skin of the scalp or other skin on the body, and then, if the chemicals eventually find a pathway to the brain, they do so through the bloodstream. Or as rain trickles down our forehead and nose, it's easy for droplets in our sinus cavities and eyes to find their way directly to the brain. Or we breathe in chemicals from the mist of rainfall, and because these agents are potent and elusive, they reach our brains too easily. None of which is to make you fear the next rainy day. Rain is also a gift to us. Rainfall is active, living water with healing properties, which means it's helpful in defusing some of these chemicals. Be aware that getting soaked in a rainstorm can mean a couple of days of worsened symptoms if you're sensitive, and take extra special care of your brain with the guidance in this book to stay healthy.

CHAPTER 27

Radiation and EMF

Common Medical and Transportation Technology

- Airplane travel

- X-rays

- CT (Computerized tomography) scans

- PET (Positron emission tomography) scans

- Fluoroscopy

- MRI (Magnetic resonance imaging)

- Food and water supply

Common Nuclear Exposure

- Current nuclear weapons exposure and current nuclear plant exposure

- Continual atmospheric fallout from past nuclear disasters

- Nuclear test sites

Common Radiofrequency Electromagnetic Fields (EMF)

- Cell phones and other technological devices

- Cell tower EMF

- Wireless Internet

- Microwaves

- Ultrasounds

We absorb radiation from many sources, some of them near constant in our lives and some of them infrequent yet potent.

Any radiation exposure instantly travels through the body and bones. In the long term, radiation shrinks organs—and the brain is an organ. It's one reason why we need to be careful with radiation: even everyday encounters with it can result in mild brain atrophy. More serious brain atrophy can occur from more serious radiation exposure. As you've read throughout this book, our brains can atrophy and shrink for other reasons too. We don't want to add one more instigator.

EXAMPLES OF RADIATION EXPOSURE

The obvious sources of radiation exposure are dental exams, X-rays, and other medical imaging such as CT scans and even (to a lesser degree) MRIs. When someone needs repeated CT scans or frequent dental work, that exposure can build up and have a more extreme effect.

Our brains sustain a milder effect from the everyday radiation we're exposed to from plane flights, cell phones and other devices, contaminated food and water, being near someone who just got an X-ray or other medical imaging test, and the continual atmospheric fallout from past nuclear disasters such as Fukushima. There's also fallout from current-day nuclear testing and nuclear weapons development of which we're unaware. Plus nuclear plants leak an "acceptable" level of radiation, by industrial standards, that's far from acceptable. Where do you think the frog with four eyes comes from? Waterways near these plants. That's definitely not acceptable.

We also inherit radiation, so if anyone in your bloodline ever got an X-ray or visited a shoe store in the days when they imaged feet using a fluoroscope, some radiation likely ended up in you. It takes time and commitment to an anti-radiation protocol—namely, the Medical Medium Heavy Metal Detox Smoothie, which is also a radiation yanker—to say goodbye to it.

MEDICAL EXAM PROTECTIVE MEASURES

Lead bibs provided for dental X-rays provide a façade of total protection. They usually don't provide enough coverage, so I recommend asking for additional protection, and try to get one bib a little higher to protect your thyroid. The same is true if you're getting an X-ray at a medical facility, whether an X-ray of the chest, neck, or elsewhere. Ask for extra gear for protection, beyond what they offer normally, for other parts of your body, not just the part of the body immediately surrounding the area being X-rayed.

So many sources of medical exam radiation are hard to avoid. It's part of the process of seeking help. When people are looking for answers, they go to the doctor with a complaint and the doctor writes a prescription for an X-ray, CT scan, or MRI. (MRI does emit a certain amount of radiation.) From chest X-rays to diagnose lung issues such as bronchitis and pneumonia to arm X-rays to diagnose broken bones, this is where our current medical system is. And yet rarely, if ever, in the X-ray and scanning world do they offer a lead helmet or protective headpiece, so our brains are left exposed. That's why it's important for us to ask for additional bibs to help shield the areas of the body we can—and to work on the radiation removal protocols in this book. Spirulina, a key ingredient in Medical Medium protocols, is essential for radiation exposure.

AIRPORT AWARENESS

Medical Medium information has always warned about radiation contamination from airports and air travel. There is so much radiation being emitted in airports that it would set off radiation detection technology. While you were walking through the rows of passengers waiting for their flights, the device would go wild picking up radiation from all the freshly scanned people and knapsacks and carry-ons fresh off the scanner conveyor belts, now contaminated. That's why it's good to be aware and proactive:

For one, luggage has to be discarded and purchased new periodically. When not in use, keep luggage that has been on a flight far away from your children and pets.

For another, when you're going through security, opt out of the full-body scanner and ask for a pat-down instead. It's perfectly safe to walk through a plain metal detector; it's the airport body scanner device you want to avoid. As you're waiting for your pat-down, try not to lean against the radiation machine that's being used to examine carry-ons. Try to stand a few feet or more away from the machine that's processing and irradiating baggage.

Extraterrestrial space travel, what some might call alien ships, also leave radiation in the atmosphere as they pass through. UFO sightings are not totally understood.

The radiation coming from these craft is not the normal radiation we experience here. Rather, it's radiation of another kind that gets into the atmosphere.

COEXISTING WITH ELECTRICITY

When it comes to electromagnetic fields, our brains can actually adapt to certain electrical currents that are around us. In the last hundred years, our brains have indeed adapted to EMF produced from electricity, electrical wiring, buildings' electrical panels, and appliances such as dishwashers, refrigerators, ovens, stoves, electric cars, lights, power strips and surge protectors, air conditioners, heaters, washing machines, and dryers. With this form of EMF, we've adapted in such a way that when the power is out, even if the temperature is comfortable, many people tend to go mad from withdrawal. And it's not withdrawal from having the luxury of an appliance or electricity; it's withdrawal from the EMF itself—because our brains have learned to coexist with this type of EMF.

As you know well from Part I, "Your Brain Story," our brain is made out of electricity. While it's not the same electricity that powers our homes and appliances, our brain's electricity has learned to coexist with this EMF emitting from all this outside electricity so that our brain can continue to function optimally. When you head to a spiritual retreat in a shack that has no electricity, or you sit in an open field with no electrical conveniences nearby, it's quite an experience. You're going through withdrawal, and your brain is learning to adjust and live without the EMF.

Now, coexisting with the everyday electricity around us is one thing. Let's not confuse that with the EMF emitting from dangerous high-voltage scenarios, such as electrical power stations. That can affect someone's health directly.

FUNNELING CELL SIGNALS

Then there's radiofrequency EMF, which is more aggressive than regular EMF. With radiofrequency EMF, we're no longer talking about simple electricity being used to power an appliance. We're talking about devices such as computers and cell phones interacting with wireless Internet and cell towers. Other sources of radiofrequency EMF include microwaves, "smart" devices, and radar facilities.

There's even cell tower exposure when you're not using your phone. You can shut down your phone and those radiofrequencies are still there, traveling through every single home and office building. So we're getting exposure that way. These radiofrequencies coming from cell towers enter our brain and hit our neurons. This exposure is a bit more aggressive than your typical appliances inside your house. Yet as aggressive as cell tower exposure is, it is not as harmful as other forms of radiofrequency EMF exposure that we'll get to in a moment.

In recent years our brains have been learning to adapt to cell tower EMF because

of radiofrequencies we're exposed to from the military. Military bases, including classified military bases, around the world send out radio frequencies that travel across the planet and away from our planet into the atmosphere. This has been developing since the 1930s, so our brains and neurons have been learning to adapt.

Our present-day cell towers are more aggressive than old-school radio frequencies (that also still exist). Whether 5G now or 6X in the future, transmission technology continues to send stronger signals. Still, these towers' mere presence is not totally where the threat lies when we're talking about EMF exposure and the possibility of compromising our brain health. Again, our brains are learning to adapt to cell towers' waves moving through the environment. What we haven't adapted to is using a device that's connected to a cell tower. When our cell phone is turned on, and especially if we're using the phone, there's additional radio frequency coming to our phone, and that's additional radio frequency to which we have not adapted. When your cell phone is off, that pinpoint radio frequency EMF has dissipated, and now you're back to being surrounded by the radio frequency everyone is surrounded by, unless you're totally off the grid, living on the side of a mountain with no cell towers for many miles.

The pinpointed radio frequency that comes to a device when it's connected to a cellular network is why, when using a cell phone, it's important not to have it pressed up to your ear. You don't want to funnel and target the radio frequency coming from the cell tower to the side of your head, where it can enter your brain in a concentrated fashion. Another reason not to press a cell phone to your ear is that the device itself emits additional forms of radiation when connected to a phone call. Try to use your phone on speakerphone.

(A headset that plugs into your phone is an option if you need privacy. With a wired headset you're at least not getting the radio frequency beam pinpointed to the side of your head. You are still getting an electrical current coming from the phone to the headset, and that mild current goes directly into the sides of the head and can be disrupting or antagonizing to brain cells. If you use a wireless headset or wireless earphones to talk on a cell phone, you'll get a moderate-strength direct cell tower signal to your headset or earphones. That would not happen with the wired version of these accessories.)

Radio frequency EMF exposure warrants taking care of your brain health—because radio frequency EMF creates a free radical toxin. A free radical toxin is made out of toxic energy that forms around brain cells and brain tissue. Especially since we can't avoid EMF altogether, the message here is to keep your neurons strong, keep your glial cells strong. Protect your brain tissue.

WIRELESS INTERNET, COMPUTERIZED DEVICES, AND THE VAMPIRE EFFECT

There are two other EMF elements in play when we're using a computerized device: (1) the computer, tablet, phone, smartwatch, or other device itself, and (2) the wireless Internet signal it may be using.

Wireless Internet signals are surrounding most all of us, whether we activate a device or not. And whether our device is connected to wireless Internet or not, or in airplane mode or not, it emits a form of EMF on its own. Many people can be sensitive to this alone when using any kind of computerized device. When the computer is connected to wireless Internet, this can be intensified. Wireless Internet competes with and opposes our body's electricity. When we're connected to wireless Internet, we get drained because our brain and body have to fight against wireless Internet to sustain their energetic position.

Radiation coming from powered-on devices, whether connected to wireless Internet or not, is one concern. There's also another issue that occurs with devices and wireless Internet signals: the EMF emitted puts a drain on the central nervous system. And not just the brain—also nerves throughout the entire body.

When you're holding your device, or your device is otherwise touching your body (for example, in your pocket), or you're using wireless accessories such as cord-free earphones with your device, an electrical current is drawn away from your body, creating a vampire effect. Instead of drawing blood out of you, computerized devices connected to wireless Internet draw energy from you:

The electrical current inside your body works in a circular continuity, swimming inside only your body. Your electricity does not power someone else's body. Your electricity is not meant to leave your body and go out in a different direction. When you're handling a device connected to wireless Internet, the electrical field that your brain and heart produce that's traveling through your body gets disrupted. Your own electrical frequency exits your brain and body into the device. Many of our computerized devices are a crude form of artificial intelligence (AI). This AI aspect can further feed off our life force as we're in contact with a device. When a computerized phone or other device is not plugged in, it's steadily losing its charge, so it creates additional drain on us. It's like an energy sucker. As we're handling the device, it's drawing from our brain's electricity in a mild way. Sometimes this electrical draw happens in small spurts, sometimes intermittently, sometimes more sustained. This is why people with neurological conditions, including EMF sensitivity, have a harder time with devices. People who are sensitive really feel this draw. They feel like they short-circuit or get drained. Many others don't feel it at all.

These devices have become a part of our everyday functioning. Our job is to reinforce and strengthen the central nervous system so we can rise up to meet the challenges that current technology faces us with in the present day.

"What people need now are answers. Answers to what actually causes brain problems, neurological problems, chronic pain problems, emotional problems, mental health problems—and answers about how to protect the brain. Because you want to protect your brain just like you want to protect anything else in your life."

— Anthony William, Medical Medium

CHAPTER 28

Brain Betrayer Food and Supplement Chemicals

Keep a close eye on food, drink, and supplement ingredient labels to avoid these brain betrayers.

You can learn about each item from the list below in this book's companion, *Brain Saver Protocols, Cleanses & Recipes.* Some of these additives, such as ammonia, won't appear on labeling, so it helps to gain the inside knowledge in that book about where these chemicals sneak into food and supplements.

1. **Aspartame and other artificial sweeteners**

2. **Monosodium glutamate (MSG)** (including seasoning with MSG, fake meats, bottled or packaged sauces, cold cuts, and hot dogs)

3. **Flavors** (natural and artificial)

4. **Alcohol**

5. **Citric acid**

6. **Soft drinks** (conventional and natural)

7. **Preservatives, ammonia, formaldehyde, and nitrates** (including sodium nitrate)

These additives creep into our lives. Often disguised as *"flavors"* or *"flavorings"* on labels, whether natural or artificial, they're much less innocent than they appear. The fact that these ingredients often appear at the end of a food or supplement's ingredient list doesn't make them unthreatening. They're that potent, even in a small amount.

Accountability still has a long way to go when it comes to food labeling. Even if you take care to buy foods and supplements that don't list preservatives as ingredients, it doesn't mean these chemicals don't make their way into your food, or haven't been present in food you ate in the past and then stuck around in your brain, liver, and body. If we're not actively cleansing these brain betrayers, they can stay in our brains, livers, and bodies for decades. For example, the additives in a hot dog and soda you ate at a sports game when you were a kid could still be affecting you today.

Food additives were never supposed to be in the brain. These problematic food and supplement chemicals heighten sensitivities and also create diseased tissue because they're so highly toxic: These chemicals can kill brain cells by eating away at brain tissue, creating pits in the brain, little crevices and craters, similar to how toxic heavy metals work. These chemicals can create lesions, white spots, gray spots, and black spots in brain tissue. These chemicals can spur along brain atrophy.

Problematic food chemicals are toxic invaders that tend to affect the emotional centers of the brain. The emotional centers of the brain are sacred spaces. Humans are constantly struggling to keep emotional stamina strong and balanced. The more aspartame, MSG, or other items from the list above that are in the brain, the more unstable someone can become. What's more, these brain betrayers are highly addictive, making us dependent without even realizing it. That's even more damaging because it means we walk around with the false perception that our brain needs these chemicals, so we consume more and more of them.

Remember, you can read much more in *Brain Saver Protocols, Cleanses & Recipes.*

"Most of us live our lives disconnected from what our brains and bodies need. That's because most of us are unaware of what our brains and bodies really do need."

— Anthony William, Medical Medium

CHAPTER 29

Brain Betrayer Supplements

Often we end up taking supplements without knowing they could be interfering with our healing process, even holding us back from the momentum we desire as we dedicate time and energy to recovery from symptoms and conditions. Below is a list of supplements to look out for to avoid continual setbacks as you're trying to get your life back.

For detailed explanations of these supplements, refer to *Brain Saver Protocols, Cleanses & Recipes.*

These supplements fall into four main categories:

A. Problematic and damaging supplements

B. Mildly problematic supplements

C. Overrated or overused supplements

D. Quality concerns

The following supplements are listed alphabetically within each category:

A. Problematic and Damaging

1. Alkaline ionizer water machines

2. Apple cider vinegar (ACV) and ACV supplements taken internally

3. Bentonite and other clays taken internally

4. Caffeine-based energy supplements

5. Charcoal taken internally

6. Chlorella

7. Chlorine dioxide (sodium chlorite)

8. Cod liver oil and shark liver oil

9. Colostrum

10. Deer antler (also called deer velvet and antler velvet)

11. Diatomaceous earth (DE)

12. Digestive bitters

13. Essential oils taken internally

14. Fat burners

15. Fish oil and krill oil

16. Gut powder blends

17. Herbal tinctures in alcohol

18. Hydrochloric acid (HCl or HCL) supplements

19. L-carnitine and L-arginine

20. Mineral oil

21. Mushroom coffee (with caffeine)

22. Oyster supplements

23. Pearl powder

24. Sodium bicarbonate (baking soda) when taken internally in large amounts

25. Turpentine oil

26. Whey protein powder

27. Zeolites

B. Mildly Problematic

28. Amino acid supplement combinations (some amino acids, such as L-carnitine and L-arginine, trigger viruses by feeding them)

29. Chicken cartilage

30. Desiccated animal organs and glandular supplements (including liver, adrenal gland, spleen, kidney, stomach, pancreas, brain, tongue, and heart; also including bovine serum)

31. Electrolyte powders and beverages

32. Herbal combination powders (low-quality mixes of many herbs and questionable ingredients)

33. Iron supplements (that are not plant-based)

34. Neem oil (taken internally)

35. Oil pulling

36. Pine needle tea

37. Pre-workout supplements

38. Senna leaf

C. Overrated or Overused

These are supplements that are heralded as highly beneficial and important. The reality is, they take up space, cost money, and don't deliver the results someone needs when they're suffering chronically:

39. CBD (cannabidiol)

40. Chlorophyll

41. Collagen

42. Fruit and vegetable powders (low-quality, dehydrated blends of common fruits and vegetables with only a few specks each of dozens of foods per capsule, which does not offer enough for the physical body to utilize)

43. Fulvic minerals, fulvic acid, humic acid, humic minerals, and shilajit

44. Maca root

45. Plant protein powder

46. Prebiotics (including inulin powder)

47. Probiotics

48. Vitamin D overuse or megadoses

D. Quality Concerns

These are supplements where it's especially important to seek out high-quality forms because they're frequently produced with low-quality ingredients or problematic additives such as preservatives:

49. Cyanocobalamin (low-quality vitamin B_{12})

50. Low-quality colloidal silver

51. Low-quality zinc

52. MCT oil (large quantities *and* low-quality versions; be especially cautious when made from palm kernel oil)

53. Multivitamins and hair-skin-nail supplements

54. Oregano oil

55. Prenatals (even when high quality, don't provide enough support on their own)

Remember, you can read details about each supplement above—and why it appears in this list—in this book's companion, *Brain Saver Protocols, Cleanses & Recipes.*

CHAPTER 30

Brain Betrayer Foods

You may look at this list of brain betrayer foods and think, *This is a list of what I should be eating.* That's how misleading food trends and food advice can be. Some of the foods in this chapter slow down, interfere with, or even stop the healing process. Some of the foods accelerate neurological symptoms and chronic illness. And some of these foods start additional health problems.

While it may seem overwhelming to try to avoid one or more of the brain betrayer foods, know that the restored health you get out of it will be more than worth it. It's not about deprivation or judgment. You're not a good or bad person based on what you eat.

Go slowly if you want:

Experiment with replacing a few of the top items on this list with some of the healing brain cell foods in Chapter 41, "Brain Cell Food and Filler Food."

Check out the Cravings Shifter Brain Shot in Chapter 42, "Medical Medium Brain Shot Therapy," for support.

Consider a 10-day Brain Shot Therapy Cleanse option from Chapter 43, or a 15-day Heavy Metal Detox Cleanse option from Chapter 45, knowing that you could someday work up to any of the longer cleanse options in those chapters if you wish.

You can also find over 100 health-promoting recipes in this book's companion title, *Brain Saver Protocols, Cleanses & Recipes.* Keeping those recipes nearby, along with the brain cell foods list in this book, will remind you that you have delicious alternatives to the brain betrayer foods in this chapter.

Find detailed explanations of these brain betrayer foods in *Brain Saver Protocols, Cleanses & Recipes.*

These foods are listed with the worst at the top. If you're sick or suffering and looking for relief, start by avoiding the foods at the top of this list. As you seek more healing, you can continue to work your way down the list.

1. **Eggs**

2. **Dairy** (including milk, cheese, butter, ghee, yogurt, cream, and kefir)

3. **Gluten**

4. **Caffeine** (including coffee, green tea, matcha, chocolate, and cacao)

5. **Alcohol** (consumed more than occasionally)

6. **Vinegar** (including apple cider vinegar, or ACV)

7. **Pork products** (including ham, bacon, sausage, pancetta, canned pork product, lard, pulled pork, pork chops, pork belly, and pork rinds)

8. **Tuna**

9. **Corn** (including corn products such as corn syrup and corn starch)

10. **Industrial food oils** (including vegetable oil, palm oil, palm kernel oil, canola [rapeseed] oil, corn oil, safflower oil, soybean oil, cottonseed oil, peanut oil, hydrogenated oils, and margarine)

11. **Kombucha**

12. **Nutritional yeast**

13. **Soy** (including tofu, edamame, soy milk, soy sauce, miso, soybeans, soy nuts, texturized vegetable protein [TVP], soy protein powder, and artificial meat products made with soy)

14. **GMO (bioengineered) foods**

15. **Bone broth**

16. **Problematic fish and seafood** (including catfish, red snapper, striped bass, bluefish, swordfish, grouper, clams, oysters, mussels, shrimp, crab, lobster, squid, octopus, scallops, flounder, tilapia, and shark)

17. **Lamb**

18. **Salt** (including high-quality varieties)

19. **Fermented foods** (including sauerkraut, pickled preserves, sourdough, cheese, and yogurt [animal- or plant-based])

20. **Grains eaten in an unproductive way** (meaning grains, even gluten-free, eaten with fats)

It's no mystery how brain betrayer foods enter our lives: we eat and drink them. What does sometimes sneak up on us is how much of them we eat. For example, it's easy to eat a high-fat diet because we've been dazzled by the high-protein trend, not stopping to think or even realizing that protein sources are almost always fat sources too. On top of which, now we're being told that lots of fat is good for us, so we pile more fats onto our plates, or into our blenders as we make our trendy smoothies, with no idea that we're doing our brains a disservice.

Some of these items, such as canola oil, nutritional yeast, and corn, frequently make it into our meals without our knowledge. Any time you see that an oil *blend* is being used, beware—there's a good chance it contains one of these brain betrayers. Even oils labeled as pure are sometimes diluted with canola or corn oil, so seek out high-quality oil whenever possible and, even better, limit your use of oil in general to keep your fat consumption lower to protect your body and brain.

The main issue with most of these brain betrayer foods is that they feed viruses in the body such as EBV and bacteria such as *Streptococcus*—viruses and bacteria that many, many people unknowingly harbor in dormant form. These viruses and bacteria can come out of dormancy if they receive the right fuel. Some of these foods don't directly feed viruses and bacteria. Instead, usually because of their high fat content, these other foods foster an environment in our body that allows pathogens to thrive. Either way, whether a food directly feeds pathogens or fosters a hospitable environment for pathogens, the food doesn't help *us* thrive. Viruses and bacteria especially proliferate when we're eating eggs, milk, cheese, butter, all other dairy products, gluten, soy, pork, corn, or an overall high-fat diet.

As you read in Chapter 4, "Your Viral Brain," publicly known medical research and science aren't aware that viruses "eat." Viruses do eat, and that's how they stay alive. They don't exist on mystical energy; viruses stay active by absorbing unproductive chemical compounds through their outer membranes. Viruses then process whatever they take in and release it as waste matter such as neurotoxins and dermatoxins. When they reach the central nervous system, these neurotoxins cause hundreds of symptoms and conditions.

Some of these brain betrayer foods themselves are also not good for the brain:

We're often told eggs are good for the brain because of their omegas. We're not told that because eggs are filled with hormones that intercept healthy hormones involved with the brain, any benefit is outweighed. Same goes for dairy. Even eggs and dairy sourced farm fresh from organic, grass-fed, pasture-raised, and/or free-range cows and chickens contain hormones that intercept and confuse the hormones involved in our systems.

Caffeinated foods and beverages are acidic, dehydrating, and hard on the central nervous system, plus they tire out the adrenals.

Vinegars are acidic and create chronic dehydration.

Brain betrayer foods with MSG, such as nutritional yeast, interfere with neurotransmitter activity and neuron strength.

Remember, you can read much more about these brain betrayer foods in *Brain Saver Protocols, Cleanses & Recipes.*

"Decades go by—generations go by—as we take the wrong steps for our health. History repeats itself, trends get recycled over and over, and every five years there's a new round of people who aren't feeling well and are ready to buy into the seemingly smart advice about our brains."

— Anthony William, Medical Medium

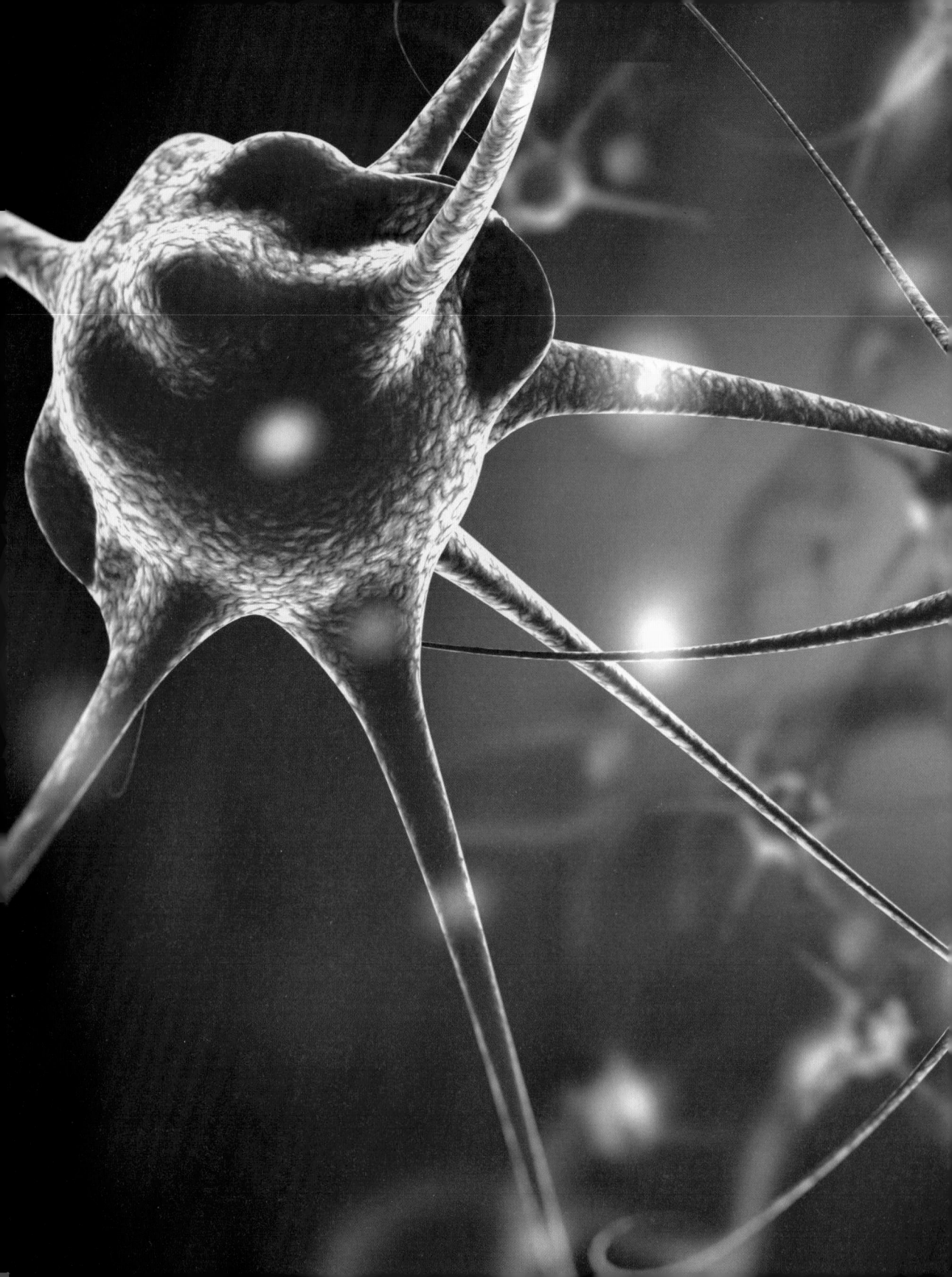

BRAIN INVASION

SACRED HEADSPACE

How to Use Part IV, "Brain Invasion"

- Anything that affects our mental health can feel like an outside source of some kind is invading our body's sanctuary. Our headspace is sacred. Our brain space is sacred. Our mind and consciousness are sacred. As we become empowered, our trust becomes restored. We have the ability to heal when we know the truth of what invades our brain.

- In the chapters that follow, you'll gain insights into several of the most common, perplexing, and complex states of suffering: anxiety, depression, eating disorders, obsessive-compulsive disorder (OCD), bipolar disorder, and Alzheimer's and dementia. For detailed explanations of dozens more symptoms and conditions, turn to Part V, "Your Pain and Suffering Enlightened."

- With the information you discover here, you can customize your own healing protocol from Part VI, "Bringing Back Your Brain," and this book's companion, *Brain Saver Protocols, Cleanses & Recipes*. Your symptom or condition isn't who you truly are. Now it's time to come back home.

CHAPTER 31

Anxiety

Not one person on the planet has anxiety that's identical to another's. Everyone's anxiety is different. Two people's anxiety may share many similarities—there could be a similar tightening of the chest, constricting of the throat, funny feeling in the stomach, feeling like they can't sit still, mouth becoming dry, nervousness, sweaty palms, overwhelmed sensation, racing heart, racing thoughts, arms going numb, feeling like they can't breathe, or shaky, weak legs. Yet even if two people share any of these symptoms, it's not possible to have the same anxiety.

For example, I often meet people who get overwhelmed quite easily. While we can all identify with what that word *overwhelmed* means, we get overwhelmed for different reasons, and even when it's two individuals becoming overwhelmed for the same reason, the anxiety is entirely different. You'll find that when they get anxious, people describe their anxiousness differently. Some call it "anxiety" without being sure that's what it is. Some live life with nervousness and other symptoms—maybe

a phobia or a sensation like they can't talk when they're around certain people—and never realize it was anxiety the whole time.

Was it anxiety? What *is* anxiety? What does the term really mean? Anxiety is a confusion in the medical industry and always has been. It refers to a set of symptoms, or even one symptom, where the root cause can't be identified. If someone is experiencing uncomfortable symptoms that are somehow interrupting their normal function on a regular basis and they've gone through medical testing looking for obvious problems and all checks out fine, they'll usually find themselves at the psychiatrist's or doctor's office being offered medication and told they have anxiety.

Interrupting normal function is a key part of the definition of anxiety. Yes, it's part of the human condition to feel some anxiousness about life. Here in this chapter, we're talking about an anxiety disorder, one that interferes with someone's life.

Anxiety can be mild to severe. With mild anxiety, it's beyond anxiousness. You're aware of mild anxiety, it's being brought to your attention enough that it's affecting some of your interactions and decisions, and yet this mild anxiety is not holding you back from most things you want to do in your life. With more severe anxiety, it's impeding life. You could be seized up, sick, or stuck in bed, shaking with anxiety.

The label *anxiety* can be applied when someone has panic attacks or shortness of breath; gets completely overwhelmed with responsibilities, uncertainties, and fears of life; or has the feeling of being seized up, where it's hard to talk, their entire body goes numb, and they have the feeling of not being able to get air in their lungs. Anxiety could be experienced as the body drenching in sweat, with arms and hands becoming freezing cold and uncontrollable shivers and shakes that eventually build to uncontrollable convulsions. Or anxiety could feel like you can't sit still, like you want to jump out of your skin, like you need to keep busy to avoid a panic attack, like you can't be alone and always have to be around someone. There are a lot of different anxiety symptoms someone can exhibit. Mild symptoms of anxiety include mild heart racing and funny sensations in the abdomen.

Many times people experience other physical symptoms with and around their anxiety, such as vision issues, eye floaters, and dizziness. In this case, they have more than anxiety—they have a virus causing additional symptoms—yet it's all bundled up as one and diagnosed as anxiety. It's very common for an anxiety sufferer to find the symptoms they experience are misinterpreted as part of their anxiety.

The true nature of your anxiety and symptoms won't be understood by today's medical research and science even when anxiety seems clear, like when you start developing symptoms at a difficult, stressful moment in life. Maybe it's a struggle you're going through, enormous stress, extreme grief over the loss of a loved one, a relationship breakup, divorce, loss of a job, or any kind of trial you can be up against in life. If anxiety symptoms start to show themselves, it seems obvious: the trauma must be the cause.

Is it? A lot of people go through some really hard times and don't exhibit any symptoms of anxiety. A lot of people go through hard times and do exhibit symptoms of anxiety. What makes them different? If trauma were the true, underlying cause of anxiety, no one would ever skate free. Every single difficult thing that happened would produce anxiety on some level, whether panic attacks, flipping sensations in the stomach, crippling stomachaches, phobias, an inability to express oneself, tightness of the chest, the feeling of your body shutting down, and on and on—we would all get that all the time from everything that challenged us.

Besides which, many people haven't had serious challenges. Life is smooth, without too many speed bumps, yet they can still be crippled by anxiety, even when everything in their life is going well.

This shows that it's not trauma or stress that's the true cause of anxiety—those are more like triggers. They can trigger some people while not triggering others. What are they triggering? A vulnerability already inside the body. It's not an illness so much as a true cause, something that's always been sitting there that finally ignites. That something could have been sitting there for six months, a year, or an entire lifetime.

WHAT CAUSES ANXIETY

For an anxiety condition to develop, there has to be an underlying physical vulnerability. Someone could go through the worst child abuse, for example, and not develop anxiety if they don't have the underlying factors we'll examine. Without those causes, anxiety would not exist. A fear would exist, a nervousness would exist, a distrust would exist, perhaps a tendency to always err on the side of caution—because we're human and we experience a range of emotions in response to our life experiences. For all of that to develop into a crippling anxiety condition is entirely different.

When it's true anxiety, the kind that limits us and keeps us from optimally functioning and making the choices we wish we could make, there's something else happening inside the body affecting the brain.

Many people experience anxiety on and off through life, even when everything is fine. They're going along, financially stable, traveling, loving their work—maybe they don't even have to work—and then they get their first panic attack and then their second panic attack, and they're off to the doctor's, ending up with medication and a diagnosis of anxiety. That's without trauma or stress, so what's the trigger? It's different

altogether. Triggers can come in all shapes and sizes. They can be elusive, deceptive, mysterious, undetectable, or they can arrive in the most obvious forms. You'll read more about triggers soon. For someone to develop the mysterious, chronic condition that eventually becomes labeled as anxiety, there needs to be at least one core, foundational neurotoxic cause present.

In the past, I've always said that chronic anxiety is caused by toxic heavy metals and/or viruses, with emotional injury sometimes acting as a trigger to these underlying causes. This is still true. It's also time to broaden this definition of cause, as chemical exposures in our world are now evolving to such a degree. Anxiety is caused by neurotoxic exposures, which include toxic heavy metals and viruses—as well as toxic chemicals and other exposures that are injurious to our nerves.

Neurotoxic chemicals are in high production at this time. They're being placed into fragrances, perfumes, colognes, scented candles, air fresheners, detergents, fabric softeners, and cleaning products. Neurotoxic chemicals also include pesticides being dropped over communities worldwide for mosquitos and other insects; herbicides being sprayed in yards, properties, buildings, parking lots, communities, towns, villages, agricultural land, highways, and roadsides; and fungicides being sprayed on all new clothing, blankets, sheets, bedding, pillows, couches, furnishings, fixtures, and car interiors. Caffeine, MSG, and radiation can also be harsh on the nerves.

Emotional upheaval can cause acute, temporary anxiety due to fight-or-flight adrenaline surges. (Read more in Chapter 5, "Your Emotional Brain.") Yet on its own, emotional upheaval does not cause chronic anxiety. If the anxiety lasts and becomes chronic, it means that at least one of these underlying physical causes is present.

INTERCONNECTED CAUSES

Anxiety is often caused by a mix of factors. Someone could have all three causes of anxiety at once, or a combination: toxic heavy metals, a viral load, and/or other neurotoxic exposures.

For example, if someone has mysterious tightness of the chest with their anxiety, this could be caused by viral or toxic heavy metal or chemical irritation, or all three, inflaming a region of the vagus nerves.

The causes of anxiety are often interconnected:

Many neurotoxic exposures contribute to anxiety in two ways: (1) the substances themselves are toxic to the nerves as they touch the nerves and the nerves become allergic, *and* (2) the substances feed and trigger viruses.

And many toxic chemicals, such as fragrances and pesticides, are toxic in two ways: (1) because the substances contain toxic heavy metals in their chemical formulas, *and* (2) because the chemical formulas themselves are injurious to nerves and feed and trigger viruses. Some of these chemicals, even without containing toxic heavy metals or acting as viral triggers, can be enough to create a neurotoxic reaction, and eventual nerve injury, that causes anxiety.

There are dozens of examples of different variations in each individual's cause of anxiety. The combinations are endless: different amounts of toxic heavy metals, different viruses, different toxic chemicals, different viral fuel, different locations of these exposures in the brain and body, different triggers, different challenges. In each person there's a variability in exposures, even on the most minute level, which makes each person's anxiety unique.

Toxic Heavy Metals Interfering with Electricity

People with anxiety can have toxic heavy metals residing inside the brain, and these metals weaken neurotransmitters and interfere with electrical impulses driving through the organ, which creates an automatic vulnerability.

As you read about in Chapter 3, "Your Alloy Brain," these metals enter into the brain before birth, throughout childhood, and even in adulthood. In every single person, there's a different combination of metals in a different area of the brain—different on the most subtle levels—and this accounts for each person's anxiety being different in sometimes the most subtle ways. Some people's anxiety may amp up at night, in the morning, or only every other day. There are so many variables to what triggers it.

Take note: The toxic heavy metals that reside inside our brains are not a trigger for anxiety. They're a cause. We can't get confused about that. What the medical industry should be identifying as a true *cause* of anxiety is the presence of toxic heavy metals sitting inside the brain that oxidize over time. When they oxidize, the toxic heavy metals outgas, leach, and corrode. That corrosion saturates adjacent brain tissue, interfering with electrical pathways—the electricity of the brain—as well as diminishing neurotransmitter chemicals by draining the electrical grid inside the brain and altering hundreds of chemical functions that reside inside the brain.

Viruses Creating Inflammation

The body harboring viruses is another cause of anxiety. These pathogens can live in the liver and other organs and from there, affect the cranial nerves such as the vagus, trigeminal, and facial nerves, as well as the phrenic nerves and the central nervous system. Viruses can also get into the brain, directly causing brain inflammation, although most people with anxiety don't have viruses inside the brain. Almost all viral-related cases of anxiety are caused by viruses in other parts of the body such as the liver. In many cases a virus will also inhabit cranial nerves. For example, shingles and herpes simplex 1 can be harbored in the facial and trigeminal nerves, while EBV can be in the vagus nerves.

Toxic heavy metals are the main creators of anxiety. Yet viruses and toxic heavy metals often go together—because viruses feed off heavy metals: consume them, absorb them, and release waste matter called *neurotoxins*, which you read about in Chapter 4, "Your Viral Brain," and Chapter 6, "Your Inflamed Cranial Nerves." Viruses eat. They eat toxic heavy metals and other toxic chemicals that shouldn't be in the body, and they even feed on the unproductive foods we eat.

Once they're excreted by virus cells, these viral neurotoxins enter the bloodstream, float around, and become allergens to nerves close to and even inside the brain. Viral neurotoxins have an extreme saturation rate because today's toxic chemicals that a virus is eating and processing are different from the toxic chemicals of yesteryear, absorbing easily into tissues and nerves. Viruses are eating much more toxic substances than they ever did. Even the smallest amounts of viral neurotoxins can make a nerve sensitive, which can trigger any form of anxiety. Viral neurotoxins can enter into the brain with ease, causing an allergic response there too. Mild headaches, dizziness, and brain fog are common allergic responses to neurotoxins in the brain. This is one reason why additional symptoms often accompany anxiety.

You don't have to be high in toxic heavy metals or toxic chemicals to get viral neurotoxins. You just need viral fuel. Viruses simply feeding on brain betrayer foods in our diet such as eggs can still produce neurotoxins that can cause anxiety. While it may not be the most potent form of neurotoxin creating the most debilitating version of anxiety, it's still anxiety.

Once again, viruses are not triggers for anxiety; they're causes. Keep this in mind because when publicly known medical research and science find Medical Medium information about viruses playing a role in certain conditions, they will classify viruses as triggers, not causes. Remember this: viruses are a true cause of anxiety all on their own.

Chemical Brews Fueling Viruses and Irritating Nerves

As a result of chemical innovation, anxiety is one of the biggest symptoms people are struggling with right now. Viruses are adapting to the new chemical creations, feeding on the chemicals and creating new varieties of viral neurotoxins that saturate and aggravate nerves.

The chemicals in fragrances (such as scented candles), chemical industry domestic invaders (such as cleaning products), and chemical neuroantagonists (such as pesticides) can also be neurotoxic themselves. These chemicals can affect nerves directly by physically attaching to nerves and becoming nerve irritants. In order for these chemicals to create anxiety on their own like this, there has to be long-term or large amounts of exposure, or an already sensitive nervous system from viruses, toxic heavy metals, and/or radiation.

These new chemical industry brews are becoming so potent that eventually they'll overthrow stand-alone toxic heavy metals. Chemical formulas on their own, even without toxic heavy metals in the recipe, are becoming as damaging and problematic for the central nervous system as toxic heavy metals, if not more so. On top of this, many new chemical concoctions contain both these dangerously advanced chemicals *and* toxic heavy metals.

Radiation Weakening Nerves

Depending on the situation, radiation can be a trigger or cause of anxiety. Although the effect of radiation from an X-ray or CT scan could be immediate, it could also contribute to anxiety years later. Radiation has a tendency to slow-cook nerves over time, even over decades, eventually weakening those nerves so that the person is more susceptible to anxiety. Even if someone's radiation exposure was years ago and has been slowly minimizing in the body as time has passed, that radiation still has the ability to weaken nerves. Someone having many X-rays and CT scans 10 years ago could be the cause of their anxiety today. Plus other forms of radiation exposure that we encounter on a daily basis can build toxicity—for example, airport scanners and cell phones. While radiation is not a fuel for viruses, radiation lowers the immune system because it gets deep into our bones.

If someone is exposed to *minimal* radiation on and off over the years of their life, that's when it can just be a trigger for anxiety problems by affecting already weakened nerves. When someone gets a larger amount of radiation exposure, whether all at once or accumulated over the years, that's when radiation can actually damage the nerves, taking it from a trigger into a cause of anxiety.

ANXIETY TRIGGERS

The term *trigger* is a tricky one. It's being used right now in the alternative and conventional medical industry in a way that makes someone believe they've found the cause of anxiety and yet never identifies the cause. With the main focus staying on triggers, it means no one's going to get down to the root of anxiety. Instead they're stuck playing the triggers game. They're trying to treat the triggers, *thinking* they're fixing the causes, thinking they have it under control. The anxiety keeps coming back again because they're not fixing the real, physical issues.

Confrontation with a coworker in the workplace, creating stress, is a *trigger* for anxiety because it prompts surges of adrenaline to enter the brain and alter brain chemistry, intensifying heat around neurotransmitters and electrical impulses. The *cause* of someone's anxiety is the presence of toxic heavy metals such as mercury and aluminum in the brain, weakening neurotransmitter activity and hindering neuron strength. The toxic heavy metals in the brain (cause) set the stage so that when adrenaline is released from any kind of stress in the workplace (trigger), the adrenaline intensifies heat, placing stress upon already compromised neurotransmitters, electrical impulses, and neurons inside the brain. Note the cause-trigger difference.

Similarly, social anxiety is a common experience. Trying to socialize can be very difficult when struggling to manage anxiety. If you start to feel that your communication is coming across as uneasy to others, it can be a confidence breaker, giving you the feeling that your intentions in the conversation are misunderstood. Plus social functions often occur in very stimulating environments such as parties. Still, socializing itself is not the cause of the anxiety. It's a *trigger*. Neurotoxic exposures that have disrupted the brain and nervous system are the *cause* of the panic attack someone may have upon walking into a party.

Exercise can *trigger* someone with anxiety if their vagus nerves are inflamed from viral neurotoxins fueled by toxic heavy metals. The virus and toxic heavy metals are the *cause* of the anxiety.

A food somebody is eating could trigger off a bout of anxiety—whether in the form of a panic attack, tightness in the chest, a strangulation sensation in the throat, dry mouth, or the like—as soon as that food enters the stomach or even the mouth. The food is only a *trigger* because the food is causing peristaltic action, which sets off sensitive, inflamed vagus nerves. Once again, toxic heavy metals, other neurotoxic exposures, and/or viruses are the *cause*.

Lack of the right food can also be a trigger: low electrolytes, low trace mineral salts, B_{12} deficiency, low glucose uptake because of insulin resistance, adrenal fatigue from caffeine use, and low critical chemical compounds can all act as anxiety triggers. (Read more in Chapter 7, "Your Burnt Out, Deficient

Brain.") When what we consume isn't rebuilding and replenishing neurotransmitters and other chemicals inside the brain, anxiety can start to show itself. Deficiency is only a *trigger* to a bigger underlying problem that's the *cause*, whether toxic heavy metals, a high load of neurotoxins from a virus, a high level of radiation exposure through the years, or a high load of other toxic chemicals that we can encounter in our daily lives.

If the industry does connect the dots and realize that toxic heavy metals, viruses, and other toxic exposures are involved with anxiety, both alternative and conventional medicine will mistakenly identify them as only triggers. That minimizes what's really happening and can intrude on your ability to heal.

Examples of Anxiety Triggers

Here are a few examples of anxiety triggers. This is not an exhaustive list:

- Blood being drawn for blood tests

- Donating blood

- Intermittent fasting done wrong

- New relationships

- Running on adrenaline all day

- Not eating consistently

- Not sleeping enough

- Having a newborn baby

- Cosmetic procedures

- Surgeries

- Emotional ups and downs

- Food poisoning

The Fine Line between Trigger and Cause

In some cases an exposure can act as either a trigger or a cause of anxiety, or both, depending on the circumstance. As you read earlier in this chapter, that's because some exposures are neurotoxic themselves, and at the same time, they can lower someone's immune system and/or directly fuel viruses. Here are a few examples:

- Perfume, cologne, air fresheners, and scented candles

- Dental work

- Medical treatments

- Pesticides, herbicides, and fungicides

- Consuming caffeine

- Consuming MSG

Anxiety Triggering Anxiety

Anxiety has the ability to compound on itself: anxiety can trigger anxiety. This is because during a bout of anxiety, the adrenals get triggered into fight-or-flight. Someone can become nervous or anxiety-ridden over having anxiety, prompting a vicious cycle that creates more intense anxiety. When this happens, anxiety can take on a life of its own.

This is a type of posttraumatic stress disorder (PTSD) that can develop around having anxiety. If you have difficulty breathing during an anxiety attack, then breathing in general can become fear-inducing, which means you have a certain level of PTSD. Many people fear passing out during a panic attack. They fear they're going to die because the panic is so intense and difficult, or because it feels like the panic takes control over their body as they're hyperventilating to the point where they get dizzy, can't breathe, and feel like they're dying. If this happens to you, remind yourself that if you ever do pass out from a panic attack, you're not going to die. You're going to wake up shortly after passing out, start to stabilize, and catch your breath. Your breathing will even out, and you'll be okay.

If anxiety is chronic, meaning the bouts of fight-or-flight adrenaline happen persistently, it can eventually create some mild adrenal fatigue. Adrenal fatigue is not uncommon with someone who's battling long-term, chronic anxiety.

When Triggers Change

Triggers of anxiety can also change—which is another indication that they're merely triggers and not causes. That triggers change and shift is a confusing aspect when someone is trying to make sense of anxiety.

A food, for example, that seems to be triggering panic attacks at one point may not do it again, yet that person could continue to experience anxiety on and off. The food trigger goes away yet the anxiety stays: it means the food trigger didn't create the anxiety. Triggers can shape-shift. A trigger can disappear and appear as something else. It can change direction: it once was this food, and now it's something completely different.

When triggers such as foods, people, events, circumstances, and fears change, it shows that they weren't the original source of the anxiety. Some people start having panic attacks the moment they enter a car, and they can't drive anymore. Professionals may claim that an association with the car is the problem, and they should stay out of the car. Then sometimes a car ride won't do it anymore. Here's what's really going on beneath the surface with driving anxiety: many car-ride panic attacks come from the cranial nerves getting overstimulated when driving. For example, optic or facial nerves endure a level of stress as you're looking through a windshield or window from within a moving car. All cranial nerves receive information about your surroundings as you're driving or riding as a passenger in a vehicle. Someone crossing the street, catching a STOP sign in time, going through a yellow light, someone behind you flashing their headlights, someone cutting you off, somebody waving their hand and letting you go, merging, driving at high speeds, and then the processing of where you're going and the time needed to get there all weigh in as factors. This is all part of the overstimulation process of the cranial nerves. When these cranial nerves are inflamed, it becomes overload. Alarm bells ring as neurons are beginning to generate more heat than normal. The cranial nerves were already inflamed beforehand, and then the stimulation of driving became the anxiety *trigger*. One car ride could be less stimulating than another on any given day, or the nerves could be less inflamed, in either case leading to less anxiety.

ANXIETY AND OCD

Anxiety is not OCD, and OCD is not anxiety. They are two very different things. A person can have OCD and not have anxiety, and a person can have anxiety and not have OCD. Or a person can have both OCD and anxiety. It's important to understand them each in their own right. Read more in Chapter 34, "Obsessive-Compulsive Disorder."

THE EBB AND FLOW OF ANXIETY

Our brain and body fight for us and have the ability to overcome obstacles. Our brain and body find ways to compensate, to hold some form of systemic balance, keeping us as operational as possible under the circumstances we're given. New cells are produced, old cells die, and someone's bouts of anxiety may come and go, no longer triggered by the same factors, because our cells that held the underlying toxins have changed. That said, having new cells doesn't automatically erase old symptoms. When old cells die and new cells are produced, the new cells still carry a level of toxins left from the old, dying cells in the brain and nervous system if we're not actively working on extracting the toxins.

Part of the reason why anxiety can ebb and flow is due to this brain and nerve cell renewal, along with our brain and body's adaptive ability. It may be that someone's anxiety is only with them for a short time in college, and then they don't see anxiety for another couple of years until a stressful time occurs, like a breakup in a relationship or a pregnancy—where they're using all their reserves to create a baby so those reserves aren't there anymore to keep their brain at the strength needed to overcome the toxic heavy metals or viral neurotoxins in the brain. All along, they still had a level of toxic heavy metals or viral neurotoxins, and they were able to cope. Then came a trigger that affected their resources and strength.

Our brain and body's ability to adapt is especially present when we're younger. As we age and we're not filling our brain up with the critical components it needs, we worsen. With new awareness we can change that. We can overcome anxiety. When somebody removes toxic heavy metals from the brain and restores the brain and nerve tissue—which can be done—anxiety will diminish. The many different varieties of symptoms can disappear. Or some anxiety symptoms may persist, at reduced levels, because a person is still viral. In that case they can work on getting rid of viruses that are living inside their body and nervous system. To heal from anxiety, we want to free ourselves of *any* neurotoxic factor, whether toxic heavy metals, viral activity, or other toxic exposures such as fragrances and chemical neuroantagonists. Finding relief from anxiety takes this understanding of the big picture.

For specific anxiety support beyond what's offered in Part VI, "Bringing Back Your Brain," refer to the Anxiety protocol, Cranial Nerve Inflammation protocol, and/or PTSD protocol in *Brain Saver Protocols, Cleanses & Recipes*.

For specific support for anxiousness (milder and less disruptive than anxiety), refer to the Anxiousness protocol.

"Everyone is under so much pressure from so many directions. Our emotions are getting invaded and manipulated like never before from factors that are clouding and disrupting and unsteadying and toying with what our emotions are meant to communicate."

— Anthony William, Medical Medium

CHAPTER 32

Depression

When we hear someone has depression, we often have a sense of what that means. They may feel hopeless. They may feel like their existence is worthless. They may feel guilty even though they haven't committed any crime. Nothing they do feels like an accomplishment. They may feel lost, even if they're where they're supposed to be. Many people who have depression could be around a loved one they want to be around and still feel like they're supposed to be somewhere else. A lot of people with depression feel like they're missing out on life, even if they can't put their finger on exactly what they're missing.

Along with these experiences of depression, there can be an inability to receive any relief. Depression compounds upon itself because part of the person's consciousness knows they tried so many avenues to get relief, so many suggestions from friends and family members and loved ones, that the feeling of failure sets in, which adds to the depression. If someone works hard to find a way to change the depression, alter it, find a way to navigate through it, find relief, and none of that alleviates the depression, that person can feel like they've let down the people around them who care. They can even feel they've let down their psychiatrist, counselor, and/or other health professional.

Then there's the word *depression* itself. Having depression is one thing. Being labeled with the term can feel like a curse because depression is not a physical diagnosis of a physical problem that can be seen by a physician. So then the burden falls on the person suffering with depression, where the depression is unexplainable, it's mysterious. This is why depression is so difficult, why it eats at the core the fabric of someone's heart and soul. To have a feeling of doom, a constant feeling of dissatisfaction, a feeling of fear and guilt and shame—it all muddles up and becomes one big feeling, and that feeling can only be described with this phantom word that everybody uses: *depression*.

MORE THAN A STATE OF MIND

Just like anxiety, everyone's depression has a different feeling, a different sensation involved. It's also easy to use the word *depressed* casually when you don't suffer seriously from depression. It's a word that people adopt who have very low levels of depression at certain times of life, which is difficult all on its own. Then there's the experience of someone who's gravely emotionally ill from suffering with depression. This range of how depression exhibits itself creates confusion for health authorities.

Depression is not just a state of mind that someone's purposely keeping themselves in. Yet to this day, many consider that to be what depression is. That's another reason why it's so hard to live with the illness. Depression is still sometimes viewed as a state of consciousness someone's deciding to stay in, maybe even to manipulate others around them, such as family members, friends, and loved ones. If depression is coupled with any other mental conditions, the depression is usually taken more seriously by the people and professionals around that individual. If depression is not coupled with other mental conditions and it's just depression on its own, that makes it most difficult to be taken seriously, especially if the depression is severe.

People who have depression know they have depression. Depression is instantly understood by an individual. While the why or how of the depression may be baffling, and depression may be hard for a person to describe, it's a knowing. They know what the feeling of depression is, and they know the feeling is real.

The lack of understanding about depression in the wider world reveals itself in the mixed messages out there about depression. On the one hand, there can be a hesitance to take depression seriously. On the other hand, it's commonplace to say, "If you are a depression sufferer, these may be your symptoms, and take this drug." Antidepressant medications are frequently prescribed, even if depression is not what someone is suffering from.

People with depression become desperate. If they're in the stage of fighting for relief and fighting to rise out of the depression, they'll try anything. Then sometimes the depression becomes so severe that they lose their sense of fight, losing even the desire to want treatment. This can often illustrate whether a case of depression is mild or severe. In a mild case of depression, the person will fight like a fish that was just pulled out of the water. Someone with more severe depression instead becomes that fish weakened on the dock, gasping for air, the sense of fight gone.

Depression is like having something inside you that's foreign or alien to your existence and who you are as a person. No one wants to be depressed, just like no one wants to be physically sick. Depression is like an alien that has entered the body, taken over, and reprogrammed the person so they can't feel anymore. So they can't regulate what they're feeling. So they feel numb, lose control over their lives, and feel like they're not in their own body. This is an out-of-body experience that's not pleasing, not happy, not a result of being overwhelmed with joy. Instead it's an out-of-body experience of dread, with feelings of loss and even hatred for oneself.

AN UN-NAMEABLE KNOWING

The best way to understand depression is to know there *is* something else taking up space inside a person's head. Something is in the way of a person's brain, their consciousness, their subconsciousness, their mind. If the initial reason for someone's depression is partly identifiable—for example, if a very big letdown has occurred in their life, or a grave loss, or if an extremely difficult situation is happening—then that event is taking up space inside their consciousness. It can feel impossible to overcome, and severe depression can take over.

Then there's depression that's not identifiable. When depression and deep sadness sneak up and creep in with no cause we can pinpoint, we have an outside source that should not be in the body inhabiting the body and the brain. The individual doesn't even know that anything has entered their brain, let alone *what* entered their brain. Without being able to name the cause, they're experiencing brain sabotage.

If your depression comes on right after a form of contamination or toxic exposure, and you're very aware of that contamination or exposure so you connect the dots quickly, you'll have something to hold on to while struggling with that depression.

You'll be able to reference, "I believe it was because of that exposure I had." Having an answer to refer back to about when it started can greatly help someone suffering from depression. That rarely happens, though. And even if someone does have the suspicion at first that their depression arrived after an exposure or contamination, it's easy to forget that eventually because depression can become like a vast, dark hole that's hard to climb out of as more and more time passes, doubt settles in, and someone loses trust in their memory.

Depression isn't a chemical imbalance in the brain, as the medical world has been known to identify it. Depression isn't someone avoiding life, being lazy, ignoring responsibilities, or hiding from the world, as we've sometimes been led to believe. And depression isn't someone just giving up on life because they're weak, as society has often alluded to. Someone suffering from depression will often describe a state of numbness, not having any feelings at all, not caring if the world ends tomorrow. This doesn't make them heartless or soulless. People suffering from depression are far from that.

POWERFUL SOUL DETECTION

The biggest reason depression is one of the hardest struggles for so many is that the soul is involved. The place where foreign contamination or exposure ends up—inside the brain—is the very place where our soul also resides. People who suffer with depression are the opposite of soulless. Instead, they happen to be more in touch with their own soul in that moment in their lifetime than many others who are not suffering with depression. People with depression have become soul sensitive. This is a strength, not a weakness. Depression is the soul detecting that something is wrong.

In lasting cases of depression, the soul is detecting a foreign body, a foreign invader, a foreign substance inhabiting the same place the soul is living in. Depression is a form of misunderstood enlightenment that something is wrong inside the body. It's not the person's fault. That "something" should never be inside the body. The soul is saying, "The temple has an invader."

The soul of a depression sufferer is telling that person there is a problem and a purification process needs to happen. The soul is sending signals and warning signs to the subconsciousness and consciousness. Because we aren't shown how to interpret these signs and signals of contamination and exposure, we don't know what's wrong.

Traumatic Loss, Traumatic Stress, and Adrenal Stress

After we experience high-volume adrenaline release from emotional conflict, emotional injury, or trauma, the soul becomes hyperaware of adrenaline release, even if that adrenaline release is the fight-or-flight kind produced artificially from everyday caffeine use. The brain now correlates any level of fight-or-flight adrenaline with trauma:

After the fact of the loss or hardship, even though the severe trauma is over, a person still has to go through the ebbs and flows of life, which means that fight-or-flight occurs often, including caffeine-infused fight-or-flight. The soul now associates any fight-or-flight adrenaline releases, even at the mildest levels, with past hardships at the highest levels. This occurs even if someone is not actively thinking about the original trauma, because the soul is connected to the subconscious. This is soul sensitivity at work, and it's a strength. Your soul is detecting sadness from overused adrenals and/ or your soul is detecting adrenaline saturation in the brain cells—that is, your soul is detecting a struggling brain that's trying to overcome constant adrenaline surges.

If depression starts at the time of an emotional blow and then continues in a grave way, that serious continuation is a sign that there's another source responsible for the depression. Either the emotional injury triggered another of the following causes responsible for the depression, or the emotional injury occurred at the same time as one of these additional exposures.

Pathogenic Presence

Many people experience depression as the result of the soul detecting a pathogen in the body. For instance, viruses that enter the body create toxins that can enter the brain and elevate inflammation. The soul is detecting and sensing that brain and nerve inflammation.

Here's another reason you can experience depression from pathogens: when a pathogen is transmitted from person to person, it can carry information from person to person. When you contract a pathogen such as a virus, that pathogen could already have a history of residing in many others before it entered you. The pathogen could have been passed along through many individuals for many years, even decades. Along the way, the pathogen collected information on other people's struggles or losses, including emotional experiences.

A virus records someone's emotional state that triggers their adrenals. If anybody who had a virus before you—whether the person who transmitted it to you or any other person who had the virus before that—suffered from depression for any reason at all, the virus brings along that information. The virus essentially takes on each person's energy, something like an imprint.

A sensitive soul can detect a pathogen radiating energy and frequency going back as far as 30, 50, 80 years, sometimes even 100 years. (Some of these pathogens can be really old.) Not everybody's soul can detect this. Yet for many people suffering from depression, the soul can. A sensitive soul can sense the fight-or-flight environment a pathogen lived in with previous individuals, and a sensitive soul can read the energy of these pathogens and even some history.

Toxic Heavy Metals and Toxic Chemicals

Toxic heavy metals hold weight, even in their smallest particle form, which means they are heavy on brain tissue. Some individuals are extremely brain-sensitive. This doesn't mean they're weak, by any means. It means that when there is a foreign invader such as a toxic heavy metal residing inside the brain, it can be more detectable by their soul.

Toxic heavy metals also short-circuit the electrical grid inside the brain, even if not at a noticeable level. Certain individuals' souls can detect that there is something malfunctioning in the brain's electrical grid, and this detection can show itself as depression.

For certain individuals, the soul even understands how these metals arrived. The soul can detect the arrival of toxic heavy metals through pharmaceutical injuries, whether from childhood or adulthood.

The soul also senses the cost to human life of mining metals in some of the most dangerous mines on the planet, going all the way back to mercury and other metals mined centuries ago. These metals have been passed on from generation to generation through exposures. When foreign invader heavy metals, mined in any era, sit inside the brain, a very sensitive soul can pick up on the suffering and lives lost in the metal's industrial history.

When toxins such as pesticides, solvents, fragrances, cleaning chemicals, and brain betrayer food chemicals reside inside the brain, a sensitive soul can also detect that these toxins are penetrating and staying in brain cells.

Sometimes toxic heavy metals and/or toxic chemicals have been present in the brain all along, with no depression. Then an emotional trauma occurs that triggers the brain betrayers to create grave depression. How does this work? For one, the adrenaline rush that accompanies trauma creates a highly acidic condition in the brain, which means metals corrode faster. At the same time, significant amounts of nutrients and other brain supplies are required to power through emotional turmoil. Previously, a strong brain with all the supplies it needed was overriding problems such as toxic heavy metals. Trauma can burn out those reserves of nutrients, phytochemical compounds, and brain hormones quickly, leading to a deficient brain. As the brain weakens from acidity and deficiencies, problems and contaminants that already existed in the brain can show themselves.

Deficiencies

Even without emotional trauma burning out reserves, we can experience brain deficiencies, which you read about extensively in Chapter 7, "Your Burnt Out, Deficient Brain." People who struggle with depression often feel like they're missing something, missing out on something, missing a part of themselves. They may feel emptiness and dissatisfaction. This is indeed the soul detecting something missing in the brain—the soul is detecting deficiencies in critical brain supplies such as electrolytes.

GET YOUR BRAIN BACK

When someone is suffering from depression, especially if it's mild and they haven't lost their sense of fight, they'll often look for ways to remedy the depression by boosting their mood. They'll try to keep living their lives, supporting themselves, making themselves happy. They'll go out to ride a bike, spend time with friends, talk to a counselor, take a vacation, take time off work if they can. They'll listen to advice: "Why don't you do this? Why don't you go here? Take a break, take a sabbatical, search for yourself." People start soul-searching, looking for something, thinking they have to find something. What's really happening is that they're trying to heal their soul—because their soul is detecting a physical problem in the brain.

Now that you know what the physical problems in the brain could be, you can assist your soul in another way. You can address the adrenaline saturation, exposures, contaminants, and deficiencies directly, and in the process find the sense of wholeness you've been missing. If your depression has taken you past the point of fighting, if it's serious and long term and has taken you to a place where you feel like there's no way out, you've seen now that there's a whole new way to think about what you've been through. You can reconnect with your soul, feel like yourself again, find yourself—by addressing your brain's physical needs. This is how you get your fight back.

For specific depression support beyond what's offered in Part VI, "Bringing Back Your Brain," refer to the Depression protocol, Chronic Mystery Guilt protocol, and/or Seasonal Affective Disorder (SAD) protocol in *Brain Saver Protocols, Cleanses & Recipes*.

CHAPTER 33

Eating Disorders

We can all become consumed by what we're eating. Are we eating too much? Are we eating too little? Are we eating when we're not hungry? Do we eat so much we make ourselves sick? Are we into portion control? Are we micromanaging our eating on a daily basis? Do we convince ourselves that we're eating in moderation or eating balanced? Do we tell ourselves we don't need much food? Are we eating the wrong things? Do we punish ourselves for eating the wrong things? Do we eat the wrong things to reward ourselves? What constitutes the "wrong" things? Who's right, who's wrong?

Eating disorders are rampant; they can exist in every one of us. We're all consumed about food. If we weren't, it wouldn't make sense because we *have* to be concerned about food. It's how we live, work, play, function—if food doesn't enter our body, we will eventually cease to exist. That's always been a part of our history as humans. What makes it a food disorder in today's modern world is the amount of unhealthy conditioning all around us combined with

contaminants in our brains. And so what we have to do is learn how to *eat in order*, not have an eating disorder.

EATING IN ORDER

"Eating in order" can have a few meanings: eating in order to heal, eating in order to live, eating in order to survive, eating in order to thrive, eating in order to function, eating in order to succeed.

A focus on food is not, on its own, unhealthy. Often when we're trying to take care of ourselves holistically and heal from symptoms and conditions—buying the right foods, consuming fruits and vegetables, eating less processed food, looking after ourselves in general—we can feel like we're trapped, alone, and worried about food in a bubble of our own world, unless we find others like us. Even when we're doing it right, life becomes all about what to eat, how healthy it is, where to find it. We can get lost, wondering, *Does anyone else have to worry about this?*

Yes, every single person on the planet has to worry about food. It's natural.

When you're trying to heal particular illnesses and diseases and conditions and symptoms, it's especially natural. You do have to be extra mindful about what you eat. If that mindfulness about food is done the wrong way, it can contribute to an eating disorder. If it's done the right way, it can correct an eating disorder and teach you how to eat properly.

Eating the right items at the right time can still feel as if you have an eating disorder because of how others view it. When you're trying to eat healthy, others often see it as too rigid. They may even label it *orthorexia*, which you'll read about later in this chapter. You can get blamed for "too much fruit," "not enough protein," "too many carbs." It's endless. Bringing your own food to holidays, not eating at events where the menu doesn't work for you, always packing snacks, orienting your life around the farmers market, or making special requests at restaurants—none of this should be considered an eating disorder when what you're doing is eating in order to truly heal.

Now, don't we want to feel normal? To go out and eat a pizza or some fried food or cheesy pasta or a grass-fed burger or maybe some sushi? To go over to a friend's house and eat whatever they're serving and have ice cream afterward? To eat whatever's on the table at a family holiday without worrying about how it's going to affect us with bloating, stomach cramps, gastritis, diarrhea, constipation, heartburn, acid reflux, indigestion, and acne? We all want to

feel normal. The irony is that all the people who seem normal actually normalize dysfunctional eating and have eating disorders themselves. They don't eat correctly. No one has ever been taught what our brain and body need, what foods our organs need, what foods to eat for our physical, spiritual, emotional, and mental health. We're left to our own demise.

In order to heal, you have to get your foods figured out. You have to understand your foods and get them in order. When your foods are in disorder, that's when you get an eating disorder. Everyone has been there, wondering what to eat, and everyone is guessing.

Many times food contributes to not feeling well; eating foods that are not appropriate for healing can contribute to developing a condition, illness, or disease. So what seemed to be normal—eating normal, acting normal, being normal with food—wasn't a good "normal." It might have seemed like a good normal because you were with family and friends. It might have seemed like a good normal because the food seemed tasty and satiating. It might have seemed like a good normal because it was convenient. It might have seemed like a good normal because it offered comforting sensations that connected you with past memories in life. Still, it wasn't good for other reasons.

People who try to use food to heal, especially young people, will frequently be blamed for disordered eating. In the older days, it was even more common. Particularly if it was a young adult trying to heal from chronic illness by eating fruits and vegetables, they could be taken to a clinic and force-fed, prompted by well-meaning family members who were actually the ones with the eating disorders, or who were very scared because the young person's diet was very different from what they believed was normal.

We're in a better, safer place now with food than we were just two decades ago. Bringing in more plant foods is more accepted—not fully accepted, just becoming more accepted. A lot of confusion around eating disorders and healthy eating remains, and rightfully so. There are many trends in the health field that aren't right for the body, and they can rain on the parade of better approaches in holistic health. Some health professionals become reckless, and it ends up looking bad for everyone in the natural health field. People venturing into certain cleanses, certain detox programs, and certain diets already have eating disorders. And when they do these reckless diets and cleanses, it worsens their eating disorders, creating more confusion, fear, and frustration. This could give healthy eating a bad name and even start a new eating disorder—because the makers of these diets and programs have no idea why anyone is sick to begin with, so the information they are giving others to use is not in order.

EATING IN DISORDER

There are different levels of eating disorders, so many different levels. Not eating all day, just getting by on coffee, and then eating at night: that's an eating disorder. Overeating at every meal, whether becoming uncomfortably full or eating until you can hardly breathe: that's an eating disorder. Trying to portion-control at every meal without regard to your hunger: that's an eating disorder. Counting every single calorie and excluding healthy foods because of calorie count is an eating disorder. Enrolling in trendy dietary programs and following all the rules without regard to how they make you feel is an eating disorder. Injecting yourself with trendy hormones or taking pills with hormones in them while eating 500 calories a day is an eating disorder. Going on radical cleanses where you eat and drink virtually nothing for weeks or even a month is an eating disorder.

There are less obvious forms too. Trying to peer pressure others into eating not-so-good foods because you don't want to feel bad about eating those foods: that's an eating disorder. Eating foods in front of loved ones that you know will tempt them and sabotage their healthy eating plans: that's an eating disorder. Consuming diet soda on a regular basis: that's an eating disorder. Thinking about food all the time is an eating disorder. Not thinking about food—pretending you don't need it, consistently letting your blood sugar drop, not planning ahead about what you're going to eat—is an eating disorder. Having a meltdown if your food doesn't come exactly the way you ordered it is an eating disorder. Eating everything that someone throws in front of you is an eating disorder. Eating only while you're driving is an eating disorder. Always having to sit at the table to eat is an eating disorder. Only eating while standing up is an eating disorder. Wolfing down food and clearing your plate in record time is an eating disorder. Painstakingly spacing out each bite without a medical reason is an eating disorder. Foods that set you off emotionally because of something that happened with those foods along the way in your life—that's an eating disorder. It's endless.

Food Conditioning

What causes these everyday eating disorders? Often, conditioning. For example, when kids go to camp, boarding school, or a friend's house, many rules around food tend to be in place. With set mealtimes when you're only allowed to eat what's being served and have no easy access to food outside those windows, it's common to get into a habit of squirreling away treats and goodies like candy bars and potato chips—a habit that can continue later in life, even when the same limits are no longer in place.

Then there's the example of someone being raised in a family where there's only so much food on the table at every meal, so if you don't fend for yourself and gobble down what you can, you're not going to get food. The faster you eat, the faster you may be able to get another serving.

Those are just two examples; there are hundreds more ways we can get conditioned around food. Even if your circumstances change, the fear and habits can stick around.

With conditioning like this, your brain receives messages that you're not going to be able to eat what you want, eat when you want, find the food you really want, or find food at all. And then often, those messages don't get resolved and refreshed as life changes. People end up in adulthood still living with that childhood feeling that they may not be able to get enough. It's like being burned by a hot stove. Once you learn that early lesson that you can get hurt by the hot surface, you're always cautious near one. If you went to bed hungry a lot in your youth, it was like getting burned. Your brain stored that information, so that going near a dinner table may have the same charge as approaching a stove—it may put you on alert and give you that same sense of wariness—and you can carry that through life.

Unless, that is, you recognize it and recondition your brain. While the memory of that injury will always be there, you can still build a new database, a new foundation around eating.

Tainted Taste

Here's another contributor to everyday eating disorders: taste. When two people eat the same food, they tend to think they're experiencing the exact same thing. They're not. When you're sitting next to someone eating the same mac and cheese, the same biscuit, and the same soup—even when you both like it all—what you're each tasting is entirely different. Our taste buds and palate are controlled by our central nervous system.

That is, our brain controls our experience of flavor. The tongue is just a tool.

Often people think the mouth is controlling flavor. That's not entirely false. If you put a cough drop or stick of gum in your mouth, that would alter the flavor of whatever you ate next. Taste buds can become saturated with anything toxic, pungent, spicy, or acidic, and that can alter what you taste. Cigarettes, for example, can alter someone's sense of taste, and so can artificial flavors. That's taste contamination coming through the mouth and even the nose.

That type of flavor contamination aside, what controls our experience of taste and flavor is the brain. Signals travel back and forth between the mouth and the brain via the hypoglossal and glossopharyngeal nerves, which come out of the brain stem. It's those nerve messages in the brain that really determine someone's experience of, for example, bitterness. It's part of the reason why people have certain food preferences: the brain causes people to perceive the experience of consuming foods in certain ways. Any interference in the brain on any level—anything toxic inside the brain—can alter how we perceive flavors inside the mouth because the cranial nerves either become poisoned or neurons sending messages to these nerves become poisoned. So if the brain has any kind of solvents, MSG, toxic heavy metals, petrochemicals, pesticides, herbicides, other toxic chemicals, or viral neurotoxins stored up in its brain tissue, that can affect whether someone likes or dislikes certain food and drink. For example, when someone has elevated levels of mercury or other toxic heavy metals inside the brain or brain stem, cilantro (also called coriander) won't have a pleasing flavor. Instead that person will dislike cilantro, or even consider it repulsive. As they're minimizing the toxic heavy metals, the taste of cilantro changes and becomes tolerable, even pleasurable.

It's not just about flavor. Which troublemakers have taken up residence in the brain and where can also determine whether people like or dislike specific consistencies of food. For example, you'll hear people say, "I don't like the texture of avocado," "I don't like anything mushy," "I only like crunchy things," or "I like something I can sink my teeth into"—that's because of what's going on in the brain.

Often the toxins in the brain plus conditioning from early life go hand in hand to shape our experience of food. Being told as a child that you have to eat something or having a bad experience at a friend's house with a certain food can lead to a lasting aversion. Sitting at your friend's dinner table, for instance, while their parents are demanding they clear their plate and eat all their meat before they can have a dessert can lead to a food pressure disorder. Add to that any kind of toxins inside the brain contaminating its messages to our tongue and nose, and you can see how everyone ends up with unique variations of taste in food.

Did you ever wonder why one family member doesn't like a food that you love? Or why a friend can find the flavor of a dish so incredible that they can't get enough, while you'll try it and say, "Eh, it's okay"?

How is it possible that one person finds a food so delicious, comforting, and good, while a parent, sibling, partner, boyfriend, or girlfriend doesn't like it? Because again, they're tasting two different things. Maybe one of the tasters had a bad experience like food poisoning and won't go near a certain type of food anymore. That's an emotional and physical wound in the brain. It's not as simple as "Oh, people have different tastes," or "We just have different palates." It's so much more than that; it's all brain-related. It's "Whoa, that person might have a lot of different levels of brain contamination," or "Wait a minute, *I* might have contamination." It's "That person might have emotional wounds," or "Hold on, *I* might have wounds from growing up." It's the sort of mental conditioning and brain betrayer interference that can lead to someone refusing to eat anything other than oatmeal. Put a leafy green or celery juice in front of them, and they won't eat or drink it—it has to be oatmeal, until the hypoglossal and glossopharyngeal nerves start to receive fresh messages from the neurons that are cleaning up.

Wake-Up Calls

Sometimes a life event will wake you up out of an everyday eating disorder. For example, what happens when you go to the doctor's office and, out of nowhere, she says, "You're type 2 diabetic"? Often the experience will scare a person into eating new foods, ones they might never have tried before, breaking out of a certain comfort zone. Instead of only having coffee all morning and then going for a double cheeseburger and soft drink at lunch and greasy takeout at dinner, being rocked by the threat of this diagnosis helps you make different choices. It's almost as if the shock of the doctor handing you bad news helped disrupt your eating disorder.

Sometimes that won't do it. Some people are told they have type 2 diabetes or are prediabetic, and they just can't change the way they eat even if they have the resources, asking instead for whatever medications it takes to compensate. Which way it goes depends on how strong the eating disorder is, how deeply embedded it is in your central nervous system and way of life. It depends on what happened along the way—what abuses and hardships—and how saturated the brain is with toxins.

Whichever everyday eating disorder you're dealing with, whether it's an aversion to foods you know would help you heal, an eating pattern that doesn't serve you, or a similar struggle, you can alter it if you detox your brain. When people start getting toxic heavy metals and other brain betrayers out of their systems, they start liking different foods, and day by day, it starts to get better.

FOOD FEAR

Oftentimes an eating disorder develops because of a symptom. A symptom related to not being able to swallow correctly, choking, nausea, pain in the stomach, a feeling of tightness in the throat or chest, or losing the sense of taste and smell. This is where someone is living their life and they're eating just as anybody else would be eating, and then these symptoms start to develop.

In some cases—if it's a chronic nausea, for example—then foods become pick-and-choose, a game of *What's going to help ease this nausea? What's not helping this nausea? Do any of these foods I'm eating contribute to the nausea? How come when I'm not eating, I still have the nausea?* Then our mind consciousness starts to pick up patterns and habits because of small bursts of PTSD developing. You eat something and you're nauseous, so you identify that food as being the problem, so you learn to avoid that food. Just as you get comfortable eating another food, thinking you're safe and good, you get nauseous again. So then that's another food you're uncomfortable eating, suspecting it's contributing to the problem. This can carry on into other foods as well. Nausea doesn't usually receive a diagnosis besides nausea, or maybe nervousness or anxiety. If everything checks out okay in the abdomen, it's usually passed off as someone "just being sensitive."

This mysterious nausea can bring about serious eating disorders, even when reaching out for help, even when searching for a doctor or practitioner to help ease the nausea, to help find out why you have the nausea. Every day becomes "What do I eat? And what time do I eat it? Is the nausea better in the morning? Better in the afternoon or evening?" Some cases of mysterious nausea make it so someone can barely eat anything. Even if the cause and the nausea

go away, the eating disorder that arose from them can be lasting. The same goes for mysterious swallowing difficulties or mysterious tightness of the chest. If your condition is diagnosed as anxiety, that still doesn't take away an eating disorder.

And then if somebody notices the eating disorder, for instance a friend or family member, and they don't understand what you're feeling or struggling with, that can contribute to a bigger eating disorder, making it more complex. Now you have an audience. Even if the audience was agreeable to start with—they were worried about your symptoms as you were doing your doctor search—it can eventually start to feel like a spotlight is on you: What are you eating and how much are you eating? Then the PTSD can start, and the feeling that you're never understood.

Regardless of what your symptoms are, regardless of how many doctors you've seen, all eyes are on what you're eating and swallowing and how much you're eating. Your original symptoms that had you seeking out doctors and help are often long forgotten by the audience. The focus has all gone to "You're not eating enough," "You're getting too skinny," "You're looking sickly," "You need to put some meat on your bones," "Are you getting enough protein?" and "You're not eating the right things." Then the fear of eating occurs, or intensifies.

Even if you're diagnosed with a named physical condition right off the bat, it's easy to develop an eating disorder, in part because there's still not a medical understanding of what causes the condition, so it's not getting healed. Somebody with a simple case of heartburn (acid reflux), for example, can develop an eating disorder because it's always on their mind: What foods are going to help? What foods aren't going to help? "Oh, this is going to hurt when I eat this." Eating a food that seems to be working gives you a sense of security. Then if it isn't working anymore and the acid reflux or nausea returns, it's like an old friend letting you down.

Sometimes it's not about the symptoms someone experiences when they're eating a food. It's about what they're told about that food. So many people are trying to figure out how to heal. In the process they're told certain foods are bad, and they become afraid of foods that are actually good for them. There's so much confusion, and people experience so much pressure as they're trying to get better.

Food has an ingrained connection to our physical being, our physical understanding, even if we aren't dealing with ongoing health complaints. If someone is home one evening, gets some chest pain, and gets on the phone with family and friends, the first thing everyone says is, "What did you eat tonight?" If that person decides to go to the ER, the doctor asks, "What did you eat tonight?" The question always comes up. That's how interconnected we are with food in general. It's one of the details that patients first volunteer. "I was sitting at home and I'd just had my dinner, I had this terrible pain in my stomach"—or back or chest or lower abdomen—"and I thought it best to come to the ER."

Oftentimes we're looking at our food for answers. "Does it have anything to do with this?" We're so consciously connected to our food that if you're someone who goes plant-based or vegan and you're starting to feel a little bit better—you've cut out processed foods, you believe animal proteins aren't something good for anyone to eat—the first symptom you get after changing your diet will cause confusion to take over. Whether you've been plant-based for a shorter or longer amount of time, you'll doubt your plant-based diet. You'll listen to mental replays, flashbacks, memories of a certain doctor or practitioner telling you that you need protein, that you shouldn't be on plant foods only. You'll remember a family member doubting your newfound plant-based diet. And now you're back to being worried about what you're eating, asking yourself, *Am I doing everything right? Am I doing anything right?*

And yes, there could be something wrong with any given plant-based diet, and it could be contributing to a health issue. Yet going on an animal protein diet isn't going to fix that. Because as you read in Chapter 14, "Food Wars," nobody, no matter what diet they're on, knows what's truly wrong with their mystery symptoms and conditions. Nobody knows how diet contributes or doesn't contribute. That very food confusion can lead to an eating disorder.

Physical symptoms that look emotional create some of the most difficult eating disorders. Mysterious nausea, tightness of the chest, tightness of the throat, difficulty swallowing, and stomach pain that don't have a definitive diagnosis will often be labeled as emotional symptoms, even though they're physical. And when we're dealing with physical symptoms misconstrued as emotional and those symptoms interfere with food, that's when it can be much more difficult on us. Breaking your jaw and then not being able to chew or have the normal foods you like for a month while your jaw is wired shut is different. While the experience of a known injury such as a broken jaw and a liquid-only diet can lead to PTSD and disordered eating in its own way, the experience of mystery, unexplained symptoms is bewildering. It can flip a switch. Just sticking your fork into food can become emotionally charged when you're dealing with these other mysterious physical, neurological symptoms that get labeled emotional. It can become so emotional that eventually the fear around food can take over the mind consciousness of both yourself and the people around you, while you're still struggling with a physical symptom that started it all. All too frequently people in this position get the message that this mysterious condition they've been seeking help for is really just all in their head, or an emotional condition that they're creating.

ORTHOREXIA

Back in the 1980s, "eating healthy" was merely counting calories. Even counting calories at the time was unaccepted by the mainstream. If you were someone who counted calories, you were going to get some serious stares across the table. On the other hand, eating too much, or what someone else thought was too much, has always been up for ridicule. There has always been concern about self-indulgence.

Yet if you were someone who went a little further than concern about caloric intake—meaning that you steered away from fried foods, greasy foods, processed foods, or even canned foods, and you were bringing more salads into your life, more fruit, more vegetables, and you maybe even thought about going vegetarian—well, you would be considered someone who'd gone too far. You could easily be diagnosed with an eating disorder, one that was considered almost dangerous to your mental health, not just physical health.

The term *moderation* was going strong back then. Forty years ago, it was that scientific-driven theory—a scientific excuse: "It's okay to have a little bit of everything, whatever your heart desires. As long as it's in moderation, it's okay." If you were someone who ate light, it would raise concerns. If you were someone who was choosy about what you were eating because you were concerned about your health, this would raise red flags. We have this fear in society that if you're choosing a different path with your food, then something must be terribly wrong.

In health today we have more freedom in how we eat. A plant-based mom can be not only plant-based but plant-based raw and feed her babies plant-based raw and not have her children taken away. There was a time not so long ago when any state in the U.S. could intervene if too many whistles were blown about a plant-based mom feeding her children too much lettuce, nuts, seeds, and avocado. Make no mistake: a lot of families were destroyed because of moms being judged for taking care of their children. As every half decade goes by, history gets scrubbed. Very few people are allowed to tell their stories, if they're even around to do so. We take for granted what it took to get to this place, and how many people were hurt along the way fighting for health rights. Nowadays it's much more accepted to eat in different ways, whether vegetarian, vegan, plant-based, or a non-processed, non–fast food animal protein diet. People can pretty much do as they please. To a degree. These people may still end up with the label *orthorexic.*

Orthorexia is a term that's being weaponized to make people feel bad for eating well and pick on people for avoiding certain foods. Basically, if you're someone who's been sick for too long, has seen multiple doctors with no results, and you're losing your quality of life, so you have to take your health in your own hands by choosing a certain way to eat, you could be labeled *orthorexic.* When weaponized like this, it's a label that's truly demeaning, disempowering, and really injuring.

We act like everyone has the health freedoms to eat and do what you want, and even though this has improved over the years, there's still some form of darkness around every corner, trying to rob and steal your chance to heal. When we pathologize someone's attempts at a healthy diet, there's so much we don't see. What was that person going through? How many doctors did they see? How many nutritionists, dieticians, health professionals? What is their real health problem? Are they living with mystery digestive issues, mystery fatigue, mystery brain fog, mystery skin conditions, mystery weight gain? Does anybody even know? None of this is looked at.

There are so many things wrong with someone throwing out blatant labels and terms at someone else. The individual labeling someone else doesn't even know what it took for that chronically ill person to get where they are, how much struggle was in their journey with food as they tried to find answers to heal. It's a sacred process someone goes through when they're trying to heal themselves because no one else can heal them.

The stage you're at when someone labels you with orthorexia makes a difference. If you've found some answers, followed your path, gained more strength, and gotten comfortable with moving forward, it's probably a little easier to digest that label. What if you've just discovered eating a certain new way that's starting to move you forward after being let down over and over again? Being accused of being orthorexic can send you off on a path without hope and light. It's like an explosion occurs in your mind.

No one gets it when they haven't been in your shoes. The hardships, the potholes, the struggles, the other people in your life you're dealing with or even having to battle for your health freedom and rights. So if you're ever given this label out of nowhere from a health professional or anyone else, you can easily doubt everything you're doing, or get angry inside because you're being misunderstood once again.

Even though we're at a place now where it's much more accepted to eat a certain way to gain your health, at the same time, ghosts from the past still come out to haunt people. The ghosts come out when you're halfway up the ladder to health and safety, at which point those ghosts start to shake the ladder as you try to climb, disorienting and destabilizing you with whispers of *orthorexia*. When you're making your smoothies and you're concerned about what goes in your smoothies and you're taking your herbs and you're choosing what fruit to eat that's helping you heal and you're cautious about what you're eating in a restaurant, when traveling, or at a friend's house, never think for one minute you're doing something wrong as far as taking your health and healing choices about food too far. Health means everything. You should never be ashamed while pursuing it.

You could be called orthorexic no matter where you are with what you're eating. You could be vegetarian eating bread and be called orthorexic, not just plant-based and eating fruit. You could be called orthorexic for eating any which way. There are so many types of eating disorders, most of them unrecognized by the industries. Of the very few eating disorders that are defined, orthorexia is one of them. If you're someone trying to heal with food, you'll often be tagged orthorexic. No one's journey with

how they're eating should ever be viewed in a negative light while they're trying to heal.

It's one thing to point out obstacles that could be in the way of healing, information that's critical about the food you're eating. That's very much different from saying, "You know, you're obsessed with food," because everyone's obsessed about food. Anyone who thinks they're not obsessed about food is in denial. Everyone wants to enjoy what they're eating, choose what they're eating, and have options. Sometimes circumstances can make it so we have to adjust what we're eating due to resources or availability—if we're in a difficult situation and can't get ahold of what we want to eat, or if we're financially held back from what we want to eat. If circumstances and resources allow us to have options, then we want those options.

No one should be punished for wanting to take good care of themselves using food as a tool, regardless of what direction they're going. If someone wants to be a carnivore, for example, sure, they're missing all of the fruit they need. They're missing critical starchy foods such as potatoes for healing. They still shouldn't be called out or blamed or labeled orthorexic because they're obsessed about eating meat and meat only. They should never be shamed for it or told they have an obsession or eating disorder based on that choice. The same goes for someone who only wants to eat fruit. Sure, they're missing their leafy greens, their critical herbs such as celery juice. They shouldn't be blamed or shamed or called orthorexic while trying to fix a problem or told they have an eating disorder just because they like to eat fruit.

Younger people especially who are trying to express that they have real symptoms—anxiety, weird feelings throughout the body, tiredness—keep on getting told, "You're physically fine. It's all mental." They start working on their food and they're getting better, and then they're told, "No, you're obsessed with food." Once you're told you have an obsession with eating healthily, it throws you off your game. This detracts people from taking health into their own hands. It keeps them reliant on the medical system and pharmaceuticals.

For some people, the term *orthorexia* has offered validation for the challenge of feeling they have to be "perfect" with food. It's true that no one should be blamed or shamed for not being "perfect" with food. There is no perfect. There's only what's right for you that allows you to eat in order: in order to heal, in order to live, in order to survive, in order to thrive, in order to function, in order to succeed. If you heal yourself with food, and then you to start to branch out with what you eat, and then you find yourself declining again, you aren't a failure with food. You can always go back to the way of eating that helped you be well.

ANOREXIA, BULIMIA, AND OVEREATING

If you live with an eating disorder, take comfort that you're not alone. As you've just seen, everyone has hang-ups around food.

You're not different or "other," the way you may have been made to feel. You were just handed a particular mix of life events and brain betrayers. Whatever has held you back with eating up until this point doesn't have to define you. You get to move on from this. To do that, first you get to discover what's been going on this whole time.

Control

Often there's an emotional side to it. When someone experiences turmoil—whether difficulties within family life or friendships, whether a breakup or betrayal, whether loss or abuse—it can cause them to feel like they have no control over the situation that's causing them pain. For certain people this leads to trying to control what enters their mouths. Because they can't stop what's happening on the outside, they may fall into a rhythm of exerting control over their bodies—whether by essentially starving themselves, getting into a pattern of bingeing and purging, or trying to numb out by overeating.

It could start with someone feeling so much unrest that food seems completely uninteresting. It's common to want to eat when we're feeling safe, relaxed, comfortable, and at peace—and therefore to feel an aversion to food when we're going through trust issues, relationship upheavals, intense pressure, workplace toxicity, financial strain, emotional attacks, harm, dread, grief, or something like siblings or other family members turning against us. Through these types of experiences, many people may withhold food or eat very little, feeling like they at least have control over food when they don't have control in other ways. Withholding food can become an addiction if more hardships come or the same hardships are repeated. Addiction to withholding food often feels like a survival mechanism, and if the cycle isn't broken, it can lead to a brain-related eating disorder such as anorexia where someone ends up essentially starving themselves.

On the flip side, it's also common to binge and overeat when you don't feel safe. When people are under emotional duress, they may take control in the opposite direction by eating to suppress emotions—bingeing or overeating to feel comforted or numbed during times of confrontation, challenge, or struggle.

With these different emotional brain-related eating patterns, age doesn't really matter. There's no saying that one type of eating pattern only comes on in someone's teens and another only develops in someone's 30s, 40s, or 50s. Emotional turmoil can come at any age. When difficult times visit, if they're not rectified in a short period and instead they stick around for weeks or months or even years, then a survival eating pattern can develop. If it's not resolved quickly enough, a survival eating pattern can turn into the type of eating disorder that disrupts life.

Adrenaline

These survival mechanisms are brain-related—though not brain-related in the sense that it's all made up in someone's head, or their mental thoughts are causing it. Eating disorders don't develop because someone was just "imbalanced" or sensitive. When a pronounced eating disorder takes over, a dependency and addiction can follow.

Many people who try to keep control of a long-term emotional crisis by eating very little may feel a sense of defeat when they do eat. They can't stomach the feeling of food inside of them. When they eat, they may feel guilty, shameful, disappointed in themselves, like they're losing control. Those feelings can lead to longer bouts of not eating, like a punishment. Simply seeing food could make them feel nervous, like it's the enemy, triggering the adrenal glands to release adrenaline. That adrenaline rushing through the body can become addictive; that sensation adrenaline provides can feel like it takes the place of eating, which can cause someone to withhold food even more and feel more in control. For some, the cycle continues like this: trying to cope by not eating, adrenaline surging from the sight of food (and also being used to replace food), allowing themselves very small portions when they do eat, and feeling distress or shame about even a few morsels passing their lips.

There are different variations of eating disorders. Bingeing and purging is one of them. It becomes addictive to those who want food out of their bodies after they've eaten. In this case, people often eat larger portions—what's called binge eating. Then, feeling like they've lost control, they'll try to take back power by vomiting up the food, which sends larger surges of adrenaline through the brain. A brain high occurs. (Other variations of purging, which are used on their own or in combination with vomiting, include taking laxatives or overexercising. These other purging methods have the same effect of triggering adrenaline surges.) The adrenaline from purging can be even more addictive than the adrenaline from bingeing, because purging triggers larger adrenaline spurts as a protection mechanism to expel the contents of the stomach in case something toxic was swallowed, whether pathogen or poison. As a result, someone can get trapped in a cycle of bingeing and purging. When we vomit, our brain needs to send a signal into and through our vagus nerves, reaching our stomach, prompting our stomach to ready itself for an emergency evacuation. Then the vagus nerves bounce the abdomen with an emergency pulse and at the same time send a message back to the brain to access an adrenaline surge.

When someone eats a lot under stress, using food to comfort themselves or suppress emotions—whether that overeating is followed by a purge cycle or not—there are often hidden, underlying reasons. One reason is to soak up adrenaline. Excess adrenaline, especially when it's triggered by emotional pain, is harmful when it's running through the brain and body. Without our realizing it, our brain will often send us the signal to eat carbohydrates to offset that adrenaline because with carbs comes extra glucose to bind onto and capture this adrenal hormone, hindering the

intense adrenaline from causing damage. The adrenaline and the glucose get used up together: the glucose attaches to the adrenaline, allowing the hormone to be eliminated through urination.

The glucose from carbs also calms down the nervous system, which is why someone so often reaches for pizza or potato chips to give themselves a little safety zone. We're not taught to reach for pure carbohydrates; instead we reach for these combinations of fats and carbohydrates, and these combination foods end up trapping the adrenaline into fat cells instead of leaving the body.

If the intense stress that's causing someone to overeat is short term, then that person will often go back to their old norm. If the emotional situation in someone's life is long term, with very little relief along the way, then the eating pattern will often continue.

Excess adrenaline can be very abrasive on the central nervous system. As it saturates the brain, this adrenaline can heighten nerve sensitivity that can lead to anxiousness developing. Eating disorders aren't always solely about the brain, though. Too much adrenaline can irritate the stomach and intestinal linings, making them hypersensitive, almost like raw wounds. Adrenaline makes nerves sensitive in general, including the vagus and phrenic nerves, which travel to the gut, and as a result this area around the diaphragm, stomach, and intestinal tract can become hypersensitive, whether food is traveling through them or not. These adrenaline effects alone can contribute to an eating disorder, often prompting someone to not eat at all for a while, or eat too fast—to try to soothe that uncomfortable feeling by eating.

Toxic Heavy Metals

Some eating disorders aren't caused by difficult emotional circumstances. These are cases where life is going along normally with its usual upsides and problems, and a severe eating disorder develops, seemingly out of nowhere. If a counselor comes in to evaluate, they won't find upheaval, bullying, family issues, relationship battles, or work-related confrontations bringing on intense stress. What's really happening in these cases is that something else is affecting the brain: toxic heavy metals.

Mercury, aluminum, and copper are the predominant metals behind these types of eating disorders that seem to come out of nowhere. Toxic heavy metal exposures can build up in brain tissue through the various sources you read about in Chapter 20, "Toxic Heavy Metals," causing eating disorders in a wide range of ages, as early as childhood, teenage years, and young adulthood or happening in someone's 30s, 40s, or later. Toxic heavy metals in certain areas of brain stem tissue can create a sense of having no appetite because the metals interfere with messages of hunger traveling between the brain stem and the stomach through the vagus nerves. Toxic heavy metals in the brain can also create momentary difficulty in swallowing that makes someone not want to eat, because the metals are interfering with vagus nerves' messaging

to the esophagus and throat. This puts the person into panic for a moment, cutting off their hunger. Not eating can then create a major conflict with someone's elemental impulse to eat for survival.

If this is happening in a young one, concerned family members will often go on red-hot alert, tracking when their loved one is eating and not eating, making it a major point of focus and concern. While this isn't the emotional harm we were talking about earlier—these are loving responses—relatives' concern, worry, or even dreadful alarm can still be hard for the person who is suffering. Already confused about why they have no appetite and maybe even feel nauseated, when they are told on repeat that they need to eat, this can start to create a little bit of an emotional wound around food for a child, teen, or young adult.

When someone is struggling with an eating disorder where they won't eat enough, professionals and loved ones will often try to change up their diet, pressuring them to increase their comfort foods like mac and cheese or pizza or waffles or bagels or fast foods. This can compound the situation, causing its own emotional trauma. Young people often have an added level of peer and societal pressure around weight, and when combined with toxic heavy metal poisoning in the brain and family members demanding that they eat—and eat certain foods at that—an anxiousness can occur.

This can be a recipe for teens or young adults to vomit up their meals as they experience acute, first-time bouts of bulimia. If the heavy metal toxicity is more severe, bulimia can develop even without any family pressure. An external trigger is not needed. The toxic heavy metals themselves sitting in brain tissue in and around neurons are both the cause and the consistent trigger.

As we touched on earlier, one issue with bulimia is that when you vomit up food (or purge in any other way), you experience the adrenaline rush to offer relief. When toxic heavy metals are in the brain, they tend to impede electrical impulses and dampen neurotransmitters, so people who suffer with toxic heavy metal–caused eating disorders also tend to develop mild to severe focus and concentration issues, fatigue, hypersensitivities of various kinds, ADHD, Tourette's syndrome, seizures, OCD, depression, tics, or anxiety. When someone is throwing up and adrenaline is released, it acts as a drug, creating a clarity, peace, or even euphoric feeling. The adrenaline rush is a temporary antidote to their suffering, basically placing a temporary patch over neurons in the brain that are saturated with toxic heavy metals. Adrenaline ignites electrical impulses, allowing them to burn hotter, without pain or discomfort, to override mental and physical symptoms by numbing them out. Adrenaline is a complex steroid composition that can be temporarily soothing at first. Then, as it wears off, symptoms can worsen, which can make it hard to be without the adrenaline. It prompts the need for more of this complex steroid. This is why some eating disorders can feel inescapable. These adrenaline rushes of bulimic purges are extremely addictive. It's very easy for

a pattern to develop that feels impossible to break.

Meanwhile, no one sees the true source of the problem: toxic heavy metals in the brain. Sometimes when a brain is still developing, new growth forms around the toxic metals over time, and someone can naturally grow out of the signals that were causing unhealthy eating patterns because electricity driving through the brain reroutes itself into the newly developed brain tissue. A person can skate along for a while and then suddenly—say, in their 30s—symptoms can redevelop because the toxic heavy metals in the original brain tissue went through accelerated oxidation, spreading into other areas of the brain. Eventually, the toxic heavy metal oxidative runoff can spread into the more newly formed brain tissue. Additional toxic heavy metals from other exposures could also inhabit the newly formed brain tissue. Sometimes, on the other hand, a person develops heavy metal toxicity later in life and experiences their first bout of anorexia or bulimia or undiagnosed bingeing with occasional purging when, perhaps, they're 40.

With bulimia, the adrenaline addiction can still have a very strong hold, so that even if the underlying cause of heavy metal toxicity is gone, it can be very difficult for someone to switch gears from the purge cycle and reverse the disorder. With any toxic heavy metal–caused eating disorder, there are different combinations in play and different levels at which the toxic metals come to affect someone's life. With anorexia, the cases where someone has toxic heavy metals in the brain plus outside sources of emotional pain can make for the most difficult variety.

Many people who have severe eating disorders are on amphetamines and other stimulants prescribed for ADHD and brain fog. These medications also trigger adrenaline that acts as a temporary patch for heavy metal toxicity, which is one way amphetamines and other stimulants offer relief, allowing someone to function, focus, and concentrate. Meanwhile, there are toxic heavy metals in the stimulants, adding to the problem. These medications create additional wear and tear on adrenal glands, eventually adding newer symptoms that can heighten an eating disorder.

Recovery: Beyond Crisis Intervention

When it comes to recovery from eating disorders, the medical system is designed around crisis intervention. When an eating disorder is recognized, the recommendation is usually to eat anything and everything the person's heart desires. The hope is that eating all the comfort food you want will break the eating disorder. The psychological conditioning is "Be happy and do not feel guilty and do not punish yourself." This is considered the best, most advanced medical technology and strategy. It's actually a grandfathered, old clinical approach that was put in place half a century ago that keeps people stuck.

They're right to say you shouldn't feel ashamed or guilty or hate yourself for eating the fun foods and comfort foods they

hope you're eating. Yet you also shouldn't be punished if you want to be mindful, intuitive, and caring about what you're eating to benefit your body and health. Everyone changes. As you grow as an individual and move past the crisis state, you'll learn about your body and your health. You'll discover healthier ways to eat. You shouldn't be made to feel guilty for being extremely mindful about your choices. Caring about what food you put in your body should not be boxed up as "You may have your eating disorder back."

The old clinical strategy that's still in practice today is based on a lack of understanding about how eating disorders develop in the first place and how to heal those eating disorders. This strategy ends up training people to eat foods that are far from healthy—foods that eating disorder patients may have been fearful to eat during or even before their eating disorder. (Another strategy is to eat these foods around others. There are some valid reasons why this strategy exists—for example, to ensure someone is actually eating and to find comfort in a shared meal.) The industry doesn't account for problems that develop because of this eat-all-comfort-foods strategy. One problem occurs if the person has a health problem that's separate from their eating disorder. If that person hadn't been diagnosed with an eating disorder, then nutritionists, dieticians, and doctors would likely recommend that the patient or client eat a healthier version of the standard American diet or avoid processed foods. The person would get the opportunity to keep themselves healthy. Yet nutritionists, dieticians, and doctors are often trained to avoid those healthier approaches when it comes to treating a patient or client with a history of an eating disorder. It's as if healthy eating is off the table for a person with an eating disorder. Suddenly, healthy eating is a serious eating disorder. It's taboo.

This leads the person with an eating disorder to fall into a new trap, which is declining health and nowhere to go with their diet. That declining health may include diabetes, obesity, severe depression, body pain, chronic fatigue, ulcers, acid reflux, IBS, Crohn's, colitis, celiac, and any number of autoimmune diagnoses. During that recovery process from an eating disorder, the system isn't looking ahead at the person's future. The patient isn't hearing, "We have to train you to eat more healthfully during your eating disorder recovery so you don't become chronically ill or deathly ill and lose any opportunities to heal using your foods." Instead individuals recovering from eating disorders often feel pressured to eat the junkiest, unhealthiest foods to prove to counselors, family members, and friends that they are eating, even if it's declining their physical health. Those recovering from an eating disorder don't feel they're allowed their own free will to discover a new approach and use foods to get healthy because it will be seen as a sign for someone in their life to blow the whistle that their eating disorder could be back. Onlookers who have lost trust get suspicious.

This is one of the big misunderstandings of the industry based around eating disorders. It's why eating disorder recovery strategies fail time and time again. We need to allow people room to grow as they get past crisis intervention and continue with their recovery. We can't sabotage them with a new form of shame around food—shame around finding a diet that helps—and expect them to watch their health decline as they eat fried, greasy, processed foods until the end of their life. There should always be an option for individuals to shift gears if their health is declining and they're seeking help. They should be allowed to change up their diet into healthier choices and not be ridiculed or punished or seen as if their eating disorder hasn't improved.

SUGAR ADDICTION

When someone is hooked on processed sugar, it's an indication of a glucose deficiency, sometimes going back to early insulin resistance in childhood. That feeling of a desperate hunt for processed sugar comes from looking for the fastest way to get glucose to the brain. It's not so much that someone is addicted to the sweet flavor; it's that their brain is seeking out a direct line of sugar to correct a deficiency.

The Hidden Factor

If that sugar could really reach the brain as intended, the person would become content and not sugar-crazed afterward. Sugar is not an addictive substance. The reason why it seems addictive is that excess fat in the bloodstream prevents much of the sugar from entering the brain, which leaves the person with excess sugar floating around the bloodstream and the fat from the food causing insulin resistance. It's a vicious cycle.

Seeing it as just a "sugar high" or "sugar crash" is not enough information for anyone to understand how sugar truly interacts in the brain and body. The real reason why someone has a crash, grows cranky or tired, or falls asleep after a sugar high is that they're dealing with insulin resistance due to fat in the bloodstream at the same time as the sugar.

It's very uncommon to consume sugar without some form of fat alongside it. Cakes, cookies, cupcakes, ice cream, chocolate bars, doughnuts—what we think of as sugary or carb-loading treats—all contain fat, even if they're vegan, even if they're healthier versions of treats. Peanut butter and jelly, chips made with high-quality oil, avocado toast: these are all fat and sugar combined. Or we eat dessert after a meal that contained dietary fat. Or when we consume sugar, we still have fat floating around in our bloodstream from an earlier snack or meal. We blame sugar highs and lows on the sugar. The real reason for the highs and lows is the fat.

Craving sugar is not a weakness. It's a human need. We're always in need of glucose for the brain. That's why anyone craves sugar in the first place, and why someone who's been off sugar eventually finds themselves reaching out for it again. While processed sugar is not the ideal way to get that glucose (we'll talk about more productive forms of glucose in Part VI, "Bringing Back Your Brain"), we can use a sugar craving as a window into the brain's needs. Even with insulin resistance occurring from fat in the bloodstream, *some* sugar is getting through, enough to give someone a quick moment, maybe even an hour or so, when they feel relief because that glucose is addressing a long-standing deficiency. It can even feel euphoric.

Trouble is, remedying a glucose deficiency with processed sugar is remedying it the wrong way. Processed sugar isn't supposed to be used in this way—and again, we're normally combining the processed sugar with fats, or there's fat in our bloodstream from earlier in the day. Very few people, if any, are eating straight sugar only and no fats at all in their diet. Even if someone does consume sugar cubes or straight sugar packets, whether a whole-food version of unprocessed raw sugar or processed sugar, there's almost always an overt, radical fat involved—either in something else they're eating or drinking at the same time or in something else they ate or drank that day. You only feel a tease of relief in the brain from the sugar, a flash, before the fat gets in the way. Now you want more. You're perpetually caught in a processed sugar addiction. That addiction isn't coming from processed sugar in the end. It's fat in the way of sugar that's creating a feeling of sugar addiction.

If someone were off fats and they used processed sugar without adding fats to it, they wouldn't get caught up in a sensation of being addicted to the sugar. They'd be just as content to have some pure maple syrup, raw honey, fruit, or sweet potatoes, and they wouldn't feel the need to reach back to the straight processed sugar. Without fats in the way, our brain can get the glucose it needs, especially when we feed our brain the best forms of glucose. We can reach a place of satiation. On the other hand, with oils, milk, cheese, butter, eggs, avocado, nuts, nut butters, cacao, and/or animal products in someone's system, these fats change the dynamic. Suddenly, processed sugar becomes almost weaponized, and the addictive cycle can kick in.

Sugar Highs and Lows

When you're coming down off a processed sugar high, it's not actually the sugar that gives you the experience of withdrawal and the temptation to binge once again on sugar. Again, you go through a withdrawal process because of fats that are in the bloodstream. Fats in the bloodstream trigger an adrenal response because adrenaline is a blood thinner. One of adrenaline's roles is to thin out fat in the bloodstream, allowing for enough oxygen and, ideally, glucose to get to the brain, two resources that are critical for brain function.

Adrenaline is a steroid that can bring good feelings, strength, clarity, and/or energy. There is also a withdrawal process with steroids. Once you start coming down off the fat you consumed combined with processed sugar, your adrenals release less adrenaline. They reduce the crisis-management levels of adrenaline they had released to thin out blood fat. That's when you can experience adrenaline withdrawal, which can bring about sadness, loneliness, a feeling of guilt, even shame. These sensations can prompt you to reach for comfort foods.

It's a vicious cycle that can lead to bingeing more and more on processed sugar, which almost always has some variety of fat involved. And if the processed sugar isn't combined with fat in what you're eating, then surely you're going to be eating fats that day, close to when you're eating the sugar, so fat is going to be in the bloodstream, blocking the sugar from getting into the cells and creating insulin resistance.

Even though we associate sugar with mood swings, it's really all about the adrenals' release of the adrenaline steroid to address fat in the bloodstream—plus insulin resistance from fat in the bloodstream. That's the real story behind the sensations and feelings such as mood swings and crashes that we associate with processed sugar addiction.

Here's another key piece of information: when you are losing weight, fat is dissolving and floating through your bloodstream on its way out of your body. The fat that's dissolving is not converted and used as fuel, as some believe. The dissolved fats coming out of organs or from underneath your derma have a different consistency and viscosity than fats that are floating in your bloodstream from a meal you just consumed. The fats dissolving and leaving your body during weight loss can still create insulin resistance—a milder form of insulin resistance than fats from food you just ate.

The mild insulin resistance from dissolving body fat can happen when someone is starting to lower fats in their diet as they are trying to lose weight or heal a chronic illness. This is why healthy carbohydrates and trace mineral salts in your diet are important as you're healing, to keep you and your blood sugar stabilized as the fats are leaving your bloodstream. Eventually, you get rid of all your insulin resistance.

For specific feeding and eating disorder support (including for anorexia, bulimia, overeating, binge eating, purging, pica, and many more) beyond what's offered in Part VI, "Bringing Back Your Brain," refer to the Eating Disorders protocol, Mystery Hunger protocol, and/or Stomach Problems protocol in *Brain Saver Protocols, Cleanses & Recipes*. For specific orthorexia support, refer to the Orthorexia protocol.

"So many people are misunderstood. Their actions, their words, their intentions, their emotional state—they're misunderstood by the people around them who know them, barely know them, or don't know them at all."

— Anthony William, Medical Medium

CHAPTER 34

Obsessive-Compulsive Disorder

The medical industry has trained health professionals to try to speak the language of people with OCD by naming all of its specific and rare symptoms. This makes an individual with OCD believe the industry knows all about their specific condition. Digging into the fine print tells a different story. That's when you find that the textbooks, studies, and conferences say OCD is caused by genetics, with the implication being that you're the cause of your OCD. Meanwhile, the medical industry knows less about OCD than any other symptom or condition. The truth is that people with OCD have taught the industry everything it knows so far, which boils down to a complicated, sometimes unique, and vast array of symptoms with which someone may suffer.

The medical industry's cataloging of OCD symptoms has gone so far that the industry has compiled virtually every mental health disorder, condition, and symptom into the list of OCD symptoms. If you have anxiety, they claim it's your OCD. If you have unexplained sadness, it's your OCD. If you worry about anything at all, you're not called a worrywart anymore; it's your OCD. If you struggle with any of hundreds of symptoms people struggle with emotionally, mentally, and spiritually, it's packaged up as OCD.

Even when serious mental disorders have led to horrible crimes, some of those crimes have been packaged up as "These individuals have OCD" as the cause. The individuals who commit such atrocities do not have OCD. They have other mental conditions that caused them to commit diabolical crimes. For some reason, the medical industry, coupled with the psychiatric and mental health industry, have by design created a massive OCD umbrella and included every mental health condition in it. I say this to protect anyone who's learning the truth about their OCD. People with OCD are not harmful people. They're not bad people. When you hear dangerous, predatory mental illnesses categorized as OCD, realize you're not under that umbrella. You don't purposely do terrible things to others. You're a good individual who's struggling with something you're about to learn more about here.

Depression, tic disorders, confusion, anxiety, harming yourself, attempting suicide, bipolar disorder, ADHD, schizophrenia, explosive anger attacks: these are also not OCD. What's happening is that the younger generations are struggling with so many emotional and mental disorders that the industry has created an OCD funnel to place them all into the OCD machine. If someone exhibits the simple nature of doubting themselves, it can be funneled into the OCD category. If someone has a lack of confidence, they claim it's OCD. The medical industry, including the alternative health medical industry, is mixing all these individuals up into one.

The industry has created subcategories of OCD so you can find a place where you fit in. This is to make you feel heard and safe when meanwhile, the industry is far from ever solving or fixing the problem. Your true OCD is still under the OCD umbrella with a whole lot of other subcategories that have nothing to do with OCD.

Yes, OCD is real, and it can rise to the level of being completely debilitating and disabling for some people. And yes, many people have mild forms of OCD and many have severe forms of OCD. It's not the compassionate, caring therapists' fault that so much else is getting lumped in with OCD. It's not the fault of the compassionate, caring psychiatrists, doctors, or counselors either. It's the industry above these professionals, training them to see OCD the way the industry wants them to see it. This has led to a tremendous amount of confusion for an OCD sufferer.

The medical industry says that people with OCD are only a tiny fraction of our population. Yet lumping so many symptoms and conditions into the diagnosis of OCD has made it so that over 95 percent of our population could be labeled with OCD. It's contradictory. They're even claiming now that being concerned about germs is OCD. If that's the case, then billions of people on the planet who have been concerned about the recent plague have OCD. Being concerned about germs is not OCD.

Meanwhile, it has become unpopular to classify constantly checking that the stove is off or doors are locked as OCD. These conceptions of OCD, along with excessive hand washing, are now deemed inaccurate stereotypes. The truth is that these are still forms of OCD, and people who struggle with this type of OCD should not be ridiculed, undermined, or declassified and told they don't count.

TOXIC HEAVY METALS OCD

The most predominant cause of OCD is the presence of toxic heavy metals in the brain, with symptoms increasing due to the release of new chemical industry products. More specifically, OCD often results from a mix of mercury, aluminum, and copper. If you have very mild OCD, you may have less metal (both fewer types of metal and lower quantities of it) in fewer places inside the brain and brain stem. Mercury is the key ingredient for creating notable OCD.

Mercury is the most brain-altering toxic heavy metal.

If someone is experiencing another illness caused by toxic heavy metals at the same time—anxiety, depression, brain fog, bipolar, ADHD, a severe eating disorder—the conditions compound on each other, creating a form of OCD that's much harder to manage or harness.

Toxic heavy metals in the brain, as you've read, could be inherited in part. We can also receive significant exposure to heavy metals in our environments. The placement of the metals, what kind they are, and what combination they're in play a profound role in whether someone develops OCD, anxiety, depression, or all three. It also affects whether the condition is long-standing or temporary, continual or involving episodes once a year or periodically throughout life.

What distinguishes OCD is that it tends to result from larger pockets of metals versus smaller metal particles scattered throughout the brain. OCD is about a concentration of toxic heavy metals in brain tissue. The larger the deposits, the more severe the OCD. The smaller the deposits, the less severe. With depression or anxiety alone, when an electrical impulse travels down a neuron on a neurotransmitter chemical and reaches brain tissue, the toxic heavy metals won't be such large blockages that they create barriers for the current. Instead the impulse will be able to travel into the brain tissue. It may be diminished because with depression and anxiety, you often have scattered toxic heavy metals and perhaps neurotoxins in the brain, so the electricity

may not be firing quite right. Still, the electricity won't be stopped completely. Or someone with anxiety or depression could *also* have a larger deposit of metal in the brain, creating OCD at the same time. This is why these conditions so commonly get bundled together.

Why OCD Cycles Happen

With OCD, the "larger nugget" of heavy metals is a relative term—this deposit is still on such a minuscule scale that it's impossible to see with the human eye. As the electrical impulse carrying a thought runs across the neuron and attempts to enter brain tissue that has a deposit of metals, the impulse hits the metal directly and starts to bounce back the other way. This reversal of the electrical impulse is what sets the scene for OCD.

Heading down the same pathway toward that reversing electrical impulse, there's already *another* electrical impulse carrying the same thought or another similar thought, like a little ball of fire. It can take more than one electrical impulse to carry a completed thought. This succession of electrical impulses is like if you were driving down the road at 65 miles per hour with other cars behind you and you suddenly slammed on your brakes, threw the car into reverse, and started traveling backward at the same 65 miles per hour while the car behind kept coming at you. Both electrical impulses carrying the thoughts slam into each other in the middle of the neuron highway. As a result, either the electrical impulses explode or the impact causes one electrical impulse to project off the neuron entirely.

Because the electrical impulse that held the thought someone was thinking just exploded or got derailed and therefore did not reach its destination, the person feels unsatisfied. This becomes unfinished business in the mind. It prompts the person to obsess because the thought did not finish its journey, so the thought wasn't completely processed. If the electrical impulse doesn't explode and instead bounces off the neuron and dissipates along with the information within it, high levels of frustration can occur that accompany the OCD.

Meanwhile, there's yet another electrical impulse heading down, which hits that same metal deposit wall and heads back the other way, and the same pattern repeats itself. This cycle will repeat itself over and over again until an electrical impulse carrying the thought finds its way around the metal deposit and continues its travel.

The variety of repetitive thoughts varies depending upon the variety of metals. What type of metal or mix of metals and in which various places in the brain they're located can determine if the thoughts are more reckless or scary and if these more difficult thoughts have a longer duration. For example, if it's a mercury deposit, mercury tends to bounce electricity farther than other metals. Mercury can project electricity back up the neural pathway with more vigor and strength, creating a larger explosion with the next electrical impulse.

An OCD cycle can create enormous stress. After enough minutes or even hours of someone struggling with this repetition, the human brain has the miraculous ability to temporarily withhold the next electrical impulse from running down that neuron. This is because, due to the fever pitch of intense stress upon the brain during an intense OCD cycle, the brain is registering there is a problem and trying to decode it. The brain will wait for the last current to bounce off the metal wall and head back into the brain tissue from where it came and attempt to find another pathway.

A prime time for the brain to do this decoding is when someone falls asleep. Falling asleep can be hard when someone is in the fever pitch of an OCD cycle. It usually happens, eventually, through exhaustion. When someone is sleeping, the brain can rebuild reserves and find the strength to implement this decoding safeguard. Sometimes upon waking, the same thought can restart down the original pathway, leading to another cycle of OCD. Yet for many who struggle with OCD, the sleep allows the thought path to shift completely so that upon waking, a person gets a fresh start, temporarily free from OCD.

What OCD Feels Like

The repeating actions of OCD have everything to do with electrical impulses slamming into the metal wall of a deposit. It creates an unfinished feeling, a dissatisfaction with whatever task, thought, or action you're doing at the time it's happening.

Everybody's OCD is different. Whatever daily thought or action, whether wanted or unwanted, you are trying to conceive or achieve, ignore or avoid—if an electrical impulse is obstructed by a heavy metal deposit while you're thinking or doing it, you're going to get the sense that your thought, action, or intention is unfinished. That leads to the urge to redo or rethink it, even if it's already complete. We may repeat a thought, task, intention, or action again and again, even if it's displeasing, even if it seems to feel frightening.

Heavy metal deposits, particularly shape-shifting mercury, could be anywhere in the brain, and that affects what someone feels the need to repeat because different areas of the brain may produce different thoughts. One example of an OCD compulsion can take the form of feeling that you didn't completely express a thought—it can feel like you didn't say everything you needed to say or like you weren't heard—prompting the need to turn around and tell someone what's on your mind. This can happen over and over again as the result of a mercury deposit in an area of the brain used for communications with others.

Another example is when a heavy metal deposit is in a part of the brain used for creative expression. This could leave you with the feeling that your paintings are never finished, driving the need to work feverishly on trying to perfect one part of it, or the feeling that you can't get a clothing design out of your system so you have to remake it over and over, never really feeling it's finished.

You could also have more than one variety of OCD at once due to heavy metal deposits in multiple areas, leading to different types of unfinished feelings, thoughts, or actions, both wanted and unwanted.

With obsessive and compulsive thoughts and actions, it can feel almost impossible to move forward without repeating them. If someone is interrupted from continuing a repetition, they will often feel anxious because it's unfinished. On top of this, someone with OCD could also have a separate anxiety condition that could get triggered by having OCD.

Knowing the frustration that OCD behaviors can cause others in your life probably creates a frustration all its own for you. It doesn't mean there's something wrong with who you are. The truth is that you can become a prisoner of your OCD. The medical industry wants to call OCD a mental illness. This is not accurate. Someone could have a serious mental illness, where they're dangerous to themselves and dangerous to others, and also have OCD. Yet OCD is not a mental illness. OCD is an obstructive physical injury. When people are shot with a bullet, they're not considered sick; they're considered injured—sometimes critically so. A bullet is identified as a foreign body; it's an impediment from an outside source. A toxic heavy metal in the brain is an impediment from an outside source too, not a chronic illness per se.

OCD can coexist with chronic illness. For instance, if someone with a mercury deposit in the brain creating OCD also has an autoimmune disorder or any other condition at the same time as the OCD, it could make the OCD much more complicated and difficult to live with. Obsessive loops can orient toward worries of "Are my symptoms back?" or "Are my symptoms worse?" so that someone almost seems like a hypochondriac. Doctors are more aware of chronic illness now and aren't labeling patients as hypochondriacs as often, at least. Still, if someone has a history of OCD and starts to develop symptoms, they may not be taken so seriously, especially if they start to talk about those symptoms a lot. Not being believed can cause more frustration, anger, and anguish, which doesn't help the OCD survivor heal and instead gives them more unease.

EMOTIONAL TRAUMA OCD

A severe emotional blow can also cause OCD. Depending on an individual's sensitivities, even mild emotional injuries can account for this type of OCD. When you feel intense emotional pain or repeated stress, it creates electrical charges in certain areas of the brain that are being overused due to the emotional strain. The intense heat from these electrical impulses burns a cluster of brain cells and neurons. Neurons become hypersensitive around the area of the burned cluster of brain cells—and that lays the foundation for emotional trauma OCD.

This injured cluster of cells develops a callus-like texture in a small area of affected brain tissue, which can occur in various regions of the emotional centers of the brain, depending on the stressor. This callus formation is in place to protect your brain from worse damage, such as an ischemic stroke, because instead the callus becomes a thin layer of tissue over the injured area. Your brain runs on electrical nerve impulses that dart around billions of nerve pathways. When cell injury occurs, the resulting callus hinders those pathways. The impulses can no longer travel easily and properly through the area on their way to their destination.

When electrical impulses can't travel through an area of the brain on their first attempt, they try again—and again—and again. Over and over, the impulses try to move forward on a path that has worked in the past yet is now partially blocked, both physically and energetically. You experience this as racing thoughts that obsessively repeat over and over. Eventually, those impulses drive into the blocked tissue, which can change the obsessive pattern. By then the impulses have lost their strength and their vitality has dissipated. Then new electrical impulses start hitting the blocked tissue repeatedly all over again, and a new cycle of OCD begins.

Emotional trauma OCD can often be outgrown as the years go by. Many people do outgrow it. Then the OCD can come back years later if triggered by a new emotional trauma. Calloused brain tissue can heal naturally over time. You can facilitate the healing process by following the guidance in Part VI, "Bringing Back Your Brain," and in this book's companion, *Brain Saver Protocols, Cleanses & Recipes*.

HEALTHY NEURAL PATHWAYS

We're habit-prone creatures, so even if the underlying problem in the brain that's causing OCD is resolved, that doesn't mean repetitive thoughts and actions will automatically correct themselves right away. It takes time, trust, and willpower.

When someone has been living with OCD, sometimes the brain adapts, or new tissue growth helps electrical impulses find a different route around a metal deposit. The ultimate way to help the brain is to remove the metals with the Heavy Metal Detox and accompanying cleanses in Chapters 44 and 45. Once heavy metals are absent, healing can begin. Many OCD symptoms will minimize. Some may linger and still need more time. Learning to trust the process and focusing on the progress of what symptoms have healed or minimized can help. It really is attainable and doable.

Coupled with removing toxic heavy metals, one of the most potent ways to heal OCD is to create new experiences. Many times people with OCD try to isolate themselves in their routines so they can avoid temptation, fear of acting on unwanted thoughts, unknown variables, or embarrassment. As you cleanse yourself of toxic heavy metal blockages in the brain, you'll want to allow for healthy neural pathways to establish themselves by changing your surroundings and/or shaking up old habits. If possible, relocate yourself, even if it's temporary. Even staying at a friend's house for a day or two can result in substantial improvement in brain health for OCD sufferers.

If you have OCD symptoms, trust in your ability to heal this state of being. Know that you can and will be free from this confusing and difficult life circumstance. Now that you know the true, real causes of the disorder, you're that much closer to resolving it. Have patience and ease of heart. You will finally be empowered to break out of the OCD cycle.

For specific OCD support beyond what's offered in Part VI, "Bringing Back Your Brain," refer to the Obsessive-Compulsive Disorder protocol in *Brain Saver Protocols, Cleanses & Recipes*.

"The light does appear at the end of the tunnel, and health freedom is possible."

— Anthony William, Medical Medium

CHAPTER 35

Bipolar Disorder

Bipolar disorder isn't nearly as sound a diagnosis as it may seem. Today's medical explanations of bipolar disorder, while they may appear convincing, are still theory. If you or someone you're close with has been diagnosed with bipolar, take heart that it's not the fixed and fated condition that we've been taught.

One main ongoing theory is that bipolar is a result of "malfunctioning hormones." *Chemical imbalance* has also been a popular term for decades and is still used today. Seeing a family member acting in a way that seems irrational or manic, being up and then down, low and then high, energetic and then lethargic, depressed and then happy—whatever those ups and downs and struggles and difficulties are—it's easy to hear "malfunctioning hormones" or "chemical imbalance" and think that fits the bill. When you hear either of these terms, know that they indicate a complete misunderstanding about what's really going on in the brain. They're terms that segue naturally into prescriptions for pharmaceuticals that, while they may help some people manage symptoms in the moment, don't remedy the underlying problem.

It's always uncertain whether medication will bring improvement to bipolar disorder or not. In most cases of mild bipolar, the non-sedative medications prescribed in those situations don't bring any results. The condition stays the same or can even worsen. In cases of serious bipolar disorder, where mania reaches a life-threatening level, the extreme pharmaceuticals applied are mostly used for their sedative nature, to get someone to shut down on a certain level to stop the episodes. Coming off those medications takes weaning a little at a time so that person can try to move forward slowly while avoiding another bout of mania. Nowhere in any of this is an understanding of a chemical imbalance. And nowhere in any of it is an understanding of the real cause.

The term *diagnosis* sounds very credible and serious, like it must be based on advanced technology, centuries of medical science, and billions upon billions of dollars invested in the medical world, all of it leading to a deep understanding of the human body.

Meanwhile, if you stop to think about the terminology given to someone who is emotionally struggling with the particular symptoms of bipolar, it means no more than up and down, high and low. A bipolar diagnosis only echoes and oversimplifies how patients themselves describe the experience. The name should go a step further, to explain the why of what's happening. A diagnosis of bipolar disorder should more accurately be called *heating-cooling disorder*, or HCD.

BIPOLAR TRIGGERS

Most mysterious conditions, depression and anxiety among them, require a trigger. It could be a trigger outside the body or inside the body.

First, let's be clear that a "chemical imbalance" is *not* a trigger for bipolar disorder.

One trigger that *can* bring about a manic episode is an emotional experience activating the adrenals into releasing excess adrenaline to be delivered to the brain. Trauma is one example that stimulates the adrenals, causing this surge of adrenaline. The sudden death of a loved one, a contentious divorce, receiving bad news, being betrayed by someone you love and not getting a chance to process it, other life events that are difficult to handle—these can direct a tremendous amount of adrenaline to the brain. When you come down from this adrenaline surge, that's when a depressive episode occurs.

Emotions are not the only trigger for bipolar disorder; chemical exposure can trigger bipolar as well. You could be standing out in front of an apartment building while a city chemical truck drives by spraying tick spray, mosquito spray, or caterpillar spray. Maybe your chemical exposure even happened from something toxic you ate in a fast food meal. Maybe you had your mercury fillings removed. Maybe you got medical treatments that were recommended for travel.

Often people who suffer from bipolar are afraid to get emotional. They know they may be seen as reactive—or overreactive—and so they may try to hide from society to some degree, not communicating as much as they need to or should. Their depression and reclusiveness are often seen by the people who know them as part of the bipolar disorder when they're not; distancing is a way of navigating how the world reacts when you've been called out as having bipolar. Parents, spouses, partners, or other people who live with bipolar folks often get nervous for them, out of a caring and loving place, and get extra sensitive and receptive to what could be a moment of struggle. They get nervous, for example, if the bipolar individual is on a high, accomplishing a lot, because they're familiar with the crash that could be coming. Meanwhile, those with bipolar often sense their loved ones' nervousness and feel they need to hold back their emotions.

Everybody has an emotional state. Everyone. And everybody has triggers to their emotions. The difference with someone whose symptoms have gotten them a bipolar diagnosis, whether mild or severe, is that there's something else going on inside the brain that's trigger-able. We could hide the truth about what that is and go along with the theory that it's hormonal or genetic or a chemical imbalance. We could do that. We're not going to.

METALS RETAINING HEAT

Toxic heavy metals are the underlying cause of bipolar disorder. As we've covered elsewhere in the book, when someone has an elevated amount of metals such as mercury in the brain, their brain runs hotter. With bipolar, the heating is different because the combination of metals—the alloy—retains heat longer.

Generally, the alloy behind bipolar is composed of mercury, copper, toxic calcium, arsenic, toxic platinum, and nickel. The levels of each metal are different for everyone, and the combination can vary—for example, a person may be missing or have very low levels of one or two of these metals. Another person may have higher levels of one or two metals. When someone experiences bipolar disorder, higher levels of toxic calcium and copper especially are present.

When certain combinations of metals are fused together and these metals get heated up, the heat can last for a longer period of time because the metals hold on to the heat. That's how it works with bipolar alloys. This heat is constant, occurring all the time, yet its temperature is always fluctuating.

When toxic heavy metals are in the emotional centers of the brain, impeding

electrical impulses and neuron activity, increased heat occurs on an ongoing basis, making someone highly emotional even when life is seemingly okay—and even during sleep. Someone with bipolar disorder who's not on medication will often be in a heightened dream state for much of the night, experiencing a barrage of dreams because of that continual, fluctuating brain heat without medication suppressing neuron activity.

People with bipolar disorder often liken the condition to having somebody else inside their head controlling them. They can't stop their depression, their manic behavior, their highs and lows, because it's as if that someone else, an entity or alien almost, has taken over. Those who know a bipolar sufferer can often identify a look in their loved one's eyes or a way of talking fast and not listening that says they're struggling to fight off being taken over by the condition.

As the metals in the emotional centers of the brain heat up, it's not a quick acceleration of heat that's followed by a quick de-escalation of the heat. Instead the lasting heat radiates from these metals into brain cells and neurons in the emotional centers of the brain. As a result, brain cells and neurons in the region around these metals dehydrate and burn out and atrophy because of the excess heat. That alone is enough for someone to experience what I call low-grade renditions of bipolar disorder. For more distinctive, heightened bipolar disorder, someone needs a trigger, and the ultimate trigger is adrenaline.

ELECTRICAL STORMS

Every single person has hardships and struggles and confrontations and difficulties at one point or another in life, and with them comes more intense adrenaline and more of it. That's not an imbalance—it happens to all of us. For someone with bipolar disorder, that flood of adrenaline is a trigger.

Here's why: Someone with toxic heavy metals in the emotional centers of the brain needs a little bit more adrenaline. If they're going to exercise or exert themselves, for example, they need a little more adrenaline to do that than the next person. This is because the emotional centers of the brain are sending a signal to the adrenals for help. Our body uses adrenaline as a remedy in times of any kind of crisis, from mild to extreme. When the metal alloys behind bipolar disorder are present in the brain's emotional centers, causing a continual heating process, it warrants the call for additional adrenaline to keep the electricity balanced and flowing through the emotional centers of the brain. Compromised, dehydrated brain cells and neurons in this area require adrenaline to alter and change the course of the electrical pattern and the heat that's being produced.

When adrenaline enters an already hot brain, it helps that person function and get what they need in one sense. It also ignites electricity on an explosive level. When it's happening day after day, an adrenaline rush to an environment that's already hot due to heavy metals ignites an electrical storm that's very disruptive. The acute, excessive heating from the excess adrenaline can't be cooled until burnout occurs.

This is when a person works for 72 hours and then crashes for days. It's when someone goes on a long jag of talking rapidly without listening and then afterward, goes quiet. It's when someone makes an impulsive, irrational decision that's not healthy for them, followed by a depression, deep sadness, and feeling of guilt and shame, accompanied by a fatigue and absence of motivation and drive. The bipolar electrical storm and its aftermath can display themselves in so many ways, to so many different degrees.

Adrenaline rushing to treat compromised areas of the brain can also lead to emotional sensitivity that varies in every single person struggling with this condition. For example, they may easily become triggered by anything that is stressful.

NOT ONE SIZE FITS ALL

Bipolar is not one size fits all. It's not as simple as bipolar I disorder, bipolar II disorder, and cyclothymic disorder. It's bipolar I through bipolar 1-million. Everyone's toxic heavy metal load is different.

Bipolar is not a genetic disorder. Having someone else in the family with similar symptoms does not mean it has to do with genes. It has everything to do with toxic heavy metals traveling through the bloodline. Heavy metals get passed along from generation to generation for hundreds or even thousands of years and find their way to different parts of the body in every person. Sometimes they end up in the emotional centers of the brain, which is how brothers, sisters, aunts, uncles, or parents can exhibit similar bipolar characteristics. It's not genetic predisposition.

Bipolar can also change over time for the person experiencing it: At a certain point, a bipolar sufferer's adrenals can shift and change. The metals can shift and change too. As a result, symptoms can alter in any direction as someone ages with this condition.

Oxidation is one reason the metals shift and change. In part because individuals with bipolar tend to have less aluminum in their alloys, the oxidation that eventually occurs in bipolar alloys tends to intoxicate brain cells and neurons differently from the heavy metal oxidation in other brain conditions. With the alloys behind bipolar, the oxidation process tends to last longer due to the continual heat. While this oxidation doesn't necessarily spread to adjacent brain tissue like with other conditions, a certain level of oxidation does occur as the years go by from the group of metals that causes bipolar disorder. This can affect the symptoms someone is living with, and that doesn't automatically mean for the worse. The brain is an incredible organ, and electrical patterns constantly being altered as the years go by can sometimes even work in someone's favor when they're struggling with a condition such as bipolar.

The metals are still there in the brain, creating bipolar, only now it may be less mania and more depression. That numbed, depressed experience of life will last until the adrenals recover, at which point the adrenaline surges, and with them, the manic episodes may start up again. The most effective way of treating this disorder is to remove the toxic heavy metals from the brain and the rest of the body.

SOOTHING, COOLING RELIEF

Your brain uses sugars to protect itself, so glycogen storage in the brain plays a big role in how severe someone's bipolar disorder is. The more glycogen storage, the less someone is going to suffer from bipolar because the less they'll get injured by an electrical storm in the brain or the brain's inability to cool itself. More glycogen forming in brain tissue that neurons run through is critical for helping someone with bipolar.

The brain is amazing. Its adaptive ability allows it to shift according to circumstances so that we can shift and adapt too. With metals gone from the brain, and specifically gone from the brain's emotional centers, the brain can cool itself to prevent emotional meltdowns. And when someone is getting enough glucose—enough natural sugars and healthy carbohydrates to fortify the brain—it can regulate its temperature even better. Your brain bringing in glucose is like rain rolling in to die out a fire after lightning.

For specific bipolar disorder support beyond what's offered in Part VI, "Bringing Back Your Brain," refer to the Bipolar Disorder protocol in *Brain Saver Protocols, Cleanses & Recipes*.

CHAPTER 36

Alzheimer's and Dementia

How does someone get a diagnosis of Alzheimer's disease or dementia? Usually the label is given when a lot of forgetfulness starts to occur. The type of forgetfulness plays a role in diagnosis. Is someone just forgetting where they left their car keys? Or are they forgetting what occurred during an eventful day and starting to forget what they used to remember from the past?

Many people become paranoid about having Alzheimer's when they start to struggle with short-term or even long-term memory loss. Are these really the first signs and signals of developing Alzheimer's and dementia? Are they even signs? Were there earlier signs that no one detected?

We all have the right in our busy lives to be forgetful. We all have the right to not remember everything. So much depends upon what you're doing in your work, how much you're taking on, how much brain space is being used, and how consumed you may be with a life event that's taking its toll mentally and emotionally.

Sometimes it's not passing forgetfulness due to overload; sometimes everything

seems to be perfect, all's happy, you have your routine, and suddenly you're getting confused, forgetting about certain events you have on your calendar, and you or someone close to you feels there's obviously something going on. Some people experience episodes of delusions, spaceouts, or truly losing all sense of time. These symptoms may come and go for years, with long stretches passing with no episodes and then sudden disorienting experiences. Someone may visit the doctor because a family member or friend suggested it, noticing unusual behaviors, and the doctor doesn't really know if there is a problem or not. Then when the symptoms start happening more often, the doctor will diagnose it as Alzheimer's or dementia.

What does this all mean? What constitutes a real Alzheimer's or dementia diagnosis? The truth is, it's all a gray area with gray matter. Doctors often rely on brain scans such as MRIs, looking for what they believe are inconsistencies in the images. If someone is becoming more forgetful, their personality is changing unusually, they're exhibiting mood shifts, attitude shifts, or changes of demeanor and it's alarming to the people around them, and then an inconsistency shows up on a brain scan, they may get a diagnosis of early Alzheimer's or dementia. Only in certain cases is anything seen on a brain scan. Besides which, the type of inconsistency that shows up on the brain scan of someone with forgetfulness may very well show up on the brain scan of someone who isn't having forgetfulness too. In the majority of Alzheimer's diagnoses, there's nothing unusual in the brain image. Diagnosis is really based on theories and guessing games. Maybe a doctor will ask a couple of colleagues in their medical group, and together they'll determine that Alzheimer's or another form of dementia is developing.

The picture painted about Alzheimer's and dementia, and especially about Alzheimer's itself, is that medical research and science understand it completely—that there's really nothing more to uncover besides a cure. If they understand it fully, why don't they have a cure? How is it possible to wholly comprehend a disease without also knowing what the antidote is? What it really means is that the disease is completely misunderstood. If the medical establishment truly understood Alzheimer's and dementia on any level, we would be at a place where they also have the answer. The same is true of any chronic illness.

ALZHEIMER'S ANSWERS

When an Alzheimer's patient benefits in some way from changing their diet or taking supplements, it doesn't mean any of it is understood, even if an expert in the field of medicine feels they stumbled across a helpful remedy to temporarily slow down the disease progression. We can throw around "improve your gut health," we can throw around "top brain foods," and someone can toss out their old lifestyle and past ways of eating, start on supplements, and see their memory get a little better as some confusion and brain fog start to temporarily ease off. It still doesn't mean the disease is grasped on any level. Medical industries, both alternative and conventional, are still completely in the dark about Alzheimer's. What medical professionals are really looking at in a brain scan, and what it means about what's occurring in the brain, is still a mystery to them.

It's going to remain a mystery. Millions of people will continue receiving Alzheimer's and dementia diagnoses with no real answers for years into the future—because the answers aren't fruitful to the medical industry. They threaten its foundation. And so a pretending will continue: a pretending that medical communities know what Alzheimer's and dementia are, how to diagnose them correctly, and how the diseases work, and that the only missing piece is a cure. The fact that some patients show improvements with changes in diet makes both alternative and conventional medical professionals feel closer to knowing what the problem is inside the brain and the body. They have no idea that they'll run up against an impediment to real knowing.

Why are the answers about Alzheimer's and dementia so frightful for the medical industry? Because in part, they're industry-caused. When an "answer" about Alzheimer's surfaces, it won't be the truth. It will be a classic decoy. Because the truth—the all-too-threatening truth—is that Alzheimer's is a collection of toxic heavy metals, many of which have entered the patient from medical treatments right from the start, beginning with babyhood, or have been passed down through the bloodline from medical treatments of old that our ancestors received. Specifically, Alzheimer's and dementia are mercury-caused, with enough aluminum also present in the brain for these diseases to form.

These toxic heavy metals that enter the brain can cause a lot of early warning signs along the way, starting in childhood and young adulthood. It's simply that no one knows these symptoms are indeed possible signs of someone, one day far in the future, losing their memory, forgetting who they are, forgetting their loved ones, and losing the ability to function. The precursors to memory loss that show up early in life are never really, truly seen—because the medical industry has to practically ignore much that's brain-related. Instead many issues are blamed on someone having mental or emotional problems. Some end up feeling that they're simply dysfunctional. Prescription antidepressants, antianxiety medications, stimulants, and mood stabilizers are being handed out at levels never before seen in history. At the same time, Alzheimer's and dementia are on the rise, and because they tend to happen later in life, a connection isn't made to earlier struggles.

Not that Alzheimer's and dementia are always preceded by obvious mental struggles. Many individuals may not show early signs of mood destabilization or the need for antidepressants. They still display other early signs that are missed along the way. These signs aren't easy to read. Doctors don't witness what we say and how we act in every moment of our lives—it's impossible—so signals go by unnoticed.

A DIFFERENT KIND OF AGING

Here's what's occurring: toxic heavy metals inside the brain are aging. That's right—we're not talking about someone aging naturally; the metals themselves age.

Over a lifetime, we collect more and more metals if we don't know how to watch out for them or detox them. And metals in the brain attract metals—that's especially true with mercury. As more mercury enters the body and circulates through, it can find old deposits of mercury within the brain, connect, and join on to the deposits, forming larger deposits over the years. The mercury expands. When that expansion occurs, the older mercury that has aged, oxidized, and corroded loosens up and breaks free, with oxidative discharge and runoff saturating adjacent brain tissue. This can be the straw that breaks the camel's back, with someone waking up one morning, not realizing where they are, and taking a half hour to shake out of it and realize that they're home. That was when that aged, oxidized mercury runoff expanded into adjacent brain tissue. The dam broke.

More oxidation can occur when it's not just mercury present in the brain. As I mentioned, aluminum may also be present. Those aluminum deposits in the brain must be fairly close to the mercury deposits for symptoms to accelerate, although aluminum deposits don't need to join mercury deposits to rapidly kill and destroy brain cells that harbor memories. What happens is that aluminum oxidizes too, at a faster rate, and problems occur when aged, oxidized aluminum debris and runoff travel and collapse into a mercury deposit—causing faster expansion of the mercury pocket.

This process can take years and years—although it can also be accelerated at this point in history. At younger and younger ages, people are feeling like they're losing their minds; you'll find more and more people in their 40s and early 50s getting diagnosed with Alzheimer's or a condition that starts out with a different diagnosis and eventually leads to an Alzheimer's diagnosis down the road.

We can have as many Alzheimer's charities, benefits, and fundraisers as possible, and they're not going to help in finding the cure they desire. They can certainly be helpful in some ways—in caring for the people who suffer from this disease, in raising awareness of it, in supporting caregivers—so we must keep them going. Still, they'll be blocked from uncovering the mercury-aluminum connection because the medical and pharmaceutical industries employ these two

metals. They're not the only industries. The cosmetics industry, too, has used them for years and years and years. The food industry has a history of using aluminum. The chemical industry has been putting aluminum in conventional cleaning products. If the truth comes out that aluminum plays a role, that some Alzheimer's patients are struggling in part because they used aluminum-based products all throughout their early years, there's going to be trouble. And what about aluminum-based deodorants? What about any kind of pharmaceutical drug packed with toxic heavy metals such as aluminum? What about the chemical industry making pesticides, herbicides, and other products packed with toxic heavy metals?

No one can go there. Going there—exploring why people really suffer with Alzheimer's and dementia—awakens a beast that no one wants to contend with. That beast is truth. It's why industries pay people to shift and hide and alter the truth; they pay people to control and calm the beast.

We have to see it like it is. In Alzheimer's and dementia, someone has a high level of mercury and aluminum in the brain already oxidizing, and as the years go on, oxidative debris from these aging metals expands and accelerates. The excess byproduct becomes runoff that saturates brain tissue, sequestering areas of the brain where electricity is supposed to run fluently and freely. Another way to see it is that dead patches form in the brain—low-voltage areas where electricity cannot function at the level it needs to. Electricity helps keep brain tissue active by stimulating brain cells, so a lack of electricity in an area of brain tissue can cause it to deteriorate and atrophy. That's what's behind so many of the symptoms of Alzheimer's or dementia.

Now, not all Alzheimer's and dementia cases display themselves in the same way. Personalities differ, people's souls differ, where the toxic heavy metals lie in the brain differs, how much toxic heavy metal is present differs, just how the toxic heavy metals eat away at tissue differs, how much oxidation is occurring differs, and how deficient someone's brain is differs.

If you're wondering about the difference between Alzheimer's and other forms of dementia, they are basically one and the same. They're both caused by the same metals, mercury and aluminum. It's just that symptoms can vary because of where those metals sit in the brain. When metals are a millimeter this way or that way in someone's brain or brain stem, they can create completely different symptoms, ranging from delusions to severe tantrums to the need to walk for hours with no direction. It varies in every way. Alzheimer's and other types of dementia are the same disease. They're both severe brain tissue damage from large deposits of metals that have oxidized.

POWER OVER ALZHEIMER'S

What we can all take away from this is to prepare way ahead of time. All of us have these metals inside us, in different places in the brain and body, at different levels and to different degrees. This is why removing

heavy metals from the brain, which you'll find cleanses for in Part VI, "Bringing Back Your Brain," is so critical and should be taken so seriously. The goal is to minimize any new toxic heavy metals coming into your body systems while eliminating any old metals you already have, ones you might have been born with or received as a child. If you start at age 20, great. If you start at 30 or 40, great. If you start at 50, 60, 70, or later, it's still powerful and can still help.

If someone who was dealing with an early onset of Alzheimer's or dementia symptoms starts eating better and taking supplements, and they're starting to see improvements, a few things happen. First is that they're getting additional nutrients to the brain to offset some of the damage being done by the toxic heavy metals. Second is that they're starting to detox many other poisons and toxins that have gotten into the bloodstream and are circulating through the body. Third is that their liver health is improving, because a stagnant, sluggish, overburdened, toxic liver contributes to a toxic brain. Fourth is that, without their realizing it, the additional antioxidants they're receiving are helping slow down the toxic heavy metal oxidation process.

What medical professionals should be trained to ask themselves when they look at an Alzheimer's patient's brain scan is "Where are the metals?" As they consult other doctors for help, they're supposed to be asking, "What kinds of metals are present? Can you see them? Are there any inconsistencies on the brain scan that could be toxic heavy metal damage? Is that what's causing these symptoms the patient is suffering with?"

If you have a loved one with Alzheimer's or dementia, the goal is to be aggressive about removing heavy metals so the condition doesn't worsen. Some brain rot can be reversed, enough to back an Alzheimer's patient out of the woods. It may not make them perfect again, depending on how severe it is. Still, it can bring them out of the dense, dark forest and into a safe clearing, or it can slow down or stop the progression of the disease. And if you're worried for yourself because you have someone with Alzheimer's or dementia in your family line, you don't have to live in dread. Your fate is not decided.

For specific Alzheimer's, dementia, or memory loss support beyond what's offered in Part VI, "Bringing Back Your Brain," refer to the Alzheimer's Disease protocol in *Brain Saver Protocols, Cleanses & Recipes*.

For specific forgetfulness support, refer to the Brain Fog protocol.

"No matter what alloys reside inside us and where in the brain those toxic heavy metal blends lie, we need to take action to remove the toxic heavy metal alloys so we can set ourselves on the course of healing. We truly must save our brains. While removing toxic heavy metals takes time, when we put that time and energy into it, the rewards are beyond imaginable."

— Anthony William, Medical Medium

"People are blamed for 'projection.' They're told they're projecting their pain and anger at others. They're told, 'Stop projecting.' So they try self-care hacks and trends for betterment, try to become better people, and then the minute they pop, they're blamed for projecting their pain onto others. What they're really doing is showing that their brain's physical needs aren't being met."

— Anthony William, Medical Medium

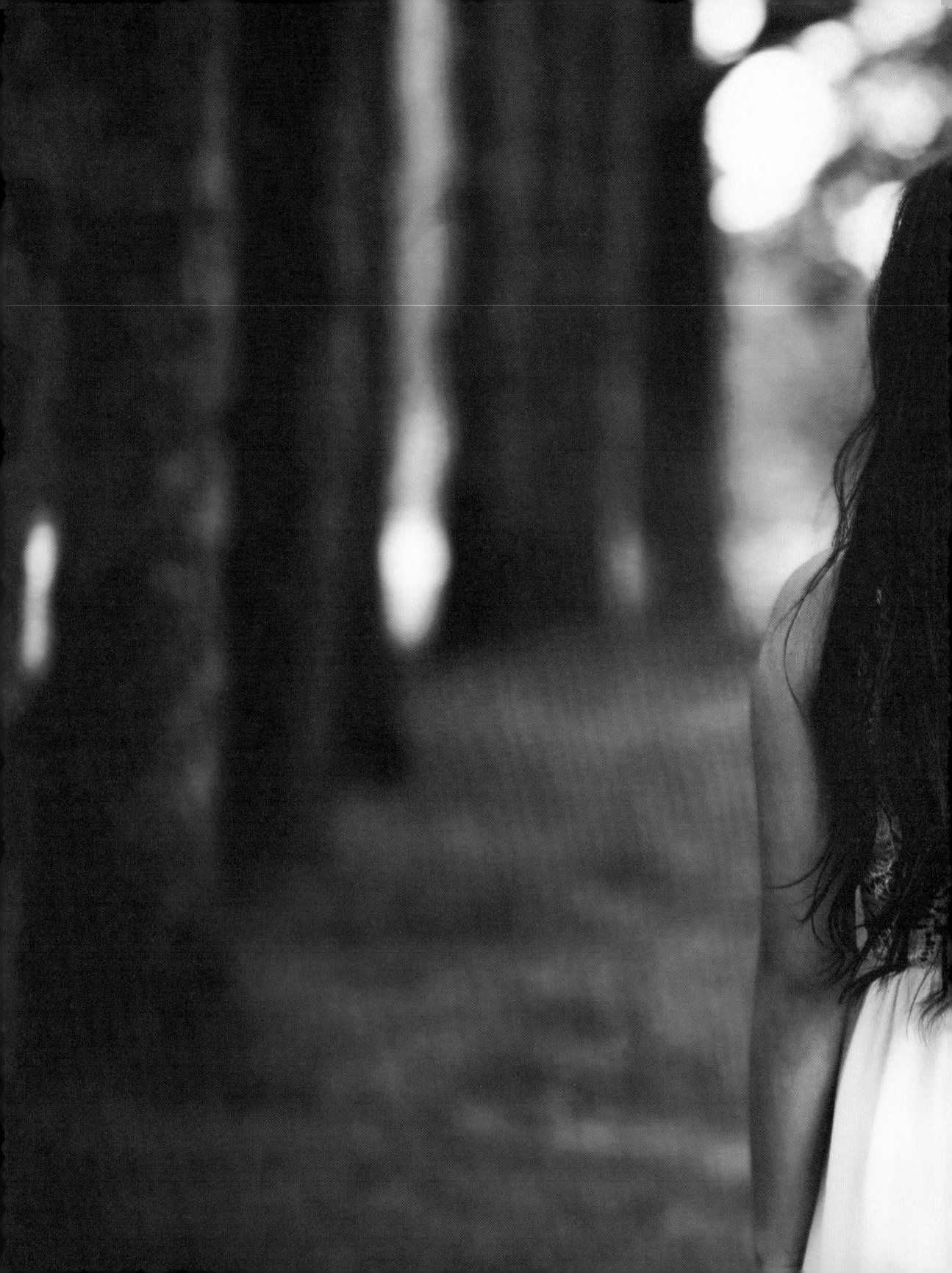

PART V

YOUR PAIN AND SUFFERING ENLIGHTENED

"In today's world, getting a symptom or condition—becoming chronically sick—is the new normal. We're at a place in the world where you're either not-so-sick or very sick. Everyone is dealing with something. Everybody is facing at least one symptom, whether they'd call it a 'symptom' or not, whether they realize their health is challenged or not."

— Anthony William, Medical Medium

CHAPTER 37

How to Find Your Way

The symptoms and conditions in this section of the book cover a wide range of experiences. To help you find your answers, I've used the conventional medical names in most cases.

If you have one of the conditions in the next chapter and yet you've never identified with the name given to it, don't let that throw you. Chronic health issues, including chronic neurological symptoms and conditions, remain a mystery to medical research and science, so the terminology given to them often stays on the surface. Once you start digging into the explanations to come, you'll see that diagnosis names are simply labels. When you find out what's behind your experience, you can start to rebuild your relationship with your health.

If you feel there's repetition regarding some of the symptoms and conditions, the reason is that the medical industry creates the repetition with hundreds of overlapping symptom and condition labels, because they don't know the true causes. You'll often hear "cause unknown" from the medical industry when it comes to chronic and neurological illness. While the medical industry offers life-saving medicine for organ failure, heart failure, and surgeries, it's unfortunate how much they don't know regarding symptoms and conditions in chronic illness. "It could be this." "Inconclusive." "Researchers are still looking for a gene." "Researchers believe."

The information in this section of the book is not repetitious; it exposes the repetition of the medical naming system and how this can be deceiving. Getting multiple labels can make you believe you have everything wrong with you. Not to mention that creating label after label for overlapping, nearly identical symptoms or conditions allows the industry to make a drug for each label.

Here, you will find answers of which the medical industry is unaware. The reality is that the same causes can create dozens of symptoms. One cause can be the answer for several symptoms and conditions that were given different names by the medical industry. Heavy metal toxicity, for example, is responsible for hundreds of diagnoses in the psychiatric world, and that's unknown.

The medical industry has yet to comprehend this set of common causes that you'll see come up often in this section. When you read each symptom and condition closely, you will notice subtle differences across these causes and what is occurring inside the brain and body that makes different symptoms and conditions unique.

If you don't find your precise symptom or condition here, or you don't have a name for what you're suffering with, don't let that deter you. Reading through these explanations can help you pinpoint your own situation. If you've flipped directly to this section of the book, you'll want to make sure you also get a chance to go back and read the rest of the book for the full context. In particular, Part I, "Your Brain Story," offered an extensive look at how our neurological struggles come to be. With the knowledge in this book, combined with your expertise on your own experience, you have the tools to put the pieces of your health in place.

You can find healing. With a focus on removing toxic heavy metals, reducing viral loads, reversing chemical exposure, healing emotional and physical trauma, and repairing and restoring injured nerves in the brain and body, symptoms and conditions can be reversed. Use the information you discover here to customize your own healing protocol from Part VI, "Bringing Back Your Brain," and this book's companion, *Brain Saver Protocols, Cleanses & Recipes*.

One vital resource in *Brain Saver Protocols, Cleanses & Recipes* is its extensive section on supplementation. There in "Supplement Gospel," you'll find information on nine Medical Medium Shock Therapies to help you through times of acute suffering, along with detailed protocols geared for even more health concerns than there was room to include in this book:

- Everyday Brain and Health Maintenance

- Aches and Pains

- Acute Disseminated Encephalomyelitis (ADEM)

- Addiction

- Addison's Disease

- ADHD (Attention-Deficit/ Hyperactivity Disorder)

- Age Spots

- Alcohol Withdrawal

- ALS (Amyotrophic Lateral Sclerosis, Lou Gehrig's Disease, Motor Neuron Disease)

- Alzheimer's Disease

- Amnesia

- Anemia

- Aneurysm

- Ankylosing Spondylitis

- Anorexia

- Anxiety

- Anxiousness

- Aphasia

- Apraxia

- Arrhythmia

- Arteriosclerosis

- Arthritis (Reactive)

- Arthritis (Rheumatoid)

- Atheroma

- Atherosclerosis

- Atrial Fibrillation (AFib)

- Auditory Processing Disorder (APD)

- Autism

- Autoimmune Disorders and Diseases

- Avoidant Restrictive Food Intake Disorder (ARFID)

- Ayahuasca Recovery

- Balance Issues

- Balo Disease

- Bell's Palsy

- Binge Eating Disorder

- Bipolar Disorder

- Bloating (Severe)

- Blood Clots

- Blood Draw (for one week directly before)

- Blood Draw (for one week directly following)

- Blurred Vision

- Body Buzzing and Humming

- Body Dysmorphic Disorder (BDD)

- Brain Abscess

- Brain Aging

- Brain Cancer

- Brain Fog

- Brain Inflammation

- Brain Lesions

- Brain Tumors and Cysts

- Breast Implant Illness

- Bulimia

- Burning Hot Feeling with No Fever

- Burning Sensations inside Mouth

- Burning Sensations on Skin

- Burnout

- Bursitis

- Buzzing in Ears

- Caffeine Withdrawal

- Calcifications on Brain
- Canker Sores
- Carpal Tunnel Syndrome
- Castleman Disease
- Celiac Disease
- Cerebral Atrophy
- Cerebral Hypoxia
- Cerebral Palsy
- Cerebrovascular Disease
- Chemical and Food Sensitivities
- Chest Tightness (Mystery)
- Chewing Difficulty
- Chocolate and Cacao Withdrawal
- Chronic Anger Disorder
- Chronic Fatigue Immune Dysfunction Syndrome (CFIDS)
- Chronic Fatigue Syndrome (CFS)
- Chronic Inflammatory Demyelinating Polyneuropathy (CIDP)
- Chronic Mystery Guilt
- Coffee Withdrawal
- Cold, Flu, and COVID
- Cold Hands and Feet
- Cold Sensitivity
- Cold Sores
- Concussion Recovery Side Effects
- Connective Tissue Disease
- Cranial Nerve Atrophy
- Cranial Nerve Inflammation
- Crohn's Disease
- Crooked Jaw Feeling
- Cushing's Syndrome (Hypercortisolism)
- Cyclothymic Disorder
- Cystic Fibrosis
- Dark Spots on Brain
- Dark Tongue Discoloration
- Dementia
- Depersonalization
- Depression
- Dermatitis Herpetiformis (DH)
- Devic's Disease
- Difficulty Coping
- Dizziness
- Drooping Face
- Dysautonomia

- Dyslexia
- Dysphagia
- Dysphoria
- Eating Disorders
- Ectopic Heartbeat
- Ehlers-Danlos Syndrome
- Electric Shock to the Head Feeling
- Encephalitis
- Encephalopathy
- Energy Issues
- Epilepsy
- Epstein-Barr Virus (EBV) (Early Stage)
- Epstein-Barr Virus (EBV) (Late Stage)
- Epstein-Barr Virus (EBV) (Reactivated)
- Excessive Sweating
- Extreme Fatigue
- Eyeball Unusual Movement (including difficulty with muscles around eyes)
- Eye Floaters (Visual Snow)
- Eye Focus Issues
- Facial Pain

- Fainting
- Fatigue
- Fever Blisters
- Fibromyalgia
- Flu
- Fluttering in Ears
- Focus and Concentration Issues
- Food Poisoning
- Food Sensitivities
- Forgetfulness
- Frozen Shoulder
- Gas Pain
- Gastric Spasms
- Gastritis
- Gastritis (Autoimmune)
- Gastroparesis (Mild)
- Gastroparesis (Severe)
- Green Tea, Matcha Tea, and Black Tea Withdrawal
- Guillain-Barré Syndrome
- Gum Pain (Mystery)
- Gut Pains and Spasms
- Headaches
- Hearing Loss (Unexplained)

- Heart Palpitations (Neurological)
- Heart Palpitations (Non-neurological)
- Heat Sensitivity
- Hemispatial Neglect
- Hepatitis (Autoimmune)
- Herpes Simplex (HSV) 1 and 2
- HIV (Human Immunodeficiency Virus)
- Humidity Sensitivity
- Huntington's Disease
- Hyperhidrosis
- Hyperpigmentation
- Impulse Control Issues
- Inflammatory Myopathy
- Influenza
- Inner Ear Disease
- Insomnia
- Intracranial Hypertension
- Irritability
- Itching and Burning (when no rash is present)
- Jaw Pain (Mystery)
- Joint Pain

- Learning Disabilities and Disorders
- Left Neglect
- Liver Spots
- Long-Haul COVID (also called Long COVID)
- Long-Haul Flu
- Loss of Face Movement
- Loss of Smell
- Loss of Taste
- Low Vision
- Lower Back Pain (Mystery)
- Lupus
- Lyme Disease
- Mania
- Marijuana Withdrawal
- ME/CFS (Myalgic Encephalomyelitis/Chronic Fatigue Syndrome)
- Melasma (Chloasma)
- Memory Issues
- Memory Loss
- Ménière's Disease
- Meningitis
- Migraines

- Mind-Body Syndrome

- Mitochondrial Myopathy

- Mononucleosis (Mono)

- Mood Changes and Mood Swings

- Motor Skills Disorder (also known as Developmental Dyspraxia)

- Multiple Sclerosis (MS)

- Muscle Pain (Mystery)

- Muscle Spasms

- Muscle Weakness

- Muscular Dystrophy

- Myasthenia Gravis

- Myelin Nerve Sheath Damage

- Myocarditis

- Mystery Fears and Worries

- Mystery Hunger

- Narcolepsy

- Nausea (Mystery)

- Neck Pain (Mystery)

- Neuralgia

- Neuritis

- Neurological Fatigue

- Neurological Gastroparesis

- Neurological Lyme

- Neurological Symptoms

- Neuromuscular Disease

- Neuropathy

- Neurosis

- Numbness

- Obsessive-Compulsive Disorder (OCD)

- Occipital Neuralgia

- Optic Nerve Atrophy

- Optic Neuritis

- Orthorexia

- Other Specified Feeding and Eating Disorder (OSFED)

- Overeating

- Pain in Back of Head (Mystery)

- Pain inside or around Ear(s)

- Pancreatitis (Autoimmune) (AIP)

- PANDAS (Pediatric Autoimmune Neuropsychiatric Disorders Associated with Streptococcal Infections)

- Panic Attacks

- Paralysis of Facial Nerves (Temporary)

- Paraneoplastic Cerebellar Degeneration (PCD)
- Parasites
- Parkinson's Disease
- Parsonage-Turner Syndrome (PTS)
- Peristaltic Issues
- Personality Disorders
- Pica Eating Disorder
- Polymyalgia Rheumatica
- Popping in Ears
- Post-polio Syndrome
- POTS (Postural Orthostatic Tachycardia Syndrome)
- Pressure in Chest (Mystery)
- Psychedelic Mushroom Withdrawal
- Psychosis
- PTSD (Posttraumatic Stress Disorder) / PTSS (Posttraumatic Stress Symptoms)
- Pulling Sensation in the Face (such as nose, eyes, or forehead)
- Pulsating Sensations in the Head
- Recreational Drug Withdrawal
- Repetitive Strain Injuries (RSI)

- Restless Legs Syndrome
- Restlessness
- Rheumatoid Arthritis (RA)
- Right Neglect
- Ringing in Ears
- Roving Pain
- Sadness
- Sarcoidosis
- Scar Tissue on Brain
- Schizophrenia
- Sciatica
- Seasonal Affective Disorder (SAD)
- Seizures
- Sense of Not Digesting Well
- Shingles
- Sjögren's Syndrome
- Sleep Apnea
- Sleep Issues
- Slurred Speech
- Spasms
- Speech Difficulties
- Stiffness (including Stiff Person Syndrome)
- Stomach Burning

- Stomach Flipping

- Stomach Pain

- Stomach Problems

- Strokes

- Sun Sensitivity

- Sunspots

- Swallowing Difficulty

- Systemic Exertion Intolerance Disease (SEID)

- Tendonitis

- Tennis Elbow

- Throat Pain, Pressure, or Tightness (Mystery)

- Tics

- Tingles

- Tinnitus

- TMJ (Temporomandibular Joint Dysfunction)

- Tongue Pain (Mystery)

- Tooth Grinding

- Tooth Pain (Mystery)

- Tourette's Syndrome

- Transient Ischemic Attack (TIA)

- Trembling Hands

- Tremors

- Trigeminal Neuralgia

- Trigger Finger

- Twitches (including twitching around head and face)

- Ulcerative Colitis

- Ulcers

- Unspecified Feeding or Eating Disorder (UFED)

- Vagus Nerve Problems

- Vasculitis

- Vertigo

- Vibrating Face and/or Head

- Vibrating in Ears

- Viral Infection Fatigue

- Visual Disturbances

- Vomiting (Mystery)

- Weakness of Limbs

- White Spots on Brain

- Whooshing Sounds in Ears

- Willis-Ekbom Disease

- Wilson's Disease

When you've lived with any kind of brain- or nerve-related symptom or condition, you've gained a new view of the world. You've gained compassion. You can bring those insights with you as you gain health freedom and move on into the next chapter of your life.

CHAPTER 38

Symptom and Condition Answers

Remember:

- The same causes can create dozens of symptoms and conditions. Often, these symptoms and conditions receive different medical names even when the health challenges are similar. Take note of the sometimes subtle variations from answer to answer.

- You don't need to be able to find your precise health concern in this chapter to find answers. Look for the explanation of the closest symptom or condition listed here and combine that with your knowledge from Part I, "Your Brain Story," about the foundations of our physical, emotional, and mental health struggles.

- Find vital healing tools such as Heavy Metal Detox, Brain Shot Therapy, cleanse options, and a guide to brain-supporting food in Part VI, "Bringing Back Your Brain."

- If you want to take your healing further, this book's companion, *Brain Saver Protocols, Cleanses & Recipes*, is available as an additional resource. On top of offering over 100 brain-nourishing recipes, nine Medical Medium Shock Therapies, an in-depth look at the foods that hold back healing, and a selection of soul-soothing meditations, that book offers supplement protocol support for hundreds of symptoms and conditions— more than there was room to cover here.

ADDICTION

See Chapter 8, "Your Addicted Brain."

ADHD (ATTENTION-DEFICIT/ HYPERACTIVITY DISORDER)

Here's what ADHD isn't: genetic or gut-related. Neither of these popular explanations addresses the true underlying cause of attentional, focus, hyperactivity, impulsivity, or even executive function or self-regulation issues. What really causes ADHD is mercury and aluminum settling in the brain's cerebral midline canal, which divides the brain's left hemisphere from the right, along with some additional metals scattered in other areas of the brain. It's the same cause as autism (more soon), although in ADHD, the ratio is a little more aluminum and a little less mercury. When these metals take up residence in the midline canal, they block internal communications within the brain. As a result, the brain must adapt, and electrical impulses must find new avenues, traveling on neurons that wouldn't normally be used for talking, listening, and other forms of action and communication. This is why you'll often find a child with ADHD behaving in one manner when you're asking them to behave in another. The evolving domestic chemicals that children are up against in today's world are triggering and worsening this condition. You'll find much more on ADHD in the revised and expanded *Medical Medium*.

For specific healing support beyond what's offered in Part VI, "Bringing Back Your Brain," refer to the ADHD protocol in *Brain Saver Protocols, Cleanses & Recipes*.

ALS (AMYOTROPHIC LATERAL SCLEROSIS, LOU GEHRIG'S DISEASE, MOTOR NEURON DISEASE)

When someone is handed an ALS diagnosis, it often leaves the patient and loved ones feeling hopeless. If this is you, take heart. As with so many chronic illnesses, ALS is only a label, not an explanation. The label of ALS alone—the fear, panic, and lost sleep it causes—is often partially responsible for someone's sudden health decline. Understanding the true cause of ALS brings insight into how it can actually get better, because the reality is that it's not a death sentence.

Also keep in mind that you may get diagnosed with ALS when what you're really experiencing is any of a multitude of other symptoms and conditions that aren't true ALS. Even some of the most debilitating neurological symptoms that mimic ALS may not be ALS.

It's unknown to medical communities that true ALS is a viral inflammatory illness, caused by a severe infection of the virus HHV-6 along with a few other herpetic virus strains that vary from person to person. This is one of those rare times when a viral infection is actually present in the brain or brain stem and even sometimes the spinal cord. What makes the disease so severe is that toxic heavy metals—usually including a high level of copper and aluminum—are present in the brain and body at the same time, providing potent viral fuel.

All that viral activity can affect neurons because the neurotoxins produced by the viruses behind ALS are extremely potent and destructive to the central nervous system, causing symptoms such as muscle twitching, stiffness, numbness, and muscle loss. In many cases the brain stem can become highly sensitized and less responsive due to inflammation, making symptoms more mysterious and complicated. It's important that people with ALS stay away from the toxic chemicals listed in this book; these brain betrayers tend to worsen ALS symptoms.

It's not inevitable that ALS will lead to someone losing control of their body. If you commit to removing heavy metals from your system, while avoiding as many chemical exposures as possible while reducing viral activity with the protocols and techniques in Part VI, "Bringing Back Your Brain," and *Brain Saver Protocols, Cleanses & Recipes,* you can finally start gaining back your health.

For specific healing support, refer to the ALS protocol in *Brain Saver Protocols, Cleanses & Recipes.*

ALZHEIMER'S DISEASE

See Chapter 36, "Alzheimer's and Dementia."

ANOREXIA

See Chapter 33, "Eating Disorders."

ANXIETY

See Chapter 31, "Anxiety."

ANXIOUSNESS

Anxiousness appears here separately from "Anxiety" because many people walk around feeling extra sensitive and extra anxious without attaching the label *anxiety* to it. Many people wouldn't say they have anxiety, and yet they do have an underlying sensitivity in the central nervous system that's a precursor to anxiety. If someone is going up on stage for a school play, about to see a friend for the first time in a year, or about to hand in a big project, those are all very natural, explainable, and temporary forms of anxiousness. The same goes for emotional stress, mental abuse, or extreme stress from loss, betrayal, or a broken relationship—those challenges can fully explain a bout of anxiousness.

If, on the other hand, you repeatedly find yourself in everyday situations (such as having a conversation while driving around in the car with friends or taking a walk with family) with extra sweating or anxiousness rising up that you can't explain, this is often an unrecognizable swelling, creating a sensitive central nervous system due to mild levels of toxic heavy metals in the brain coupled with low-grade viral activity. Turn to Chapter 31, "Anxiety," for more insights.

For specific healing support beyond what's offered in Part VI, "Bringing Back Your Brain," refer to the Anxiousness protocol in *Brain Saver Protocols, Cleanses & Recipes.*

ARTERIOSCLEROSIS, ATHEROSCLEROSIS, AND ATHEROMA

When we think about vascular plaque buildup, we're often worried about the major arteries and the heart, and right-fully so. What warrants almost more of our concern is buildup within the brain's blood vessels. Larger arteries in the body have more room, so they can narrow for years without causing incident. In the brain's many blood channels, there isn't much room to narrow and still let blood through, so a smaller blood vessel in the brain can become blocked more quickly. Often when someone experiences a tran-sient ischemic attack (TIA) or mild stroke, it's an early sign that fats, toxins, and viral waste are building up and clogging these blood vessels—and that a more severe event could be on the way. This is one very important reason why lowering fats in your diet, keeping your immune system strong to ward off viruses, and reducing your toxin exposure are so critical.

You'll hear arguments that only bad fats cause atherosclerosis. Don't be persuaded by this inaccurate reasoning behind trendy high-fat, high-protein diets. A diet high in even beneficial, healthy fats can cause arte-rial hardening, fat deposits, plaque depos-its, and blockages inside the brain.

For specific healing support beyond what's offered in Part VI, "Bringing Back Your Brain," refer to the Arteriosclerosis protocol in *Brain Saver Protocols, Cleanses & Recipes*.

AUDITORY PROCESSING DISORDER (APD)

This disorder is caused by toxic heavy metals in or around the auditory cortex of the brain. While someone could experi-ence APD at the same time as hearing loss, APD itself is not a hearing or ear problem. Rather, metals in the auditory cortex block electricity from entering neurons, disrupt-ing someone's ability to process what was communicated. Exactly where in the cortex those metals are and in what quantity deter-mines how mild or severe someone's audi-tory issues are.

For specific healing support beyond what's offered in Part VI, "Bringing Back Your Brain," refer to the Auditory Process-ing Disorder protocol in *Brain Saver Proto-cols, Cleanses & Recipes*.

AUTISM

Autism is caused by toxic heavy metals (mercury and aluminum especially) settling in the cerebral midline canal as well as other areas of the brain. In autism larger amounts and proportions of mercury are involved, and regions of the brain additional to the midline canal are more saturated, result-ing in a more extreme condition. In partic-ular, heavy metals heavily dispersed in the speech, language, communication, move-ment, and motor control areas of the brain (in addition to the midline canal) are behind the symptoms associated with autism.

The variability in autism's severity—that is, the autism spectrum—is due to the variability in quantity of metals in someone's brain, how much mercury is present, and exactly where in the brain those heavy metals have deposited themselves.

Recently the diagnostic rate of autism on the milder end of the spectrum has increased greatly, leading us to sometimes forget about the people and families struggling with autism on the severe end of the spectrum. When parents have a child with severe autism and they mention their child is autistic, someone else may assume everything is fine because so many people now are diagnosed with mild autism. What onlookers aren't seeing are the exhaustion, the lack of sleep, the parents not being able to find help, the system not being set up to help parents dealing with severe cases of autism.

Parents and family members of someone with severe autism, once they learn the cause, can understand that their child or loved one is dealing with severe heavy metal toxicity. On the other hand, parents and family members of a child or loved one on the lower end of the autism spectrum, with very mild symptoms (many of which can't be seen), tend to be less open to the toxic heavy metal connection. Very mild autism allows life to move forward without the grave search and need for an answer. It's that need for an answer that opens the door to the understanding of what really happened to create autism symptoms,

whether mild or severe: injury from toxic heavy metals.

If someone with autism experiences tics, spasms, and fatigue, there could be a viral load in play too—see "Tics and Spasms" and "ME/CFS" later in this chapter. For more on autism in general, refer to the revised and expanded *Medical Medium*.

For specific healing support beyond what's offered in Part VI, "Bringing Back Your Brain," refer to the ADHD protocol in *Brain Saver Protocols, Cleanses & Recipes*.

BALANCE ISSUES AND DIZZINESS

Chronic balance issues and dizziness are a result of vagus and even phrenic nerve inflammation—and that's a result of viruses such as EBV feeding off toxic heavy metals and other food sources, such as chemical toxins, eggs, and dairy, and then releasing neurotoxins to which the central nervous system becomes allergic. Also, EBV can actually directly infect the vagus nerves, resulting in the same symptoms. Because the vagus nerves run into the cranium, swollen vagus nerves can even lead to brain stem swelling, which—even though it's on such a minute scale that brain scans won't detect the swelling—can compound balance issues and make them more constant.

For specific healing support beyond what's offered in Part VI, "Bringing Back Your Brain," refer to the Vertigo protocol in *Brain Saver Protocols, Cleanses & Recipes*.

BELL'S PALSY

This mysterious form of facial paralysis, when not a result of an obvious head trauma, develops from a viral infection releasing large waves of neurotoxins that saturate and inflame facial nerves, trigeminal nerves, or even other cranial nerves. The specific virus is shingles. Someone can have a Bell's palsy variety of shingles and another of the over 30 undiscovered varieties of shingles at the same time. It's not uncommon for someone to have more than one variety of shingles. In extreme cases, the shingles virus can be so close to nerves that the virus inhabits or sits on the nerves. Most of the time, the virus's neurotoxins alone are enough to cause the facial pain, weakness, numbness, drooping, or even trigeminal neuralgia. For more on shingles, see the revised and expanded *Medical Medium*.

For specific healing support beyond what's offered in Part VI, "Bringing Back Your Brain," refer to the Shingles protocol in *Brain Saver Protocols, Cleanses & Recipes*.

BIPOLAR DISORDER

See Chapter 35, "Bipolar Disorder."

BRAIN ABSCESS

An infection of the brain that causes fluid to collect and form an abscess can be viral, bacterial, or both. While this condition doesn't necessarily cause a lot of neurological symptoms the way many of the illnesses in this list do, it can put someone in a mysteriously weak state. What sets the stage is an extremely weak or sensitive immune system. (A weak immune system doesn't mean that person is weak or genetically flawed, by the way. It means that brain betrayer toxins have compromised their immune defenses.) Viruses that can be behind brain abscesses are anything from a rare variety of EBV to HHV-6, HHV-7, HHV-10, HHV-12, HHV-14, HHV-15, and HHV-16—the last several of which are undiscovered by medical research and science. Bacteria that can cause brain abscesses include a range of specific mutated groups of strep or MRSA that are also undiscovered by research and science.

For specific healing support beyond what's offered in Part VI, "Bringing Back Your Brain," refer to the Brain Abscess protocol in *Brain Saver Protocols, Cleanses & Recipes*.

BRAIN FOG

Severe cases of brain fog can be devastating, making people feel like they're losing their minds. Even mild brain fog is very challenging on the person's mental and emotional state. One major factor behind brain fog is a liver that's saturated with toxic heavy metals, scented candles, air fresheners, fragrances, pesticides, herbicides, and other toxins that are providing fuel to the Epstein-Barr virus. When EBV feeds on these poisons, the neurotoxins it releases explode through the bloodstream and spinal fluid, and from there, they can cross the blood-brain barrier due to their unique infiltration quality, enter the brain, and short-circuit neurons and/or damage neurotransmitters. These neurotoxins have the ability to diminish neurotransmitter activity and neurotransmitter chemicals themselves, meaning that when an electrical impulse tries to run down a neuron, the electrical impulse can misfire as it's approaching any kind of contamination or inconsistency. The electrical impulse was carrying messages, thoughts, and information, so when it misfires, confusion and brain fog is the result of these messages becoming fragmented.

Another factor in brain fog is a high toxic heavy metal load within the brain itself. When those metals oxidize over time, their corrosive waste saturates adjacent brain tissue, glial cells, and connective tissue, with the corrosive waste eventually contaminating neurotransmitters, similar to how viral neurotoxins affect neurotransmitters.

For specific healing support beyond what's offered in Part VI, "Bringing Back Your Brain," refer to the Brain Fog protocol in *Brain Saver Protocols, Cleanses & Recipes*.

BRAIN INFLAMMATION (ENCEPHALITIS)

Millions with chronic illness live with some level of undetected or undiagnosed brain inflammation. You could be sick with over 50 different symptoms, most of them neurological, to the point where you're in debilitating pain, and as you consult a number of specialists and experts, it's most likely that not one will consider brain inflammation.

There are three main varieties of brain inflammation. The first is the easiest to identify, and it's the one the medical establishment does tend to recognize: the result of injury. Whether you bang your head in an accident or experience head trauma, the brain can become inflamed on a short-term or longer-lasting basis, depending on the severity of the internal injury.

The second type of brain inflammation can seem more mysterious. Here, symptoms stick around past when the individual is expected to heal from a head injury. Brain inflammation persists, becoming chronic. This is a sign that a virus is present in the body or even the brain, and that the virus is taking advantage of the vulnerable state the brain is in. When an injury affects nerves by weakening them, nerves become more sensitive, exposing nerve root hairs, especially in the brain stem, and the nerves can be triggered easily from a virus creating neurotoxins, whether in the brain, near the brain, or somewhere else in the body. What is known by the medical establishment is that there can be a delayed aftereffect of head injury. This is where someone gets injured yet seems to be okay—no internal damage is detected inside the brain, they're walking and functioning normally or just a little sore—and then days or weeks and sometimes even months later, symptoms arise. While the delayed symptoms are mysterious to the doctor, the doctor is normally open to affiliating the symptoms with the original injury. What is not known is that this is a late injury response of the brain stem due to viral inflammation of the cranial nerves exiting the brain stem.

The third type of brain inflammation is when a virus creates brain inflammation without an initial injury that becomes a trigger. In rare cases, viruses attach themselves to nerves close to or even inside the brain, including the brain stem. The viruses that do this are usually undiscovered varieties and mutations of herpetic viruses such as HHV-6, EBV, shingles, and herpes simplex 1 or 2, and normally there must be a lowered immune system and elevated toxic heavy metal load at the same time for a virus to be encouraged enough to make a home in the brain area. Direct viral infection of the brain will often lead to the brain becoming so inflamed that someone experiences an acute attack of encephalitis that leads to hospitalization for viral encephalitis.

In most cases, it's a virus in *another* part of the body that remotely causes milder, mysterious, chronic brain inflammation. Many people live day to day with a chronic, low-grade viral load. As you read about in Chapter 4, "Your Viral Brain," and Chapter 6, "Your Inflamed Cranial Nerves," when a mutated strain of a virus such as EBV, shingles, or HHV-6 camps out in an organ or gland such as the liver, spleen, or thyroid, the virus will start releasing neurotoxins that travel throughout the body. If that virus is thriving, a large amount of neurotoxins will be released into the bloodstream, and from there, they can enter the brain and pollute it, creating a mild level of brain inflammation that is undetectable. This is the type of brain

inflammation that people living with chronic illness so often experience undiagnosed.

Many people are sensitive to viral neurotoxins, allergic to them, developing tingles, numbness, headaches, dizziness, weakness in their arms and legs, abnormal sensitivity to heat or cold, difficulty handling a hot, humid day or being exposed to cold for too long, tiredness even after sleeping enough hours, fatigue, or even severe fatigue, which I call *neurological fatigue* (see "ME/CFS"). When these symptoms of viral neurotoxin–induced brain inflammation are debilitating, it's usually a result of *more than one* herpetic virus sitting inside the liver or even spleen. For example, it could be two varieties of EBV, one or two varieties of shingles, herpes simplex 1 or 2, and HHV-6 all at once—along with a lowered immune system and lots of pesticides, herbicides, fungicides, chemical fragrances, eggs, dairy products, and gluten in the body systems, which all serve as viral fuel. The high quantities of aggressive neurotoxins that the combination of toxins and viruses create lead to suffering for many people that's often difficult to decode.

Toxic heavy metals usually have to be present, too, for someone to develop brain inflammation from a chronic viral infection elsewhere in the body. Toxic heavy metals create a specific variety of neurotoxin that's particularly inflammatory for the central nervous system.

For specific healing support beyond what's offered in Part VI, "Bringing Back Your Brain," refer to the Brain Inflammation protocol in *Brain Saver Protocols, Cleanses & Recipes.*

BRAIN LESIONS, WHITE SPOTS, DARK SPOTS, SCAR TISSUE, AND CALCIFICATIONS

Little do we know that so many of us are walking around with less-than-perfect brains. I don't say that to spook you. I say it to make you feel better if you already know about a brain issue that's shown up on a scan—and to make anyone who feels it could never happen to them aware that it could already be happening, so our brain needs precious care.

Our best technology, such as CT scans and MRIs, can only spot imperfections in the brain if they're large enough to stand out. Even when white spots, dark spots, shadows, and gray spots do appear with imaging, a doctor may not know what they mean.

Here's a common experience: Someone visits the doctor, perhaps after a concussion, either complaining of other symptoms or not, and requires a routine MRI—which ends up catching an abnormal spot on the brain. That's how these issues are often first detected. The doctor will say, "You have what seems to be a little dark spot in the brain tissue. Let's do additional tests and scans, and blood work. We should keep our eye on that along the way," and not offer any immediate solutions. Many doctors become concerned, in part because they don't know what is causing the imperfection. If they had answers in an ideal world, they'd be able to tell you instead, then and there, that toxic heavy metals, toxic chemicals, aspartame, MSG, salt, pharmaceuticals, recreational drugs, and/or pathogens inside the brain are creating these imperfections in the form of calcifications, crystallizations, scar tissue, stains on brain tissue, or lesions.

Again, imperfections aren't always prominent enough to show up on scans. A doctor in that ideal world would be able to tell you that even if your brain imaging appeared clear, you could still be dealing with an abnormality. And in a truly ideal world, that imaging would be advanced enough to pick up even the early-stage imperfections.

Some people have what seems to be a lighter spot on the brain. Some have a darker spot. Some have gray areas. And there can be multiple spots. They all have particular meanings.

Dark spots on the brain can be dead or damaged brain tissue that turned dark due to toxic chemical exposure, pharmaceutical exposure, or recreational drugs. Oxidized metals interacting with each other are a common alternative cause of dark spots.

Toxic heavy metals are one of the main causes of brain abnormalities, with different heavy metal interactions creating different abnormalities. For example, when mercury and copper react, their oxidative runoff is a mucky color, and gray or dark spots in the brain can result. Other examples of heavy metal interactions include mercury reacting with aluminum, mercury reacting with nickel, or aluminum reacting with copper. These all create different stains on the brain, which can show up as any variety of shadow or dark spot. Many people walk around with this issue, whether completely unaware or with spots that are showing up on a brain scan with no one able to identify the cause. It can start out small and very slowly at the beginning of life, developing along the way and remaining undiscovered until someone reaches their 50s or 60s and by chance gets an MRI.

Lesions can also show up as dark spots, and they can have different shapes than other shadows and dark spots. Lesions are damaged tissue. Many times, lesions are on the myelin nerve sheath and occur from chronic viral infection, primarily an infection of one of the many mutations of EBV, shingles, or HHV-6. A virus can either create a lesion on contact, or a virus can create a lesion in brain tissue inches away from where the virus itself is located, if the virus is creating high quantities of neurotoxins that travel to a nearby region of the brain. You could have a lesion in the brain from a past viral infection. The lesion could be there for years afterward—the lesion could be there forever, even—with the virus long since gone and out of the brain. Viruses can create lesions of different sizes and shapes when they're feeding on toxic heavy metals such as mercury or even aluminum or industrialized, toxic copper.

White spots in the brain can be pockets of aluminum, calcifications from calcium deposits, crystallizations from salt, or clusters of MSG. Aluminum tends to oxidize differently from mercury, nickel, copper, or lead; it also has a brighter metallic coloration

that easily reflects off magnetic resonance imaging (MRI). Aluminum's oxidative rate and color lead to these white spots. Now, you can have mild levels of aluminum in the brain and not have any white spots show up on an MRI. That doesn't mean they're not there. Many of these spots are so subtle that doctors don't yet have the technology to discover or diagnose them.

Another cause of calcifications (which show up as white spots) is the interaction of aluminum with calcium in the body. Disruptive food-based forms of calcium from milk, cheese, and butter can be aggressive to the brain because they tend to react with aluminum, causing toxic calcium deposits, which are calcifications. There are even toxic industrial forms of calcium that are toxic heavy metals themselves, detrimental calciums that we're exposed to in our environment from industries. Different calciums that find their way to the brain tend to react with each other, causing a hardening expansion of calcium deposits there.

Scar tissue in the brain (which can show up as extreme shadowing or gray spots, or may not appear at all) can occur for a lot of different reasons. You do not have to have a stroke or mini stroke in order for scar tissue to be produced. Even emotional injury can cause scar tissue. Hardship, betrayal, broken trust, or loss can be so intense and so damaging for connective brain tissue that scarring can occur from the extreme heat the experience generates in the brain's emotional centers, especially if someone was not prepared for particular news. Adrenaline from emotional experiences also saturates the brain, which can create scar tissue in those emotional centers. If emotional injury occurs over and over, such as in an abusive relationship, a callus tends to form in brain tissue. While electrical impulses can still surge through these calluses, it takes more power and repetition. Tiny pockets of scar tissue can form from these micro calluses, because these cells within the calluses are trying to survive, so the cells group together and start to grow into something different (scar tissue) from what they were before. Scar tissue can also occur from viral infection; viruses can make micro adhesions in the brain.

Mysterious spots in the brain vary because we all have such varied exposures and experiences. Different metals, toxic chemicals, pharmaceuticals, and pathogens make their way into our lives. Whether an exposure is daily, yearly, or a one-off makes a difference. Stressful situations are unique from person to person—two people faced with a situation will react differently because of their unique brew of exposures.

For specific healing support beyond what's offered in Part VI, "Bringing Back Your Brain," refer to the Brain Lesions protocol in *Brain Saver Protocols, Cleanses & Recipes.*

BRAIN TUMORS AND CYSTS

Tumors and cysts are not genetic, as theorized. Brain tumors of any kind, both benign and cancerous, have the same cause: viruses and toxins. What type of growth develops depends on what virus

is present as well as what toxins and poisons and problematic foods have accumulated in the body, particularly in the liver and the brain itself, to fuel that viral activity and accelerate its development. Some viral strains in the herpetic family are behind brain cysts and tumors. HHV-6, HHV-7, the undiscovered HHV-10 through HHV-16, and EBV all have specific mutated strains that can create these growths in the brain.

To be clear, having one of these viruses does not automatically translate to getting cancer or a tumor. It takes specific, aggressive viral mutations *plus* the right brew of toxins for cancer and tumors to develop. That means that if you're interested in prevention, you have solid steps to take: (1) avoid whatever brain betrayers you can from Part III, and (2) protect your brain with protocols from Part VI, "Bringing Back Your Brain."

For specific healing support beyond what's offered in Part VI, refer to the Brain Tumors and Cysts protocol in *Brain Saver Protocols, Cleanses & Recipes.*

BREAST IMPLANT ILLNESS

Breast implant illness is a term for a broad spectrum of symptoms, many of them neurological, such as fatigue, tingles, numbness, restless legs, heart palpitations, dizziness, eye floaters, brain fog, anxiety, and weakness of the limbs. People suffering with breast implant illness have spent decades trying to be validated, trying to be heard.

In science there are two sides when it comes to breast implant illness. One side believes it's not possible for breast implants to cause sickness. The newer side believes if the implant is broken or leaking, it could be harmful and create a variety of symptoms. In the past no one was open to the idea or possibility that it could occur. Breast implants are medical devices. The world of medical devices, just like the world of drugs, is covenanted, protected. Proving that a medical device is causing sickness is not an easy feat. It has taken hundreds of thousands of women over the years to fight to be heard that this type of medical device—breast implants—has caused harm. Now we're in a place where it's accepted more. Still not enough is spoken about it. It's still a topic that's purposely avoided out there in the health world, both conventional and alternative.

Those in the medical industry who believe in breast implant illness theorize that the treatment is to just get the implants removed, and then everything should go back to normal. There's more to it than that. The neurological symptoms that come with breast implant illness don't simply go away when you remove the implant. This causes a tremendous amount of confusion. This is where the naysayers of the medical industry say, "See? The implants were never the issue." It's why breast implants still stay on the market.

What really happens when breast implants cause trouble? It starts with the surgery itself. Many women have not gone under general anesthesia before. The anesthesia alone is traumatic and can be a trigger to something else deeper inside them that eventually becomes breast implant illness.

Then they're inserting foreign objects (implants) into the body. This alone can lower and weaken the immune system. It's similar to metal plates that are used inside the skull for head injuries, or titanium nuts and bolts and rods used in knee replacements and hip replacements, or marker plates that are put inside breast tissue to monitor cysts, nodules, and calcification growths. Anything implanted in the body can create a reaction inside the body, and everyone is different as to what reactions occur. The presence of a breast implant, even without leaking, can slowly lower the immune system in many women. Residue from the outside surface of the implant—again, even without the implant filler leaking—can lower the immune system. The surgical procedure itself lowers the immune system too. You don't have to have a leaking implant to create problems.

Let's look more closely at the residue from implants. That residue can start to slowly outgas and leach because of ammonia gases and acids inside the body touching the implant. This is still not the contents of the implant leaking; it's the outer implant material leaching. Most people are extremely acidic. Their bloodstream is filled with fat from eating a high-fat diet. They're on vinegar and caffeine. Their blood acids are extremely high, and their blood fat is extremely high. Fat is absorbent. When fat is inside your bloodstream, it absorbs anything and everything like a sponge. Blood fat has the ability to draw chemical toxins from an implant casing. This, in turn, can lower the immune system. The high fats don't allow the toxins of the leaching implant to leave the body; the chemicals circulate until they find a destination to settle.

Triggers from outside sources in life such as betrayal, an overabundance of stress, broken relationships, divorces, financial stress, hardships, and losses can also lower the immune system because these experiences are stressors on the adrenals. At the same time, when someone's adrenals are in fight-or-flight, the adrenaline can be extremely corrosive and also start to weaken the outside of the breast implant, leading the implant casing to leach.

When breast implants do start leaking their inner contents, they leak in one person faster than they leak in another, depending on the acidity of the person's body environment and the amount of adrenaline in their bloodstream from fight-or-flight. These factors can even determine if an implant is going to leak in someone and not at all in another person.

Whether breast implants leach or leak (or both), the lowering of the immune system at the same time is a key factor in breast implant illness. The leaching and/or leaking causes the immune system to struggle because immune cells are trying to gobble up any of the toxic contents or materials. That lowered immune system is what allows viral and bacterial problems to occur—and viruses such as EBV are the number one cause involved in breast implant illness. Many people can experience breast implant illness from this effect of a lowered immune system from leaching alone, without the implants even leaking. Or, if their implants

do end up leaking, they could have started experiencing symptoms such as fatigue, brain fog, weight gain, bloating, eye floaters, dizziness, or body pain before the leak occurred because the implants had been leaching before the leak.

We also have to factor in the routine lowering of the immune system during the menstrual and reproductive cycles. Eighty percent of the immune system already goes to the reproductive system during menstruation, lowering the immune system in the rest of the body during that time. During ovulation, 40 percent of the immune system goes to the reproductive system. During pregnancy, 50 percent of the immune system goes to the baby. During childbirth, 90-plus percent of the immune system goes to the birthing of the baby. When breast implants are also drawing from the immune system, we have more possibilities of pathogenic problems such as viruses occurring.

Again, viruses are the number one reason for breast implant illness. Without breast implants, women already struggle with EBV-caused, shingles-caused, and herpes simplex–caused symptoms and conditions such as Hashimoto's thyroiditis, tingles and numbness, vertigo, tinnitus, eye floaters, body pain, fatigue, lupus, fibromyalgia, neurological Lyme, and many more. So the susceptibility to develop illness *with* breast implants is higher, because implants are another immune system–compromising trigger to chronic neurological problems caused by EBV and shingles.

Chronic fatigue syndrome from breast implant illness, for example, is really a viral infection that has gone awry because the immune system is so compromised from breast implants leaking or reacting to high fats in the bloodstream. This is why some women who do not have multiple EBV strains, shingles, cytomegalovirus, or even simplexes—that is, women who are only low-viral—can have leaching, leaking breast implants and they're still playing tennis, swimming at the beach in 90-degree heat in the sun, going for runs, drinking wine, drinking coffee, and living their life without knowing an implant is leaching or leaking. The implant filler could have leaked and traveled inches from the implant, the implant could be leaching into the bloodstream, and it could even be years without that person knowing. Eventually, if they have an EBV inside them that becomes awakened—or they contract a new EBV, shingles, or herpes simplex from eating at a restaurant or a new relationship—that's when the immune system gets pushed overboard, and these viruses take advantage of the compromised immune system.

When breast implants corrode, seep, break, and leak, the immune system is compromised even more from the toxins inside breast implants. The filler inside normally contains toxic heavy metals, solvents, and formaldehyde. When these toxic substances travel into the bloodstream, they can become fuel and food for viruses. This fuel and food can feed the fever blister virus, which is herpes simplex 1, resulting in trigeminal neuralgia, neck pain, mouth pain, tooth pain, gum pain, or shoulder pain (with or without a fever blister). Or breast implants' toxic filler can feed the shingles virus, leading to jaw pain, burning mouth, tooth pain, gum pain, neck pain, head pain, or shoulder pain. Or breast implants' toxic filler can feed EBV, resulting in body pain, fatigue, tingles and numbness, ringing in the ears, eye floaters, burning skin, and brain fog. The toxic substances such as toxic heavy metals inside breast implants can either feed viruses that are already actively causing symptoms, making those symptoms worse or adding new symptoms to the list, or ignite and launch viruses that were dormant, creating symptoms for the first time.

On top of fueling viruses, these toxic substances also are harmful to the body outright. They lower the immune system, place stress on organs such as the liver (making it stagnant and sluggish and causing weight gain), and put stress on the adrenals because toxins of any kind create an internal allergic response that prompts adrenals to release adrenaline, which in return can slightly raise heartrate. All of this can quicken symptoms that otherwise would have come much later. A woman suffering from breast implant illness at age 30 who's also now getting diagnosed with neurological Lyme, lupus, Hashimoto's, weight gain issues, or skin conditions most likely would not have started developing these conditions until her early 50s. Breast implant illness can shorten the timeline, speeding up a viral condition that otherwise would have taken years or decades to develop into a neurological problem.

If you have breast implants that seem to be stable and symptoms are not developing, you can leave them in, unless it's your decision to take them out. If breast implants are not ruptured or leaking or causing symptoms, you can work on strengthening your immune system as a preventative measure and using any of the Medical Medium cleanses to remove toxicity. And if you and your health-care provider believe there is a leak with your breast implants, you're welcome to try any of the tools in this book and its companion while working on a solution with your doctor. These tools are also an option if you've had breast implants removed and you're still exhibiting symptoms.

For specific healing support beyond what's offered in Part VI, "Bringing Back Your Brain," refer to the Breast Implant Illness protocol in *Brain Saver Protocols, Cleanses & Recipes.*

BULIMIA

See Chapter 33, "Eating Disorders."

BURNOUT

See Chapter 7, "Your Burnt Out, Deficient Brain."

CEREBRAL ATROPHY

While brain atrophy can occur in all ages, from young to old, it's most common in people over 40. Medical research and science often believe that injuries, strokes, or a natural process of aging are what lead to this brain shrinkage. That's not entirely accurate. In truth, the main cause of atrophying of the brain is the inability of brain cells to receive adequate sugars and restore glycogen reserves to sustain brain tissue.

Connective brain tissue is mostly made out of glycogen (stored glucose). Glucose is not only the food for brain cells; it's the birthing environment for them. A brain cell needs an environment with ample available sugars in order to be produced. That's why atrophy in any area of the brain means that glucose deprivation is occurring. If sugar isn't entering into brain cells to feed, sustain, and replenish them, it means the glucose storage is diminishing. As a result, brain cells start to decrease in size and eventually die off rapidly.

Often years and years of a high-fat, high-protein diet create insulin resistance in the brain—fats blocking sugars from entering brain cells. We don't need to have diabetes for this specific type of insulin resistance to occur. When the brain isn't getting the glucose it needs, it also means it's being deprived of the vitamins, minerals, antioxidants, phytochemical compounds, oxygen, and other nutrients that natural sugars deliver to the brain. Nutrients and sugars enter the brain as one, and fats can't deliver those nutrients. So when precious glucose is blocked from being put to use in the brain, other precious building blocks are too, which contributes further to brain atrophy.

For specific healing support beyond what's offered in Part VI, "Bringing Back Your Brain," refer to the Cerebral Atrophy protocol in *Brain Saver Protocols, Cleanses & Recipes*.

Lack of oxygen is another factor in brain atrophy. Read more in "Cerebral Hypoxia."

CEREBRAL HYPOXIA

The brain can't be without oxygen for long. Even the shortest amount of time without oxygen can cause some kind of harm. The same goes for when the brain is getting *low* oxygen, as in hypoxia. Here, the direct result of what's going on is well known: a lack of oxygen to the brain causing any number of issues, including brain cells dying, brain tissue atrophying, and stroke.

What's unknown is that many people walk around every day eating diets that create chronic, low-grade cerebral hypoxia. It's not enough to cause damage in any one moment on a substantial level. Rather, it adds up over time—the brain can be harmed if years go by with someone eating a diet consistently high in fat. The higher your blood fat, the lower your oxygen levels. While it's true that oxygen is still getting to your brain on a high-fat diet, many strokes occur from years of buildup in arteries and small blood vessels. That buildup—caused by fats and toxins that have hardened into plaque—reduces blood flow to the brain. So excess fat in the diet translates to both lower oxygen levels in the brain and less blood getting to the brain, which means less oxygen.

Almost any person you meet is on a high-fat diet in one way or another, causing unknown reduction of oxygen to the brain. Even if an oxygen test shows your oxygen level is adequate, the test isn't detecting subtleties of diminishing oxygen to the central nervous system; it doesn't mean the brain is getting the full amount of oxygen that the brain needs. It's true that exercise can get more oxygen into our bodies. That doesn't erase what's happening with a high-fat diet. As fats invade the bloodstream, they reduce the available room for oxygen, and so oxygen begins to eddy and pool in places rather than being evenly dispersed. Where the oxygen eddies is random; it's not predetermined as it's being pushed around and squelched by fats.

For a long time, the brain can adapt to this uneven oxygen distribution and to receiving overall low levels of oxygen—to a degree. And then, over time, atrophy occurs. With this type of undiscovered, chronic hypoxia, rather than brain cells dying rapidly and aggressively, it's a slow progression of brain shrinkage. Not getting enough oxygen over years and years, the brain has no other choice than to reduce in size to match up with the lower levels of oxygen it's been trained to receive. Not to mention that glucose, which helps deliver oxygen to the brain, is not as present in a high-fat diet, compounding the issue.

For specific healing support beyond what's offered in Part VI, "Bringing Back Your Brain," refer to the Cerebral Hypoxia protocol in *Brain Saver Protocols, Cleanses & Recipes*.

MEDICAL MEDIUM BRAIN SAVER

CEREBRAL PALSY

In unexplained cases of cerebral palsy—that is, instances that are not explained by a documented and diagnosed injury to the areas of the brain that control movement—toxic heavy metals are the cause. When heavy metals such as mercury saturate regions of the brain such as the primary motor cortex, they can damage neurons responsible for the symptoms of cerebral palsy.

For specific healing support beyond what's offered in Part VI, "Bringing Back Your Brain," refer to the Cerebral Palsy protocol in *Brain Saver Protocols, Cleanses & Recipes.*

CEREBROVASCULAR DISEASE

Although brain- and heart-related, cerebrovascular disease stems from the liver—and is primarily caused by a high-fat diet. When the liver gets oversaturated with fats, it loses its ability to protect you by absorbing toxins and controlling viruses. As the liver weakens, viruses start to gain control, releasing their poisonous waste matter into the blood, which dirties a bloodstream already congested with toxins the liver can't contain. If someone keeps eating high levels of fat, regardless of what diet they choose, then the blood maintains a high blood-fat ratio. That causes chronic dehydration, high blood pressure, or dirty, thick blood, which eventually leads to buildup of rancid fats, cholesterol, and plaque in the veins and arteries. This, in turn, constricts blood flow to the brain. At the same time, the blood that gets to the brain is consistently high in fats and toxins such as viral neurotoxins, which leads to brain inflammation. This combination can eventually result in weakness in the limbs, TIAs, or even strokes.

For specific healing support beyond what's offered in Part VI, "Bringing Back Your Brain," refer to the Cerebrovascular Disease protocol in *Brain Saver Protocols, Cleanses & Recipes.*

CHRONIC ANGER DISORDER

If posttraumatic stress disorder (PTSD) has been ruled out—which is to say, if it's been determined that trauma from past abuse or suffering is not the cause of someone's chronic anger, and rather, it's unexplained—then toxic heavy metals saturating emotional areas of the brain and a stagnant, sluggish liver are the underlying causes.

You can also have a mix of all three: trauma, metals, and an overloaded, overworked, stagnant, sluggish liver. If someone had a sluggish liver and went through mental abuse and toxic heavy metal exposure at roughly the same time, chronic anger will often be expressed more aggressively and more frequently. For example, if someone went and got their mercury dental fillings removed (which destabilizes the metal) and also got the worst news that day or week, the emotional impact of the difficult development plus the mercury exposure can lead to more severe symptoms of frustration and anger if the mercury saturates the brain's emotional centers.

Mercury saturating other areas of the brain can lead to other neurological symptoms, such as fatigue. Most often, chronic anger stems from toxic heavy metal exposures long ago, in childhood. As someone gets older, the metals age and oxidize, causing chronic anger to worsen through later years.

When people aren't feeling well physically, it can be angering. If you're chronically sick plus you're also experiencing any of these factors—trauma, heavy metals, or an overloaded liver—that feeling of chronic unwellness can act as a trigger for these underlying causes of chronic anger.

For specific healing support beyond what's offered in Part VI, "Bringing Back Your Brain," refer to the Chronic Anger Disorder protocol in *Brain Saver Protocols, Cleanses & Recipes*.

CHRONIC MYSTERY GUILT

In the emotional centers of the brain, certain areas of nerve tissue are partly responsible for the way we feel. It's not only the tissue itself. The brain's emotional centers are intertwined greatly with our soul. If someone feels guilty for something they've done and that's appropriate for the circumstance, the soul is tied in to this emotional response in the brain. If someone never feels guilty even when they should—when it would help them learn and grow and give others resolution—there's a disconnect. For one, there's a disconnect between the soul and the brain's emotional centers; the soul has pushed away from the brain. For another, there's usually been some sort of toxic exposure in the emotional centers of the brain causing a disconnect in electrical signals. When toxic heavy metals such as mercury and aluminum take up residence there, it can interfere with the empathy, sympathy, compassion, and guilt that are supposed to arise upon causing harm to others. It can mean that someone never apologizes for what they've done. That's because heavy metals can derail electrical impulses, never allowing them to reach the guilt region of the brain, which is one of the places where the soul connects to nerve tissue. It's the part of the brain that allows someone to have heart.

What about when someone's guilt is overactive? When toxic heavy metals saturate a different area of the brain's emotional centers, they can cause electrical impulses to surge into adjacent tissue, and if that's the area that governs guilt, it heightens guilty feelings. The littlest thing someone does, like borrowing a penny from the penny dish at a convenience store, can fill them with regret. Getting so busy one day that they aren't able to call back a friend, even if that friend would completely understand, can make someone feel terribly guilty, to the point where it hurts, and they're saddened and depressed. Then, when something happens where guilt is the appropriate response—if that person makes a particular mistake—their attempts to learn from it can be heightened to the point of obsession or danger, even approaching harming themselves in some cases. If that person's soul is injured from abuse, hardships, betrayal, or trust breakage, it can compound the situation and make the guilt reaction worse. Or the reaction can go the opposite direction, where anger and numbness settle in and displace all feelings of guilt completely, until the numbness and anger wear off and the guilt returns.

For specific healing support beyond what's offered in Part VI, "Bringing Back Your Brain," refer to the Chronic Mystery Guilt protocol in *Brain Saver Protocols, Cleanses & Recipes*.

CUSHING'S SYNDROME (HYPERCORTISOLISM)

A number of symptoms that could be given a number of diagnoses have been lumped under the Cushing's umbrella, regardless of whether someone has a pituitary gland cyst or not.

Actual Cushing's is more rare than we think. Cushing's is really a result of a long-standing viral infection: EBV is the virus that creates a cyst or tumor on or near the pituitary gland, causing it to produce an excess amount of adrenocorticotropic hormone (ACTH). This overstimulates the adrenals, often causing them to create excess cortisol.

Why could someone be misdiagnosed with Cushing's? Why else do cortisol levels rise, if it's not Cushing's? To begin with, let's not forget that in many cases, the adrenals are already producing excess cortisol due to diet and lifestyle alone. Also, a high-fat diet and weakened liver causing high blood pressure, weight gain, skin conditions, and muscle loss can look like Cushing's.

Further, EBV can create cysts and tumors on the pituitary gland or the pituitary cavity that do not trigger ACTH production—and yet cortisol levels can be elevated due to that pre-existing viral infection weakening the liver, which can confuse the doctor into thinking an individual has Cushing's. The EBV creating a non-Cushing's pituitary cyst or growth in the brain also lives in the liver and other areas of the body such as the spleen, releasing large amounts of neurotoxins that put stress on the central nervous system, causing fatigue, and forcing the adrenals to work harder and increase cortisol output.

Medical research and science tend to blame all this excess cortisol on the pituitary gland producing too much ACTH without realizing what else could be in play—a chronic viral infection combined with a laboring, stressed-out liver that can't absorb excess cortisol (or adrenaline) anymore, causing these stress hormones to float rogue through the bloodstream.

For specific healing support beyond what's offered in Part VI, "Bringing Back Your Brain," refer to the Cushing's Syndrome protocol in *Brain Saver Protocols, Cleanses & Recipes*.

DEMENTIA

See Chapter 36, "Alzheimer's and Dementia."

DEPERSONALIZATION

No one wants to be depersonalized. Being numbed out is not something someone wants to portray to others or feel inside. People with depersonalization often don't feel as though they've experienced what they've just experienced. It's almost like a numbness or inability to connect occurs for those with depersonalization. They could be standing next to a friend with whom they just took a hike to watch a beautiful sunset, and they could feel a disconnect from it all. It can be experienced as a disconnect from oneself, a spiritual disconnect. They're seeing life from a perspective as if they themselves weren't there. If you've experienced depersonalization, you may have been told you need to "find yourself."

One person's depersonalization could be much different from someone else's. It's a large gray area bordering the threshold of depression and anxiety. The classic variety of depersonalization is the inability to feel emotionally. You're completely numb, nothing excites you, nothing gets you upset, nothing matters, nothing interests you, and you feel like you're not inside your body and you don't exist. Even within this classic variety of depersonalization, there can be plenty of variables.

The reason for so much variability in the experience of depersonalization is the range of causes. These causes range from emotional injury to toxic heavy metals to adrenal burnout to brain burnout to low-grade viral infections to all of the above. Each cause can vary too. For example, when it comes to toxic heavy metals, there are differences from person to person in what type of metal or metals are in the brain, where the metals reside, how close they are to the emotional centers of the brain, how fast the toxic heavy metals are oxidizing, and whether there are any other poisons, solvents, or exposures involved that can partly contribute.

Is brain fog present with the depersonalization, or is brain fog not present? That's another variable. A low-grade viral infection such as EBV can worsen brain fog, adding to the depersonalization. The combinations are almost endless. How much toxic heavy metal is involved? Is there a low-grade viral infection present? What kind of emotional injury has someone sustained?

Depersonalization can also happen without emotional injury, without emotional trauma. Someone could have what seems to be a perfect life, with no financial concerns, no stress, no pressure, no worry, a loving support system, and yet have severe depersonalization. Someone else could have extreme emotional abuse, hardship, and emotional trauma and no toxic heavy metals, no low-grade viral infection, and they could sustain depersonalization from the emotional injuries alone, if they're severe enough. Someone else can sustain emotional injuries and not have depersonalization. Everyone's threshold for emotional injuries differs.

The majority of people with depersonalization have a combination of emotional injury, even if mild, plus toxic heavy metals such as mercury and aluminum in the brain. When the toxic heavy metals are removed, the person can actually relive the missed experiences and feel them for the first time.

For specific healing support beyond what's offered in Part VI, "Bringing Back Your Brain," refer to the Depersonalization protocol in *Brain Saver Protocols, Cleanses & Recipes*.

DEPRESSION OR DYSPHORIA

See Chapter 32, "Depression."

DIFFICULTY COPING

People should never be blamed for a struggle to cope. What's really happening is a sensitive central nervous system and neurotransmitters that are weakened. The *person* is not weak. You could be the strongest person with the strongest will, spirit, personality, and nature—and when neurotransmitters are affected in some way, it makes it tough to deal with some of life's challenges. Neurotransmitter disorders are common for anybody dealing with ME/CFS or any kind of autoimmune condition. Toxic heavy metal loads and viral loads combined create a lot of neurotoxins, which weaken neurotransmitters. When this is coupled with adrenal issues and other symptoms, it can be difficult to cope with any additional stressor that comes your way.

Not that you need to be diagnosed with a condition to have trouble coping. Toxic heavy metals in the areas of the brain that help us process emotional information and maintain equilibrium when navigating

challenges can make difficult times in life even more difficult. Heavy metals dampen and hamper neurotransmitter activity. That could cause someone to retreat or procrastinate during a time of emotional stress, which can lead to not feeling able to look at a document they're supposed to look at, contact someone they're supposed to contact, or generally "deal."

There are also cases where someone can be very accomplished, with incredible grit, in one area of life and yet have an emotional sore spot or a soul injury with a PTSD pocket. Consider a super athlete with a strong personality, for example, who wakes up early every morning to run 20 miles, and yet you bring up a particular subject, and they can't cope. Once again, that's from heavy metals in certain areas of the brain creating little blocks. That will happen especially if someone has an emotional wound around the subject. Heavy metals and emotional wounds can cluster together in the brain by happenstance, making the wound or injury that much easier to trigger.

For specific healing support beyond what's offered in Part VI, "Bringing Back Your Brain," refer to the Difficulty Coping protocol in *Brain Saver Protocols, Cleanses & Recipes*.

DYSAUTONOMIA

This chronic inflammatory condition is caused by neurotoxins produced by viruses such as EBV saturating areas of the brain that affect the autonomic nervous system.

In many cases, the inflammation is extremely mild, causing symptoms as simple as nervousness or excess sweating. Some cases are a little more intense, with neurotoxins saturating the central and autonomic nervous systems to the extent that they cause heart rate issues and sporadic fluctuations of blood pressure, whether causing blood pressure to be extremely low or even elevated.

Most people with dysautonomia experience many other symptoms of EBV too, including Raynaud's syndrome, dizziness (which is inflammation of the vagus nerves), tinnitus, or even thyroid issues. Medical research and science are unaware that these are all EBV-related, so when they classify dysautonomia as a specific set of symptoms separate from someone's other struggles, they don't realize that all of that person's health complaints could be connected to the same viral cause.

For specific healing support beyond what's offered in Part VI, "Bringing Back Your Brain," refer to the Dysautonomia protocol in *Brain Saver Protocols, Cleanses & Recipes*.

DYSLEXIA

Every case of dyslexia is different; each person's experience of it is unique. That's because of its cause: exposure in early life, even before birth, to toxic heavy metals such as mercury that saturate a combination of language areas of the brain, which could include learning, visual, and recognition regions. As you know from reading Chapter 3, "Your Alloy Brain," heavy metals never settle and interact in the brain in the same way. For example, one child could have less aluminum and more mercury, or more aluminum and less mercury, and they could be in different areas, and that will all influence how their reading and writing issues take shape.

Often, if a child has too much mercury in processing areas of the brain, if heavy metal exposure is ongoing, or if dyslexia isn't diagnosed until teens or young adulthood, someone will have a more difficult time with dyslexia, and it will stay with them in life if no steps are taken to remove the heavy metals. In other cases, if the heavy metal exposure is firmly in the past and was not too severe, children can grow out of the dyslexia to a degree as new neurons are created and the brain adapts. It makes a big difference if dyslexia is identified early and a child receives specific tutoring, because that helps a young brain grow around the heavy metal impediments.

Brain scans on children with severe dyslexia combined with OCD and ADHD can sometimes reveal a mysterious shadowing in the brain. What's the cause? Toxic heavy metals coupled with lower levels of electrical activity. If doctors knew how to interpret gray matter and shadowing on scans, this could be a gateway into seeing larger deposits of toxic heavy metals with the eye.

For specific healing support beyond what's offered in Part VI, "Bringing Back Your Brain," refer to the Dyslexia protocol in *Brain Saver Protocols, Cleanses & Recipes*.

EATING DISORDERS

See Chapter 33, "Eating Disorders."

ENCEPHALOPATHY

Encephalopathy describes symptoms resulting from a brain experiencing some sort of problem with no clear, definitive cause. Medical research and science have not yet pinpointed what causes general dysfunction of the brain. Encephalopathy is an umbrella for many mystery symptoms and changes within the brain. If someone suffers from a stroke or brain tumor and then develops central nervous system symptoms where they're struggling with what looks like brain problems, then the stroke or tumor will be seen as the cause of encephalopathy.

No matter the seeming source of encephalopathy, whether diagnosed as a result of stroke or tumor, there are always underlying foundational roots of encephalopathy. These roots can occur on their own, or in combination with each other: (1) severe brain deficiency, (2) viral infection, (3) toxic heavy metals, (4) chemical toxicity.

(When a viral load is causing encephalopathy, that viral infection can be directly in the brain, although the virus is more often somewhere else in the body, affecting the brain from afar with neurotoxins, creating a low-grade chronic brain inflammation.)

When two people have a stroke or develop a tumor and only one person experiences symptoms of encephalopathy, that's because the affected patient has an underlying viral load, toxic heavy metal load, brain deficiency, or chemical toxin load (which could also be from pharmaceuticals).

In many people, encephalopathy develops years after a brain trauma or injury to the brain. Someone else can have that same brain trauma or injury and not develop encephalopathy. Their brain tissue isn't dying as fast as the other individual's post-injury. The difference depends on these other underlying causes present in the brain—severe deficiency, viral infection, toxic heavy metals, and/or chemical toxicity. Brain tissue recovery could be more difficult for one individual versus another because of these factors.

For specific healing support beyond what's offered in Part VI, "Bringing Back Your Brain," refer to the Encephalopathy protocol in *Brain Saver Protocols, Cleanses & Recipes*.

EXCESSIVE SWEATING (HYPERHIDROSIS)

This condition occurs as a result of a part of the brain overexerting itself due to tiny impediments of the brain in the form of blockages in and around neurons, plus weakened neurotransmitters within areas of blockages.

The tiny blockages in the brain are normally toxic heavy metals. They can also be a combination of metals, MSG pockets, and/ or chemical toxicity from anything from pesticides to air fresheners. The dominating toxic heavy metal that contributes to this condition is copper. Copper is in most chemical formulas, and it is impossible to detect in the brain. Copper toxicity is hard to diagnose or discover with today's medical technology.

Copper is a conducting metal and also a grounding metal. Copper draws and guides electricity. This interferes with messages that are being delivered to the brain. Copper in the brain tissue will guide messages off the beaten path due to its radical grounding effects. For example, if someone is speaking to you, you may become distracted in some situations because copper draws energy from the neurons that are supposed to be receiving the message, which in turn triggers a sympathetic nervous system response such as sweating. Copper also interferes with messages being delivered out of your brain. For example, if you're talking to someone, as you're retrieving thoughts from electrical impulses traveling through neurons, copper is drawing energy from the neurons delivering the information. You'll still be able to communicate the information, yet the sympathetic nervous system will become triggered as you do. As you sense this physical draw, it heightens your awareness that something is draining your nervous system. Copper toxicity saturates neurons and weakens and even destroys neurotransmitter chemicals, grounding them out. Depending on what part of the brain copper is in, copper can run cold inside the brain, so when electricity touches microscopic copper deposits, more cooling occurs in that part of the brain, weakening the electrical fire that messages travel on.

Because copper is the number one toxic heavy metal responsible for interrupting messaging and signaling through the sympathetic nerves, the presence of toxic copper can create what seems to be constant fight-or-flight.

Nerves throughout your body receive the messages delivered from the brain. Your brain is the voltage. Electricity going through your brain is being driven by neurons and electrical impulses that have the strength to deliver and shoot out messaging throughout all the nerves in the body. Some nerves are more grounding than others, meaning they convert that electricity to a more grounding frequency and energy. The sympathetic nerves are grounding nerves. They are smaller nerves and also denser (whereas the nerve material of larger nerves is not as dense). When copper is in the brain, it disrupts this grounding function of the sympathetic nervous system. The copper is already grounding those messages heading down the sympathetic nerves, which flips a switch. The sympathetic nerves have lost stability and are no longer grounding. These disrupted signals from the brain are enough to cause extra sweating.

The adrenals can also contribute. The brain detects a problem with the instability of the sympathetic nerves and sends a message to the adrenals that there's a problem. The resulting adrenal response can heighten the sweating.

Almost all individuals with hyperhidrosis experience a form of anxiety with the condition, with some of that anxiety coming from PTSD that has developed from the experience of excessive sweating itself. Anxiety around not being able to express oneself can compound the situation, firing up the adrenals. When someone is in a situation where they're struggling to express themselves, and anxiety kicks up because of PTSD around the concern that they're going to embarrass themselves by sweating when they don't want to sweat, the adrenals release adrenaline—which tends to make them sweat more. This adds to the complications of hyperhidrosis. You can sweat simply from the thought of saying something, even if you don't end up speaking.

Low-grade viruses such as shingles can also play a role in hyperhidrosis. Individuals with the shingles virus anywhere near the cranial nerves such as the vagus or trigeminal nerves, in combination with having high copper, can make hyperhidrosis a more difficult or even severe condition. Neurotoxins created by the shingles virus feeding off copper also add to the complications of this condition. Additional chemical toxicity and MSG in the brain can add to the already existing copper and viral condition.

Many people with hyperhidrosis opt for surgery called endoscopic thoracic sympathectomy (ETS). A successful surgery, which is rare, can minimize or reduce sweating—and can also have unintended side effects. Surgery doesn't address the underlying problem that caused the hyperhidrosis to begin with. The copper isn't eliminated from the brain; the chemical toxins and MSG in the brain aren't minimized. After surgery the condition can rise to a new level, causing or worsening other symptoms such as elevated anxiety, depression, and fatigue—which raises an important point. Most people with hyperhidrosis, even if they don't get surgery, don't just have this excessive sweating condition. They also live with fatigue, brain fog, anxiety, depression, and/or unusual body sensations, to name just a few.

For specific healing support beyond what's offered in Part VI, "Bringing Back Your Brain," refer to the Excessive Sweating protocol in *Brain Saver Protocols, Cleanses & Recipes*.

FATIGUE

See "ME/CFS."

FIBROMYALGIA

See "Neuropathy," "Neuralgia," and "Joint and Muscle Pain." For more information on fibromyalgia, see the revised and expanded *Medical Medium*.

For specific healing support beyond what's offered in Part VI, "Bringing Back Your Brain," refer to the Fibromyalgia protocol in *Brain Saver Protocols, Cleanses & Recipes*.

FOCUS AND CONCENTRATION ISSUES

One source of focus and concentration issues is along the lines of what you read about in the ADHD section: heavy metals such as mercury and aluminum in the cerebral midline canal, "sprinkled" throughout the brain, or both. When metals reside in the brain, they often dampen electrical activity, causing the brain to try to adapt by increasing electrical output, which brings on temporary bouts of clarity. That results in overheating, so then the brain must go into extreme cooling, which ends up reducing electrical activity, leading someone to flip-flop back to moments of poor concentration.

Focus and concentration issues can also come from a chronic viral infection, where a virus such as EBV is feeding off toxic heavy metals such as mercury and aluminum, releasing neurotoxins that float through the bloodstream to the brain, saturating neurotransmitter chemicals that are around or sitting on neurons. When this occurs, the electrical impulses running across neurons short-circuit because of the polluted neurotransmitters, resulting in trouble staying tuned to a task or conversation.

What's now occurring is a new wave of dangerous chemicals being produced every day by the chemical industry and pumped into our environment for our children and pets to ingest and inhale. These toxic chemical substances are adding to the viral fuel while also adding to neuron toxicity, complementing the toxic heavy metals already present and exacerbating focus and concentration issues from which people already suffer.

Sometimes focus and concentration seem to improve randomly on their own, and sometimes they get worse. One theory is that the gut has everything to do with the brain, and so cleaning up the gut automatically improves mental clarity. This theory is misleading. The real reason that someone can focus more easily when they start eating better is that removing unhealthy foods removes viral fuel, which in turn results in fewer neurotoxins to interfere with brain activity. It's not all about cleaning up the intestinal tract and restoring bacterial balance to the gut. This is why so many unhealthy people with very messy intestinal tracts filled with unproductive yeast, mold, fungus, and bacteria don't have a focus and concentration issue. Someone else could get a clean bill of intestinal health from their gut health doctor—their stool samples aren't raising any alarms, they're eating a very healthy diet with no processed foods, and they show no signs of what doctors would say is parasitical activity or a *Candida* problem—and still, the person could have debilitating focus and concentration issues.

For specific healing support beyond what's offered in Part VI, "Bringing Back Your Brain," refer to the Brain Fog protocol in *Brain Saver Protocols, Cleanses & Recipes*.

GASTROPARESIS

See Chapter 6, "Your Inflamed Cranial Nerves."

GUILLAIN-BARRÉ SYNDROME

This condition is still highly misunderstood by medical research and science.

The theory goes that in Guillain-Barré, the body's immune system attacks its own nerve cells, causing damage that can eventually lead to paralysis. This autoimmune misconception is a mistake made across hundreds of symptom and condition labels in the medical industry. In reality, the body doesn't attack itself, and the body's immune system doesn't attack nerves. The true cause of Guillain-Barré is viral. Specifically, certain varieties of EBV often cling to nerves or enter the brain, and when a virus latches on to a nerve or nerve cell, it creates chronic swelling, which can lead to temporary bouts of paralysis; tightening of the face; difficulty moving the jaw; severe body stiffness; the feeling of pulled muscles when doing very little physically; difficulty doing any tasks with the hands because the wrists are giving out; pain of the elbows, wrists, shoulders, legs, or neck; or seizures. For extensive nerve *damage* to occur, a specific mutated strain of EBV must be present. To be clear, the EBV is not a trigger for Guillain-Barré. It is a cause.

The majority of people dealing with chronic Guillain-Barré are also living with the effects of viral neurotoxins, and the neurotoxins aren't necessarily only coming from EBV. Shingles, HHV-6, cytomegalovirus, and herpes simplex 1 and 2 can be involved here too. Dozens of mutations of these viruses love to feed on toxic heavy metals, solvents, pesticides, fungicides, fragrances, and petrochemicals, as well as eggs, milk, cheese, butter, and gluten—and produce neurotoxins as waste matter. These neurotoxins find their way to nerve tissue throughout the brain and body, resulting in symptoms such as tingles, numbness, aches, pains, weakness in the limbs, tremors, and even mild bouts of temporary paralysis. The health effects of viral neurotoxins can lead to dozens and dozens of other diagnoses too, including multiple sclerosis (MS), ALS, neurological Lyme, and even diabetic neuropathy.

For specific healing support beyond what's offered in Part VI, "Bringing Back Your Brain," refer to the Autoimmune Disorders and Diseases protocol in *Brain Saver Protocols, Cleanses & Recipes*.

HEADACHES

There are many different causes of headaches. One type is caused by a low-grade strep infection embedded in the sinus cavities, whether short term or long term, from *Streptococcus* bacteria that someone has been carrying around for a lifetime. When the immune system drops, strep can gain strength, swelling the sinus cavities and placing pressure on the trigeminal nerves, facial nerves, and optic nerves. It's common for this sinus swelling to happen when someone is going through their menstrual cycle or a hormonal change, because the body will put its resources into their reproductive system at that time, which results in a lowered immune system.

Chronic headaches can also result from chronic dehydration. People are more dehydrated than anyone realizes, running around with toxic livers and thick, dirty blood.

Dehydration reduces electrical activity and neurotransmitter support, causing overheating of the brain that can allow headaches to occur randomly at any time.

People also live on high-fat diets, consuming fats more than once per day. As you've discovered, the constant presence of fats in the bloodstream causes chronic insulin resistance in the young and old, which interrupts precious glucose absorption. The constant presence of fats in the bloodstream also stops water, mineral salts, and oxygen from quickly restoring brain cells and connective tissue. The resulting deficiencies in brain supplies can cause periodic headaches.

Look out for headache triggers such as fragrances, caffeine, aspartame, preservatives in processed foods, alcohol, smoking, and vaping. Also look out for foods like gluten, eggs, and dairy products, which will feed pathogens such as EBV, shingles, and herpes simplex 1 and 2 in your body systems. Viral neurotoxins can go to the brain through the bloodstream and create periodic and sometimes chronic headaches. When low-grade viral infections themselves are close to critical nerves, they can create headaches. The trigeminal, facial, and vagus nerves are highly sensitive cranial nerves that run variously through the chest, neck, and face—and even connect to the brain stem—so viral activity in their vicinity can be highly agitating.

Sensitive nerves in general caused by toxic heavy metals, excessive caffeine, fragrances, MSG, insecticides, nicotine, chemical toxicity, and more—separate from or in addition to a viral infection—can also cause mild to moderate headaches. Some people can't handle certain scents because scents are so highly toxic. Without someone realizing it, the fragrances are irritating their nerves. Everyone is becoming oversaturated by toxic chemical soups. Fragrances coming from scented candles are becoming one of the biggest causes of headaches now.

Some people get a headache from trying to wear contact lenses, because their optic nerves are sensitive. Some people's eyeglass prescription might not be as up to date as it needs to be, so they strain their eyes and get headaches. Some people stare at screens all day long and develop headaches. These are all slight nerve sensitivities that hundreds of millions of people experience.

Toxic heavy metals in the brain can cause headaches, sometimes for a lifetime if the metals are not removed. Heavy metals such as mercury and aluminum dispersed throughout the brain, interacting with each other and oxidizing, can create lifelong headaches. (Read more in "Migraines" and Chapter 3, "Your Alloy Brain.")

Headaches can have an emotional component—which isn't to say they're "all in your head." When there is emotional or mental strain or confrontation—for example, with a difficult coworker or partner, or connected with a loss, hardship, or struggle—the brain can overheat, in turn causing emotional meltdown. After a long period of being upset, we often shut down to a degree, and then headaches can occur afterward as the brain tries to heal and recalibrate following the extensive overheating or emotional storm. If there are other underlying factors, such as metals or low-grade viral infection, and cranial nerves are mildly sensitive already, emotional struggles can bring on uncomfortable, painful headaches and even migraines.

Another cause of headaches can be mild fluid buildup from edema. This fluid buildup can place pressure on trigeminal, facial, and optic cranial nerves, causing discomfort.

Headaches can worsen over the years and eventually become migraines.

For specific healing support beyond what's offered in Part VI, "Bringing Back Your Brain," refer to the Migraines protocol in *Brain Saver Protocols, Cleanses & Recipes*.

HEMISPATIAL NEGLECT (RIGHT NEGLECT, LEFT NEGLECT)

In obvious injury-related cases, hemispatial neglect occurs from damage to brain tissue from accidents, strokes, or even chemical or radiation exposure. There's also temporary hemispatial neglect, which you probably won't hear about in discussions of the condition. In this case, the issue with processing input from the right or left isn't always there. Episodes may occur periodically, whether once in a lifetime or six months apart.

One reason for temporary hemispatial neglect is food poisoning. Foodborne microbes and toxins, whether dead or alive, can enter the brain, saturate certain areas of brain tissue, and cause hallucinations and

delusions that lead to temporary moments of hemispatial neglect.

Or the temporary version of the condition can occur when someone becomes extremely ill from a viral infection that goes to the brain—for example, a strain of HHV-6 or the undiscovered HHV-10 through HHV-16, or even an aggressive variety of EBV. Upon first entering the brain, the virus can release a tremendous amount of poisons, and if the poisons saturate brain tissue in a specific area that controls the ability to navigate without obstruction, it can cause a temporary version of hemispatial neglect that's milder than brain injury–related hemispatial neglect. Often people hospitalized with viral infections in the brain will experience small bouts of hemispatial neglect that never get diagnosed.

For many people with chronic illness, hemispatial neglect can become chronic, going beyond temporary and periodic and instead seeming like the condition could go on indefinitely. When viral hemispatial neglect lasts like this, it's due to an underlying injury, stroke, accident, or chemical exposure *plus* a viral condition.

For specific healing support beyond what's offered in Part VI, "Bringing Back Your Brain," refer to the Hemispatial Neglect protocol in *Brain Saver Protocols, Cleanses & Recipes*.

HUNTINGTON'S DISEASE

Medical research and science believe that Huntington's disease is a genetic, inherited condition that runs in families. Even though this theory is completely incorrect, there is some indirect merit to the observation that *something* here is passed down from generation to generation to generation: toxic heavy metals such as mercury. Medical research and science also believe that in Huntington's, brain cells are dying in specific regions of the brain that control emotions, movements, and cognitive abilities. While only a theory, this also holds some merit. It's true that brain cells are dying. Why, though? What are brain cells dying from? Why is someone's cognition failing? Why are involuntary movements occurring, disrupting their motor functions? What's the cause? That all remains a complete mystery to medical research and science. A gene defect does not cause brain cells to die.

The undiscovered cause of Huntington's is a specific blend of mercury with a lesser amount of aluminum interacting and oxidizing around the brain's ganglia. As you know by now, mercury looks for more mercury. So as someone goes through childhood, exposed to heavy metals along the way, new mercury finds established mercury deposits, and they join together.

As heavy metals oxidize around the ganglia, cells rapidly die. Also, the ganglia form a hot spot for viruses and viral neurotoxins when they're saturated with heavy metals. If someone contracts a herpetic virus such as EBV along the way, that virus will likely seek out that hot spot, feeding off those metals and releasing their poisonous waste, which accelerates the oxidative rate and kills more brain cells more quickly. That's when Huntington's symptoms progress rapidly. In most cases, it's caused by metals alone, which result in a slower progression of the disease.

For specific healing support beyond what's offered in Part VI, "Bringing Back Your Brain," refer to the Encephalopathy protocol in *Brain Saver Protocols, Cleanses & Recipes*.

INFLAMMATORY MYOPATHY

Inflammatory myopathy is caused by a viral infection feeding on toxic heavy metals, although their signature viral neurotoxins don't affect nerves in the usual way. Here, due to the specific brew of heavy metals and the types of viruses that are present, the neurotoxins that are excreted inflame muscles first and foremost rather than nerves. Generally, neurotoxins aggravate nerves. In this case, while some direct nerve aggravation can occur, the nerves mostly become inflamed secondarily, by default, because the nerves are inside the muscles. When a muscle becomes inflamed, it affects the nerves inside it.

Different viral strains of EBV, herpes simplex, and cytomegalovirus tend to have appetites for different metals. When someone is experiencing myopathy, it tends to mean two or more metals are feeding a virus or viruses. There are a lot of different "recipes" and "brews" of metals. Some people experience myopathy and neuropathy combined. That's from different types of neurotoxins being excreted by the virus or viruses, leading to different effects and symptoms. When both skin and muscles are affected in myopathy, that's also from different types of viral waste being produced at once. For example, one virus may have an appetite for copper, nickel, lead, and aluminum, inflaming muscles with its neurotoxins, while another virus has an appetite for copper and nickel, producing more of a dermatoxin, resulting in what's essentially derma-myopathy.

While the brain itself may not get inflamed in myopathy, oftentimes, the muscles around the skull, face, and neck can become flared, putting pressure on the brain. Not to mention that the brain is a group of nerves, and nerves often telegraph pain, so if muscles elsewhere in the body are inflamed, which inflames the nerves inside them, the brain can be affected. When this happens, fatigue and depression can occur alongside a person's struggle with myopathy.

For specific healing support beyond what's offered in Part VI, "Bringing Back Your Brain," refer to the Cranial Nerve Inflammation protocol in *Brain Saver Protocols, Cleanses & Recipes*.

INSOMNIA

Trouble sleeping can sometimes be as simple as a racing mind that's trying to solve a problem, stress, or worry in your life. We don't need to stress ourselves out over a bad night or two. When sleeping problems become chronic, that's when there's more going on. Neurotransmitter chemicals are one critical part of being able to sleep. Electricity is running through every neuron as we're sleeping. If neurotransmitters are diminished, electrical impulses have a tough time traveling throughout the brain. Low neurotransmitter chemicals or weakened ones can cause the brain to have difficulty finding balance so you can ease into sleep and stay there.

Someone may also have a sensitive nervous system due to a chronic, low-grade infection in the liver of a virus such as EBV or shingles, which often goes undiagnosed. Neurotoxins breaking out of the liver and traveling through the bloodstream can reach the brain, where they saturate, pollute, and diminish neurotransmitter chemicals. This is especially true if someone's diet is not conducive to protecting them from viruses and building up neurotransmitter activity.

Often people with toxic heavy metals inside the brain have difficulty sleeping from toxic heavy metals oxidizing and affecting neurotransmitter chemicals. In cases of very chronic, serious insomnia, it's usually a combination of both toxic heavy metals in the brain and a low-grade viral infection in the body. Toxic heavy metals and viruses weaken the central nervous system just enough to constantly disturb someone's sleep or to make it very difficult to fall asleep in the first place.

Body aches and pains from low-grade viral infection or injury can also create insomnia. So can pharmaceuticals that make a liver sluggish and stagnant while feeding a low-grade infection of a virus such as EBV.

For specific healing support beyond what's offered in Part VI, "Bringing Back Your Brain," refer to the Insomnia protocol in *Brain Saver Protocols, Cleanses & Recipes*.

INTRACRANIAL HYPERTENSION

Women, who are affected more often than men by intracranial hypertension, are also the group more likely to experience viral infections. That's no coincidence. Intracranial hypertension is viral.

Commonly, intracranial hypertension is associated with pharmaceutical use. Yes, it's true that some pharmaceuticals can increase fluid buildup in the body or between the brain and the skull. And yet given that's the case, why wouldn't everybody taking the medication get ringing in the ears or other symptoms of intracranial hypertension? The difference is whether someone has an underlying viral infection. Pharmaceuticals are a perfect food for viruses. From antibiotics to benzodiazepines to anti-inflammatory steroids to antidepressants, the list goes on of medications that have the potential to feed chronic, low-grade viral infections.

These medications are used to address health issues already underway. So many people, whether diagnosed with idiopathic or secondary intracranial hypertension, are already dealing with a diagnosis such as MS, rheumatoid arthritis, Hashimoto's thyroiditis, Lyme disease, lupus, fibromyalgia, or ME/CFS, or struggling with various symptoms,

such as floaters in the eyes, heart palpitations, or dizziness. If they haven't been diagnosed with an additional condition besides their intracranial hypertension yet, it's highly likely they will eventually get an autoimmune diagnosis at some point in their life. These autoimmune diseases are not, in truth, the body attacking itself; they're viral infections. The viral activity behind these illnesses creates a lot of lymphatic fluid buildup—edema—inside the body. The viral activity can also swell cranial nerves, creating more pressure between the skull and the brain.

How many viruses and which strains and mutations are present, along with which toxic heavy metals and other chemical exposures are present, have an effect on how much lymphatic fluid builds up, creating headaches with mild intracranial hypertension. This low-grade viral edema can also cause someone to hold an extra 15 to 20 pounds of water weight, which is toxins overflowing from a stagnant, sluggish liver that's having a difficult time doing its job properly. The fluid buildup is a protection method to try to suspend and dilute the viral toxins. You don't have to be overweight to experience the viral edema version of intracranial hypertension. You can have fluid buildup between the brain and skull due to viral infection feeding off toxic heavy metals and toxic exposures closer to the head.

Spinal fluid buildup and lymphatic fluid buildup are two different things. When you're swollen from lymphedema, it will often swell up to the brain, creating pressure that's often mistaken for spinal fluid pressure.

Low-grade viral infections inside the brain or spine can create additional spinal fluid. Viral infections elsewhere in the body can also create more spinal fluid. Even though this causes worrisome symptoms, it's your body's reaction to protect you, like when your knee gets hit and swells up like a balloon and you can't walk. In that moment, it doesn't feel great that you can't walk, yet that's how the body responds to injury, and it's protecting you by not letting you further injure it.

Certain viral infections in the body prompt more spinal fluid production to protect the brain. "More" is not much at all—it's just a fraction of an elevation in some cases, and it may not cause intense symptoms. Most people with autoimmune disorders walk around with extra cerebrospinal fluid as a natural protection for the brain because they're experiencing viral swelling from neurotoxins affecting the brain stem, and extra spinal fluid helps dilute this. As the spine, brain stem, and nerves swell, cerebrospinal fluid pressure increases. One reason is that there's less room for the cerebrospinal fluid to be housed. This tends to make people with conditions such as MS, rheumatoid arthritis, Hashimoto's, Lyme, lupus, fibromyalgia, or ME/CFS more sensitive to heat and humidity, because heat and humidity swell the body, adding to the pressure.

People with intracranial hypertension often get spinal taps. The problem is that this procedure is not good at identifying pathogens. It's nearly impossible for a spinal tap to detect a stealth pathogen, a viral sleeper cell, considering the various herpetic mutations that are not on record with medical research and science. You can't find what you don't know could be there. There are so many of these undiscovered strains of herpetic family viruses that 99 percent of them are virtually impossible to detect through a spinal tap. It's why viral meningitis remains such a mystery to research and science: because spinal taps can't detect viral infections. They don't detect the actual virus or viruses present; although doctors will guess that there could be a viral infection causing viral meningitis, they will not know what kind of virus it is.

For specific healing support beyond what's offered in Part VI, "Bringing Back Your Brain," refer to the Cranial Nerve Inflammation protocol in *Brain Saver Protocols, Cleanses & Recipes*.

ITCHING AND BURNING

Everybody is unique in the brew of poisons, toxins, and viruses they carry in their systems. The number of varieties and mutations in the EBV family alone, never mind the varieties and mutations of other viruses, means that the effects they cause from person to person also vary widely. Some toxins are more toxic to peripheral nerves, so when a virus feeds on them and releases them in neurotoxin form, those neurotoxins are more inflammatory to peripheral nerves that are closer to the skin, and that can cause an itchy-burning feeling. People often find it's an itch that can't be scratched—no matter how hard they try, they can't remedy it from the surface. Many people experience moving itches, sometimes going from the legs to the feet to the arms to the hands, with no eczema, psoriasis, or dermatitis present.

If someone has the shingles virus, whether diagnosed or not, its neurotoxins usually cause itchiness or burning on the feet that doctors may mistakenly diagnose as foot fungus, mites, the wrong shoes, or an allergic reaction. Really, it's peripheral nerves reacting to a poison. Neurotoxins can also inflame deeper nerves, creating aches or pains or roving pains that get diagnosed as fibromyalgia.

Viruses can also release dermatoxins, which go to the skin's surface and create eczema and psoriasis. Medical communities believe this is an autoimmune reaction—that is, that it's the body's immune system attacking its own skin. That's not correct. Again, this itching and burning is from viral dermatoxins inflaming the skin. Mild dermatoxins that don't create rashes can also inflame peripheral nerves, accounting for unexplained itching, pinching, and burning.

All of these toxins can also float to the brain, causing it to send burning signals throughout the body too. Someone can also have a combination: both viral neurotoxins creating nerve inflammation in, say, an arm while viral nerve inflammation in the brain sends a burning sensation to the legs. Medical research and science still have decades to go in understanding this information.

For specific healing support beyond what's offered in Part VI, "Bringing Back Your Brain," refer to the Cranial Nerve Inflammation protocol in *Brain Saver Protocols, Cleanses & Recipes*.

JOINT AND MUSCLE PAIN

If someone falls on a knee or twists an ankle and experiences acute pain, it is usually straightforward. Some pain comes from injury, accident, or incident, and there's no mystery involved. What's very different is if somebody experiences chronic pain in the joints or muscles with no discernible source. Even if a doctor diagnoses someone with rheumatoid arthritis, Lyme disease, or fibromyalgia, giving the struggle a name, it is still mystery joint and muscle pain.

The real cause of this chronic pain is viral infection, sometimes acute, although mostly long-term infection of a virus or viruses sitting in the liver, feeding on its favorite foods. People often notice less joint and muscle pain when they cut out gluten (and other brain betrayer foods) from the diet, although the why of it is unknown to medical research and science. You'll hear that they're just generally inflammatory foods. The truth is that it's because they give viruses fuel.

Regardless of your diagnosis, ongoing joint and muscle pain is viral, caused by one or more of the many varieties and mutations of EBV, shingles, HHV-6, herpes simplex 1 and 2, or cytomegalovirus. Once again, viral neurotoxins are to blame, inflaming nerves and causing pain. Often what feels like muscles hurting is the nerves inside muscles hurting. Often what feels like joints hurting is the nerves around the joints hurting. Neurotoxins float through the bloodstream, entering muscles, and inflaming nerves inside them and also landing on nerves around the joints. Certain strains of EBV can attach themselves to nerves, causing direct contact inflammation. There are also occasions when joints themselves become inflamed from viral-created nodules; the pain is still arising from the nerves all around those joints.

When neurotoxins from viruses enter the brain, this can cause nerve pain in different areas of the body. If a long-term, chronic viral infection somewhere in the body releases enough neurotoxins that end up saturating the brain, those neurotoxins can eddy and pool, creating clusters of neurotoxins in pockets of the brain where there are pain receptors that receive pain signals from other areas of the body when someone gets injured. Yet in this case, someone isn't getting injured in those areas of the body; the pain receptors are being switched on by neurotoxins in the brain. This can send pain signals throughout the body via nerves, creating phantom body pain. I call these *brain pains*. "Phantom" doesn't mean the pain isn't real. The pain is from a signal coming from your head. It's very real pain with a very real source, and it's common with many neurological conditions such as fibromyalgia. Certain varieties of viruses, for example mutations of EBV, can create neurotoxins that are more toxic when they enter the brain, creating more brain pains throughout the body.

Someone can have all of this happening at once. A brain affected by neurotoxins can send signals that cause nerve pain, viral neurotoxins can float through the bloodstream and inflame nerves, a mutated variety of a virus such as EBV can cause nerve inflammation from direct contact, and a virus itself can enter into joints, causing them to inflame and swell, putting pressure on those nerves around the joints. Or someone can experience one, two, or three of these causes.

When people are sick and weakened from conditions such as Lyme disease, rheumatoid arthritis, fibromyalgia, or ME/CFS, basic everyday household chores and functions can be difficult, and they can't exercise or use their body the way they would normally want to in order to build up or sustain muscle strength. Sometimes when they do move or exercise, they experience heightened joint and muscle pain. It can become a catch-22, making it more difficult to sustain or build muscle because you're in pain and discomfort. The more neurotoxins floating in the blood, the more difficult it makes it to exercise, with your pumping heart sending that blood rushing around, with the potential to cause more bouts of fatigue and joint and muscle pain.

For specific healing support beyond what's offered in Part VI, "Bringing Back Your Brain," refer to the Joint Pain protocol and/or Fibromyalgia protocol in *Brain Saver Protocols, Cleanses & Recipes*.

LEARNING DISABILITIES AND DISORDERS

Learning disabilities and disorders can start at a young age, with toxic heavy metals such as mercury and aluminum settling in the cerebral midline canal. They can also result from toxic heavy metals "sprinkled" throughout different areas of the brain. One area where heavy metals commonly reside and impede function is the processing center of the brain, the region that receives information. Heavy metals also commonly reside in regions of the brain where processed information is then delivered; this can affect someone's ability to answer questions on an exam or express thoughts and feelings.

A brain that's not yet fully developed tries to adapt quickly to the presence of toxic heavy metals by rerouting electrical impulses that the metals would otherwise block. Children's brains don't yet have a large abundance of connective brain tissue or neurons because they're still developing, so electrical impulses tend to travel around the toxic heavy metals in very creative ways. That's part of adapting and surviving when toxic heavy metals saturate young brain tissue.

Unless there's been physical injury to the brain, every person with a learning disability or disorder, whether child or adult, has had some form of toxic heavy metal exposure. Every single case is unique. No learning disability or disorder is identical to another because no toxic heavy metal exposure is identical. As children's brains grow and develop, more connective tissue is created, along with more brain cells and more neurons, often allowing them to grow out of some, if not all, of their learning challenges. What often causes a learning disability or disorder to stick around is continual toxic heavy metal exposure through medical treatments or other common avenues of exposure.

For specific healing support beyond what's offered in Part VI, "Bringing Back Your Brain," refer to the Learning Disabilities and Disorders protocol in *Brain Saver Protocols, Cleanses & Recipes*.

LONG-HAUL COVID AND LONG-HAUL FLU

A lowered immune system from COVID or flu reactivating EBV and/or other herpetic viruses that are already present in the body.

No one's ever had their eye on the reality that the flu virus has done this every year. Long-haul flu has been around for decades, reactivating EBV in people's body systems, leading to post-flu EBV-related symptoms such as brain inflammation, chronic fatigue, and neurological symptoms. The cause of the long-term symptoms isn't the flu itself. Rather, flu acts as a trigger, lowering the immune system so that a herpetic virus such as EBV can take advantage, grow in numbers, and burden the body systems chronically, keeping someone sick long term. Long-haul COVID (also called long COVID) works the same way.

Read more about the reactivation of EBV in Chapter 4, "Your Viral Brain," and the revised and expanded *Medical Medium*.

For specific healing support beyond what's offered in Part VI, "Bringing Back Your Brain," refer to the Autoimmune Disorders and Diseases protocol and/or Mononucleosis protocol in *Brain Saver Protocols, Cleanses & Recipes*.

LUPUS

The cause of lupus is viral infection. When someone exhibits symptoms of what medical communities label as lupus, the underlying cause is EBV. Lupus can cause many different varieties of rashes, including the classic butterfly rash. Lupus rashes are caused by a combination of neurotoxins and dermatoxins released from EBV that's feeding specifically on toxic heavy metals, mostly mercury—because people struggling with lupus are dealing with high levels of mercury in the system. The presence of that mercury and the chronic, ongoing EBV infection lead to a lowered immune system.

In lupus, the dermatoxins from EBV circulate in the bloodstream, surfacing through the skin and creating various rashes, along with joint pain in many cases. EBV's neurotoxins circulate through the bloodstream and inflame the central nervous system, which then telegraphs out to the peripheral nervous system. EBV's neurotoxic waste and byproduct create hives or unidentified mystery rashes that can come and go in various places on the body. This byproduct and waste create an allergic reaction within the body because the byproduct and waste are overloading the immune system, which is already overloaded by the Epstein-Barr virus to begin with.

EBV causes the neurological symptoms of lupus, ranging from headaches and migraines (which are caused by inflamed trigeminal, facial, optic, and sometimes phrenic nerves) to dizziness, anxiety, fatigue, and balance issues (inflamed vagus nerves) to frequent urination and bladder pain (inflamed pudendal and sciatic nerves) to elbow, wrist, and shoulder tendonitis and finger and hand pain (inflamed ulnar nerves) and more, as various other nerves throughout the body can become inflamed too.

Neurological fatigue can also result from central nervous system inflammation—that's often a big part of lupus. People with lupus normally have a host of other diagnosed conditions, such as thyroid problems and Lyme disease, which stem from the same EBV infection. Lupus is also a prime example of a label given to a set of symptoms that could be diagnosed as other conditions. There are blurred lines, contradictions, and inconsistencies when it comes to lupus diagnosis, which confuses individuals. Meanwhile, all of these conditions and labels are different ways of describing the same, original viral problem.

For specific healing support beyond what's offered in Part VI, "Bringing Back Your Brain," refer to the Autoimmune Disorders and Diseases protocol in *Brain Saver Protocols, Cleanses & Recipes*.

LYME DISEASE

Lyme disease has caused great suffering for many people over the past decades. Most medical communities still believe that Lyme is caused by a bacterial infection from a tick bite. The truth is that a tick bite is only a trigger to an underlying condition that's already there. That underlying condition is viral. And in almost all cases, someone with Lyme was never bitten by a tick; instead, they experienced another trigger. Here are the most common triggers of Lyme symptoms. Note that a tick bite is at the very bottom of the list:

1. Severe COVID

2. Extensive blood draw

3. Mercury-based dental amalgam fillings (especially filling and removal processes)

4. Mercury in other forms

5. Continual toxic mold exposure

6. Pesticides, herbicides, and fungicides

7. Insecticides in the home

8. Flu

9. Mild COVID

10. Death in the family

11. Broken heart

12. Taking care of a sick loved one

13. Virus-feeding prescription medications and medical treatments

14. Overprescribed medications

15. Recreational drug abuse

16. Physical injuries

17. Summer swimming where toxic runoff occurred

18. Professional carpet cleaning

19. Spider bite

20. Bee sting

21. Financial stress

22. Fresh paint

23. Insomnia

24. Tick bite

For some people, it's EBV causing the neurological symptoms of Lyme. Someone can also have multiple EBV strains, along with the shingles virus, herpes simplex 1 and 2, cytomegalovirus, and/or HHV-6 or HHV-7, making the body extremely burdened. What's known as Lyme bacteria cannot create neurological symptoms. Lyme bacteria do not produce neurotoxins, and only neurotoxins can create the myriad neurological Lyme symptoms. Herpetic family viruses such as EBV are what produce some of the most aggressive neurotoxins, the ones that can lead to fatigue, brain fog, tingles, numbness, aches, pains, fevers, ringing in the ears, dizziness, floaters in the eyes, insomnia, and much more.

There is misinformation regarding Herxheimer reactions when it comes to antibiotic treatments for Lyme. Medical communities believe that the symptoms a Lyme patient experiences when taking antibiotics is a Herxheimer reaction from the medication killing off Lyme bacteria. The true reason for someone's discomfort isn't bacterial die-off. Instead, the discomfort is a reaction to antibiotics and harsh supplement concoctions that are abrasive on sensitive, inflamed cranial nerves.

Again, Lyme symptoms are not bacteria-related. They're the result of neurotoxins produced by herpetic viruses such as EBV. Those neurotoxins can chronically inflame the central nervous system. The symptoms that someone experiences depend on how low their immune system has been, how toxic their liver may be, their toxic heavy metal and chemical exposure and load, and what kinds of stress-related and other viral triggers are occurring in their life, their diet, and their environment. It all plays a role in someone's individual case of Lyme. It's a very real struggle with very real answers. For extensive, detailed, life-protecting information about Lyme disease, refer to the revised and expanded *Medical Medium*.

For specific healing support beyond what's offered in Part VI, "Bringing Back Your Brain," refer to the Lyme Disease protocol in *Brain Saver Protocols, Cleanses & Recipes*.

ME/CFS (MYALGIC ENCEPHALOMYELITIS/CHRONIC FATIGUE SYNDROME)

Also known as Neurological Fatigue, Chronic Fatigue Syndrome (CFS), Chronic Fatigue Immune Dysfunction Syndrome (CFIDS), Systemic Exertion Intolerance Disease (SEID), Extreme Fatigue, Viral Infection Fatigue

Sometimes fatigue is easy to explain. If someone has been excessively exercising and not getting enough downtime or not taking in enough calories to balance it, if someone is overworked mentally or physically, if someone is fasting, or if someone has experienced an acute sickness such as the flu—these are just some examples of temporary fatigue that the world tends to understand.

Extreme fatigue that's not from lack of sleep, on the other hand, has an air of mystery about it. While it can last for a shorter time, extreme fatigue is often long term, sometimes lasting for years or even decades. Its undiscovered underlying cause is a chronic, ongoing viral infection starting in the liver. Sometimes the fatigue comes from multiple viruses at once—anywhere from one to three or more varieties of EBV and/or shingles, herpes simplex 1 and 2, or cytomegalovirus. Most of the time, the fatigue stems from the Epstein-Barr virus. Having other viruses can add to the EBV fatigue.

Rather than calling it "chronic fatigue," I often call this condition *neurological fatigue* or *viral infection fatigue* because it's caused by a central nervous system that's chronically inflamed. For a virus to stay active, there usually has to be viral food present that feeds it. That leads to the virus producing neurotoxins, creating an energy draw on the nerves, which in turn weakens the nerves, creating the neurological fatigue. This is when the central nervous system gets saturated with neurotoxins, and nerves become highly allergic and inflamed—not that this brain and nerve inflammation is going to be detectable by technology we use today. Viral fuels such as toxic heavy metals are at the top of the list for creating antagonistic neurotoxins. Other foods that can be big instigators are ones you found in Part III, "Brain Betrayers." When the brain or brain stem is swelling, pressure increases to all other nerves close to and traveling from the swelling. These other nerves receive a message from the central nervous system that there is a problem occurring. This creates a tension on the nerves, causing further energetic draw.

Often with viral infections, adrenal fatigue—which is different from neurological fatigue—can occur at the same time. That's because when viruses release neurotoxins and the central nervous system becomes stressed and inflamed, the adrenals must work harder. The person with fatigue must also work harder to function, pushing the adrenals further. Or someone can have adrenal fatigue from an emotional trauma that weakens the immune system, allowing a viral infection to start, creating

viral infection fatigue. Yet they still can have adrenal fatigue from that emotional trauma, so now they have adrenal fatigue and viral infection fatigue combined.

There are cases where adrenal fatigue can occur independent of viral infection fatigue (aka neurological fatigue)—where adrenal fatigue is caused, for example, by excess stress, excessive caffeine, drug use, overexertion, or intense heat or cold exposure alone. Improvement from adrenal fatigue on its own will be ongoing, so that someone feels that they're on an upswing, getting a sense of encouragement from continuing to get better. With fatigue that persists longer and stays the same or gets worse, more is going on beneath the surface: a chronic viral load. Adrenal fatigue itself is never as drastic.

Your fatigue doesn't mean there's a genetic issue or spontaneous adrenal malfunction, as it's so often misdiagnosed, prompting doctors to put someone on cortisol steroids to try to correct the hormonal loss or imbalance they're detecting. In truth, it's very often a viral issue causing weak adrenals in the first place.

Some people struggle with certain scents, because the fragrances are so highly toxic and irritating to the nerves. Fragrances from scented candles, for example, can compromise someone already battling fatigue.

For specific healing support beyond what's offered in Part VI, "Bringing Back Your Brain," refer to the ME/CFS protocol in *Brain Saver Protocols, Cleanses & Recipes.*

MEMORY LOSS AND FORGETFULNESS

There are different levels of memory loss and forgetfulness. It's perfectly normal to forget some things. It's perfectly normal for some older memories to fade as new experiences replace them. Maybe you remembered something that was important to you for a long time, and then as the years have gone by, more important experiences and memories have taken precedence so that once treasured detail has become more vague. If you're having a busy day or week, with a lot on your plate, it can be easy to forget things on a daily basis. Many people who don't have brain disease, Alzheimer's, or dementia rely on lists to remember everything they need to get done. With so many expectations, it can be easy to get distracted, drift off task, or forget.

Memory loss and forgetfulness can be a little more persistent and disruptive. For example, someone can regularly forget to write down the list of what they don't want to forget, or forget important birthdays for pets and family members that they used to remember, and that can start to interfere with life to the point of being a problem. When true memory loss and chronic forgetfulness occur, something more is going on in the brain. If injury or trauma is not a factor, toxic heavy metals are the reason for memory loss. Viral infection can play some part. If viruses are consuming toxic heavy metals such as mercury, releasing neurotoxins that interfere with neurotransmitter chemicals, that can cause some forgetfulness

and mild memory loss. Nothing compares to the direct effect of toxic heavy metals in the brain.

Often the problem is heavy metals interacting with each other in negative ways. Metals such as mercury and aluminum reacting with one another send corrosive discharge into adjacent brain tissue, weakening or even destroying neurons and saturating areas of the brain where memories might have been stored. When someone loses their older memories and yet can remember new occurrences in the present day, it often baffles medical communities. They don't realize the true cause: toxic heavy metals corroding in areas where long-term memories are stored in the brain. The reverse can also happen: toxic heavy metals' oxidative runoff saturating areas where memories of the moment are supposed to be stored. *Where are my keys? What neighborhood do I live in? What store did I just visit?* When short-term memory is affected like this and yet older memories remain easy to access, it's an indication of this different toxic heavy metal placement.

There are subtleties to all of this, and it can take decades for symptoms of memory loss or forgetfulness to develop. If oxidative runoff flows one way, it could affect an area of the brain that stores memory of what happened a few minutes ago, meaning someone could remember what happened a year ago and not what happened in the last five minutes. Toxic heavy metals are never in the exact same amount, same combination, and same place among different people, which means the symptoms they cause are never exactly the same from person to person.

If someone has additional symptoms from other health problems, such as a viral infection causing more neurotoxic exposure to neurons and neurotransmitter chemicals, the effects of these other instigators will contribute to that person's unique symptomology, making their health all the more confusing to medical communities.

For specific healing support beyond what's offered in Part VI, "Bringing Back Your Brain," refer to the Brain Fog protocol and/or Alzheimer's Disease protocol in *Brain Saver Protocols, Cleanses & Recipes*.

MÉNIÈRE'S DISEASE

For decades medical communities claimed that Ménière's disease was a result of calcium crystals or stones becoming disrupted in the inner ear. Now medical communities have altered their theory, saying that Ménière's is fluid buildup and a possible viral infection, and in the same sentence saying cause unknown. Original Medical Medium information has always stated that Ménière's is a viral infection and not calcium crystals.

Ménière's is a chronic viral infection of EBV—essentially a version of vertigo, which is inflammation of the vagus nerves. When the vagus nerves are inflamed by EBV's neurotoxins, they swell. That swelling creates pressure, oftentimes in the neck and ears. This can cause chronic or recurring balance issues, where you feel as if you're on a boat. It won't necessarily be pronounced; it could be subtle. When the brain stem is inflamed, the

informational signal changes as the signal is exiting the brain stem into the vagus nerves, prompting the vagus nerves to spasm. Vagus nerve inflammation can also cause a range of experiences of dizziness, from a slight dizzy sensation to a feeling that the room is spinning so much that you can't move an inch without vomiting. EBV can also directly enter the brain stem, where the vagus nerves are exiting, and cause inflammation this way. (Read more about dizziness in "Vertigo.")

It's also common for those with Ménière's to experience a version of tinnitus, whether mild or severe. This is because viral neurotoxins tend to affect the labyrinth of the inner ear, creating a ringing, buzzing, or humming. If someone experiences an internal popping sensation in the head, that's from neurotoxins inflaming the vagus nerves, putting pressure up against the inner ear, plus neurotoxins directly swelling the labyrinth of the inner ear. EBV can also enter the nerves of the inner ear, causing tinnitus. (Read more in "Tinnitus.")

When EBV enters the labyrinth of the inner ear, it can create fluid production. Fluid production does not cause chronic vertigo and dizziness. Rather, fluid production causes pressure, which can create a whooshing or popping sound. Sometimes, if the fluid production is severe in both ears, a person can get a sensation like their head is floating. If someone with fluid production gets dizzy, the dizziness is from vagus nerves that are inflamed at the same time, not from EBV's fluid production. Someone else could have fluid production and no dizziness because vagus nerves are not inflamed.

For specific healing support beyond what's offered in Part VI, "Bringing Back Your Brain," refer to the Vertigo protocol in *Brain Saver Protocols, Cleanses & Recipes.*

MENINGITIS

Medical communities believe that meningitis can be either bacterial or viral. The truth is that meningitis is always viral. The virus can be anywhere in the brain itself, or many times the virus is nowhere near the brain; it's in the liver, another organ, or the bloodstream, causing high fevers and other symptoms. Meningitis can be the result of a chronic viral infection that's been in the body for a long time (sometimes decades), yet for the most part, meningitis is the result of a brand-new onset of an acute viral infection. Meningitis is like an awakening reaction of the body to a new invader.

You'll notice that we hear a lot about college students contracting meningitis. That's because when they're away at school, students tend to experience weakened immune systems from staying up late working hard on papers, stressing out, and partying, often engaging in physical contact or sharing bedrooms and bathrooms, passing around viruses in the process. Another reason why you'll hear about meningitis in college is medical treatment campaigns taking advantage of the lowered immune systems college students have, and these medical treatments don't address the viral aspect of meningitis. The viruses students are exposed to in college could be brand-new strains and mutations of EBV (that is, mono) or brand-new varieties of shingles, herpes simplex 1 or 2, HHV-6, cytomegalovirus, or HHV-7. Brand-new exposure can cause a viral cytokine storm, where the immune system goes into rapid fire trying to destroy the invader, sometimes causing a fever to spike at an extremely high level.

Someone experiencing meningitis could be diagnosed with meningitis, or they could be diagnosed with the flu or receive no diagnosis at all. Spinal taps are never fruitful in diagnosing it, because it's extremely rare for a virus behind meningitis to be discovered with the test. Even if a pathogen such as a bacterium is discovered in the spinal fluid, that doesn't mean it's responsible for someone's symptoms of what's truly viral meningitis. Bacteria are common cofactors to viral infections. Bacteria are present in the body of someone reacting to a fresh, acute viral infection, so it makes sense when bacteria show up once in a blue moon in spinal taps—if a test was even accurate and outside contamination didn't occur. Bacteria showing up in a spinal tap doesn't make bacteria the cause of meningitis. Further, someone could be carrying around undetected bacteria in their body and spinal fluid for years that doesn't affect them. If they contract a viral infection that causes meningitis symptoms and receive a spinal tap, the bacteria could show up in the results and be mistakenly blamed for the illness. Bacteria cannot cause the brain inflammation that's behind meningitis because bacteria lack neurotoxins. Often spinal taps don't reveal anything when someone has a severe viral infection, so many doctors have become wise enough to diagnose meningitis regardless of what a spinal tap says.

As we covered, a new viral infection behind meningitis is often in the liver or bloodstream, remotely causing symptoms of brain inflammation and high fever by releasing neurotoxins that saturate the brain and cause high fever and inflammation. New viral infections can induce an aggressive war between the immune system and the virus, producing large quantities of byproduct, which contributes to elevating the fever. Sometimes the virus is even in the spleen. Only in rare and extreme cases does the virus end up in the brain itself. In some cases, a virus can end up infecting liver, spleen, and brain all at the same time.

For specific healing support beyond what's offered in Part VI, "Bringing Back Your Brain," refer to the Meningitis protocol in *Brain Saver Protocols, Cleanses & Recipes*.

MIGRAINES

So many varieties of migraines exist, and so many triggers. Two underlying causes set the stage for most migraines, and then a multitude of triggers can take that vulnerability and turn it into a migraine.

Toxic heavy metals, which set the stage for many migraines, can be dispersed in different areas around the brain. Wherever they are, that's where an electrical storm can surge, and when an electrical storm occurs inside the brain, migraines can come in all different shapes and sizes. Some people get a migraine where they see an aura, whether pain has started yet or not. This is from mild swelling of the optic nerves, which can happen even when the nerves are perfectly healthy, with no injury or disease. Heavy metals in different parts of the brain can create pain in those areas, such as the top of the head, either side of the head, the back of the head, or the face, from an electrical storm surging in that area.

Viruses are the other main cause that set the stage for migraines. Chronic infections of EBV, shingles, and herpes simplex are the most common creators of viral migraines—when their neurotoxins float through the bloodstream and land on vagus, trigeminal, facial, or other cranial nerves, the nerves can swell easily and headaches or migraines can result. Heat exposure from being in the sun too long can put inflamed nerves over the edge and prompt a migraine. Breathing in toxic air—smoke from someone's chemically saturated campfire, perfume, cologne, detergents, scented candles, gasoline, pesticides, or air freshener—is another major trigger. These are overlooked, and our air is getting more contaminated by the year from these exposures. Somebody can even become chemically sensitive and get an instant headache that turns into a migraine from walking into a store scented by candles, toxic cleaning supplies, air fresheners, potpourri, or incense. Pharmaceuticals can trigger migraines too. In our current environment, fragrances are going to the next level. Their toxicity is becoming a cause of its own because the toxic level of the fragrances is starting to damage nerve tissue directly.

Or a trigger can *seem* like the cause of a migraine. In this case, what's really happening is that triggers such as heat exposure or certain foods are setting off an underlying cause of toxic heavy metals in the brain and/or chronic, low-grade viral infection somewhere in the body that make the central nervous system sensitive. Other underlying causes can include large calcium deposits, large salt crystallizations, and large MSG deposits in the brain, creating toxic blockages and allowing any trigger to set off a migraine.

When stress triggers a migraine, it's not stress itself creating a migraine—someone else with the same level of stress may not get a migraine. The person who does get a stress migraine usually has mild impediments from toxic heavy metals, which cause the brain to run hotter at times: if those heavy metals are in the emotional centers of the brain, they'll get hot when someone is feeling under pressure, and that can easily be a trigger for a headache or migraine. Electrical impulses running through the brain can also become derailed by toxic heavy metals, often setting the stage for ongoing, chronic migraines. Medical research and science remain completely unaware of toxic heavy metals causing migraines.

Some people develop a more sensitive central nervous system from multiple viral infections at once. One variety of shingles plus one variety of EBV or two varieties of

shingles plus two varieties of EBV or one variety of EBV and one variety of herpes simplex 1, and so on. *Streptococcus* is a common cofactor to viral infection and can play a role too. Alongside EBV or shingles, someone could have chronic sinusitis from strep bacteria residing in the sinus cavities, creating mild inflammation there. When there's pollen in the air, they may develop a migraine and think that pollen itself was the cause. It wasn't. The pollen was merely touching the inflamed sinus cavity walls. Pollen was only a trigger; low-grade strep in the sinus membrane was really responsible.

There are countless migraine triggers, and most people experience more than one trigger at the same time. They may point to only one trigger, not realizing that other triggers are present too. For example, someone could have low electrolytes from chronic dehydration while eating viral-feeding foods such as gluten, milk, cheese, other dairy, and eggs that cause viruses to release more neurotoxins that agitate and inflame nerves, or feed strep bacteria, inflaming the sinus cavities—and they may not know that any of this is going on. They may say that it was only the computer or phone that started a migraine.

One reason chronic dehydration is a migraine trigger is that it doesn't allow the body to flush neurotoxins or toxic chemicals, toxic substances, or pharmaceuticals out of the bloodstream, so they build up. Almost everybody is walking around chronically dehydrated, and that deprives neurotransmitters of the microminerals they need to stay strong, which means toxic heavy metals in the brain can also do more harm and instigate more migraines. For even more on migraines, check out the chapter on this subject in the revised and expanded *Medical Medium*.

For specific healing support beyond what's offered in Part VI, "Bringing Back Your Brain," refer to the Migraines protocol in *Brain Saver Protocols, Cleanses & Recipes*.

MITOCHONDRIAL MYOPATHY

Mitochondrial cell injury is caused by chronic viral infections, toxic heavy metals, and chemical toxins. The medical industry blames mitochondrial cell damage on genes, and they've conveniently lumped almost every condition and disease together under a mitochondrial myopathy umbrella.

Yes, cell damage can occur from viruses and toxins. That said, when viruses—specifically, viral neurotoxins—damage mitochondria (parts of cells), the mitochondria are not what cause the multitude of symptoms and conditions associated with mitochondrial myopathy. Cell damage on its own does not cause neurological symptoms, unless it's *nerve* cell damage. Viruses and toxins killing off cells throughout the body faster speeds up aging—which is different from experiencing neurological symptoms. It's when a viral infection damages or inflames nerves and nerve cells that neurological symptoms develop.

With the over 60 varieties of EBV, over 30 varieties of shingles, HHV-6 through HHV-16, and dozens of other herpetic family viruses, there are a vast number of viral strains and mutations with different appetites. Most viruses choose one variety of toxic heavy metal to consume, such as mercury. Many viruses, in addition to toxic heavy metals, are also choosing to consume synthetic chemical agents that the chemical industry is producing. Some viral mutations like to dine on different brews of two or three heavy metals, chemical toxins, pharmaceuticals, and/or insecticides, resulting in a much more destructive type of neurotoxin. As those neurotoxins saturate muscles and land on nerves and in organs, they can create damage themselves. Some viral strains will enter cells and injure them directly.

Again, for somebody to experience a neurological symptom associated with a mitochondria problem, the virus would have to irritate, inflame, or enter a *nerve* cell. The only real condition that happens when the mitochondria are damaged in cells is faster aging because cells are dying. This is already happening in society today. Humankind is aging faster than ever—because viruses, toxic heavy metals, and chemical poisons are causing this quicker aging process by killing cells. The myriad of symptoms such as muscle weakness, pain, numbness, and any other neurological symptoms throughout the body are caused by inflamed nerves from a viral infection, not mitochondria cell problems. Just because someone is experiencing numbness, atrophy, muscle weakness, limited mobility, or even seizures does not automatically mean they have mitochondrial myopathy.

For specific healing support beyond what's offered in Part VI, "Bringing Back Your Brain," refer to the Autoimmune Disorders and Diseases protocol in *Brain Saver Protocols, Cleanses & Recipes*.

MOOD CHANGES

We often hear mood changes being blamed on hormone imbalances. Whether puberty, a menstrual cycle, or menopause, hormonal shifts are an easy target. The truth is that there's much more to mood changes than hormone fluctuations. When someone's altered state of mind isn't the result of something emotionally challenging or traumatic happening in life, one common cause of irritability or the blues is toxic blood. Even if something difficult is going on, if that person's blood is also toxic, they'll be more sensitive and susceptible to triggers from confrontation and conflict or even the demands of the daily grind.

This is what I call *dirty blood syndrome*. When blood is toxic, it's dirty. This is the result of a liver overloaded and overburdened by toxic heavy metals, adrenaline, viruses, other pathogens, and other brain betrayers that you'll find in Part III, "Brain Betrayers." As the liver, the body's filter, gets sluggish and stagnant, the blood can get more toxic. Where do these toxins go? They float around the bloodstream and often find their way to the brain.

Everyone has different toxins in different amounts, so exactly how they affect different people varies. These toxins saturate brain tissue and neurons, diminish neurotransmitter chemicals, and can alter somebody's mood. Toxic heavy metals such as mercury and aluminum can sit inside the brain and cause mood changes all on their own, without the liver being toxic and the bloodstream filled with toxic waste and poisons. Viruses inside the liver can feed off toxic heavy metals and release different brews of neurotoxins, some more potent than others, which can enter the brain and short-circuit electrical impulses on a very mild level, resulting in frustration, agitation, and irritation.

Everyone is different in how their body handles a toxic load. One person may not be swayed too easily to a dark place when their liver, blood, and brain are overloaded with toxic waste and poisons. Another person with a similar toxic load can go to a very dark place and struggle. When someone is highly toxic, mood changes can fluctuate up and down, high and low, and this can lead to a diagnosis of bipolar disorder, depression, seasonal affective disorder (SAD), Tourette's, or OCD.

Why does mood express itself differently in two people with similar toxic loads? Childhood can play a role. If someone grew up with tremendous family stability in early years that gave them confidence and emotional support, that can strengthen their path and journey. Someone else might have lacked that emotional support growing up. One person might have had all the resources they needed when they were young, and another person might have struggled with very few resources or unpredictability. That tends to change people.

Then there's an individual's soul itself, which is unique to each of us. It could be fragile from being tattered along the way. Many people become wounded in life, and soul wounds can make a person more sensitive, affecting how they cope, process, or deal with circumstances involving other people. That can reflect itself in mood.

Someone can be dealing with all of the above. They could be experiencing toxic heavy metals in the brain, a highly toxic liver filled with pathogens and poisons that's caused it to become stagnant and sluggish so that dirty blood develops, and a tattered soul from a journey through life that's been very difficult—all at once. Or they could be dealing with one factor, or some combination. Everyone has a different variation. Mood is so much bigger than chalking it all up to hormones.

For specific healing support beyond what's offered in Part VI, "Bringing Back Your Brain," refer to the Mood Changes and Mood Swings protocol in *Brain Saver Protocols, Cleanses & Recipes*.

MOTOR SKILLS DISORDER (ALSO KNOWN AS DEVELOPMENTAL DYSPRAXIA)

Childhood exposure to the toxic heavy metals mercury and aluminum is behind this disorder. When these heavy metals saturate areas of the brain related to coordination, speech, movement, or carrying out instructions for basic tasks, electrical activity gets derailed as it's traveling down neurons.

Motor skills disorder is often outgrown or can improve because the brain can adapt to heavy metal toxicity to an extent. New brain tissue grows and new neurons develop in a child on a daily basis, allowing electrical activity to move around deposits of mercury and aluminum. If, on the other hand, the heavy metal exposure is ongoing during crucial periods of brain development, growing out of it can be much more difficult, and setbacks can occur.

For specific healing support beyond what's offered in Part VI, "Bringing Back Your Brain," refer to the Motor Skills Disorder protocol in *Brain Saver Protocols, Cleanses & Recipes*.

MULTIPLE SCLEROSIS (MS)

There are two major groups of MS. In one group of MS, EBV is releasing neurotoxins from the liver that are inflaming the central nervous system, causing various symptoms that lead to a diagnosis of MS. In the other group of MS, EBV itself goes to the brain or brain stem, causing brain inflammation and sometimes causing brain tissue abnormalities such as lesions. There are also dozens of symptoms that can prompt a doctor to believe a patient could have MS when it's not necessarily MS.

It's important to note that developing brain lesions does not mean those lesions are what's causing symptoms. Sometimes a doctor discovers a lesion, and that person isn't feeling any symptoms. When someone with a lesion is exhibiting MS symptoms, the symptoms are usually still from EBV's neurotoxins inflaming the central nervous system. That's because if you have an EBV infection that moves to your brain or brain stem, (1) EBV can release neurotoxins from its new residence in the brain or brain stem, (2) some EBV is still living in your liver, sending neurotoxins into your system, plus (3) there's usually a large storage of neurotoxins in the liver that had accumulated throughout the years, and the overloaded liver is releasing these old neurotoxins. Neurotoxins from any combination of these sources will compound neurological symptoms.

If you have a brain lesion, you can still take care of your viral load and get rid of your symptoms. Your lesion can also stop progressing. Many people had an EBV infection many years ago, and the lesions are there like old war wounds. You can move on with your life and heal. A brain lesion is not a deciding factor in how you're going to feel. In rare cases brain lesions are severe and there's a larger amount of EBV in the brain or brain stem, which can lead to more advanced symptoms of MS. Even then, once the virus is addressed, they can stop experiencing symptoms even if brain lesions are still present. No matter your form of MS, the key is going after EBV. The true cause of MS was published in the first edition of the first Medical Medium publication and has been used by many doctors and health professionals as a reference for MS.

For specific healing support beyond what's offered in Part VI, "Bringing Back Your Brain," refer to the Multiple Sclerosis protocol in *Brain Saver Protocols, Cleanses & Recipes*.

MYELIN NERVE SHEATH DAMAGE AND CHRONIC INFLAMMATORY DEMYELINATING POLYNEUROPATHY (CIDP)

Many people with this condition will receive multiple diagnoses as they try to figure out what's wrong. What's considered to be known is that chronic inflammation and damage to myelin nerve sheaths are occurring, and often these are mistakenly pegged as autoimmune disease. This is not accurate. What's really occurring is chronic viral infection creating chronic inflammation—specifically, aggressive herpes-family virus strains attaching themselves to nerves, which is what causes that myelin sheath damage.

People with myelin nerve sheath damage or CIDP have often been exposed to high levels of some of the most potent industrial chemical pesticides and herbicides, household cleaners, detergents, air fresheners, scented candles, solvents, and nano sprays. These are potent forms of food for the viruses that create myelin nerve sheath damage. As they fuel themselves, viruses produce large amounts of highly inflammatory neurotoxins. The central nervous system becomes allergic to these neurotoxins, creating chronic inflammation in large nerves deep within the body as well as peripheral nerves.

Symptoms of myelin nerve sheath damage or CIDP depend on whether the viruses themselves are actively attaching themselves to nerves, creating that myelin sheath injury, or whether inflammation from viral neurotoxins is more of the problem. Some people could have a lower viral load overall, resulting in lower levels of neurotoxins, and yet the viral strains they do have could be more aggressive, clinging to the nerve sheaths, irritating them, and causing a slow breakdown of myelin.

For specific healing support beyond what's offered in Part VI, "Bringing Back Your Brain," refer to the Cranial Nerve Inflammation protocol in *Brain Saver Protocols, Cleanses & Recipes.*

MYSTERY FEARS AND WORRIES

Sometimes we know exactly why we're afraid or worried. Sometimes it feels like it comes out of the blue. Those unexplained cases of fear and worry are often due to a past experience that's been triggered without us knowing—because in times of pain, our brains put up healthy, productive emotional walls to help us cope. These are boundaries that we're not meant to knock down; these walls allow us to get through our days without being constantly reminded of what's happened to us. Unresolved experiences remain recorded in our brains, so when we have an encounter in our present that invokes the past, it can trigger emotions we've felt before, even if we don't understand why.

Much of the time, those unresolved episodes involved other people who didn't rectify or recognize their wrongdoings. Sometimes what happened was terrifying, extreme, or unthinkable. Sometimes it didn't seem upsetting to outside observers, and yet we had our reasons for finding it deeply hurtful. When someone new appears in our lives who reminds us—even subconsciously—of a person from the past, mystery fears and worries can surface. A gateway in an emotional wall opens because that new person awakened a memory in the emotional centers of the brain, behind the wall.

Another source of pain that can come back to visit is the trauma of once being sick or injured. After we heal, feeling a hint of a symptom or any sort of twinge again can put us into fear and worry mode without our registering that it's because we're afraid of being ill again. The same goes for those who've watched loved ones suffer. If that person close to you gets overtired or develops a cold or even a sniffle, seeing them impaired can bring up subconscious panic that the difficult times are happening all over again.

Finally, if someone has been busy all their life—pushing through every day in survival mode from a young age without much help or support—and some of the stress finally dissipates and circumstances improve because of a windfall, new job or career, opportunity to take time off, or nourishing friendship or relationship, it will take some time to process past experiences. Because that person's not running away anymore, healing can start to happen, which means letting go of some of those difficulties. As the body is releasing hurt and hardships, whether through dreams at night or unexplained emotional surges and tears during the day, worries and fears may surface on their way out. It usually takes a year in that new relationship, job, place, or other improved circumstance for healing to happen within emotional walls.

For specific healing support beyond what's offered in Part VI, "Bringing Back Your Brain," refer to the Mystery Fears and Worries protocol in *Brain Saver Protocols, Cleanses & Recipes*.

MYSTERY NAUSEA AND VOMITING

When someone is experiencing nausea or vomiting, the first thing almost everyone assumes is that it's stomach-related. Someone who visits the doctor complaining of nausea will grip their stomach because that's where they're feeling uncomfortable. It's true that these symptoms can originate from the stomach and intestinal area, when food poisoning or stomach flu are behind the symptoms. In some cases, stomach cancer can also cause nausea and vomiting, although in many cases they're not symptoms of the disease.

Most cases of unexplained nausea and vomiting have everything to do with the central nervous system and nearby nerves. The vagus nerves, which originate in the brain stem, are the most important nerves regarding anything to do with the stomach. If the vagus nerves are inflamed or irritated

on any level, whether up in or near the brain itself or down closer to the stomach, then nausea can occur. The vagus nerves can even go into spasm, resulting in vomiting. Often the reason for vagus nerve inflammation is a chronic, low-grade viral infection that's releasing neurotoxins.

Toxic heavy metals inside the brain, close to the vagus nerves, can also cause nausea. Brand-new exposure to a heavy metal such as mercury can cause nausea and vomiting. It's not uncommon for someone to get all their dental amalgam fillings removed and be overcome by these symptoms afterward due to the mercury exposure. Other varieties of mercury exposure from medical treatments can cause nausea and vomiting too.

Further, migraines and other headaches related to viral infections or toxic heavy metals can make the vagus nerves sensitive, leading to the mystery stomach symptoms. Emotional trauma is another cause of nausea and vomiting. When the brain experiences an emotional blow or upset that makes us sick in the gut or heart, that's all vagus nerve–related. Sinus infections from strep that's been in the walls of the sinus cavities for years can also cause chronic nausea as a result of sinus nerves affecting facial nerves and other cranial nerves, eventually placing pressure on the vagus nerves.

There are certain situations where someone can have acid reflux due to a toxic liver and overload of strep or *H. pylori* in the intestinal tract, creating SIBO, and this can create nausea too. That's an instance of the vagus nerves and other nerves associated with the gut getting a signal from the ends of the nerves, rather than getting a signal up at the brain.

For specific healing support beyond what's offered in Part VI, "Bringing Back Your Brain," refer to the Vagus Nerve Problems protocol and/or Stomach Problems protocol in *Brain Saver Protocols, Cleanses & Recipes*.

NARCOLEPSY

Narcolepsy, or what seems to be narcolepsy, can have different causes. One example that the medical industry doesn't know is when someone has a chronic viral infection causing neurological fatigue, forcing them to shut down neurologically at unplanned times during the day and search for a spot where they can lie down and restore. Specifically, that's from the viral neurotoxins inflaming the central nervous system, causing a neurological weakness, especially if there's not enough of an electrical charge surging through the brain and brain stem, driving down to the cranial nerves. Not all viral infections that cause chronic fatigue lead to sleep. In many cases, restlessness and insomnia can occur alongside that extreme fatigue. Viral narcolepsy is a specific, unknown category in which neurotoxins saturate the area of the brain that controls sleep, which is the center of the brain that partially encompasses left and right hemispheres and frontal and occipital lobes. It's a ball-shaped area that combines the physical and the spiritual together. To cope with viral narcolepsy, some people have to take breaks every couple of hours throughout the day and find a couch, chair, or corner where they can rest their eyes and fall asleep, or else they find themselves constantly dozing and entering a partial sleep-like state.

Another cause of narcolepsy is toxic heavy metal saturation in the brain. As with viruses, heavy metal exposure here can go two ways. It can cause an inability to sleep, or it can cause the need to sleep at random times, sometimes with the feeling that it could happen at any moment. If sleep doesn't happen at that critical moment, a mild seizure or what feels like a complete shutdown can begin, including slurred speech and severe muscle weakness. The toxic heavy metal that's mostly responsible for narcolepsy is aluminum. Higher levels of aluminum in certain areas of the brain can create a disruptive, sedative effect. When aluminum saturates the sleep center of the brain, it causes the sleep time clock to become confused. Someone with this type of narcolepsy may not sleep through the night and then may sleep on and off all day. Or they may sleep at night and still sleep on and off throughout the day. Either way, the clock is never balanced, especially if they have both viral inflammation and heavy metals inside the sleep center of the brain.

Medical research and science believe it's a gene that's causes narcolepsy, and they're still searching for it.

Electrical activity that controls sleep is different from the electrical activity in other avenues of the brain because sleep's electrical activity is not governed by our wants, needs, and daily intentions and interactions. When we're asleep, we're not the boss anymore.

Mercury plays a small role in narcolepsy too, although it's mostly aluminum saturation; aluminum has an extremely sedative effect when it's in the sleep area of the brain. Aluminum slows down brain cell activity. If there's too much mercury present in this area of the brain, someone will experience less sleep time clock problems and more overall insomnia. Aluminum here dies down the sparks of electrical impulses, dampening electricity to the point where at a given moment, someone will need to sleep no matter where they are. While it can come unexpectedly, many people with narcolepsy learn to expect its ebb and flow and find its rhythms predictable to some degree.

For specific healing support beyond what's offered in Part VI, "Bringing Back Your Brain," refer to the Narcolepsy protocol in *Brain Saver Protocols, Cleanses & Recipes.*

NEURALGIA (INCLUDING OCCIPITAL NEURALGIA)

The term *neuralgia* is associated with a wide range of struggles, from fibromyalgia to neuropathy and everything in between. One cause of neuralgia is a physical injury to a nerve from an outside source—and that's a definitive cause that medical communities can identify. Most neuralgia cases are not so clearly traced to a cause. The true cause is internal and therefore a mystery to medical research and science.

Neuralgia is caused by one, two, or a combination of three viruses: herpes simplex 1 or 2, EBV, or the shingles virus. Note that someone doesn't have to have experienced a herpes zoster rash to have shingles. There are over 30 varieties of the virus, many of which don't display rashes, and those mutations keep increasing. Certain varieties of shingles cause a lot of deep, insatiable itching, stabbing, pulsing, burning, and jabbing pain. Certain varieties of EBV can cause peripheral itching, moving or roaming pain, tingles, numbness, and burning. Certain varieties of herpes simplex 1 or 2 can cause continual aching, burning, throbbing, or tingling pain. Most people who have one, two, or three of these viruses are dealing with severe neuralgia that could show up anywhere in the body at any given time, especially if their immune system is lowered through other various triggers discussed in this book.

Shingles-predominant neuralgia tends to show itself in the hips, back, legs, feet, and shoulders. Occipital neuralgia is when shingles or herpes simplex 1 or 2 is the predominant virus, and it's affecting nerves in the back of the neck, the side or back of the head, and the face. Many times, shingles resides in the shoulder and neck area, releasing neurotoxins that affect nerves in the back of the head as well as the phrenic and facial nerves. EBV can play a role in some of those symptoms too. EBV-predominant neuralgia tends to surface in the arms, hands, back, chest, and neck. Medical communities do not know herpes simplex or EBV can cause neuralgia.

One of the confusing parts about neuralgia is that because so many different symptoms can occur, so can many diagnoses. It depends on the doctor. One doctor may interpret symptoms to be one condition, and another doctor may label them differently. Neuralgia is not a condition that can be tested for with certainty. Often it requires repeat visits to the doctor and one inconclusive test after another to determine what could be wrong, and the answer is always a guess about what is truly causing a patient's pain, matching complaints of discomfort to a textbook diagnosis. If only doctors were trained to recognize neuralgia as an aggressive viral neurotoxin brew.

For specific healing support beyond what's offered in Part VI, "Bringing Back Your Brain," refer to the Herpes Simplex 1 and 2 protocol and/or Shingles protocol in *Brain Saver Protocols, Cleanses & Recipes.*

NEUROLOGICAL ASTHMA

See Chapter 6, "Your Inflamed Cranial Nerves."

NEUROMUSCULAR DISEASE (INCLUDING MYASTHENIA GRAVIS)

This group of conditions that lead to muscle weakness and loss of neurological control is caused by an inflamed nervous system. Often viral neurotoxins floating from the liver to the bloodstream cause

nerves to inflame in any part of the body, including the extremities. If a specific viral strain or multiple viral strains of EBV or even shingles, HHV-6, herpes simplex 1 or 2, or cytomegalovirus feeds on certain toxic combinations of metals and synthesized industrial chemicals in the liver, the virus can release potent neurotoxins with specific neuromuscular effects. In rarer cases, an aggressive, mutated strain of any of these viruses is what's behind these neurotoxins.

Many viruses only have an appetite for a few poisons that reside inside the liver. Some have a more sophisticated palate and enjoy a wide variety of poisons. Fueling themselves on more brain betrayers such as fragrances and other chemicals makes these viruses more aggressive and injurious. Most of the people suffering from neuromuscular disease have an extremely toxic liver filled with just the right recipe of toxic heavy metals and other poisons, as well as more than one virus residing in the liver and feeding off these toxins and poisons. The resulting neurotoxins can saturate the brain, invading neurons, diminishing neurotransmitters, and inflaming connective tissue such as glial cells in the brain. Inflamed connective tissue in the brain puts pressure on the other nerves that stem from or are close to the brain, such as the vagus, optic, trigeminal, and facial nerves. This can lead to drooping in the face and neck, weak limbs, and even digestive paralysis. Muscles can become weak because the nerves inside the muscles are temporarily paralyzed by the neurotoxins and prevent someone from functioning fully.

Many cases of neuromuscular disease are extremely mild, and some instances are more severe. This depends on what viral mutations someone has, what degree of brain betrayers are in their system, how strong their immune system is, how depleted they are, what *types* of betrayers are present, and how actively hungry the mutated viruses are.

For specific healing support beyond what's offered in Part VI, "Bringing Back Your Brain," refer to the Autoimmune Disorders and Diseases protocol in *Brain Saver Protocols, Cleanses & Recipes.*

NEUROPATHY (NEURITIS)

Neuropathy and *neuritis* are broad terms, sometimes used interchangeably, for diagnoses people get ranging from neurological Lyme to fibromyalgia to neuralgia to rheumatoid arthritis to psoriatic arthritis. These are all viral, all connected to certain varieties of neurotoxins and/or dermatoxins, and they all end up creating some variety of neuropathy or neuritis, even if only on a mild level.

Many cases of neuropathy are experienced in the legs, feet, and toes. This is when the peripheral nerves seem to become damaged after a period of mysterious inflammation. Most of the time, the nerves aren't truly damaged. The numbness, burning, and/or pain someone experiences with neuropathy is not necessarily from dead nerves. Rather, it's from nerves that have been chronically inflamed long term. The nerves can be injured to a certain degree; they usually haven't died, though.

Many varieties of shingles cause most lower-body neuropathy. Herpes simplex 1 or 2 and EBV can cause some lower-body neuropathy cases. These viruses release multitudes of neurotoxins that chronically inflame the nerves. This is often confused with diabetes, since some diabetics develop neuropathy. The truth is that more people without diabetes develop lower-body neuropathy than people with diabetes do. Shingles itself can also cling to and inflame nerves high in the hip, lumbar, piriformis, and gluteal areas. Shingles has an ability to inflame the sciatic nerves, whether vertebrae are also impeding the nerves or not. And not only the sciatic nerves—shingles can inflame the pudendal and tibial nerves too, causing sensations of neuropathy in the lower body.

Different varieties of shingles behave differently—there are over 30 undiscovered varieties. Some shingles varieties cling to certain nerves, causing irritation and inflammation there, while also releasing neurotoxins that cause neuropathy in peripheral nerves elsewhere in the body. Shingles or herpes simplex can be in the neck or jaw area, causing trigeminal neuralgia, which is a form of neuritis where the face becomes so sensitive that nerves all around the face, head, and neck feel painful or on fire. Someone could also have EBV, shingles, and herpes simplex all at once. The viruses could be creating neuritis by releasing neurotoxins and dermatoxins after gobbling down poisons that they find sitting in our liver or elsewhere in our body.

Optic neuritis is a result of the optic nerves becoming inflamed or showing some type of lesion or impediment. People with optic neuritis often get diagnosed with MS at the same time. The reason people can experience the two conditions together is that the same virus, EBV, is behind both optic neuritis and MS symptoms. (Read more about MS under "Multiple Sclerosis.") The virus can inflame the optic nerves directly in two different ways: (1) If it's a certain variety of EBV, it can latch on to the optic nerves, creating a temporary home there and directly inflaming the nerves. This can cause some visible damage that's often treated with steroids. (2) In most cases, EBV isn't attaching to a nerve directly; rather, neurotoxins from the virus are inflaming nerves all through the body. This leads to millions of MS diagnoses. Certain neurotoxins can become intense irritants to certain nerves in the body. The optic nerves are particularly sensitive, so in cases where a particular strain of EBV is feeding on particular poisons, the optic nerves can be affected. Eye problems often develop from EBV—glaucoma, for instance, is caused by the virus. In other cases, it's EBV feeding on different toxic heavy metals, pesticides, fungicides, fragrances, or other brain betrayers, creating different neurotoxins that affect, say, the vagus or phrenic nerves instead. Everybody is unique in what they're harboring, which makes everyone's symptoms unique.

For specific healing support beyond what's offered in Part VI, "Bringing Back Your Brain," refer to the Shingles protocol in *Brain Saver Protocols, Cleanses & Recipes*.

NEUROSIS

See Chapter 31, "Anxiety," Chapter 32, "Depression," Chapter 34, "Obsessive-Compulsive Disorder," and/or Chapter 35, "Bipolar Disorder."

NUMBNESS AND TINGLING

Numbness and tingling can come about because of direct inflammation, which is swelling of nerves throughout the body, or inflammation of the brain or brain stem that's affecting other nerves. One way these symptoms can occur is if a virus (such as EBV, shingles, herpes simplex 1 or 2, HHV-6, HHV-7, or the many other undiscovered varieties and mutations of human herpesviruses) creates neurotoxins. Most people dealing with numbness and tingling are dealing with EBV neurotoxins. EBV is the most common neurotoxin-creating virus; it creates neurotoxins by gobbling up mercury, aluminum, and other toxic heavy metals and toxic substances that it finds in places like the liver or spleen. Once it releases the neurotoxins as waste, they saturate the bloodstream and can find their way to muscles throughout the body.

Other than in the case of inflammatory myopathy (read more in "Inflammatory Myopathy"), neurotoxins don't tend to affect muscles as much as they affect nerves inside muscles. These nerves become sensitive and allergic to the neurotoxins, and that's what makes them swell, causing symptoms that may be diagnosed as neuropathy. When someone's experiencing numbness, it can be easy for a doctor to think the nerves have died when in most cases they're only inflamed.

Before someone develops numbness, tingling happens. That tingling may be so mild the person doesn't notice it, or it may be obvious. The sensation, whether registered or not, comes from a nerve starting to expand and inflame within the muscles, under the derma, or around and in organs because of viral neurotoxins. Tingling can happen anywhere. It can happen on the back of the neck, the arms, hands, legs, feet, toes, fingers—anywhere on the body, even on the nose. While it can recur in a single place, the tingling doesn't necessarily keep coming back to the same spot. It could be a roving tingling, where some days, weeks, or months it's in one place and at other times in another place in the body. This is because nerves can swell and de-swell, coming out of inflammation, depending on where neurotoxins happen to land. If tingling occurs in what feels like the inside of the head, that means neurotoxins could be landing on nerves between the brain and the skull, or landing on the cranial nerves. If the virus itself is in or near the brain or brain stem, it can create more pronounced tingles that are impossible to ignore, because the neurotoxins don't have far to travel and they don't get diluted.

It's not always the case that numbness follows tingling. In many cases, though, it does, with either mild or extreme numbness alternating with tingling or taking the place of tingling. If the neurotoxin is highly potent, then the swelling of the nerve will be greater, which could pinch or put pressure on the nerve to the point where part of the body goes numb (for example, when falling asleep). If someone has trouble drinking, chewing, or speaking and it's not a stroke, it could be from neurotoxins saturating the nerves that control the mouth and speech, creating numbness that they may or may not even be able to feel, because certain nerves are associated more with movement than sensation. If neurotoxins saturate the area of the feet instead, that's a type of numbness that's usually easy to feel because you stand on your feet, whereas you don't stand on your hands. Some mutated viral strains, such as those of EBV or shingles, may latch on to nerves themselves, causing tingles and numbness directly rather than only through neurotoxins.

Tingles and numbness are almost universal symptoms for most Lyme disease patients. As we covered under "Lyme Disease," that's because people who suffer from Lyme are dealing with viral infections, not the cofactor bacterial presence mistaken by the medical industry as Lyme's cause. Lyme patients' neurological symptoms are viral, which is why tingling and numbness occur so commonly for Lyme sufferers.

For specific healing support beyond what's offered in Part VI, "Bringing Back Your Brain," refer to the Cranial Nerve Inflammation protocol in *Brain Saver Protocols, Cleanses & Recipes*.

OBSESSIVE-COMPULSIVE DISORDER (OCD)

See Chapter 34, "Obsessive-Compulsive Disorder."

ORTHOREXIA

See Chapter 33, "Eating Disorders."

OVEREATING

See Chapter 33, "Eating Disorders."

PARKINSON'S DISEASE

Parkinson's is no longer seen the way it was in yesteryear. More doctors are prone to diagnosing Parkinson's today based on symptoms that never would have been identified as the disease in the past. The playing field has widened. In the old days, Parkinson's was fairly limited to symptoms like a tremor and a shake. Now a combination of symptoms such as general stiffness, aches and pains, confusion, depression, and anxiety may be miscategorized as Parkinson's.

Medical communities don't realize they're mixing up conditions. Because a patient is shaking and tremoring, they're lumping all of the patient's other conditions into a Parkinson's diagnosis. This widening of the Parkinson's definition has gotten to the point where even if a patient *isn't* shaking or tremoring and is instead exhibiting other symptoms, such as confusion or brain fog, they could mistakenly get a Parkinson's diagnosis. We need to take care here. Parkinson's diagnoses should only apply when a patient is exhibiting severe tremors and shakes. Medical communities should also stay open-minded that a Parkinson's patient could be experiencing additional conditions at the same time.

If doctors were handed the tools and training they needed, they would discover that the true foundation of Parkinson's is the toxic heavy metals mercury, aluminum, and copper interacting with each other in the brain and oxidizing there, causing corrosive runoff that spreads into adjacent connective tissue in the brain. The toxic heavy metals' discharge injures neurons, defuses electrical impulses, and starves neurotransmitters of the electricity and fuel they need in order to stay healthy and active.

That's part of what causes the severity of Parkinson's patients' involuntary shaking and tremors. Another part is that there are large deposits of toxic heavy metals and other contaminants spread out in many areas of the brain, surrounding neurons. The neurons become hypersensitive to pesticides, herbicides, fungicides, fragrances, scented candles, air fresheners, colognes, perfumes, and gasoline, worsening already weak neurotransmitter chemicals. Neurons become dysfunctional, and neurotransmitter chemicals defuse and dehydrate.

In Parkinson's, toxic heavy metals are concentrated deep inside the brain. While someone may have higher or lower metal levels, it must be just the right blend of mercury, aluminum, and copper touching each other to cause the tremors and shakes of "classic" Parkinson's. If that Parkinson's patient also experiences anxiety and forgetfulness, these other challenges are caused by toxic heavy metals spread out in different areas of the brain, in different amounts.

Still, publicly known medical communities are operating without the knowledge that toxic heavy metals are classic Parkinson's real cause. They also don't realize that viruses can lead to false Parkinson's diagnoses. When a virus is feeding off toxic heavy metals in the body, releasing neurotoxins that saturate the brain, this can cause tremors, confusion, and brain fog—and this chronic viral load can be mistaken for Parkinson's.

For specific healing support beyond what's offered in Part VI, "Bringing Back Your Brain," refer to the Parkinson's Disease protocol in *Brain Saver Protocols, Cleanses & Recipes*.

PERSONALITY DISORDERS

The medical industry has created a massive umbrella of personality disorder symptoms, just like they've done with OCD. They have lumped every single human trait, human behavior, human action, and human personality under the personality disorders umbrella and then blamed it on your family's genes.

There's a fine line between personality changes and personality disorders. Somebody shouldn't be shamed for changing in some way. Many people like to try new experiences in life that could seem abnormal to family or friends. We're also allowed to be moody. Life is not an easy road, and the world is not always a fun place. Daily hardships and the daily grind can be daunting and difficult for so many. "Midlife" crises can occur, whether in your 20s, 30s, 40s, 50s, or later. Mood changes, interest changes, and personality changes can be alarming to those around you who are used to knowing how you beat your drum. If the rhythm of that drum changes, everyone gets alerted. *What's that new sound I'm hearing?* We give teenagers space to explore different music and start dressing and acting differently. Sometimes we need that later in life too.

Let's set all that healthy self-exploration aside. What if something noticeably toxic is occurring in somebody's mood or in how they perceive themselves or the world? It can cause confusion for observers. Is the person depressed? If they're always angry, how come? Personality disorders can be classified in so many different ways that it can feel virtually impossible to keep your finger on the pulse of them. Everyone has the right to get angry. To what degree? Everyone has the right to be moody. To what degree? Is it vastly different from how they'd normally act or behave? Does it seem like they could be destructive and hurtful to the people around them or even themselves? This is some of what must be monitored to determine if someone has a personality disorder. Quite frankly, every person on the planet could be diagnosed with a personality disorder at some point in their life. When it's extreme and pronounced and becomes chronic and even disturbingly dangerous to anyone, that's when someone is most likely dealing with a true personality or other psychiatric disorder.

What's the cause? To begin with, someone could be suffering from emotional wounds in the brain. When someone experiences an emotional blow or continual emotional blows, one after another throughout life, adrenaline from these emotional blows has a different blend to it that can scorch the brain. Certain emotional regions of the brain can become injured, as we talked about in Chapter 5, "Your Emotional Brain." Going forward, that person can become allergic to reminders of what's hurt them before. This alone can alter someone's personality, creating a mild to extreme personality disorder.

Of course, we need to think about toxic heavy metals too. Was there recent exposure? Old exposure? Old exposure oxidizes. Toxic heavy metals break down over time and saturate adjacent tissue, and this can cause an unexpected change of heart in people, one that can be devastating and unpredictable, leading to a change in demeanor, behavior, thinking processes, and dislikes.

For some people, strep bacteria living in the liver and intestinal tract can be enough to cause ups and downs. Viruses such as herpes simplex 1 (the fever blister and cold sore virus) can also live inside people, releasing poisonous waste matter on a daily basis. If this waste matter travels through the bloodstream, it can make someone's personality change in many ways without their realizing the cause. This herpes simplex 1 viral waste matter can swell cranial nerves on a subtle

level, altering someone's personality. Or you can bite your coworker's head off because, without your knowledge, you're running a low-grade viral infection that's affecting your central nervous system and you are not displaying any other symptoms yet. If those outbursts are repeated, they can lead to a personality disorder diagnosis.

Exposure to certain chemicals can have a profound effect on personality. Someone could be experiencing no real problems and then get exposed to air fresheners, scented candles, fabric softeners, cologne, pesticides, and herbicides in their home, and they could seem to lose their mind for a week or more—not acting like themselves, making strange decisions. That's a result of being infused with brain-altering chemicals. It can also make them sensitive down the road, so that every time they get new chemical exposure, it changes their personality a little more, causing constant ups and downs that are never traced to their real source.

So many other factors can influence how we feel and act, including a sluggish, inflamed, or sick liver and a diet high in fat, whether it's a so-called healthy diet high in healthy fat or not. These alone can make someone unpredictable, shifting directions in their demeanor. As the liver becomes more bogged down, more sluggish, and loses its ability to function over time, that affects personality.

Then there's being chronically ill. When someone goes through the hardships of long-term illness, it tends to change who they are. Going from doctor to doctor looking for answers and validation; losing friends, spouses, partners; finding out who your real friends are; worrying about your livelihood; struggling with aches and pains and other symptoms on a daily basis—it can alter the way you perceive the world around you and yourself. Often those close to chronic illness sufferers feel that the sufferer's personality has changed. This is a very different situation. While dwelling in a dark place can hold us back for a time, some of the changes that come from being sick can become our greatest treasure.

For specific healing support beyond what's offered in Part VI, "Bringing Back Your Brain," refer to the Depersonalization protocol in *Brain Saver Protocols, Cleanses & Recipes*.

POTS (POSTURAL ORTHOSTATIC TACHYCARDIA SYNDROME)

People living with POTS really struggle. The unpredictability of POTS symptoms can be maddening for many. In most cases of POTS, it takes months to years of doctor shopping to get validation for their symptoms. The cause of these mystery symptoms is byproducts and toxins built up in a stagnant, sluggish liver being released and collecting around heart valves. POTS symptoms go way beyond problems with getting up, leaning forward, and leaning down— because POTS is a viral neurotoxin disorder.

One reason POTS is so difficult is that it's a chronic viral infection. In POTS, the Epstein-Barr virus has been in the liver for a long time, and it's this virus releasing the neurotoxins that causes POTS symptoms, ranging from dizziness to difficulty exercising to light-headedness to fainting, fatigue, brain fog, nausea, chest pain, blurred vision, racing heart, and unstable blood pressure. When the liver is stagnant, sluggish, overburdened, and filled with years' worth of viral toxins, various areas of the liver become blocked. This makes it harder for blood to draw through the liver to get to the heart, putting the heart under a continual strain. When someone quickly or even normally stands up, walks uphill, or exerts themselves, they can get light-headed and dizzy or faint, and they can have an increased heart rate. The heart is struggling to draw blood out of the liver, which can destabilize blood pressure.

Often in POTS, viral neurotoxins are also floating around, saturating and inflaming nerves such as the vagus. Depending on which areas of the nerves are saturated, viral symptoms can vary. If the vagus nerves are inflamed higher up, closer to the brain, that inflammation from those neurotoxins can create symptoms when someone is just getting out of bed, picking themselves up off the ground, standing up quickly, bending down, trying to climb a hill, or exerting themselves. For some people it feels like having sandbags on their legs, full-body weakness, or even the feeling of collapsing.

Everybody's POTS symptoms vary because everybody's immune system varies, everybody's viral load or mutations of viruses vary, and everyone's liver capacity for toxins varies. Often these days, people don't get a POTS diagnosis by itself.

Someone with POTS has often seen multiple doctors and received other diagnoses. Often POTS gets wrapped into Lyme disease, fibromyalgia, lupus, vertigo, and/or ME/CFS because someone is experiencing various symptoms of the same virus (EBV). The distinction is that in POTS, the liver is more stagnant and sluggish, more overloaded with neurotoxins, which means that certain areas of the vagus nerves end up more puffed out and inflamed, so that certain movements or any kind of exertion can prompt dizziness, light-headedness, vertigo, struggle with breathing, or tachycardia. The combination of a liver that has blockages along with viral infection creates the unpredictability.

The tachycardia aspect, in many cases, is neurological tachycardia, especially if the doctor can't find an actual, physical ailment with the heart. Messages from the brain can get derailed as they're traveling through the brain stem out into vagus nerves and to the heart. Meanwhile, the heart is physically okay. These derailed nerve messages can create a neurological tachycardia that means any quick movements, such as turning your head, getting up off the ground, or trying to run, can send an incomplete signal to the heart, causing an increased heart rate.

Any antibody detected with POTS is not an indication that your immune system is attacking your body. The antibody is actually created by your body to fight Epstein-Barr virus. Rather than fighting against you, its entire job is to help you fight off the pathogen behind POTS.

For specific healing support beyond what's offered in Part VI, "Bringing Back Your Brain," refer to the POTS protocol in *Brain Saver Protocols, Cleanses & Recipes*.

PSYCHOSIS

Psychosis can occur at many different levels. An extreme situation is when someone becomes completely disconnected from their surroundings, almost as if they were on mind-altering drugs, where you can't communicate with them, they're delusional, they're seeing things, they're lost, they're not "there." If we're keeping drugs out of the equation to explain this, whether prescribed pharmaceuticals or recreational, the other explanation is a developing illness inside the brain—for example, an interaction between toxic heavy metals and solvents. Specifically, we're talking about solvents deep in the brain *touching* toxic heavy metals there, creating chemical reactions. Psychosis doesn't normally happen as one big, acute, severe attack out of nowhere. Usually it's a buildup over years of smaller bouts of psychosis slowly worsening, leading to larger bouts.

It usually takes three or more toxic heavy metals residing deep inside the brain to set the stage for psychosis and then the "right" chemical solvents entering the scene to cause a reaction. Imagine a chemist in a lab playing around with different metals, dropping different chemical substances on them and then monitoring and studying what kind of reactions occur. Now imagine all of these elements inside the brain—when they combine in a reactive way, they can make someone more susceptible to psychosis. Cannabis often triggers psychosis. What determines the level of psychosis depends upon how the cannabis has been grown and what chemicals were sprayed on the cannabis or added to the soil. Many chemical solvents are used in growing cannabis. Pharmaceuticals can worsen psychosis. And many pharmaceuticals can create an acute episode of psychosis. Adrenaline is often part of the equation too. When someone experiences a bout of psychosis, that results in adrenaline saturating the brain, causing a fight-or-flight reaction and increasing the psychosis, and then the adrenaline with the toxic heavy metals and solvents deep within ignite the electrical grid inside the brain, and that can keep a bout of psychosis going and going.

Mild psychosis, with lower levels of metals and solvents in the brain, can even occur for someone who's been chronically ill and stuck in bed for too long. That's perfectly normal and acceptable. Someone should never be shamed for developing emotional issues, mental struggles, or PTSD while chronically ill. I've witnessed people sprain an ankle, get stuck on the couch for a month away from their busy life, and become so upset and disturbed by the isolation and change of pace that they develop a mild psychosis. Any kind of illness or disruption in our physical life can create psychosis.

On top of which, experiencing chronic illness can also be a sign of constant viral infections. This leads to a lot of viral waste and viral die-off, sending poisonous matter into the body systems that then saturates the brain. Ammonia is also present in the brain because of a sick liver causing weakened digestion. Combine this with the struggle of not feeling validated and not living the life you want to live—it could create mild psychosis in any and all of us. That isn't a delusional type of psychosis that's disconnected from reality. It's a completely sane psychosis.

Often people who have struggled with chronic illness are diagnosed with depression, anxiety, mental issues, neurosis, or even psychosis, making it feel like their struggles are in their head. Meanwhile, it's physical. Even though we just explored why psychosis is a natural emotional struggle, focusing on the mental side of chronic illness misses the mark. First and foremost, people's physical struggles need to be recognized. What they're going through is often avoided, ignored, or misunderstood—people with chronic illness or chronic injuries are almost always misunderstood. When the survival methods they call upon to get them through their struggles—what any of us would do if we were down and out—are labeled as mental issues, it can make the situation worse. We need to remember that anyone could be susceptible to feeling out of their head if they, too, were chronically misunderstood.

For specific healing support beyond what's offered in Part VI, "Bringing Back Your Brain," refer to the Psychosis protocol in *Brain Saver Protocols, Cleanses & Recipes*.

PTSD (POSTTRAUMATIC STRESS DISORDER)/PTSS (POSTTRAUMATIC STRESS SYMPTOMS)

The variations and levels of PTSD are endless, for almost any circumstance we face.

PTSD is a combination of physical and metaphysical injury:

One aspect of PTSD is an imprint in the physical brain tissue—cell damage from intense electrical surges or heat in one specific area of the emotional centers of the brain.

Another aspect of PTSD is an imprint on the subconscious and conscious mind. Physical brain tissue harbors what's literally a ball of energy filled with information, thoughts, and memories of this lifetime—that's the subconscious and conscious mind, the bridge between the physical brain tissue and the soul.

The other aspect of PTSD is a metaphysical imprint in the soul at the same time. This imprint comes from whatever occurred, ranging from a tragedy to an everyday difficult challenge. PTSD could even occur from something difficult or displeasing that we have to do repetitiously every day—for example, a job that has you completing the same identical tasks that offer no joy for an extended length of time.

Part of PTSD is the soul trying to pierce through the ball of energy of the subconscious and conscious mind in order to heal. The subconscious and conscious have a connection to the soul. With PTSD, the metaphysical soul injury is not staying suppressed or buried. Instead, the soul injury enters the subconscious and conscious mind so someone can move past the soul injury and then the subconscious and conscious mind can find resolve, which in turn can help heal the soul and physical brain tissue that are injured.

The level of PTSD depends upon the level of both soul injury and physical injury to the emotional centers of the brain. Everyone's PTSD differs. Someone may have more physical injury in the emotional centers of the brain and less metaphysical soul injury. Someone else may have more metaphysical soul injury and less physical injury.

Another aspect that makes people respond differently to life events is whether they've had any kind of PTSD at other times throughout life, or whether it's their first experience in life that prompts their first physical and metaphysical injury. This also plays a role in how someone copes with their PTSD or how fast they move past it. If someone who has never experienced PTSD before has their first crisis, it could be more devastating than someone who is somewhat used to having things fall not in their favor, with different varieties of crises throughout their life prompting different levels of PTSD. It's similar to how someone who knows what it's like to be sick can handle a new symptom much differently from someone who is down and out for the first time in life.

Common PTSD triggers and instigators include:

- Constant letdown

- Betrayal

- Broken trust

- Heartbreak

- Loss

- Mistreatment

- Abuse

- Fear

- Not being understood

- Not being heard

- Financial stress

- Family stress

- Being ignored

- Unfulfilled promises

- Having the (figurative) rug pulled out from under you

- Prolonged overabundance of adrenal stress

- Extreme adrenaline-based sports and activities

- Caffeine-related adrenaline

- Fireworks

Read more about PTSD in the revised and expanded *Medical Medium*.

For specific healing support beyond what's offered in Part VI, "Bringing Back Your Brain," refer to the PTSD protocol in *Brain Saver Protocols, Cleanses & Recipes*.

REPETITIVE STRAIN INJURY (RSI) (INCLUDING CARPAL TUNNEL SYNDROME, TRIGGER FINGER, TENNIS ELBOW, TENDONITIS, BURSITIS)

In the obvious version of a repetitive strain injury, someone is using a part of their body over and over again, usually with the same set of motions, to the point that the muscles become overused without having the time they need to heal and recuperate. Weakness and temporary injury can result. In some cases someone can even end up with near-permanent injury, if the usage was intense and sustained. These types of RSIs are common when someone's job involves physical labor without many breaks. Coaches are also careful with athletes; they learn the delicate finesse of how far to push their trainees in a session for how long, and that they need to follow the basic, fundamental rules of nature and allow healing to happen between workouts.

What's in play when someone develops the marks of an RSI and isn't engaged in repetitive activities? When someone gets carpal tunnel syndrome without writing, painting, drawing, crafting, or being on a computer or device all the time? When someone gets tennis elbow and doesn't play tennis? When someone gets tendonitis without exercising much at all? When someone gets bursitis out of the blue? When someone gets trigger finger and they're not typing on a computer all day? To begin with, when the liver is intoxicated with neurotoxins (released by EBV feeding on toxic heavy metals, fungicides, and antibiotics and other pharmaceuticals) and has to let them into the bloodstream, these neurotoxins damage nerves, tendons, ligaments, connective tissue, and muscle tissue. When someone doesn't have the proper diet to help get rid of these neurotoxins, the neurotoxins can land on tissue and nerves, clinging to them, making nerves highly sensitive and reactive. One of the ways nerves react is by getting mildly inflamed. The level of inflammation depends on what brew of toxins was consumed by which viruses in the liver. For example, someone can have a pharmaceutical-filled liver, with antibiotics, cold medicines, ADHD medicines, antidepressants, antianxiety medications, sleeping pills, and contraceptive pills increasing the liver's toxicity.

Next, the neurotoxins can enter the brain, where they rest themselves upon neurons and connective brain tissue. Neurotoxins can also rest themselves upon nerves elsewhere in the body that run either directly to or near the brain, nerves that connect to the cerebellum, brain stem, and spine. When these nerves closest to the brain become even slightly irritated or inflamed by neurotoxins, they send pain signals to other nerves throughout the body—for example in the arms, hands, or legs. This is why so many people with chronic illness have trouble exercising. It's not only that they're suffering from fatigue. It's that neurotoxins

have saturated nerves, often ones connected to the brain, or even saturated the brain itself, making nerves throughout the body hypersensitive because the nerves are spasming and tensing as they're getting a signal from the brain. This can make ailments such as back injuries and foot injuries (think Morton's neuroma and plantar fasciitis) more common. It can lead to carpal tunnel syndrome and tendonitis. It can lead to shoulder injuries that aren't joint related and instead are a result of an ulnar nerve flare causing the pinkie or index finger to hurt.

Many people with these mystery RSIs also experience fibromyalgia at one time or another. That's because EBV is responsible for both. What the virus is doing at any given time affects whether someone is experiencing more of an RSI, more general fibro symptoms, or everything at once. Many times the EBV can seek out an injured area, making that area take longer to heal.

Sleep is critical for anyone dealing with an RSI. Sleep helps restore nerves more quickly so that the immune system can gobble up and overcome the neurotoxins that are inflaming the nerves, making it so that if you use your arms to scrub your shower, use your legs to take a walk, or whatever it is that may be a struggle, you aren't set back.

When exploring RSIs we also need to talk about electromagnetic frequencies (EMFs). People with tendonitis, carpal tunnel syndrome, other RSIs, or even brain fatigue often find themselves sensitive to computerized devices. For example, someone may get a tingle or numbness in the fingers all the way up to the elbow after touching their phone or tablet for too long. This is because those with RSIs are already sensitive, and electronic devices emit frequencies, even small amounts of radiation. As advanced as our technology is, it's antiquated compared to the devices we'll have in 30 years, which will most likely not emit the frequencies or low levels of radiation that affect us now. Today we're still living with vibrations and energy that we can't see or technically feel coming out of our devices, wireless Internet routers, and cell towers. All of this can affect someone with sensitive nerves. It's one reason why your eyes can get more easily fatigued looking at a screen and why some people feel drained after using a device; modern-day computerized devices can actually draw away some of our stabilizing energy. The more sensitive you are from neurotoxins or other low-grade viral debris creating inflammation of the nerves, the more these frequencies can trigger your RSI, even if you aren't aware of it. Read more in Chapter 27, "Radiation and EMF."

For specific healing support beyond what's offered in Part VI, "Bringing Back Your Brain," refer to the Fibromyalgia protocol in *Brain Saver Protocols, Cleanses & Recipes*.

RESTLESS LEGS SYNDROME (WILLIS-EKBOM DISEASE)

Often when addressing restless legs, medical communities start with the legs first. "Is there muscle cramping?" they'll ask. "Could that be the problem? Try putting a pillow between your legs when you sleep at night." Or they'll ask, "How's your bed and your mattress? Are they uncomfortable? Are they supporting your lower back when you lie down?" Or even, "How are your feet? Are your shoes supportive? Do they fit right and have enough padding? Is one leg shorter than the other?"

If looking at the place where the symptoms are felt doesn't yield results, then the doctor may move on: "Is your mind too active when you're trying to sleep? Read a book, maybe light a candle and take a bath, listen to some calming music. Consider taking magnesium." If none of this helps, often patients are told it's time for an MRI of the lower back to investigate for a degenerative disc problem or bulging disc. And if this all checks out—no signs of a structural spine issue—the restless legs will be considered a medical mystery. There are some neurologists these days who will start looking into the brain to some degree at this stage. They may even order an MRI of the brain to try to see if anything is abnormal there, although they won't find the cause of restless legs that way. The true cause of restless legs wouldn't appear on today's MRIs. Even if the scan showed a brain tumor, it wouldn't mean that was the cause. And even if someone does have a lower back issue or anything of the sort, it doesn't mean that's the source of the problem either.

Restless legs can come from two places. First is the shingles virus releasing neurotoxins that affect the lower spine, inflaming nerves there. This is one of the undiscovered mysteries of restless legs. The neurotoxins produced by the shingles virus sitting inside the liver can settle in different places in the body depending on what those neurotoxins are filled with. Higher amounts of lead and copper being consumed by the shingles virus will result in heavier neurotoxins that tend to settle lower in the body due to their weight; they'll often drop to the lower back, legs, and feet, irritating the nerves and creating subtle spasms. Some varieties of EBV can also create these heavier types of neurotoxins. People can have restless legs all day long while standing, working, or sitting and not realize it until they're still and lying down for the night.

Here's the other way restless legs can occur: viral neurotoxins filled with the same methylated metals can enter the brain. Although blood flow goes to the brain when we're standing or sitting up all day, heavier neurotoxins don't usually flow that high with the blood. That changes when we're lying down. Now these metal-laden neurotoxins can use gravity to migrate to the brain through blood flow. Once they get there, neurotoxins can saturate brain tissue, interfering with neurotransmitters and neurons and interrupting electrical impulses. The short-circuiting and stray messages this causes are what results in those uncomfortable leg (or even arm or torso) sensations.

Restless legs won't necessarily bother someone immediately upon lying down. Sometimes it takes an hour or two to kick in. It often takes that amount of time for heavier neurotoxins to circulate and settle. At the same time, neurotoxins can short-circuit neurotransmitters and make it

difficult for someone to fall asleep within the window before the neurotoxins settle and create a fresh episode of restless legs. Falling asleep quickly helps bypass a rough restless legs night.

The second cause of restless legs syndrome—viral neurotoxins saturating the brain—is why people who suffer from restless legs often find relief by falling asleep in a recliner chair. Some elevation of the head keeps heavy neurotoxins from traveling to the brain so quickly. It's also why they'll find themselves having to get up and pace or walk to the kitchen—without realizing it, they're getting those neurotoxins to gravitate away from the brain. Even though these neurotoxins are now headed to the lower spine, abdomen, knees, and feet, getting up can allow someone with restless legs to get more comfortable because neurotoxins in the brain make restless legs a little worse.

For specific healing support beyond what's offered in Part VI, "Bringing Back Your Brain," refer to the Cranial Nerve Inflammation protocol and/or Shingles protocol in *Brain Saver Protocols, Cleanses & Recipes*.

SADNESS

With mystery sadness, a vicious cycle can occur: We can't understand our sadness, so that leads to more sadness. And if those around us are not understanding our feelings or blaming it on us, that can lead to strained relationships with friends, family, and coworkers, creating even more sadness. Then there's doubting yourself when you're sad—thinking you're not a normal or good enough person. It can lead to crankiness and irritability and even become a pattern over time.

Let's establish first that it's a human right to feel sad. It's part of our free will and existence as human beings with souls. Even though it may feel unpleasant or be tough for others to witness, we have a right to feel sadness when something difficult is happening.

Then there's the sadness that occurs when everything seems to be okay—the kind of sadness that isn't helping us process a struggle, loss, or trial. We're not talking about other people observing your life—people who may not understand you, your life, your world, or your soul completely—and telling you that everything looks agreeable, so you should be fine. Only you have the right to determine if your sadness comes with a reason or if it feels unwarranted and out of nowhere. That doesn't mean that mystery sadness doesn't have meaning behind it. Not being able to pinpoint the source of your sadness doesn't mean it's not real. We don't need to justify sadness. If we want to move through it, though, it can help to understand how it arises.

One source of mystery sadness is hurt from yesteryear. When you're going through a hard time in life, sometimes the adrenaline that goes along with those difficult emotions will get stored with toxins that the body stores away to protect you. When the body is cleansing on a daily basis, a lot of different toxins can surface, and with them can come emotional information in the form of adrenaline that was stored alongside the toxins. With the adrenaline reentering your system, you may reexperience sadness from long ago during the cleansing process. Pockets of adrenaline carrying information from yesteryear can even be stored in fat cells, and when those fat cells dissolve, releasing that adrenaline will often mean releasing stored emotional experiences and toxins too.

The organs, too, harbor emotional experiences combined with toxins and adrenaline saturated within the cells. The brain takes it to another level. The brain can harbor memories and emotional experiences within cell tissue without toxins and adrenaline stored in those brain cells. Your brain can also harbor adrenaline and toxins with stored information in it *alongside* memories and experiences. The stored adrenaline and toxins can conflict with the nearby stored memories and experiences and create additional emotional sensations and sadness. Sometimes an experience can trigger information stored from the past that makes us sad without our even realizing that trigger is what brought back a feeling of hurt, even if the hurt was many years ago.

Often it's not only stored adrenaline making us sad. Another variety of mystery sadness comes from toxins that are floating around the body and entering the brain. For example, when viruses' waste matter such as neurotoxins saturate the brain, they can dampen neurotransmitters, making them less responsive and causing an emotional numbness to occur. EBV, herpes simplex 1, and herpes simplex 2 are some of the viruses that emit poisons and toxins that saturate neurotransmitter chemicals, leading to sadness even at the mildest level.

Sometimes sadness can occur from brand-new toxin exposure in the moment that has nothing to do with viral infections or past hurt. Breathing the fumes of scented candles into your lungs can saturate your brain and allow for a sadness to occur that lasts for days or even weeks.

For specific healing support beyond what's offered in Part VI, "Bringing Back Your Brain," refer to the Difficulty Coping protocol, Depression protocol, Chronic Mystery Guilt protocol, and/or Seasonal Affective Disorder protocol in *Brain Saver Protocols, Cleanses & Recipes*.

SCHIZOPHRENIA

Schizophrenia is a physical condition. It should never be passed off as just a mental or emotional condition. If someone is severely damaged from emotional and/or physical abuse by other individuals or an institution of some sort, then yes, an emotional-mental condition can develop resembling some variety of schizophrenia. Really, that scenario is more likely a combination of severe OCD with PTSD, depression, anxiety, and inability to sleep, all mixed up in one, and there's still a physical cause. While this could accidentally lead to a schizophrenia diagnosis, it's still a misdiagnosis of schizophrenia, even if the symptoms mirror schizophrenia.

Schizophrenia on its own, without physical or emotional abuse, is another story. Passing it off as a "chemical imbalance," genes, or loss of dopamine is antiquated. Oxidation from old toxic mercury that has been passed on from generation to generation for hundreds of years plus aluminum from recent generational exposure can interfere with neurons in a specific way, resulting in symptoms of schizophrenia. Oxidation crosses neuron pathways and saturates an area of multiple neurons.

There are a thousand varieties of schizophrenia. It all depends on where and how much mercury versus aluminum is in the brain, how aged the mercury is, how oxidized the mercury and aluminum have become, and where they travel. Schizophrenia develops quickly in most cases, as opposed to dementia caused by mercury and aluminum, which develops more slowly. This is why younger people develop schizophrenia. Toxic heavy metal contamination is expanding and breaking down rapidly, leading to schizophrenia quickly and abruptly —a fast-paced contamination of heavy metal byproduct. In dementia, on the other hand, the toxic heavy metals are stable and have been slowly gathering for years, oxidizing slowly rather than fast, leaching into brain tissue as the decades go by and creating a slow advance of symptoms such as delusion, confusion, forgetfulness, angry rants, constant frustration, and an inability to navigate what's reality and what's not reality. Schizophrenia can share many of these symptoms because the same toxic heavy metals are behind it. Symptoms can occur in spurts and then disappear because the rapid breakdown of neurotoxic heavy metals leads to acute attacks, followed by the body and brain trying to recalibrate back to homeostasis. Normally an acute attack is brought on by a larger explosion of byproduct and runoff of mercury and aluminum (often stimulated by recent medical treatments that contain hidden toxic heavy metals such as mercury and aluminum) in combination with caffeine.

If someone is on caffeine while a larger deposit of mercury and aluminum is disintegrating in the brain tissue, the mercury and aluminum byproduct can have a forced saturation rate deeper into the brain tissue, near the original deposit, from the caffeinated adrenaline response. One of the reasons why people often have a schizophrenic attack while on recreational drugs is because they're also using high amounts of caffeine. Recreational drugs are filled with higher levels of chemical solvents, plus anyone using recreational drugs tends to self-administer large amounts of caffeine frequently, creating fight-or-flight, which prompts adrenaline and an accelerated heart rate to flush and move the original decaying toxic heavy metal byproduct deeper into the brain. The same goes for prescribed drugs. Pharmaceuticals have a lot of different chemical compositions and agents in them that react with the higher levels of decaying mercury and aluminum.

People with schizophrenia have accelerated oxidation. Their blood acids are high. Their diets are usually high in fat when their brain really needs glucose. Not to mention that people diagnosed with schizophrenia, or even conditions close to it, are often told by physicians to eat a diet composed of mostly fat, which accelerates the symptoms further. A fat-based diet causes an increased oxidation level of the toxic heavy metals that cause schizophrenia.

For specific healing support beyond what's offered in Part VI, "Bringing Back Your Brain," refer to the Schizophrenia protocol in *Brain Saver Protocols, Cleanses & Recipes*.

SEIZURES (INCLUDING EPILEPSY)

Intermittent onsets of severe seizures come from large deposits of heavy metals rather than the "sprinklings" of heavy metals throughout the brain that can cause some other toxic heavy metal symptoms and conditions. Sometimes there are even clusters of large deposits, although it's usually only a cluster of two deposits. What creates these seizures is the interaction of metals— specifically, an alloy of mercury, aluminum, and copper, with all three of those residing next to each other and sometimes even partially forged together through excessive heat exchange from past seizures. Most people who suffer from severe seizures were exposed to all three metals at the same time, rather than exposed to different metals at random different times. Individuals who have routine seizures often have mystery shadows appear inside their brain on MRI scans. These are markings created by metals and the interaction of metals.

Heavy metal alloy deposits or deposit clusters don't necessarily create many other symptoms because they're not interrupting signals right and left the way heavy metals distributed throughout the brain can. What brings on severe seizures is usually a chemical reaction with the alloy deposit or deposits. That chemical reaction could come from something the person's ingesting, including some medications, or even an episode of severe stress, because in that case, adrenaline will flood the brain. Whatever the chemical reaction is, it will create heat in the brain, and because metal conducts heat, it will bring *intense* heat to wherever that heavy metal deposit or cluster is located. An electrical storm will occur as the body and brain try to find balance—and that's what creates a severe seizure. After the seizure, the toxic heavy metals are intertwined more from the heat exchange.

Some seizures are not caused solely by toxic heavy metals. A number of factors and combinations can cause seizures, including MSG deposits in the brain, calcium and sodium deposits in the brain, viruses and viral byproduct and even viral neurotoxin deposits in the brain, brain tissue that's callusing or scarring, brain tissue that's dying, severe neurotransmitter deficiencies in the brain, severe B_{12} deficiency in the brain, highly toxic chemical exposure in the brain, and byproduct and waste in the brain from foodborne pathogens. This is not an exhaustive list. Most seizures have a foundation of metals combined with one or more of these other factors.

Everyone has some level of toxic heavy metals in the brain. A smaller amount of toxic heavy metals sprinkled about could be grounds for seizures someday if conditions are just right. These other factors make a brain more vulnerable to an electrical storm starting, allowing the minimal amount of toxic heavy metals to join forces in toxicity with MSG deposits, calcium deposits, sodium deposits, viral neurotoxin deposits, callusing, scarring, dead or dying brain tissue, neurotransmitter deficiency, B_{12} deficiency, and so on to create a seizure.

The variety of seizures is vast. Some people receive an epilepsy diagnosis for their seizures. In many varieties of seizures, someone can hold complete consciousness and awareness as a seizure is happening. The seizures are mild, and it's still possible to function. Some seizures are more severe, where the seizures takes hold and someone is in a state of electrical shock, having an electrical storm overheating of the brain. The central nervous system feels as if it's shutting down, and the person has to rest and heal to recover, even if it's just for a short period of time. It could be a situation where someone has more of one factor than another. Some people can have more MSG deposits, more calcium deposits, a little less toxic heavy metal such as mercury and aluminum, more viral byproduct such as neurotoxins. It also matters where these toxins are positioned in the brain and how the person handles the condition personally. Are they frustrated? Are they angry about the seizures? Have they lost all confidence? Have they lost all hope that they can heal? These play a role when living with a seizure disorder.

By the time you know a seizure is happening, you have already been having a seizure in a small part of the brain. As the ripple effect occurs, radiating into another part of the brain and then another part, eventually you feel the seizure when the entire brain is engulfed in the electrical storm.

Someone who has experienced seizures before often knows what symptoms to take as forewarning. Many people find a way to cope when they feel those first warning signs of a seizure. They have techniques they have learned so they can try to lessen or navigate the seizure and it won't be so bad or can be thwarted altogether. For some people, tremors are a sign of a seizure coming, or weakness in the legs is a sign, or tics and spasms, or severe headaches. Techniques include finding a safe space, staying calm, drinking fluids to get hydrated, lying down and resting, shutting the eyes, not speaking, relaxing the breath, staying cool or cooling down, splashing cold water on the face, taking off excess clothing if hot or adding clothing if cold, getting some fresh air, forewarning a nearby loved one that they're not going to be available for the moment they're struggling, and stopping all work to preserve cognitive strength.

For specific healing support beyond what's offered in Part VI, refer to the Seizures protocol in *Brain Saver Protocols, Cleanses & Recipes*.

STIFFNESS (INCLUDING STIFF PERSON SYNDROME)

Stiffness is a condition where acidosis plays a role. This is when an acid environment is created by foods, chemicals, radiation, and high or unbearable stress levels. Fight-or-flight creates adrenaline that's highly acidic and corrosive. When someone is under intense stress, more adrenaline is released. Or when someone is on caffeine products, more adrenaline is released, creating a blood acid state that oftentimes becomes chronic, especially when someone ages and they're not in their 20s or 30s anymore. Caffeine is just one contributor to the blood acid state that leads to stiffness. Vinegars are another contributor to blood acid. Dairy, pharmaceuticals, nutritional yeast, and kombucha tea are other common contributors.

When we're in this blood acid state, we lose calcium from our bones and teeth quickly. Calcium is our buffer, our neutralizer to keep the blood acid as balanced as possible so acid doesn't reach a dangerous level. Tiny calcium crystals end up saturating connective tissue around nerves, inside muscles, and around joints, causing a feeling of stiffness that eventually gets shaken off as you move through your day. When you're younger, you can't feel these effects so much. As the years go by, if this buildup becomes chronic over time and begins to build up in the brain and other organs, the feeling gets worse.

What takes stiffness to a chronic, problematic, and serious condition, and maybe even a stiff person syndrome diagnosis, is when viruses and toxic heavy metals are in the mix. Viruses such as EBV release neurotoxins that attach themselves to nerves. When these viral neurotoxins saturate connective tissue and nerves throughout the body, it amplifies stiffness to the next level, making it extremely uncomfortable.

And if toxic heavy metals are inside the brain, interfering with electrical impulses and neurons, that can create a variety of stiffness. That's because signals being carried through the nerves are strained by the toxic heavy metals so the signals aren't as strong as they were. If the brain and nerves are functioning optimally and someone has a strong central nervous system, stiffness from another cause could be minimal. The minute there's a strain put on electrical impulses—in this case, a strain from toxic heavy metals in the brain—nerves aren't going to have that high percentage of strength to compensate for and override existing stiffness.

If someone is dealing with multiple causes of stiffness at once—a blood acid state leading to calcium buildup, viral neurotoxins saturating nerves and connective tissue, and/or toxic heavy metals in brain tissue—plus a severe methylation issue, where the liver is not methylating or converting vitamins and nutrients such as B_{12}, stiffness can become severe.

For specific healing support beyond what's offered in Part VI, refer to the Cranial Nerve Inflammation protocol in *Brain Saver Protocols, Cleanses & Recipes*.

STROKES (INCLUDING TRANSIENT ISCHEMIC ATTACK, TIA) AND BLOOD CLOTS

One cause of strokes is when a foreign invader enters the body. That foreign invader, most normally, is a pathogen. Sometimes the invader can be a toxin or a toxic substance. If the invader, such as a virus or a type of bacteria, enters the body through the mouth or lungs, its chances of causing a stroke are minimal. More commonly the invader behind a stroke enters in through the skin, penetrating past the derma directly into the bloodstream, at which point the pathogen or toxic chemical is seen by the body as a threat. White blood cells try to attack and destroy the invader so the invader doesn't multiply and create an infection. The toxic invader isn't easily destroyed by white blood cells, and the battle goes on. More white blood cells try to come to the rescue, and eventually, a very large group of white blood cells is surrounding the invader, forming a blood clot. The size and length of the blood clot are determined by the amount of toxin. If this clotting isn't remedied before the clump of white blood cells clustered around the invader enters the brain, the possibility of a stroke is much higher. As the group of white blood cells around the invader reaches smaller blood vessels inside the brain, a jam-up can happen and we can have a stroke, ranging from mild to more severe, or if the blood clot blocks or fills up the length of an artery, a stroke or heart attack could occur.

Viral infections can cause mild strokes. These are viral infections that are not controlled early enough by your immune system. These viruses escape the immune system and stay active in the body for many years. Viruses such as EBV can also cause Guillain-Barré syndrome, which in many severe cases can mimic a stroke. Or someone could have a combination: a viral stroke plus another condition caused by the virus. If someone's immune system is chronically low and the viral load is high, chances are that the virus (or viruses) can find its way to the brain because the virus bypassed the immune system in a stealth manner, causing ME/CFS, brain inflammation, and encephalitis—which, if chronic for too many years, could lead to a stroke as the brain ages. As we age, brain tissue and vessels shrink.

We often think about stress causing a stroke. What we don't realize is, stress is lowering our immune system, allowing for a pathogenic infection to create a stroke. Blood vessels do constrict inside the brain when we're angry or under tremendous distress. Yet it takes somebody being susceptible to other problems, such as low-grade viral infections, toxic heavy metals, chronic dehydration long term, and a diet high in fat to create the foundation for a stroke. Continuously high blood fat means less oxygen gets to the brain, and when the blood gets thick, that blood moves more slowly throughout the brain's blood vessels. This sets the stage for other problems. The lower the oxygen levels in the blood of the brain, the higher-percentage chance of a virus thriving because there's less oxygen to keep the immune system strong. White blood cells need oxygen to survive and keep viruses out of the brain.

High blood fat also creates an acidic environment, since fats are acidic. Coupled with the restriction within blood vessels from high stress, anger, worry, and fear—plus chronic dehydration from high salt intake and caffeine use and not enough fruit, leafy greens, herbs, juices, or water in the diet— this acidic environment allows areas of the brain that already have scar tissue from toxic heavy metals, chemical toxins, pharmaceuticals, emotional wounds, or MSG deposits to become more vulnerable. As a result, chances increase that when a low-grade viral infection does occur—even the flu or COVID, for example—it could lead to a TIA or stroke.

In some cases, plaque deposits breaking free in the blood vessels can also cause strokes.

For specific healing support beyond what's offered in Part VI, refer to the Strokes protocol in *Brain Saver Protocols, Cleanses & Recipes.*

TICS, SPASMS, AND DYSTONIA

These symptoms are often the result of toxic heavy metals, mostly mercury and copper, inside the brain—many times in the frontal lobe or brain stem. When an electrical impulse travels across and through synapses and enters into other neurons, if it hits a deposit of copper or mercury (or a combination of copper and mercury), many times the electrical impulse will charge up, creating a quick spark that blows outward. Mercury and copper mixed together can force the spark to bounce recklessly. These quick sparks tend to radiate electricity outside the synapses, sending a charge through the cranial and other nerves—such as down the vagus, facial, trigeminal, optic, phrenic, and/or spinal nerves. A spark can send a tic or spasm to the face, arms, hands, neck, eyes, or all the way down to the back and thighs.

Everyone's tics, spasms, involuntary body movements, or jerking depend greatly on how much mercury and/or copper is in the brain, the particular mix of mercury and copper (how many parts mercury to how many parts copper), and where it is located.

Viruses that feed off copper, such as EBV, herpes simplex 1 and 2, and shingles, can contribute to the problem. Neurotoxins created by the shingles virus, herpes simplex, or EBV can amplify the situation because, as the virus feeds off copper and/or mercury anywhere inside the body, the virus releases a copper- and/or mercury-based neurotoxin. As that toxin floats through the system, it can go to the brain and add to the condition.

For specific healing support beyond what's offered in Part VI, refer to the Cranial Nerve Inflammation protocol in *Brain Saver Protocols, Cleanses & Recipes*.

TINNITUS

When decibel damage has been ruled out—and you haven't worked around heavy machinery for many years, worked in the music industry around live concerts, or had physical injury to the ear or any inner workings of the ear—then, when you receive a tinnitus diagnosis because you have ringing or humming in the ear, you're someone who's living with viral inflammation.

Tinnitus doesn't have to be ringing in the ear. It could be humming, buzzing, vibrating, popping, fluttering, crackling, or whooshing. When someone has the high-pitched ringing in the ear, it can change, alter, and dance about when a fan or air conditioner is on, or when music is playing. Some people experience what sounds like air rushing through their ear. Some people experience popping, like they're popping popcorn in the ear. Tinnitus can vary from mild to extreme. Often people get small moments when they hear a ringing in the ear and then it goes away. This has been passed off as "Someone's speaking about you," or "Angelic forces are speaking to you." What most of these people who experience passing tinnitus discover is that eventually, the ringing sticks around a little longer. They get to a point where they're past the whole phase of "It must be a ghost or a spirit or an angel or someone talking about you," and they realize they're developing a condition.

Sometimes it takes years of intermittent ringing in the ears to be diagnosed with tinnitus. Many times hearing loss can occur with tinnitus, because the ringing is so dominant. In many situations, even if the ringing isn't dominating, hearing can also be lost.

EBV is the number one reason why people have mystery tinnitus. Two things can occur with EBV:

One: neurotoxins released from the virus have an injuring effect upon the ear canal nerves and nerves of the inner ear, such as the vestibulocochlear nerves. These nerves can swell from the neurotoxins constantly saturating them. Nerves closest to a viral infection tend to react more seriously. When your sciatic nerves are inflamed, you can't hear it with your ear because the sciatic nerves are in your lower back and below. A nerve that's inflamed in your ear is a different story. That's the only situation where you hear the inflammation make noise. You're listening to the nerve spasming and vibrating.

Two: in many cases, the virus itself ends up nesting in the labyrinth of the inner ear and making a home. This is when tinnitus can get more extreme, more chronic, resulting in different varieties of symptoms—moving beyond ringing to louder ringing, popping, humming, buzzing, or whooshing. In most cases, the virus is EBV. In some cases, it's EBV, shingles, and/or herpes simplex 1 combined. In very rare cases, it's just the shingles or just herpes simplex. If the shingles or herpes simplex virus is present and active in the area of the neck, the side of the head, or even the shoulder, the neurotoxins released from the shingles or herpes simplex virus can contribute to the tinnitus. In those cases, the tinnitus can be more intermittent.

For specific healing support beyond what's offered in Part VI, refer to the Tinnitus protocol in *Brain Saver Protocols, Cleanses & Recipes*.

TOURETTE'S SYNDROME

Tourette's syndrome is caused primarily by mercury and copper, with traces of lead, impeding electrical impulses in the brain. Here's how it happens: when an electrical impulse travels across a synapse, it's something like traveling through a tunnel. If a deposit of toxic heavy metals surrounds that tunnel, the toxic heavy metals narrow the channel, creating a bottleneck. The electrical impulse traveling through gets hung up, practically stuck. In a very short amount of time (a fraction of a second), another electrical impulse follows behind. This new electrical impulse hits the impeded electrical impulse and propels the impeded electrical impulse forward. This is unlike OCD, where an electrical impulse hits a heavy metal deposit and gets propelled backward. In Tourette's the copper mixed with lead that's surrounding the synapse conducts the electrical impulses forward, even as the bottlenecking blocks the impulses physically to some degree. Sometimes both electrical impulses are even stuck together, combined, and they shoot out of the synapse together.

These electrical impulses in the brain are carrying information. They carry the messages someone is trying to articulate or deliver. And when these electrical impulses get impeded and then propelled forward, the information inside electrical impulses gets propelled forward as well, which makes the information hard to control or keep back. The information jumps ahead of the consciousness, which means an action, word, movement, or noise can occur in an uncontrollable fashion. The electrical impulses can literally go in many different directions, at quicker speeds than normal. That's why Tourette's is so vast, with so many variables. The size of the tunnel between neurons and how much toxic heavy metal is surrounding the synapse and neurons also influence the experience of Tourette's; the amounts of mercury, copper, and trace lead involved also plays a role. In many cases three electrical impulses run into each other before the first electrical impulse combined with the other two are blasted through the synapse tunnel. Basically, it's a logjam. All of these factors determine how pronounced an individual's Tourette's symptoms are.

Most of the time, Tourette's is consistent and predictable because of where in the brain the logjams consistently occur due to toxic heavy metal deposits present in those areas. When someone fights to overcome Tourette's symptoms with concentration and focus, what they're doing is redirecting neural pathways, even if they're not aware that's what they're doing. Sending electrical impulses on different pathways in the brain where logjams may not occur from toxic heavy metals can alter the experience of Tourette's, sometimes in unpredictable ways.

For specific healing support beyond what's offered in Part VI, refer to the Tourette's Syndrome protocol in *Brain Saver Protocols, Cleanses & Recipes*.

TREMORS

Tremors are usually caused by larger deposits of toxic heavy metals in the brain composed of a combination of mercury and aluminum, with some copper. These toxic heavy metal deposits don't need to have years of oxidation to create the problem. Someone doesn't need to be in their 40s, 50s, 60s, or beyond to develop tremors from toxic heavy metal deposits in their brain; they could be any age.

If someone is living with tremors and their nervous system weakens, the tremors can worsen. Extreme cases of tremors come from larger deposits of toxic heavy metals. Tremors worsening can also result from these toxic heavy metals oxidizing, with byproduct of the metals leaching into other areas of the brain, contaminating other neurons, and breaking down neurotransmitter chemicals. Eventually the worsening tremors can warrant a Parkinson's diagnosis.

Sometimes tremors can happen from a blood sugar imbalance. These tremors are called "the shakes," and they're a different type of tremor. Someone's blood sugar can be acutely low because of insulin resistance or a weakened pancreas or weakened adrenals. Blood sugar dropping like this, creating hypoglycemia, can bring on temporary, mild tremors. This is the brain firing warnings that glucose is not at an optimal level and that more glucose is needed to sustain nerve strength. A short-circuiting occurs as you're getting low on glucose. In some people, the tremors from hypoglycemia might not be so intense because their nervous system and neurotransmitters are stronger, with fewer deposits of toxic heavy metals. When someone does have toxic heavy metal impediments in the brain combined with hypoglycemia, it can make for the most severe type of tremors, which often feel more intense than a case of the shakes.

Adrenaline surges can give someone intermittent shakes similar to hypoglycemia. Adrenaline shakes might happen when someone has had a close call on the highway, received bad news, or is up against a confrontation. Their whole body could be shaking. If someone has a weakened nervous system to begin with, the shakes from an adrenaline surge could be more intense and longer lasting. Your vagus nerves literally rattle as adrenaline is surging. The corrosive nature of adrenaline can overstimulate inflamed or sensitive cranial nerves.

Viral infections such as EBV can also contribute to tremors, if the virus is releasing ample amounts of neurotoxins because the virus is feeding off toxic heavy metals. The nerves react and become irritable. When these neurotoxins saturate cranial nerves closer to the brain stem, someone can experience full-body vibrations, which are similar to full-body tremors yet are more subtle. These neurotoxins can land on nerves and even enter the brain and land on neurons, worsening the tremors.

Where the toxic heavy metals or viral neurotoxins are located in the brain or nervous system determines which arm a tremor's going to occur in, or if it's going to be a torso tremor or a leg tremor.

Tremors can occur in the lower legs stemming from the lumbar and sciatic nerves, if a virus such as the shingles virus is in the area of the lower back, inflaming nerves. These types of tremors don't tend to last long if back and leg pain are not present. If back pain and leg pain are present from spinal, sciatic, and tibial nerves inflamed by the shingles virus, then other symptoms such as tremors could be longer lasting. When pain subsides from these inflamed nerves, tremors usually diminish because the nerves are less inflamed.

When dealing with tremors, strengthening the nervous system is critical. It can help lessen tremors. Oftentimes electrical impulses will reroute themselves around a larger mercury-aluminum-copper deposit, taking a different route through a different part of the brain. This can sometimes give people relief. It's why people with a mild tremor tend to lose the tremor at times and then it comes back.

For specific healing support beyond what's offered in Part VI, refer to the Cranial Nerve Inflammation protocol in *Brain Saver Protocols, Cleanses & Recipes*.

TRIGEMINAL NEURALGIA

In the past, the majority of trigeminal neuralgia cases were caused by the shingles virus. Times are changing. Viruses are mutating. The herpes simplex 1 virus (aka the fever blister virus) is on the rise. This is why so many children have fever blisters. It was rare in the past for children to have fever blisters.

It's becoming all too common today. Herpes simplex 1 is being passed down from generation to generation, and new mutations are increasing, causing complicated symptoms. Herpes simplex 1 is now causing almost 50 percent of cases of trigeminal neuralgia. Some very debilitating cases of trigeminal neuralgia are caused by both viruses at work: shingles and herpes simplex 1.

These viruses don't have to look obviously active, where you have shingles pustules on the side of your face or body or a herpes simplex active sore or fever blister on your mouth, nose, or face. Even without these external signs, either virus can still be active internally, creating debilitating pain by inflaming trigeminal nerves. All facial and other cranial nerves can become inflamed from shingles and from herpes simplex 1. Symptoms can include pain in the jaw or teeth; burning pain on, in, and around the gums; pain on the side of the face; pain in the back of the neck; pain in the temple; and pain behind the eyes. Even burning sensations and pain on the tongue or burning sensations inside the head can occur in some cases. Millions of people have gotten root canals or teeth unnecessarily drilled or pulled because trigeminal neuralgia is often mistaken for teeth problems or dental issues.

Trigeminal neuralgia can be very difficult to overcome because of its mysterious nature. With an understanding of trigeminal neuralgia comes clarity: viral neurotoxins from the shingles and/or herpes simplex 1 are saturating the trigeminal and other facial and cranial nerves, causing them to inflame. In some cases shingles or herpes will even nest inside the trigeminal nerves, where the virus makes a home. In these cases the trigeminal neuralgia is much more severe. Many people are getting botulinum injections (of the type traditionally used in cosmetic injections) as a pain relief method for facial, neck, eye, jaw, and head pain as they search for relief in any way possible. Many people will get surgery for trigeminal neuralgia with no results, only additional problems from surgical complications and treatments.

For specific healing support beyond what's offered in Part VI, refer to the Shingles protocol and/or Herpes Simplex 1 and 2 protocol in *Brain Saver Protocols, Cleanses & Recipes*.

VERTIGO

Most cases of vertigo are caused by viral infection. Some are caused by physical injury or a growth or tumor inside the brain, or some other physical impediment that is discovered and diagnosed. If no such thing exists, then someone is dealing with mysterious vertigo. The medical industry believes vertigo is some kind of inner ear problem that may involve crystals, particles, or stones inside the inner ear. The theory goes that if you move your neck or head a certain way, it disrupts the crystals and triggers a bout of vertigo.

The real cause of most cases of vertigo is the Epstein-Barr virus excreting neurotoxins that inflame the vagus nerves. Which area of a vagus nerve is inflamed affects the variety of vertigo. Some rare cases of vertigo can be inflammation of the brain—mild, undiagnosed encephalitis or even severe brain inflammation caused by a viral infection, predominantly EBV.

Vertigo symptoms can range from feeling like you're on a boat to not feeling balanced to feeling like you're falling forward or sideways when you're walking. It can become so severe that you get what I call the bed spins: as you lie in bed, the room is spinning or rocking back and forth when you shut your eyes. Some cases of vertigo are severe, where you're vomiting and can't even move your head. These are more acute viral infections, where someone's immune system strength dropped and EBV got a good foothold into a vagus nerve or entered or attached itself to the brain stem, where the vagus nerves originate. In many cases, it's not just EBV neurotoxins inflaming the vagus; EBV itself can latch on to a vagus nerve and inflame it. In many other cases, it's only EBV neurotoxins inflaming the vagus nerve vine. Sometimes these neurotoxins inflame an entire vagus nerve, top to bottom or bottom to top.

Treatments where you're moving your head around, or physical therapy treatments for vertigo (including vagus nerve exercises), aren't always successful. In many cases, vagus nerve exercises can worsen vertigo. When they do work, it's because the vagus nerves were gently shifted. Swelling is still there, yet the vagus nerves were shifted enough to change the reaction someone was experiencing to that inflammation. A lot of times, vertigo was only going to be

temporary after all, so a week later the vertigo goes away on its own, whether someone was receiving treatment or not.

Chronic cases of EBV-related vertigo don't just go away. Someone could experience different versions and bouts for years without relief. There are rare cases of vertigo where optic nerves become severely inflamed from EBV and as a result, balance problems can occur when someone is walking or standing. In most cases the optic nerves are inflamed at the same time as the vagus nerves, with the inflammation most likely deriving from the brain stem. Vertigo can be complex.

The vagus nerves are the equilibrium nerves. They're the nerves that communicate information from the brain allowing physical stability, grounding, and stamina as you're fighting and battling gravity. The vagus nerves keep you level while gravity is trying to pull you down. When the vagus nerves are inflamed, the signal coming from the brain becomes choppy and fragmented, allowing gravity to alter your perception. The vagus nerves hold balance between all the different parts of the brain. It's why when people have vertigo and they're walking along, they're getting the sensation of being pulled down or falling forward. That's an example of when gravity takes over as the vagus nerves are short-circuiting.

Also refer to "Ménière's Disease."

For specific healing support beyond what's offered in Part VI, refer to the Vertigo protocol in *Brain Saver Protocols, Cleanses & Recipes*.

"Rather than seeing our brain as a single, isolated lump of gray matter, a better way to view our brain is as a group of neurons—because the truth is, the brain is a complex organ containing billions of neurons. Even if we called the brain *a neuron*, we'd have a better grasp of how to protect it and at the same time, a better understanding of what goes wrong with it."

— Anthony William, Medical Medium

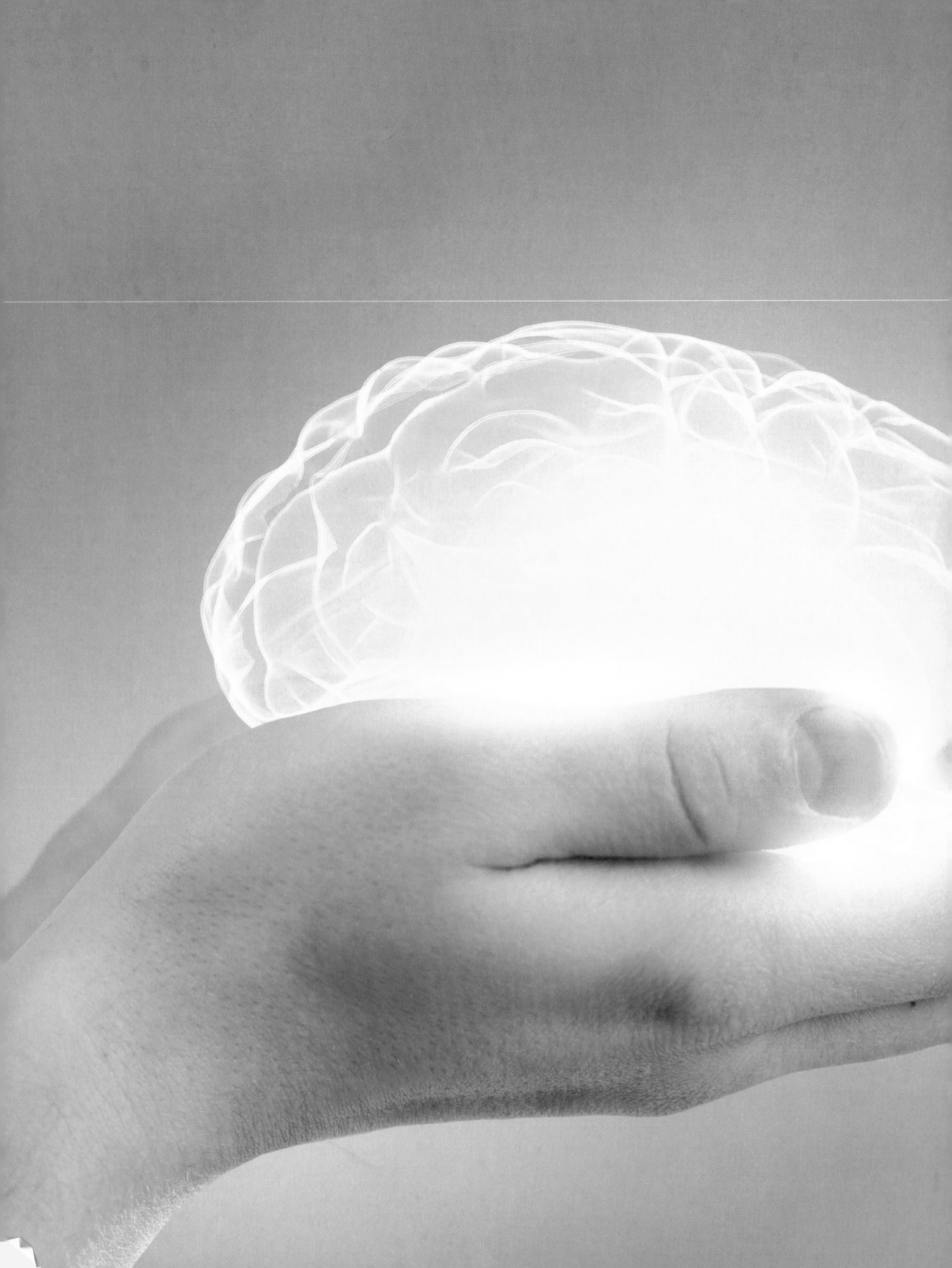

PART VI

BRINGING BACK YOUR BRAIN

"The brain is amazing. Its adaptive ability allows it to shift according to circumstances so that we can shift and adapt too. With metals gone from the brain, and specifically gone from the brain's emotional centers, the brain can cool itself to prevent emotional meltdowns. And when someone is getting enough glucose—enough natural sugars and healthy carbohydrates to fortify the brain—it can regulate its temperature even better. Your brain bringing in glucose is like rain rolling in to die out a fire after lightning."

— Anthony William, Medical Medium

CHAPTER 39

What Your Brain Is Made Of

Does it matter that we know what's inside our brains? Greatly. Why? Because if you know what your brain is made of, you can live a longer life. The knowledge can give you a more conscious, enlightened existence. It can make your world better in every way. It may not make the people who want to sell you trendy "health" ideas rich. What it will do is help you avoid disease and illness, brain rot, atrophy, inflammation, and early aging. It's vitally important that you know what your brain contains.

The trend today is to try to convince everyone that the brain is made of fat and is therefore in constant, desperate need of high-quality fats like omegas to keep us healthy. We're told that sugar hurts the brain, injures the brain, even kills the brain. We're put on no-sugar, low-or-no-carb diets.

This is in spite of the fact that conventional science already knows the brain runs on sugar. You'll see in medical textbooks that after only a short period without sugar reaching the brain, your brain is imperiled. It's a discovery that medical research and science got right—a good discovery that

can quickly go into hiding as trendy propaganda tries to teach differently. Even with the scientific knowledge that glucose is our brain's true fuel, we've all gotten the message that our brain runs on fat.

Is it true that there's fat inside our brains? Yes. And that there's such a thing as healthy fats? Yes. Other considerations are left out, though. How much fat is really inside our brains? How much fat does that mean we need to consume for our brains? What do our brains really need that we're starving them of?

Science is manipulated when it comes to food belief systems. Today's trend-makers seek out bits and pieces of science and then cut and paste what makes their case, leaving out the rest. So many people are convinced to eat almost all-fat diets under the guise of those foods being high protein. The studies that support that the brain runs on fat, or the brain needs ample fat to be healthy, are not what they seem. Behind the scenes, they're inconclusive or flawed in their methodology. Too often, a study's financing influences its outcome. Too often, what's only an article or paper gets referenced as a study. Too often, what's only a theory and opinion gets presented as fact. This can lead even experts with the best intentions to become misled.

NOT THE SUPPLIES WE NEED

Remember that hike we went on in Chapter 1, "Save Your Brain"? Let's go on another version of it.

Say that as you drive to your destination, you're drinking coffee with butter or MCT oil to give yourself a boost. You arrive, park your car at the trailhead, and begin, confident that you're fully prepared for what's going to be a great day.

Then say that as you start to hike, it's hotter than you'd realized. You heard there would be a lot more shade on the trails, so you keep walking, thinking it will get better, only to find that two hours in, you've had nearly constant exposure to the sun. You're parched. That's okay; when you finally stop, you'll dip into your high-tech provisions, including your fancy bottle of kombucha.

After another hour you're not feeling well, so when you finally find a scrap of shade, you decide to nest there for a while. Although you're overheated and starting to get dizzy, before you even open your knapsack, you feel relief thinking about what you have inside. You were taught so well about what rations to pack—you read up beforehand on all the latest literature about protein and healthy fats for endurance.

As you start to paw through your pack for something to revive you, your fingers land on a nut bar with cacao nibs. You stop just short of opening the package. It seems too dense for what you need right now. You pull out the next item: cubes of chicken. While your mind tells you it would make a great lunch, you're a little too queasy to try it quite yet. Next you find your plastic container of bone broth. The thought of that slick of fat on top doesn't sit right, so you reach for the item settled in the bottom, what you know you really need: your bottle of kombucha tea.

You pop open the cap and take a sip. Something about it doesn't seem as refreshing as you'd expected. You remember times as a kid, taking a hike with family, when you'd reach such a state of thirst that you felt like you were crawling through the desert, and how being handed a nice big bottle of spring water would bring you back to life. You remember playing in the backyard with your friends on a hot day, and how everyone would gather around the hose for the perfect refreshment of that stream of pure water. You remember a soccer game in high school on a blazing afternoon, when no one could wait to get to that water fountain for the cool jet of water. Today, it's not the same. When you opened the top of your kombucha bottle, you got a whiff of off-smelling liquid. A bubbly, fermented, acidy, slightly slimy liquid fills your mouth. As hyped up as kombucha has been, it isn't giving you relief. It's even dehydrating you further. In this 105-degree heat index, you're withering by the minute. You need to get home.

Little do we know that by following popular opinion on feeding the brain, we lead ourselves down a risky path. Taking along a knapsack full of the latest trendy foods for the brain is not so different from that knapsack turning out to be completely empty. When your brain reaches a state of strain, it becomes clearer what it really needs, and an influx of fats and dehydrating beverages isn't it.

To begin with, say you'd already been on a high-fat, low-sugar diet for months, which meant that you hadn't been getting hydration from juicy fruits or coconut water, and that you'd instead been drinking dehydrating coffee, kombucha, and matcha beverages. No one had told you to drink 32 ounces of water with fresh-squeezed lemon every morning for electrolytes, hydration, and a little glucose. And while you'd been periodically trying green juices, they weren't cucumber- or celery-based, so they weren't optimal for hydration, and most likely they were juices from the store that were HPP (high-pressure pasteurized or high-pressure processed). Eating high levels of fat (which were likely from foods advertised as high protein) thickened up your blood substantially, slowly causing parts of your brain to become critically dehydrated without your awareness. Then on the way to that hike, you drank your coffee with butter or MCT oil—or you drank matcha or black tea with oat milk, soy milk, nut milk, or cow's milk—with no idea that your beverage created substantial dehydration that morning, making your bloodstream even thicker with fat before you'd started. By the time you'd been

hiking for three hours, you had no hydration reserves left to cool the brain and body.

If something else had been in your bag, you would have been a lot better off. Coconut water, say, or even pure, regular water. Half a melon alone would sustain a hiker and keep them hydrated enough, even after months of a dehydrating diet. A big, juicy Fuji apple would have been life-saving in that critical moment of need; it could have staved off the beginnings of hyperthermia. Juicy mango or cantaloupe slices, which contain living water and glucose, are what we need for the long haul.

We're taught the opposite: that for endurance, whether to get through a physical challenge or a long day of errands or work, we need fat and protein, not carbs. We're taught that the liver gets damaged by sugar yet thrives on fat, that the brain goes haywire on sugar and needs fat to function. Only when it's too late do we find out that it was empty misinformation.

BRAIN RESERVES

Your survival depends on what reserves you have. How hydrated were you before this hike? At the same time, how thick was your blood? How much fat was in your blood? How deficient were you in glucose and trace mineral salts inside your brain?

Brain reserves are going to decide your timeline in getting home, or if you're going to get home at all. Brain reserves are going to decide the condition you're in when you get out of the weeds. "I'm up here, I'm lost,

I don't have the right provisions. The countdown is on. How much time do I have, and what determines how much time I have? What determines if I make it out of here versus someone else?"

We should also be asking, "How many toxic heavy metals do I have in my brain that require more electrolytes for functioning if I'm somebody who already has ADHD or bouts of anxiety? Am I somebody who already has mild neurological symptoms yet is completely unaware that's a brain issue?"

It's not so much "Am I out of shape? How much muscle do I have?" That's not always the determination of how long you're going to last. You can be a wiry person with not a lot of bulk and muscle and yet have more reserves in your brain to hold out longer and function longer in the heat of life without provisions.

WHAT YOUR BRAIN REALLY NEEDS

Glucose and Glycogen

Your brain is an organ that needs food just as much as your stomach needs it. Your brain relies on that food, which turns into energy, to function. What food does your brain really need? Glucose. Our brain is mostly made out of glycogen—that is, stored glucose. We get our first glucose and glycogen through our mothers, while we're in the womb and then through breast milk.

Breast milk is defined by its natural sugar content—comparatively, it has little fat and protein—and that bioavailable sugar creates the building blocks of a baby's brain. (If a newborn isn't able to breastfeed, those beneficial sugars come a bit later, from ingredients like fruits and sweet potatoes in baby food.) A portion of this early glycogen is permanently sealed off, creating actual brain tissue, stored in such a way that it will never be disturbed in the future. To a degree, your brain keeps adding to that foundational glycogen storage as it continues to develop through childhood, teenage years, and your early 20s. This glycogen tissue is the figurative meat on the brain's bone. If someone were to tear into your brain as though it were a drumstick, that gray-matter "flesh" would be made from pockets of decades-old glycogen. Sugars are your brain's place of origin. Your brain also starts to collect glycogen in storage bins to be used for fuel. The spiderweb of glycogen connective tissue is a safe haven for new brain cell development. It's how brain cells are birthed.

Is there any fat in a healthy brain that's in a healthy body? Yes, there is—extremely low levels of fat compared to what science and research theorize. The fat in the brain is a small fraction of the brain itself. The healthier the person's brain and body are, the smaller the fraction of fat that resides inside the brain. The more unhealthy the brain and body are, the higher levels of fat that reside inside the brain. The cadavers that medical science used to determine a basis for how much fat resides inside the brain were cadavers of older age and the poorest health. The cadavers' brains were atrophied, and what was replacing the atrophy were fat deposits.

The fat inside the brain of a healthy person should be roughly the same percentage of fat as in every other organ in the body. Just like when someone's liver becomes unhealthy and starts to take on additional fat and becomes a fatty liver, the brain can do the same, becoming an unhealthy brain that takes on additional fat and becomes a fatty brain. Instead of medical science understanding that the same thing that occurs to the liver can happen to the brain, they theorize that the brain is supposed to have that much additional fat. In truth, a healthy 20-year-old in good shape does not have a brain that's made of 60 percent fat.

The roughly 60 percent fat inside the brain that medical research and science claim is not all omegas. The fat that accumulates in the brain is the same as the fat that's in a sick liver, which is also not all omegas. It's fatty deposits of unproductive fat. Are there omegas inside a healthy brain? Yes, there are. Do they play a role? Yes, they do. It's a small role. The role these trace omegas play inside the brain is the same role they play inside all organs in the body: they act as insulation for cold temperatures. Omegas inside all organs, including in the brain, are there to act as a mild barrier inhibiting the body from going into shock too fast from cold temperatures. And yet glorifying the importance of fats for the brain doesn't save us. For the brain, fats are a small tool with a relatively small purpose compared to the major significance of sugar's role in keeping you alive.

The role that sugar plays in the brain is monumental compared to the significance of fats. For one, there's that glycogen storage acquired in babyhood, childhood, and young adulthood that keeps the brain healthy and prevents atrophy. Being starved of glucose for too long shrinks the brain. It's one reason why millions and millions of Americans are suffering from brain issues. As brains are degenerating and reducing in size, those in the health movement should be saying, "Whoa, we need to get diet truly right. We need to get sugars back to the brain."

The brain's electricity does not run on fat; it runs on sugars. Too much fat actually gets in the way of the brain's electrical grid system, causing it to overheat. This is why only a small percentage of fat naturally occurs in a healthy brain. Glucose helps reduce heat and keep brain tissue cool. This is why someone with toxic heavy metals in the brain causing a condition such as bipolar often has such strong sugar cravings: with the increased heat from the toxic heavy metals, the brain's own adaptive cooling nature is diminished. Plus, excess fat in the long term can lead to unhealthy fatty tissue in the brain, which increases brain heat. When that happens, the brain—which, again, is formed from glycogen—starts to shrivel up and break down as fat increases and builds up, taking what was the brain tissue's space, at the same time that heavy metals oxidize, and maladies such as strokes, Alzheimer's, and dementia can occur more easily.

Fatty tissue buildup in the brain is not the same as someone being overweight. Just because someone is overweight doesn't mean they have a fatty brain, if they're eating healthily. And just because someone *isn't* overweight doesn't mean their brain tissue is free from fatty deposits. They could still have an unhealthy brain that contains large deposits of fatty tissue. Whether someone is overweight or not, with a low-fat diet and the healthiest foods, there won't be this high increase of fat tissue in the brain.

Going on a low-carb diet for an extended time causes you to start losing precious glycogen deposits. In the short term, you may not notice. You could even feel better temporarily; if you've gotten rid of processed food, your inflammation may drop, and you may get some relief from what's bothering you. Meanwhile, you'll start losing those glycogen storage banks, first from the liver, then from the brain—because the early site of brain problems is the liver.

One way to recover from illness is to get glucose to the brain. Fevers from sickness caused by the flu, COVID, or other pathogen infections can burn away the brain's glycogen storage reserves. It's imperative that recovery after fever consists of a diet lower in fat and higher in critical clean carbohydrates such as fruits, starchy vegetables, and potatoes.

Just because the cells of the brain consume sugar to thrive doesn't mean I'm advocating that we all start eating spoonfuls of table sugar. The sugar our brain needs comes from natural sources, is unrefined, and is blended with other critical components: trace minerals, trace mineral salts, phytochemical compounds, antioxidants, anthocyanins, vitamins, and other nutrients.

Trace Mineral Salts

You need enough trace minerals in your brain to light the electrical grid and create continuity of that electrical grid so your brain is functioning at its optimum level.

The trend today is to say you can get your trace minerals if you put a pinch of sea salt in your water. That's not going to do the job. That's not going to get you the trace minerals you need. Your mineral salts have to come from leafy greens such as spinach, celery juice, and even lemons.

How do trace mineral salts work in the brain? What are they doing?

First, it's important to know that neurotransmitter chemicals sit on neurons and send out a signal and frequency throughout the brain *and* outside our body. That frequency connects above throughout the universe. Neurotransmitter chemicals are a bridge between neurons in the brain and what's above us in the atmosphere, behind the stars.

Trace minerals are not just physical, tangible minerals. They have a Godly presence. Trace minerals have connected to everything above us, beyond the earth. Our atmosphere is filled with trace minerals. Outer space is filled with trace minerals. Trace minerals can be dead, or trace minerals can be alive and active. The frequencies and signals that come down from the universe on the bridge that neurotransmitter chemicals are extending stimulate, activate, and ignite trace minerals inside our brain into life, giving them an order and direction:

to directly attach themselves to neurons and restore neurotransmitter chemicals.

When trace minerals come from plant foods and enter into our bloodstream, they start picking up on the frequency between our brain and above, and the trace minerals become activated. These trace minerals from plant foods already sustain life. They're living. Yet a new level of living activity occurs. They become supercharged and stay alive and active, versus dissipating and dying. They're now more than just living minerals, and they have a greater purpose. The living trace minerals are floating around our bloodstream looking for a place to land. They're directed with the frequency above and have an intelligence.

Both fat in the bloodstream and fatty deposits that should not be in the brain diminish the oxygen that's trying to reach brain cells. Fat in the bloodstream and fatty brain deposits also impede mineral salts from entering brain cells. In reality, fats hold on to trace mineral salts, blocking brain cells and neurotransmitters from absorbing them.

For more on your brain's needs, refer to Chapter 7, "Your Burnt Out, Deficient Brain."

FINALLY UNDERSTANDING FAT SOLUBILITY

If we want perspective on food and what's good for the brain, we need to question what we hear, such as the popular belief that eating fats alongside leafy greens and vegetables helps us absorb nutrients better. Trends are not always based on logic or

fact. Beliefs and popular sayings around fat-soluble vitamins are a prime example of taking data, spinning it, skewing it, and citing it without giving anyone a complete picture of what they're really reading. In the end, it's like a court of law. It relies on whether the jurors understand what they're seeing.

The studies in this area make assumptions. They measure the levels of nutrients in your bloodstream and conclude that the presence of nutrients means you're absorbing the nutrients. They don't say, "Just because nutrients show up in your bloodstream doesn't mean they were absorbed by your organs and cells. We still don't know if these are being absorbed."

Nutrient Absorption

In reality, when you eat a salad, your salad nutrients shouldn't be floating around your bloodstream getting ready to be excreted via your kidneys or bowels. Nutrients aren't supposed to be free-floating in the bloodstream so much. They're supposed to be absorbed quickly by organs and cells while they're still active. You don't want to pee out a salad's nutritional value like a big junky multivitamin. Urine samples should be measured to show whether vitamins are leaving right after being consumed. If someone eats a high-fat salad, you would see those vitamins in their urine hours later because the vitamins are not being absorbed. Whereas if someone ate a fat-free salad on a day they didn't eat any fat-based foods at all, you would hardly see any of those vitamins in the urine. Where did most of the vitamins go in the fat-free scenario? The organs and cells absorbed them. Even though studying urine samples rather than blood samples would still not offer the entire picture, it would at least be trying to see the situation through a different window.

When we absorb vitamins and other nutrients through our digestive tract, some nutrients need to be converted by the liver into more useful forms and then stored or released back into the bloodstream. Your liver is the storage bin for nutrients. Too much fat in your meals interferes with the liver, so nutrients such as vitamins and minerals won't find a resting place where they're supposed to be inside the liver. Some nano-sized phytochemical compounds and nutrients, such as small levels of glucose, absorb through the esophagus, stomach, duodenum, or intestinal tract walls and enter directly into the bloodstream without needing to go up the hepatic portal vein to be converted. Either way, vitamins and nutrients are best utilized when they enter cells and organs quickly from the bloodstream. Whether nutrients need to be converted by the liver or not, fats in the bloodstream suspend the nutrients, interfering with the chance for these nutrients to see their journey through.

Vitamins, minerals, and other nutrients from our foods and supplements have a shelf life in our bloodstream. Most nutrients are supposed to be absorbed into your liver, not floating around in your bloodstream for hours and hours, tangled up in and suspended by fat. It doesn't take too long

before nutrients start oxidizing and losing their strength. Fat in the bloodstream also causes insulin resistance, holding back glucose from entering into cells. Then the pancreas has to release more insulin in hopes of getting glucose to bypass some of the fat so the glucose can enter into cells. Insulin resistance is part of what stops other nutrients from leaving the bloodstream and entering cells too. When vitamins, minerals, and other nutrients are floating around the bloodstream too long, suspended there because of fat in the blood, they're not entering cells and they're really not being utilized.

In order to utilize vitamins and other nutrients, you have to have rapid absorption time into organs and cells. You have to get the minerals, vitamins, and nutrients at their peak strength and usefulness. Again, nutrients are supposed to be entering organs quickly, entering nerve cells throughout the body, and most importantly, entering the liver and the brain. Nutrients aren't supposed to be free-floating in the blood for long. Fat slows everything down, and not in a helpful way—it's not like fat sitting in the bloodstream and holding back vitamins and nutrients creates some type of beneficial time-release.

When you eat any kind of fat, insulin does not attach itself to those fatty lipids and fatty acids, driving them into cells inside the body. Those fatty lipids and fatty acids are not utilized like sugar is utilized. Glucose is the number one nutrient that takes precedence over anything else. Remember, the brain starts going into crisis within seconds of not receiving glucose. And all fat does in the bloodstream is inhibit the ability of glucose to enter cells. Glucose is a freedom ticket for a nutrient or vitamin to quickly enter a cell. Vitamins and nutrients have to be attached to sugar and insulin in order to enter cells and be utilized; nutrients don't have a way into cells otherwise. Insulin simultaneously opens up a cell and attaches itself to sugar so that sugar can enter a cell.

If someone eats a salad with papaya and berries on top of leafy greens, cucumbers, tomatoes, and fresh herbs, the nutrients from the leafy greens and fresh herbs will combine with the glucose from the papaya, berries, tomatoes, and even cucumber so that the nutrients quickly enter cells throughout the body without being suspended in the bloodstream. Insulin will easily open the door of nerve cells and a passageway to the brain if no fat is in the way. This is an example of an excellent salad for high absorption rates of nutrients in cells without insulin resistance.

On the other hand, if someone eats a salad with fat in it—such as avocado, nuts, seeds, animal protein, or oil (whether toxic canola or healthy olive oil)—the salad's nutrients won't quickly enter nerve cells. They'll get caught up in the slow, agonizing process of being suspended around fats inside the bloodstream while insulin is being pumped out of the pancreas in hopes of finding glucose trapped somewhere around the fats so some glucose can enter the cells rather than being urinated out of the body and wasted. Keep in mind that the glucose that does enter cells won't be filled with vitamins and other nutrients because the fat in the salad would have inhibited the leafy greens' nutrients from attaching to the sugar for insulin to easily open cells. Only a small portion of nutrients will survive the journey around blood fat and be brought into cells. When someone has their blood tested, vitamins and nutrients will be plentiful inside the bloodstream, creating the deception that having fat with your meal allows for better absorption.

Antioxidants are an example of what we miss out on if our bloodstream is consistently filled with fats. The brain is partially saturated with antioxidants. We rely on antioxidants to slow down oxidation of brain tissue. When we consume foods rich in antioxidants, the majority of the antioxidants are meant to be drawn into the brain, where they're needed the most. Fats consistently interfere with antioxidant absorption in the brain, minimizing the amount of antioxidants entering and even reaching the brain. Fats in the bloodstream and fats inside the brain are antioxidant stoppers and blockers.

A Source of Confusion

Alongside talk of fats and nutrient absorption, you'll hear the misunderstood term *fat soluble*. People often assume "fat soluble" means that a certain vitamin needs to be consumed with fat for the vitamin to be dissolved and absorbed in our body system. What "fat soluble" really means is that certain vitamins, such as vitamin D, get absorbed by fat cell deposits in our body when there's too much of these vitamins in our bloodstream. And the reality is that when a vitamin is stored inside a fat cell, the vitamin is not being used.

Fat solubility can also lead to unwanted accumulation of vitamins. Medical research and science stumbled upon this discovery because people were getting sick on high dosages of vitamin A supplements, and they had to understand why this was toxic to the system. The theory they landed on was that when someone consumed high quantities of a fat-soluble vitamin, the excess was not being eliminated and leaving the body. Large quantities were staying in the body. "Are the vitamins absorbing into fat cells?" researchers asked themselves. "Sounds like it."

There are indeed certain vitamins, such as A and D, that can get trapped in the fat inside the liver and the fat all throughout the body. If large quantities of fat-soluble vitamins stay in the body and aren't excreted easily, they can eventually cause high toxicity in the bloodstream and organs.

One key understanding here is that we're talking about fat cells that are in the body already. That's different from fats you're actively consuming. Fat cells change when they're stored inside our body. Fat becomes alive inside our body. That's why fat is found in tumors. Fat is not dead inside us, even if it was dead when we ate it—for example, in a piece of chicken. Even if the fat has been cooked, once it gets converted and stored around our waist or elsewhere in our body, the fat has a living force to it.

Fat-soluble vitamins getting absorbed into established fat cells in your body does not mean that *eating* fats in your meals makes nutrients more bioavailable and absorbable. When you hear the term *fat soluble*, it doesn't mean that when you're eating a dish containing plant fats such as avocado or animal fats such as chicken, the fats you're consuming are helping you absorb the vitamins from the meal. Instead, it's the reverse. Fats you're consuming inhibit vitamins and nutrients from easily entering nerve cells or organ cells. Fats slow down nutrient absorption because they suspend and block the meal's beneficial nutrients from being absorbed by your organs and cells.

The true meaning of fat solubility—that existing fat cells in your body absorb vitamins such as A and D—does not translate to vitamins A and D being utilized and absorbed into any nerve tissue, organs, or cells throughout the body as usable nutrients. The accumulation of these vitamins inside fat cells and organs has nothing to do with the vitamins being absorbed to be utilized. Instead large dosages of supplementation of vitamins A and D and other fat-soluble vitamins get absorbed by the liver to protect you—to keep you out of harm's way. The liver is the converter and storage bin for many vitamins, minerals, and other nutrients. It's also the storage bin for substances that are toxic—for example, high dosages of vitamin A. So the vitamin A will store itself in the liver's fatty cells, which are different from the fats you're actively eating.

Foods like lettuces, bananas, and potatoes do have fats in them, including traces of omegas. Their fat levels are low enough not to interfere with insulin's job of bringing glucose into cells. You will not get insulin resistance from these foods alone. It's a correct balance. Anywhere from 2 to 5 percent fat in a food, meal, day, or diet allows nutrient absorption to be rapid and doesn't create insulin resistance.

Long gone are the days of the old keto diet and the old carnivore diet, where you keep out all carbohydrates and natural sugars. Keto diets are not keto diets anymore. You can't go into ketosis on them because these diets are bringing in avocado, green apples, and berries, which have sugar in them. Carnivore diets are not carnivore diets anymore either. They bring in green juices and honey. These diet changes are happening because no one can survive without glucose for too long before they get deathly ill. Meanwhile, the diets have kept the same names, even though the diets themselves have changed.

Floating and Sinking Stools

Keeping the fat in your diet in that 2-to-5-percent range serves your digestion as well, which helps you get the nutrients you need out of what you eat—which ultimately serves your brain. Here's how it works:

A lower percentage of fat in your food allows for rapid protein and fat absorption in your intestinal tract. Less fat also means your stomach, liver, and pancreas don't need to work as hard, so they get a chance to restore. All of this means that the proteins and fats you *do* eat get broken down, assimilated, and utilized. As a result, your intestinal tract doesn't become filled with undigested, putrefying fats that otherwise

would have interfered with accessing and processing nutrients from food you've eaten.

Undigested, putrefying proteins and fats filling the intestinal tract make your stools heavy, so they sink to the bottom of the toilet. In contrast, a stool with no undigested protein or fat inside of it will occasionally float midway in the water because it's lighter and filled with more fiber, pectin, pulp, and even animal gristle if you're an animal protein eater. More fruit, leafy greens, herbs, and vegetables in the diet will eventually help bring healthy mid-floating stools.

That's not to be confused with another type of floater: some stools float because they're filled with gas and ammonia from someone suffering from chronic gastritis due to chronic fermentation of rotting proteins and fats outgassing in their intestinal tract.

It's okay to have a dense stool that sinks. You can be on a very healthy diet, even low fat, and still have a dense, sinking stool. Over time as you're healing your gut and strengthening bile reserves and hydrochloric acid, you may see some mid-floating to floating stools, which is a good sign. Healthy stools are an indication of healthy nutrient processing in the digestive system, which contributes to a healthy brain because it's a brain that's receiving more nutrients.

New Perspective on Testing for Deficiencies

If you get a blood test for a vitamin and nutrient analysis and you're on a diet that's consistently composed of fats, and you see from your analysis that you're low in some vitamins and nutrients, this means you're severely low. If you see adequate or higher levels of nutrients on your analysis, you could still be deficient and low in these vitamins and nutrients—because they're suspended in the bloodstream and not being absorbed. The best way to test for vitamin and nutrient deficiencies is to keep fats out of the diet for at least 30 days.

If the reading shows that you're deficient when you've been off fats for 30 or more days, it doesn't mean you're completely deficient. It likely means you're absorbing and utilizing your vitamins and nutrients. It's a positive sign if the nutrients are not lingering in your bloodstream. The longer you stay low-fat or no-radical-fat in your diet, the more you will restore all your vitamin and nutrient banks inside your body. Eventually, your blood test will show as non-deficient because the organs are stocking up their nutrient reserves. If your diet stays low-fat for long enough and nutrients are suspended in

the bloodstream long enough to showcase in a blood test, this is exhibiting an abundance of nutrients, versus nutrients trapped in fat in the bloodstream. This restoration of reserves could take some time for some individuals who are under immense stress or high physical demands or are chronically ill—because their nutrient banks were so low, and they're utilizing new nutrients just as fast as the nutrients are coming in.

Keep in mind that blood tests are just a snapshot of a window of time, of that hour when you got the blood test. A factor as simple as going to the bathroom prior to the blood test, something you consumed last night for dinner, or how your adrenals react to health care appointments, can change the reading in blood results. Don't rely on just one blood test to determine deficiency.

The next chapter, "Blood Draining Agenda," is also critical reading so you can protect yourself if you're getting blood tested.

"Medical Medium protocols are customizable to take you as far as you need to go."

— Anthony William, Medical Medium

CHAPTER 40

Blood Draining Agenda

Working on your healing process while trying to live your life is difficult when you're encountering stressful situations, pollution, chemicals, and other environmental disturbances and exposures every day, including exposures to the many sources of toxic heavy metals and pathogens. There are numerous obstacles in the way of healing, and those obstacles are hard enough. Trying to heal is difficult all on its own.

Then there are obstacles in medical treatments and testing that are never accounted for or considered. These obstacles can interfere with someone's healing and recovery, or with staying healthy and strong. Neurological symptoms especially can create the most mystery, which leads to more testing, which in turn leads to a greater drain on someone's system. Blood tests are at the top of the list for being a drain on the brain—literally draining all body systems of the blood that's critically needed to keep you balanced and stable. With sickness and deaths rising to levels we've never seen before in history, blood tests are going to be administered more than ever before in history.

We all find common ground with getting our blood tested. It's a window into picking up important clues so your doctor can keep an eye out for your best interest with whatever condition you're struggling with—or perhaps you're just fine, and the testing is intended to confirm that. At the same time, blood testing comes with tremendous pitfalls, from problematic to life-threatening, if we don't approach it with the proper awareness. One pitfall is that many people have mystery symptoms and yet their blood work is normal, healthy, and stable—because most chronic illness conditions are not detectable through blood work. For the other pitfalls of blood testing, keep reading. With any condition, it's important to bring awareness to the limitations of the tools we're using to diagnose and treat the illness. For anything that's brain-related, that's especially true, with diagnostic and treatment tools having even more potential to be compromising.

NOT MEANT TO GO TO WASTE

A major aspect of blood testing that's overlooked in the health industry is excessive blood draw and wastage. Our blood is treated like it's disposable. It's not respected. When someone gets a blood test, there's always too much blood drawn for what's being tested, and blood ends up discarded and thrown away—as though our blood is not actually a valuable resource. No one questions it. No one questions the excessive amount of blood taken from the human body of someone who's in a weakened state. No one questions where the extra blood goes that's not being used.

We're even told it's healthy for our body to get our blood drawn, that it cleans up our blood, that fresh blood is produced, as if this is a good thing. We're told our blood is refillable, practically instantly. We're told everything will be back to normal, almost right away. They act like our blood is refillable within minutes or hours. It's not that easy. Just because you add water to your bloodstream by drinking fluid and work on boosting your blood sugar by eating some form of sugar doesn't mean your blood is back to normal. It could take weeks or even months to restore.

A fraction of the blood taken for blood testing is used for the test itself. The blood that's left is discarded. Meanwhile, the person is in a more weakened, vulnerable state because they lost blood that was treated as disposable. Then, just as that person starts to regain a little strength as they rebuild their blood, another test is ordered and the drain happens all over again. This happens for many patients without a clue about what's really taken place and how the system is broken when it comes to blood tests and blood draws. If you're someone who's battling a chronic illness, more blood draws can lead to a more weakened condition. The sicker you become, the more blood gets drawn and the more frequently the blood gets drawn. It becomes a vicious cycle, worsening your condition more.

CRITICAL IMMUNE SYSTEM KNOWLEDGE

There's a theory going around that your immune system is all in your gut. There's no accuracy to it, no science behind this to factually determine that your immune system is in your gut. It's an alternative medicine theory that is considered pseudoscience by conventional medicine. In this case conventional medicine is right. It *is* pseudoscience. That pseudoscience aligns with what probiotic companies want us to think. Gut health product companies want you to believe your immune system is all in your gut. And to the alternative medicine world and even a portion of the conventional medicine world now trying to understand why people are truly sick, the theory seems plausible. Our immune systems are in our guts and that's the reason everyone is suffering with their health? It sounds like it makes sense.

When they say your immune system is in your gut, they're claiming that microorganisms sitting inside your intestinal tract and on your intestinal tract lining are your immune system. That's where the misconception gets pretty wonky and points to the bigger issue: Gut health products from probiotic companies are claiming you improve your immune system by installing these microorganisms in your gut. Trouble is, microorganisms and probiotics are not immune cells. Good bacteria in your gut are not immune cells. Good bacteria in your gut do not create or feed immune cells. Good bacteria in your gut do not keep immune cells healthy. Besides, the majority of your body's actual immune cells are not sitting inside your intestinal tract alongside your gut's microorganisms.

Yes, the largest portion of your immune system is in your torso, because the majority of your body is in your torso. Just because your immune system is within your midsection, though, does not mean your immune system is centered in your intestinal tract. Alternative medicine and even now conventional medicine, a little bit, are confused about this and conditioning everybody that the majority of your immune system is in your gut, meaning your intestinal tract, and that probiotic companies will help you rebuild your immune system by providing microorganisms. The whole concept is grossly mistaken.

Ask yourself this: If your immune system really is all in your gut and not in your blood system throughout your body, why do they measure your immune cell counts through blood tests? The doctors aren't taking a stool sample every time you visit to measure your quantities of immune cells. They're measuring your immune cells by doing a complete blood count (CBC) through your blood. It goes to show how much confusion there is in this area—and how the theory that your immune system is all in your gut doesn't hold up once you start to examine it.

The reality is that the majority of your immune system is in your bloodstream, so that your brain doesn't take on an infection. Your bloodstream is patrolled by your immune cells systematically looking for potential invaders, so those invaders don't get to your brain or your heart. Your brain and heart are the two top dogs that your immune system is looking out for, plus your immune system has to cover your lungs, pancreas, kidneys, spleen, and more. The majority of your immune cells are not sitting inside your intestinal tract, mingling with probiotics and microorganisms, looking for invaders. The majority of your immune cells are in your blood—your bloodstream and blood vessels all through your entire body.

Your lymphatic system also carries a large portion of your immune system, and that lymphatic system wraps around the organs of your torso, including your chest and abdomen. This does not mean your immune system is sitting inside of your gut. A portion of your immune system also resides inside your liver and spleen, although that's not to be confused with the theory that your immune system is centered in your intestinal tract either. The liver and spleen are not part of that equation.

You can't live without your brain. You can't live without your heart. You can live with most of your intestinal tract gone and still have a strong immune system—because without your intestinal tract, you can still have most of your lymphatic system, and you can still have your bones producing a variety of immune cells for your blood. So your bloodstream is where the majority of the immune system lies. If it weren't, then blood infections would be the number one cause of death at this point.

As blood tests are ordered for you, more blood than necessary is removed, which means a large portion of your immune system is removed every time you go to get blood drawn. And if you're someone who's sick, removing any portion of your immune system can make you more susceptible to anything from a relapse to worsening of old symptoms to coming down with new symptoms. Doctors don't have time or energy or awareness to single out tests and space them out, drawing smaller amounts of blood over multiple visits to cover different areas of blood testing. They like to get it all in one swoop, especially when you're sick with a condition. Oftentimes more than 3 vials of blood are drawn at a time. Normally 5 to 7. In many cases, 14 to 30 or more vials. This should all be reconsidered.

Part of the reason why the areas of blood testing, blood draw, and the immune system are so void of knowledge, void of understanding, and lacking information is because, once again, medical research and science don't know why people are sick. That's why all autoimmune disease is listed as "cause unknown" and then theories such as "It's all genes and your body

attacking itself" are thrown into the mix—or the newer one, "You're creating it with your thoughts, and you're not really sick," which is now being adopted by the conventional medical world as an option.

Why don't they seem to care as they're removing your immune system? Well, they're not really thinking about it that way. Not even doctors realize the immune system's being removed every time you get a blood draw. It's not even on their radar. And why is it critical to realize that the immune system is being removed during the blood draw? If medical research and science knew why people are sick, which is low-grade and high-grade viral infections such as Epstein-Barr virus causing chronic illness and dozens of autoimmune diseases, maybe they would think twice about removing your immune system, the very line of defense that keeps the viral infection from getting worse.

Indeed, viral infections are getting worse in patients who are getting blood drawn, especially excessive amounts of blood, sometimes landing them in bed permanently, whereas before, they were fatigued and struggling yet functioning. That's because as you get sicker, the protocol is to draw more blood. In the quest to find answers, you have to go to the hospital again, see another specialist. The sicker you are, the less functional you are, the more blood is drawn on the search for the problem. It's not unusual to get 100 vials drawn within a six-month period. After another blood draw from the fifth specialist, you could end up in bed indefinitely. There's no spotlight on this, yet it happens every day.

Blood draws accelerate the aging process because they draw from the body's reserves. The more blood taken, the more quickly someone ages. Removing large amounts of blood, especially when done frequently, drains the body of its life force, putting a strain on every organ in the body. Medical research and science don't know exactly how much blood can be drained out of someone before they die. Everyone has a different strength and limitation. The accuracy of how much blood is appropriate to take is still theoretical and debatable among medical communities—which means it's more important than ever to be cautious about how much blood is removed during blood draws and blood donations.

Irresponsible blood draw has led to millions of premature deaths. It's a slow death. It can be years of blood draws and chronic illness until you're pushed over the edge and your disease takes over. A plain old blood draw, as it's practiced today, can be enough to act as a trigger for worsening illness.

If someone has chronic illness, they are already weakened and their immune system is already fighting battles. Battles that are not seen by a microscope, battles that are not seen by medical testing. That's why chronic illness is still a mystery. These battles your immune system is fighting are a large part of why you're sick. Your immune system is exhausting reserves to try to defend you as it keeps low-grade and high-grade viral infections, as well as bacterial infections, under control while also battling exposure from toxins. Then comes the blood test. A

metabolic panel, thyroid panel, CBC, hormone panel, nutritional deficiencies, and more. And now you're in it for 5, 10, 12, maybe 14 or more vials of blood. And in all that blood, your immune cells get stolen from your body, not taken in a mindful or respectful way. This places immense stress upon your bone marrow because your bone marrow has to go into overdrive, burning out its reserves to replace your missing immune system.

If they needed all that blood to run a test, it would be one thing. Even then, it should still be done differently. Yet they don't need all that blood. Most of the blood drawn is unneeded, so it's thrown away or used in experimental testing for possibly nefarious reasons. This is an antiquated system left unchecked and unbalanced, just like other corruption in our system today, like so many outdated techniques and bodies of medical hierarchy.

THE ENDLESS CYCLE OF "WE'D BETTER ORDER MORE BLOOD"

After general blood tests, specialists may come in and order a lot more blood, wanting an extensive window into anything they can uncover and find. No one's counting! No one's saying, "Whoa, we're removing a lot of blood from you right now, blood that your body needs because you're fighting an infection, as indicated by your Hashimoto's thyroiditis"—or your multiple sclerosis, eczema, chronic fatigue, lupus. "Your chronic condition is a chronic viral infection, and we're taking your immune system out, so we'd better be careful and only remove a little at a time so your condition doesn't worsen." No one's doing that, in part because doctors don't even realize you're fighting a viral infection, unless they're starting to learn it from Medical Medium information.

Some doctors think removing your blood is helping your autoimmune condition because they believe your immune cells are attacking your organs and glands. This is why many doctors recommend sick people donate blood—they think that lowering their immune cells and rebuilding fresh blood will somehow give them a fresh start. (More on donating blood later.) This is a mistaken belief. For some reason, medical communities are overlooking an incredibly important point. You have sick patients battling autoimmune disease and you're telling them to donate blood without realizing their blood could be sick and even infectious, which is not a considerate recommendation for someone receiving the blood. Hemochromatosis is also a condition where doctors commonly recommend donating blood, with the intention of lowering your iron levels. Meanwhile, medical science doesn't know the cause of hemochromatosis. In truth, the cause is a chronic viral infection in the bones, and your immune system is a critical part of fighting that viral infection.

This is the first time you're going to hear this information about blood draw and your immune system. That is, unless you learned this information through Medical Medium teachings or through the grapevine from someone who learned it from my teachings, possibly even prior to the publication of the Medical Medium book series. I've been talking about this topic for decades because I want people to know as much as possible about how to protect their families, other loved ones, and themselves.

Excessive blood draw is another great mistake of our medical industry. Or is it a mistake? Is it on purpose? What is happening with all that excess blood? They're discarding it. Are they? No one would know. They're certainly not using all the blood drawn for a given test, that's for sure. Are they using it on the black market? Are they using it for genetic testing that's not for the greater good but geared to harm us? Is there a secret society of blood drinkers? Is there an extraterrestrial race we're providing blood for to utilize as their food source or for their own experimental testing? Are labs simply throwing the blood away? Only a portion of blood donations go to hospitals. Where do all the other millions of gallons go?

Regardless of how leftover blood is discarded, whether it's going down the drain or somewhere else, your white blood cell count takes time to rebuild. That majority of your immune system that's in your blood takes time to rebuild and replenish. It can take weeks. For many people struggling with a symptom or condition, depending on its severity, it can take anywhere from two to six months or even longer. It's like your blood's bank account is being drained, and before you can get enough money back into savings, more is taken. That is, before you can get enough immune system back into your blood, more is taken. And then the sicker you get—because a large portion of your immune system is taken from you—the more blood testing is called for to solve the mystery. Chronic illness is still a mystery, no matter how many experts think they have it pegged. It's still a mystery leading to the refrain "We'd better order more blood." This is the vicious cycle I mentioned earlier. Many people have a hard time bouncing back from the continual cycle of blood draws. Some may never bounce back.

When someone gets a bad cut—for example, from a broken glass injury or mishandling of a knife—and they lose a lot of blood, it's traumatic to the body. The shock alone from losing what would equal 10 or 14 vials of blood is traumatic to the body. Even a less aggressive cut on the body that leads to blood loss equal to seven small vials—that blood loss would be traumatizing for the body. The person would need time to recover. And yet we draw this amount of blood out of people without question. We say, "Oh, drink some fluids later, eat some food, build your blood back up," acting confident that it will happen in a few hours. "We'll see you here in two weeks."

When you go to a new doctor or specialist, they'll want to do it all over again: a whole new round of blood panels, regardless of when the last blood draw was. We lose a substantial part of our immune system every time—unless they're small blood draws for individual tests, separated out over multiple doctor visits instead of trying to get it all done in one swoop. With that more measured approach, we can preserve

our immune system, at least a larger amount of it. Otherwise, getting blood drawn can be that trigger that weakens your immune system, allowing a pathogen to rise up and make you sicker. Preserving our immune system is more important than we realize.

There's also hemorrhagic shock to consider. Medical research and science only deem certain levels of blood loss as hemorrhagic shock. The reality is that it can vary from individual to individual. Someone with a weaker constitution because of chronic illness can suffer from a mild case of hemorrhagic shock from a large blood draw. Others can suffer from mild hemorrhagic shock or even severe hemorrhagic shock from a routine blood donation. The medical industry is not monitoring the variations and variables of hemorrhagic shock as it relates to blood draw. They have their one mindset about the level of blood loss that leads to hemorrhagic shock. They don't investigate all the subtle differences of each individual and how they handle large blood draws for testing or donation. Hemorrhagic shock should have a scale, from mild all the way to extreme, with consideration of all the different amounts of blood that can create all the different levels of hemorrhagic shock. This is a one-size-fits-all approach and an unchecked area of medicine.

DRAINING OUR BRAIN SUPPLIES

The immune cells in your blood aren't all that's lost with blood draws. What about the critical electrolytes needed in your blood to keep your central nervous system, your brain, functioning? Do we think those electrolytes just appear out of nowhere? Even if you drink an electrolyte-based drink, it would take hundreds of those drinks to get those electrolytes back where they need to go. When we consume electrolytes, they need time to find their way to where they're needed. Plus people already have electrolyte deficiencies before a blood draw. We don't just drink electrolytes and find they instantly go to our reserves. It isn't an instant refilling of our bloodstream with electrolytes. It's a building process that takes time, little bit by little bit. It takes months of constantly staying with it to replenish deep electrolyte reserves. Your hamburger or pizza or keto dinner meal won't restore those deep electrolyte reserves. Everything you've read in this book about neurotransmitters becoming deficient and dehydrated applies to blood draw.

There are also nutritional deficiencies to consider. The critical nutrients that have found their way into our bloodstream from our foods and are on their way to their destinations, nutrients such as glucose (our blood sugar) that are needed to keep us in balance and sustain us and fuel our brain—they get removed as well when our blood is taken. We can get nutritional deficiencies faster from blood draws than from poor diet.

Ironically, we're often getting a blood test in the first place to see if we're nutrient deficient, and that very blood draw makes us more nutrient deficient. We won't see the extra deficiencies in those blood draw results because the deficiencies occurred from our

loss of that blood that was analyzed. As we leave the doctor's office or blood lab, we're far more deficient than we were to begin with. Our caring doctor or health care provider unknowingly made us more nutrient deficient. If another blood test were taken immediately after, it would be vastly different. Yet no one does this, seeing that you lose precious nutrients from getting blood drawn, which is just as well because they'd be draining your blood even more as they try to analyze your deficiencies.

Often, after performing a blood draw and getting back the test results, a doctor will try to "fix" us with supplements. These attempts to address deficiencies that do show up on blood testing will not fill the blood's nutritional bank faster than the nutrients are being removed via blood draw. The doctor is looking at your calcium, potassium, vitamin B_{12}, zinc, or vitamin D levels—or levels of many other nutrients—at the same time they're drawing those nutrients and more out with the blood. Then they add supplementation that may not even be of the highest quality (meaning assimilable, absorbable, and bioavailable) to meet the needs they see.

Vitamin C is imperative in this day and age in order to stay healthy and heal chronic illness. Vitamin C is an antioxidant that fuels our immune cells. When blood is taken, we lose a large portion of vitamin C reserves: after blood is drawn, any vitamin C reserves in cells, tissues, and organs are quickly released into the bloodstream to help fill in for vitamin C that had been traveling through the bloodstream. After this occurs, not only do we still have a deficit of vitamin C in the bloodstream but now we also have a deficit in the organs, including the brain. So after a blood draw, your brain loses vitamin C reserves that were keeping your brain from getting an infection while also keeping your brain tissue from oxidizing and aging.

MODERN-DAY BLOODLETTING

Back in the old days, especially the 1600s and 1700s, bloodletting was popular in conventional medicine. You got sick and they cut you and drained your blood into a pan. It wouldn't actually help you recover, and conventional medicine eventually learned that. First, it took a while for them to learn the lesson. Back then, if you didn't heal from a first round of bloodletting, you'd get cut again and bleed into a pan again. A few days or weeks later, if a doctor saw you and you weren't better yet, you'd get cut and bleed into a pan again. Eventually people would get so sick from bloodletting that they died.

Whether you like hearing this or not, whether you believe it or not, some entity in the medical industry knows that the modern-day practice of drawing excessive amounts of blood is similar to the historically outdated practice of bloodletting. It's a classified industry understanding, one not shared in medical training or medical schools. It's bloodletting continued in a fancy way without telling anyone—least of all the well-meaning professionals performing the blood draws—that it's modern-day bloodletting.

If you disagree, ask yourself this: Why do blood tests call for so much blood when only a fraction of that blood is needed? If your answer is that they may use the extra blood later to run more tests, it's important to know that's not how it works. New tests require new blood. If your answer is that they need extra blood to make a serum, that's also not how it works. You don't need to take many milliliters of blood to make a serum; you can make a serum with minimal blood. Much smaller amounts of blood are drawn from infants, yet they can still use that tiny amount of blood to test for the same thyroid panel as an adult who gets so much more blood taken.

Someone with neurological Lyme disease will usually have so many frequent blood draws that it's a miracle they can get better. It's one reason why most don't get better. Neurological Lyme is just one condition. Cancer patients are also pushed into a lot of blood draws—when one of the very factors that causes cancer is chronic infection of specific, aggressive viral strains creating cancer cells from feeding on specific, aggressive toxins. Medical research and science are aware that EBV is linked to non-Hodgkin's lymphoma, for example, yet they don't know to show mercy when they draw blood. Taking that blood is removing the immune cells that keep viral infections and viral cancer cells from spreading. Getting constant, routine blood draws can be challenging, especially to the cancer patient undergoing a bone marrow transplant, which means they already have a compromised immune system.

As we covered, your brain is meant to be safeguarded by your immune system. The majority of your immune system is in your blood, not in your gut like alternative medicine theorists love to say to sell their gut health products. Yet theories and trends take precedence over common sense. They miss the mark and don't protect the person who's struggling with symptoms. They don't have your back. They don't have your brain either. Gut health specialists in alternative medicine, whether they practice a blend of conventional and alternative medicine or simply alternative, draw a lot of blood to try to make conclusions as to the treatment or condition of someone's gut. They're presuming the gut is causing the health problem without understanding what's truly behind their patients' chronic illness. It's trendy theories like this that have allowed modern-day bloodletting to take hold—and to take someone down a darker path with their sickness.

Some people ask, "Isn't it natural to lose a lot of blood? That's what a period is." Blood draw is very different. Yes, when someone is menstruating, they often lose blood through the process of shedding the lining of the uterus. Yet this natural process still reserves and sustains immune cells, unlike blood draws. The immune system has an intelligence. As blood is being eliminated through the menstruation process, most immune cells exit the blood and stay behind in the reproductive system before the blood leaves the uterus. This is part of how 80 percent of a person's immune system guards their reproductive system during this part of their menstrual cycle. Also, there's not as much blood loss during menstruation as it seems. It isn't just straight blood being eliminated. It's mucus, the lining of the uterus, and additional fluid with that blood.

When an individual experiences heavy periods with continual bleeding that seems like it won't stop and verges on hemorrhaging, there tends to be great concern from physicians about the blood loss. They are not aware that during a regular period, the immune system works the way it does, nor are they aware that during an intensely heavy period, more of the immune system does escape and leave. They simply know that blood loss is worth their concern and could even lead to a blood transfusion. Yet they're not concerned about blood draws of five or many more full vials from pregnant women, or frequent blood draws from pregnant women, or having someone who's chronically sick give a blood donation. This is another area of disconnect.

Here's another disconnect: blood donation protocols. When someone is giving blood, the system overlooks many critical considerations. One very important consideration is whether the blood donor has a history of chronic illness. Now, they may ask the question. Yet they only pick and choose certain health conditions as a red flag for not giving blood. They generally don't see autoimmune or hundreds of other symptoms and conditions as a concern. And the majority of blood donors are women who have a history of chronic illness, many of them told to donate blood by their doctors, women who kindly and generously donate their blood in an effort to help humanity. Surprisingly, the healthiest and strongest people rarely donate blood. These blood donation protocols should be reconsidered, with screeners looking more closely at whether a potential blood donor has a history of chronic illness.

PRACTICAL CONSIDERATIONS OF BLOOD TESTING

If by this point, you're thinking that I must not believe in blood testing, know that I do. I believe in blood testing. I believe in the window it offers doctors and patients. I also believe there's a serious problem with how it's practiced that's prematurely taking people's lives away. That problem is being overlooked or purposely ignored.

If you think it's too far-fetched that the entire medical world missed this problem regarding our immune system and blood draw and that I'm the only one to bring this to people's attention, I agree with you. Someone knows. We're supposed to be so technologically advanced that we can find a murderer through a speck of blood the size of a fine grain of sugar on a pair of jeans buried in a shallow grave 40 years ago. To run a test on somebody's DNA—for example, to learn family lineage—you don't need to put a big tube of blood in a box and ship it out; you can stick a swab in somebody's mouth. This is to say that with all these medical advances, you don't need a large tube of blood to find a nutritional

deficiency. You don't need a large tube of blood to look at somebody's thyroid panel. You don't need a large tube of blood to run a test for someone's A1C. So let's keep our wits about us.

What to Ask Your Doctor

I recommend asking your doctor for the minimum blood draw needed for a test, and asking if it's possible to come back periodically, so that no more than two to three full tubes of blood are taken per visit. Ideally a blood draw should be limited to two to three *quarter* tubes or, if you have to, two to three *half* tubes. (If you notice that the phlebotomist happened to fill the tubes less than quarter or halfway with blood, even better.)

Now, if you request quarter or half tubes, the phlebotomist or blood lab will likely say they can't use them. They could say they have to have full tubes or they can't run the test or make a serum. This is not true. A blood lab can test anything using a quarter or half tube of blood or even less, and they will receive that partial tube and use it if the doctor sends it. Find a doctor who will send the quarter or half tubes. The blood lab will receive it, utilize it, and do all the testing needed with partial tubes. Even if a blood lab tells a phlebotomist they won't use partial tubes, if that phlebotomist sends quarter or half tubes, the blood lab will still accept it. The lab only needs a small fraction of blood. In reality, the blood lab only needs blood drops the size of a grain of rice or a bean, although they will refuse dosages that small.

If you're told you need to get five tubes of blood taken, get five *quarter* or *half* tubes. If it's recommended that you get seven tubes of blood taken, try to get seven *quarter* tubes (equal to 1.75 full tubes) or seven *half* tubes (equal to 3.5 full tubes) as a compromise. If they want more blood than that, ask the doctor to single out tests or divide them up and schedule you to come back so you can keep each blood draw within that two-to-three full vial maximum. Ideally, less is better, especially when someone's health is compromised.

Quarter and Half Tubes: The Standard of the Future

Blood work is important, and I recommend getting blood work when your doctor is asking for it, as long as it's done responsibly.

There are ways to protect yourself—and believe it or not, you're protecting your doctors too, whether your doctors realize it or not. Because if you get sicker, that doesn't help your doctors. Most doctors have track records of people getting sicker. It doesn't help their confidence, reputation, or career if you're getting sicker from their blood draws. It's only hurting your doctors too.

Many compassionate doctors feel the blow as their patients are getting sicker. It's why a lot of doctors struggle with drinking; it can be their way of dealing with the enormous stress and the losses. Your health going downhill doesn't help your nutritionist, dietician, or acupuncturist either, the one who's recommending a clean diet yet

is confused as to why you're getting sicker. Everybody gets the blame as you get sicker, which in turn can make everybody blame you. Your trainer, nutritionist, dietician, acupuncturist, naturopath, health coach, general practitioner, functional medicine doctor—they're likely to blame you. You're likely to blame them. Not always. It does often happen. Meanwhile, nobody's looking out for the vampire in the room—the unmonitored, unchecked, archaic medical system vampire stealing all the blood. It's not the doctors' fault, and it's not your fault. It's the system.

Any brain-related symptom or condition that's listed in this book worsens with excessive blood draw because, as we've covered, blood draws remove critical, foundational electrolytes; macro minerals; glucose; trace mineral salts; amino acids; antioxidants such as vitamin C, B_{12}, and other nutrients; plus oxygen and hormones, along with critical components of the immune system.

For instance, when someone has anxiety or depression and they get blood drawn, their anxiety and depression tend to immediately worsen that day, and then continue to worsen for quite some time afterward, usually for a week to a month, if they don't know the tools in this chapter to guard against it.

Fatigue and energy problems are also common. The day after a blood draw, someone could be fatigued and not even connect the dots to the loss of blood. That fatigue can last for two to three straight weeks in seemingly healthy people who are doing routine blood work. If the fatigue is impeding the person's life in any way, they'll often go to the doctor and get new blood drawn, and this will continue the fatigue for another month.

And for the chronically ill, the effects of a blood draw can be all the more heightened and long-lasting. Getting excessive amounts of blood drawn can be a trigger that turns any symptom or condition into a greater burden.

So far we've been talking about the effects of blood loss. There's also another aspect of blood draw with health effects: as the needle enters the vein to draw blood, a burst of adrenaline is released and instant fight-or-flight occurs, which is difficult on anyone who is chronically sick. The aftermath can be a sleepless night, rapid heartbeat for the rest of the day, and/or an elevation of neurological symptoms, including OCD, anxiety, depression, and additional fatigue.

It's not uncommon for a young woman who's experiencing chronic fatigue and brain fog to see her second or third doctor in six months, and to get 18 vials of blood drawn at one time with just one of those doctors. That's not to mention another 7 vials drawn with another doctor, and another 10 vials drawn with another doctor. It can easily accumulate, adding up to 35 vials of blood in just four to six months. And that's not the limit. Many young women get more than that. Doctors have gotten script-happy with blood draws, especially the specialists who are functional medicine doctors.

We have to find a balance. The old conventional doctor of yesteryear (20 to 30 years ago) would order a basic 3 to 7 vials to look at a complete blood count, maybe a metabolic panel, test for cholesterol, blood sugar, and maybe liver enzymes. In contrast, functional medicine doctors of today tend to order anywhere from 7 to 28 vials, and 28 is not the stopping point. Many of them order more than that—35 to over 40 vials—at one time.

With this chapter, I'm not trying to instill fear. I believe in blood testing. Let's do it responsibly. Let's get it *right*. We need to respect people and their life force that resides inside of them: their blood. When we take blood, we need to find a balance to start with, and then we need to do better. Quarter and half tubes need to be the standard of the future.

How to Rebuild Your Blood

We're supposed to be all about balance. With exercise, workouts, yoga, meditations, mindfulness, "everything in moderation" mindsets—we're always hearing that it's about staying in balance. We're practically obsessed with balance. And still, no one is questioning, "Is removing a large amount of blood out of balance?"

Does it seem balanced that for blood testing, they remove the same amount of blood from a 100-pound petite adult as from a 250-pound adult? Does it seem balanced that many blood donors pass out after giving blood, or that many patients faint when they've had more than two or three vials of blood taken?

Pregnant women get frequent blood draws without any consideration to the developing baby or the mother's immune system, which is responsible for protecting the baby and the mother. Does that seem balanced?

If someone has a weakened immune system, it can take months for them to rebuild after a larger blood draw. Before they get a chance to rebuild, they often get another blood draw. Rebuilding blood is not as simple as the recommendation of eating a cookie and drinking a cup of apple juice after giving blood. Those partially help bring your blood *sugar* back. They bring in a few electrolytes to get you started. They don't help *rebuild* your blood. That takes time. No one is saying, "Here's what to do so you can build your immune system back up—the immune system we just removed from you." That's not even on the radar after they just removed a large portion of your immune system.

There are more productive ways of bringing back blood sugar than the recommendation of eating cookies, anyway, and they're the same productive steps to build your blood back up with other nutritional components too. Eating overt, radical fats—by which I mean fat-based foods—is not a productive way to build blood back up because radical fats hinder the immune system and block cells from receiving critical nutrients. Looking for something considered "constitutional" like steak, chicken, avocado, peanut butter, oils, milk, cheese, eggs, or butter is not going to restore the immune system and build the blood faster. It's only going

to slow down the blood-building process. Instead, getting more critical clean carbohydrates (without fats at the same time) after a blood draw is more beneficial. Ideal forms of blood-building carbohydrates include potatoes, sweet potatoes, winter squash, bananas, carrots (not large amounts of carrot juice), peas, papayas, mangoes, wild blueberries, and apples.

What can you do specifically to build up your immune system after a blood draw? To assist your body with rebuilding immune cells (both red and white blood cells), you can turn to spirulina, barley grass juice powder, celery juice, leafy greens such as spinach and kale, and leafy herbs such as cilantro and parsley. Fruits such as grapes, cherries, blackberries, cucumbers or cucumber juice, and melons (such as honeydew, watermelon, and even cantaloupe), as well as coconut water (that's not pink or red), are also critical.

Keep in mind that your body knows it's missing part of its immune system after a blood draw, and so manufacturing begins. Bone marrow goes into rapid immune cell production after a blood draw, especially after donating blood (because most of the time, blood donation takes larger amounts of blood). That manufacturing requires vitamin B_{12}, magnesium, zinc, and vitamin C. Getting as much fruit in your diet as possible is critical to provide extra vitamin C. Immune cells feed on vitamin C, zinc, vitamin B_{12}, and magnesium. At the same time, know that these nutrients you take in are not necessarily going to create new immune cells instantly. Immune cells take time to produce. In the meantime, these nutrients are going to help the immune cells that were left behind after the blood draw. As the killer cells in your white blood cell count are leaving organs and entering the bloodstream in order to fill in for the loss and protect your brain and heart from infection, bringing in zinc (as liquid zinc sulfate), B12 (as adenosylcobalamin with methylcobalamin), vitamin C (as Micro-C or comparable buffered, non–ascorbic acid vitamin C), and magnesium (as magnesium glycinate) can at least strengthen those immune cells even while the immune cells are minimized in number. You'll find the best forms of each supplement in the directory on my website at www.medicalmedium.com. Read more about supplementation, including specific protocols for before and after blood draw, in *Brain Saver Protocols, Cleanses & Recipes*.

Blood Draw Protocols

The following supportive protocols offer options for before and after getting blood drawn. You're welcome to try all the options listed, or incorporate as many options as you can.

One Week Directly before a Blood Draw

A week before getting blood drawn, start preparations to strengthen your blood and lessen the blow of the shock so your blood will be able to restore at a quicker pace.

To protect yourself further, you can find a supplement protocol that corresponds with this list in *Brain Saver Protocols, Cleanses & Recipes*.

- 16–32 ounces **fresh celery juice** daily (see the end of Chapter 44 for recipe and guidelines)

- 32 ounces **lemon or lime water** twice a day (see the end of Chapter 44 for the recipe with the proper ratio and water temperature)

- 20–40 ounces **coconut water** daily (avoid coconut water that's pink or red)

- Try to incorporate as many **Brain Saver Recipes** from *Brain Saver Protocols, Cleanses & Recipes* as desired throughout the week

One Week Directly following a Blood Draw

Directly after getting your blood drawn, you can turn to this one-week protocol to help strengthen the portion of your immune system that was left behind after blood was taken. It also lessens your body's shock while it helps build your blood back up and restore the missing pieces such as macro minerals, glucose, trace mineral salts, other vitamins, amino acids, and other nutrients.

To protect yourself further, you can find a supplement protocol that corresponds with this list in *Brain Saver Protocols, Cleanses & Recipes*.

- 16–32 ounces **fresh celery juice** daily (see Chapter 44)

- 32 ounces **lemon or lime water** twice a day (see Chapter 44)

- 20–40 ounces **coconut water** daily (avoid coconut water that's pink or red)

- Optional add-ons: **Brain Builder, Brain Soother Juice,** 16–32 ounces **cucumber juice** (recipes in *Brain Saver Protocols, Cleanses & Recipes*)

- Half a **melon** (such as honeydew or cantaloupe) or 2–3 cups watermelon daily

- **Medical Medium Spinach Soup** or **Brain Saver Salad** daily (recipes in *Brain Saver Protocols, Cleanses & Recipes*)

- Try to incorporate as many other **Brain Saver Recipes** from that book as desired throughout the week

If you have questions about how to navigate food beyond the protocols offered here, the next several chapters will offer answers. Throughout the pages to come, you'll gain knowledge to help guide you on your path of physical and spiritual internal health.

"Whether you like hearing this or not, whether you believe it or not, some entity in the medical industry knows that the modern-day practice of drawing excessive amounts of blood is similar to the historically outdated practice of bloodletting."

— Anthony William, Medical Medium

CHAPTER 41

Brain Cell Food and Filler Food

People often refer to "filler foods" as bad because they associate the term with unproductive processed foods, preservatives, food chemicals, and additives. In truth these ingredients should not be called fillers. They should be called toxic processed foods, toxic preservatives, toxic food chemicals, and toxic additives. These foods and food chemicals are in the category of brain betrayers.

We don't realize that our diet is composed of three categories:

- **Brain betrayer foods:** Foods and food chemicals that actively work against our healing

- **Filler foods:** Foods that take up space and don't offer healing powers for what we're up against in today's toxic world of sickness

- **Brain cell foods:** Foods that actively help us heal

The true meaning of *filler foods* is that they take up the room of other foods—healing brain cell foods—that could help turn your life around and reverse chronic illness. Filler foods don't reverse chronic illness. They may not worsen chronic illness, but they still don't heal chronic illness. Restoring and healing the brain depends on non-filler foods: brain cell foods.

In the filler foods list you'll find later in this chapter, don't be surprised when you see whole foods listed. You might think it's a mistake that the filler foods list is not a list of processed foods. It's no mistake. Filler foods, in their true meaning, can be wholesome, pure, organic, and not processed food or food made in a lab. Filler foods can sustain us when we're not fighting chronic illness. As human beings, we can survive on filler foods. While our quality of survival may not be the best, regardless, we can still survive.

It's when we're chronically ill with any kind of condition or symptom that there are critical requirements for our food. Those requirements are antiviral compounds, antibacterial compounds, and ample amounts of nutrients such as trace minerals, vitamins, antioxidants, and helpful amino acids (not unhelpful amino acids).

There's a difference between medicinal foods and filler foods. Yes, filler foods have nutrients in them too. Filler foods have trace minerals, vitamins, amino acids, omegas, and other nutrients, yet they're present in such small quantities that they aren't easily accessible—versus medicinal, healing, brain cell foods, where these nutrients are in higher quantity and much easier to absorb and access. Filler foods are missing one of the most important types of chemical compounds for humankind to survive in this this day and age: antiviral, antibacterial, antiparasitical, and antimold compounds. Filler foods are also missing another critical set of chemical compounds: the compounds that remove toxic heavy metals and toxic chemicals. Even though filler foods contain nutrients, they don't have these abilities.

One reason we get into a rhythm of relying on filler foods is that we're taught they're healthy. We're led to believe that according to food science, our filler foods offer more than enough of what we need. It's easy to be misled, sent down a misguided nutrition path. When food science glorifies a nutrient inside a nut, fish, chicken, or bean, we tend to run with it, as if it's a golden nugget. It could even lead you to reciting in your mind, as you're eating your oatmeal, how good it is for you because of the nutrients found in oats.

We get into a habit of consuming filler foods, making our diet mostly composed of filler foods and brain betrayer foods, squeezing out opportunities for foods that are powerful for our healing process. Restoring the brain takes highly nutrition-charged food. Restoring the neurons, neurotransmitters, brain tissue, glial cells, nerve cells, brain stem, and cranial nerves takes more than grass-fed beef, oatmeal, or almond butter to accomplish.

BRAIN CELL FOODS LIST

Brain cell foods fall into five categories: fruits, leafy greens, herbs, wild foods, and vegetables. These foods are all disease fighters. They also support the growth of cells in the brain such as the glial cells, connective tissue, and neurons.

Your goal isn't to try to get as many different foods from this list into your diet as possible. Rather, if you want to heal, focus on making whichever foods you choose from this list the main part of your diet. Try to take up the space of filler foods and brain betrayer foods in your diet with brain cell foods instead. Focus on any of these brain cell foods in any way you choose to eat them. If you'd like to try mono eating for a period of time, refer to Cleanse to Heal. There, you'll find guidance on mono eating bananas, papaya, potatoes, or peas (with celery juice and optional lettuce), along with other mono protocols for different conditions.

Keep in mind that this is not an exhaustive list. For example, you may have wonderful local fruits available that aren't listed here. This is simply a representative list of examples to give you ideas about the healing possibilities available with fruits, leafy greens, herbs, wild foods, and vegetables. Also note that this list is not in order of potency.

Fruits

- Apples
- Apricots
- Asian pears
- Avocados (sparingly due to fat content)
- Bananas
- Berries (including blackberries, blueberries, raspberries, black raspberries, strawberries, and your local edible berries)
- Canistel (eggfruit)
- Cherimoya
- Cherries
- Cranberries
- Cucumbers
- Custard apples
- Dates
- Figs
- Grapefruit
- Grapes
- Guava
- Jackfruit
- Kiwis
- Lemons
- Limes
- Loquat
- Lychee
- Mamey
- Mandarins
- Mangoes
- Melons (including watermelon, honeydew, cantaloupe, crenshaw, canary, Santa Claus, galia, Charentais, and casaba)
- Nectarines
- Olives (sparingly due to fat content; seek out olives without vinegar, citric acid, and other preservatives)
- Oranges
- Papayas
- Passionfruit (lilikoi)
- Peaches
- Pears
- Pineapple
- Pitaya (dragon fruit)
- Plums
- Pomegranates
- Pomelos
- Rambutan

- Ripe peppers (not green)

- Sapodilla

- Sapote

- Soursop

- Starfruit

- Summer squash

- Tangerines, tangelos, and mandarins (including clementine, satsuma, Robinson, Ponkan, and Minneola)

- Tomatoes

- Winter squash (including butternut, delicata, sweet dumpling, kabocha, acorn, and honeynut)

- Zucchini

Leafy Greens

- Arugula

- Bok choy

- Broccoli rabe

- Collard greens

- Frisée and endive

- Kale

- Lettuce (including green leaf, red leaf, butter leaf, romaine, heirloom lettuces)

- Mâche

- Microgreens (including sunflower greens and pea shoots)

- Mustard greens

- Radish greens

- Spinach

- Sprouts

- Watercress

Herbs

Note: Additional medicinal edible herbs appear in the "Supplement Gospel" section of *Brain Saver Protocols, Cleanses & Recipes*.

- Basil

- Celery

- Chives

- Cilantro

- Garlic

- Ginger

- Lemon balm

- Marjoram

- Mint

- Onions

- Oregano

- Parsley

- Rosemary

- Sage

- Scallions

- Thyme

- Turmeric

Wild Foods

If you recognize a food in this list and doubt that it's wild, know that there's a reason it's listed: because the food is so close to its wild origin, even if it's readily available from the grocery store.

Note: Additional medicinal edible wild herbs, such as nettle, appear in the "Supplement Gospel" section of *Brain Saver Protocols, Cleanses & Recipes*.

- Aloe vera

- Burdock root

- Chaga mushroom

- Chestnuts

- Coconut (sparingly due to fat content)

- Coconut water (not pink or red; no natural flavors)

- Crabapples

- Currants

- Dandelion greens

- Heirloom bananas

- Heirloom lettuces

- Mulberries

- Mushrooms (non-hallucinogenic, non-psychedelic edible varieties such as portabella, button, chanterelle, shiitake)

- Other wild edible berries

- Persimmons

- Raw honey

- Reishi mushroom

- Rose hips

- Sea vegetables (preferably Atlantic, including dulse, kelp, and Irish moss; also nori)

- Wild blueberries

- Wild cranberries

Vegetables

- Artichokes

- Asparagus

- Beets (be cautious of GMO/ bioengineered)

- Broccoli

- Brussels sprouts

- Cabbage

- Carrots

- Cauliflower

- Celeriac

- Eggplant

- Kohlrabi

- Lentils (best eaten after soaking for a day; remove any pebbles; do not let lentils dominate your diet unless they're your only available food source)

- Parsnips

- Peas

- Potatoes

- Radishes

- Romanesco

- Rutabaga

- Snow peas

- String beans (including green beans)

- Sweet potatoes and yams

- Turnips

FILLER FOODS LIST

Filler foods won't necessarily hurt you. Many of the filler foods in this list are better than other filler foods in this list. They're not all equal. Regardless, if you dominate your diet with filler foods, whether fat-based or not, you'll be missing what you need to heal and keep you healthy and strong.

Note that that these foods are not listed in order of importance. This is not an exhaustive list either. Rather, each category lists a representative set of examples in the bullet points. Also keep in mind that this is not a list to encourage you to add filler foods to your diet, or add variety to the filler foods already in your diet. Your goal isn't choosing more of these to eat. If you're struggling with a symptom or condition, these are foods you only want to incorporate sparingly, if at all.

Remember, filler foods are missing antiviral, antibacterial, antiparasitical, and antimold compounds. Filler foods are also not detoxifiers of pathogens, toxic heavy metals, or toxic chemicals. There's a difference between medicinal brain cell foods and filler foods.

Gluten-Free Grains and Pseudo-Grains

- Amaranth

- Buckwheat

- Millet

- Oats (including homemade oat milk)

- Quinoa

- Rice

- Teff

- Wild rice

Beans

- Adzuki beans

- Black beans

- Black-eyed peas
- Butter beans
- Cannellini beans
- Garbanzo beans (chickpeas)
- Kidney beans
- Navy beans
- Pinto beans
- White beans

FAT-BASED FILLER FOODS

The filler foods in the categories that follow are fat-based foods, which inhibit detoxification. The high fat content does not allow the liver, lymph, and blood to release pathogens, toxins, and poisons, which in turn does not allow the brain or other organs to cleanse and rejuvenate. While it's true that foods such as nuts, seeds, and animal products can contain vitamins, trace minerals, and other nutrients, fat-based foods' nutrition is not abundant enough to compensate for what the human body is up against in this day and age. These foods' nutrients do not outweigh the ramifications of their high fat content. Keeping fat-based filler foods in your diet all depends on how sick you are. Fat-based filler foods should always be consumed sparingly, even if you're in a time in your life when you still consume filler foods and you're not sick with symptoms and chronic illness. If you're someone trying to recover, you want to avoid these foods.

Nuts and Seeds

- Almonds
- Brazil nuts
- Cashews
- Chia seeds
- Flax seeds
- Hazelnut
- Hemp seeds
- Macadamia nuts
- Nut and seed milks (homemade)
- Peanuts
- Pistachios
- Pumpkin seeds
- Sesame seeds
- Sunflower seeds
- Walnuts

Nut and Seed Butters

- Almond butter
- Brazil nut butter
- Cashew butter
- Hazelnut butter
- Hemp seed butter

- Macadamia nut butter
- Peanut butter
- Pistachio butter
- Pumpkin seed butter
- Sunflower seed butter
- Tahini
- Walnut butter

Healthier Oils

- Almond oil
- Avocado oil
- Coconut oil
- Flaxseed oil
- Grapeseed oil
- Macadamia oil
- Olive oil
- Peanut oil
- Sesame oil
- Sunflower oil
- Walnut oil

Fish

As with other filler foods, if you don't already eat fish, you certainly don't need to add these foods to your diet. These are the best options if you are eating fish.

- Wild haddock
- Wild halibut
- Wild mackerel
- Wild salmon
- Wild sardines
- Wild trout

Animal Products

As with other filler foods, if you don't already eat meat and/or poultry, you certainly don't need to add these foods to your diet. These are the best options if you are eating animal products.

- Grass-fed beef
- Free-range, organic chicken
- Free-range, organic turkey
- Wild game

CHAPTER 42

Medical Medium Brain Shot Therapy

Medical Medium Brain Shot Therapy offers instant relief while you're working to fix problems at a deeper level in your brain, nervous system, and body. Your brain and body have a quick response to medicinals delivered in liquid form, what I call a "shot." Designed to be highly absorbable in the mouth, these Brain Shots' valuable healing components can reach the brain fast. These specially formulated shots have the ability to reset and rewire the brain, to shock it out of patterns while at the same time reducing triggers.

Medical Medium Brain Shot Therapy is uncharted territory. These are special configurations synergistically combined just right to crack the code of how fruits, herbs, leafy greens, wild foods, and vegetables can work as medicine. While creative juice concoctions have their place, and human creativity in the kitchen should be honored, that's not what you'll find here. These Brain Shots aren't tasty delights thrown together for fun and experimentation.

The healing shots of Medical Medium Brain Shot Therapy are tools that come from above. These Brain Shots are composed of specific combinations of ingredients working together systematically for specific reasons that only a source above could know. The relationships among these ingredients are intricate and unknown to anyone. Until now, this knowledge from above has remained untapped.

THE BRAIN SHOT THERAPY LIST

Exposures

1. Pathogens
2. Toxic Fragrances
3. Negative Energy
4. Mold
5. EMF and 5G
6. Radiation

7. Toxic Heavy Metals

8. Pesticides, Herbicides, and Fungicides

9. Pharmaceuticals

10. Chem Trails

Shifters

1. Obsessive Thoughts

2. Mood

3. Nerve

4. Energy

5. Food Fear

6. Cravings

7. Anger

8. Guilt and Shame

9. Ego

10. Dreams

Stabilizers

1. Nerve-Gut Acid

2. Trauma, Shock, and Loss

3. Adrenal Fight or Flight

4. Burnout

5. Betrayal and Broken Trust

6. Relationship Breakups

7. Sleep and Recharging

8. Speaking Your Truth

9. Finding Your Purpose

10. Wisdom and Intuition

HOW TO USE MEDICAL MEDIUM BRAIN SHOT THERAPY

Medical Medium Brain Shot Therapy is highly adaptable to your needs. You have two main options:

- **Use these shots as stand-alone Medical Medium Brain Shot Therapy.** Apply the Brain Shots as needed or desired, based on whichever specific form of relief you're seeking. Just like with any other Medical Medium therapy, you may also want to incorporate various other Medical Medium tools as part of your customized healing protocol.

- **Use these shots in a Medical Medium Brain Shot Therapy Cleanse.** Systematically work your way through the Brain Shots as part of a 10-, 20-, or 30-day cleanse. Find details for how to do this in the next chapter, "Medical Medium Brain Shot Therapy Cleanses."

Choosing Your Therapeutic Tools

If you're using stand-alone Medical Medium Brain Shot Therapy, you may know simply from looking at the names which Brain Shots you'd like to try. Or you may discover what resonates once you read the suggested uses. Or you may want to explore, trying them all.

Keep in mind, the descriptions of the Brain Shots are only examples. You may be up against an issue that's not listed. Don't let that deter you—the shot still applies to you. For instance, you may decide from the names "Mood Shifter" or "Burnout Stabilizer" or "Toxic Fragrances Exposure" that these shots are supportive for your situation, then perhaps not see your exact situation in the explanations. The Brain Shots still hold just as much merit for you.

When it comes to Medical Medium Brain Shot Therapy, it's good to explore. Any Brain Shot can apply to anyone. Feel free to experiment with which shots you choose. Use them as therapeutic tools whether you're targeting a specific need or not—because whether you're aware or not, you probably do have a cause and a reason for needing these Brain Shots. For example, you may not know you have a trust issue, yet when you try the "Betrayal and Broken Trust Stabilizer," enlightenment follows.

Many people don't know what issues they have within. They don't know what's broken. With Medical Medium Brain Shot Therapy, you don't need to know what's wrong for these shots to help you. Even if you don't believe you have a need, these shots will find a way to help you. That's one reason why the Medical Medium Brain Shot Therapy Cleanses, some of which methodically take you through the different Brain Shots, can be such a revelation.

With Medical Medium Brain Shot Therapy, however you decide to use it, you venture into uncharted territory with your healing.

When to Take Your Shots

If you're doing stand-alone Medical Medium Brain Shot Therapy, you can take your shots at any time of day as long as you follow this one golden rule: **drink your Brain Shots at least 15 to 30 minutes before or after celery juice.** In other words, drink your shots separately from celery juice, waiting at least 15 to 30 minutes in between drinking the shot and the celery juice. You don't want to disrupt pure celery juice's efficacy as it does its work inside your brain and body.

Ideally, drink your Brain Shots 15 to 30 minutes apart from any other food and drink too. That is, wait a minimum of 15 to 30 minutes after consuming anything else before you have a shot, then wait a minimum of 15 to 30 minutes after consuming a shot before you consume anything else. You want to give yourself time to resonate with each Brain Shot, letting the therapy enter the bloodstream and allowing yourself to pick up the frequency of the shot metaphysically and physically.

If you're doing a Medical Medium Brain Shot Therapy Cleanse, you'll find specific guidance about when to take your shots in the next chapter.

Frequency

For stand-alone Medical Medium Brain Shot Therapy, it's up to you how often you take these shots. You may decide to take the Brain Shots daily. If your need for exposure protection, shifting, or stabilization is great or you're dealing with an aggressive situation, you can take the shots multiple times a day.

You're also welcome to try different shots within a day or different shots from day to day.

For the Medical Medium Brain Shot Therapy Cleanses, there's specific guidance about frequency in the next chapter.

Preparation and Storage

You are welcome to make your Brain Shots fresh or ahead of time. If prepping ahead, you may decide to make them the night before or to juice multiple shots in the morning for the day ahead. If you won't be drinking your shots right away, store them in an airtight container in the fridge or in a cooler or insulated lunch bag if you're on the go. Consume your shots within 24 hours of juicing.

Notes on Juicing

- While you can use any juicer for these recipes, a cold press, masticating juicer will be more effective at extracting all the juice nutrients, especially from herbs and leafy greens. If you're using a centrifugal juicer, keep in mind that you may need to increase ingredient quantities a little to get full shots.

- When juicing herbs and greens in a centrifugal juicer, you may have the most success if you wrap your leafy greens and herbs around some of the firmer ingredients, such as apples, rather than sending the greens and herbs down the juicer chute separately.

- If you feel like your juicer is not producing a full shot, you can try running a tiny bit of water or coconut water through your juicer, after the other ingredients, to top off your shot. This isn't ideal. If you can, it's better to try increasing the ingredient quantities a little if your juicer isn't producing enough when following these recipes.

- It's best to follow the listed recipes if at all possible. If you can't use or access any of the ingredients, use the listed ingredients that you can or focus on Brain Shots for which all the ingredients are available to you. If you're missing a particular ingredient because you can't source it at the moment, you may come across it another time or decide to grow it yourself. When you can finally make the complete shot recipe, that Brain Shot will be all the more precious.

Adjustments for Children

Depending on the age and size of your child, serve a small portion of a given Brain Shot, whether that means reducing to a 1-ounce serving or even as little as a teaspoon.

Exposure Shots

These Brain Shots can be administered before an exposure, during an exposure, shortly after an exposure, or even days, weeks, or months after an exposure.

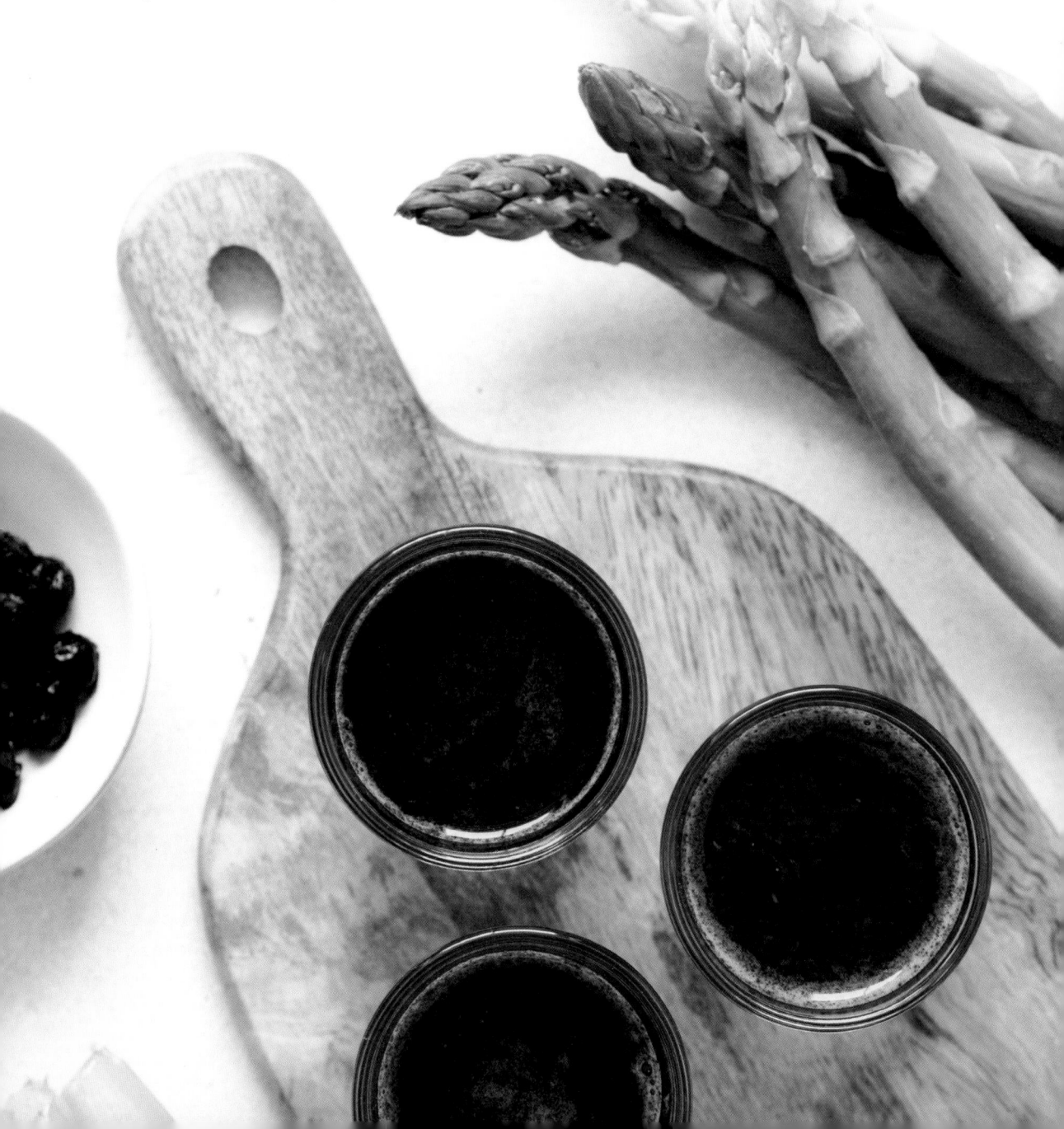

PATHOGEN EXPOSURE

(VIRUSES, BACTERIA, AND VIRAL/BACTERIAL BYPRODUCT)

Makes 1 to 2 shots

This shot can be useful if:

- You feel you've been around others who could be contagious due to COVID, the flu, or mono

- You're concerned about having shared bodily fluids with another person through shared glasses, bottles, food, utensils, or plates

- You're concerned about having shared bodily fluids through public restrooms or sexual activity

- You believe you might have been exposed to foodborne pathogens and you're concerned about getting food poisoning

Also consider trying this shot before attending an event where there will be a crowd of people and/or before eating out in restaurants.

6 sprigs fresh thyme
2 sprigs fresh rosemary
1 small garlic clove (optional)
2 raw medium asparagus spears
  (¼ cup chopped)
2 raw brussels sprouts
1 to 2 stalks celery

Run each ingredient through a juicer in the order listed from top to bottom.

Pour into a glass and serve.

TIPS

- For the fresh thyme and rosemary, if the stems are woody, you can use just the leaves. If the stems are soft, you can juice them too.

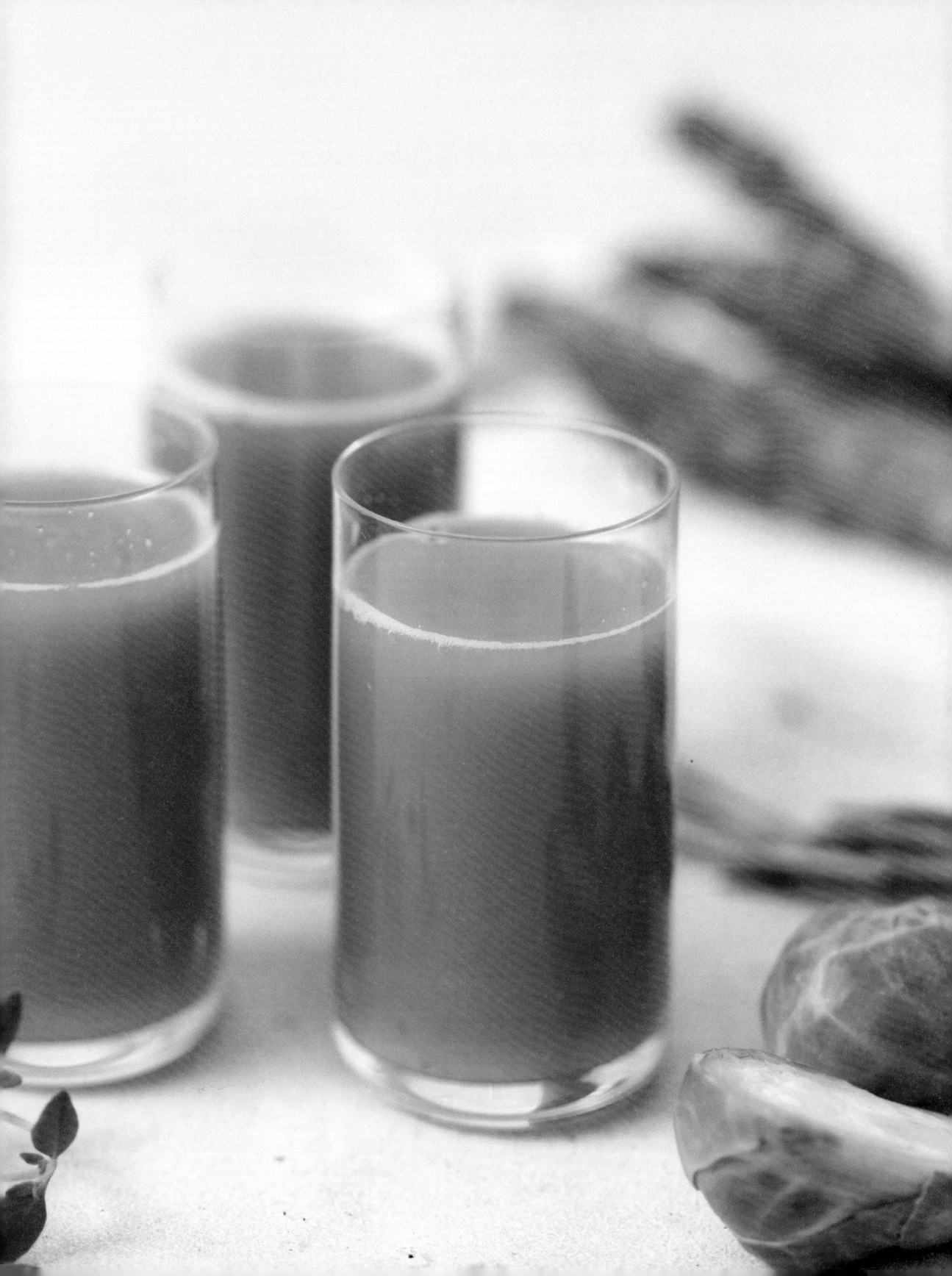

TOXIC FRAGRANCES EXPOSURE

Makes 1 to 2 shots

Try this shot when you've been exposed to toxic fragrances and scents through such circumstances as:

- Gatherings of people with fragrances coming off their persons
- Walking through department stores, grocery stores, other shops, or visiting doctors' offices where exposure to perfume, cologne, fabric softeners, scented candles, air fresheners, and other fragrances could be present
- Recently driving in a car where air fresheners are installed and/or family members saturated in perfume, cologne, laundry detergent, and other chemical toxic scents were in the car with you
- Close contact with others saturated in hair products, aftershave, cosmetics, body lotions, and body oils
- A neighbor's laundry sending dryer exhaust filled with perfumes, colognes, scented detergent, and fabric softener into the air

1 radish
1 cup roughly chopped green leaf lettuce, tightly packed
1 cup tightly packed fresh cilantro
½ apple

Run each ingredient through a juicer in the order listed from top to bottom.

Pour into a glass and serve.

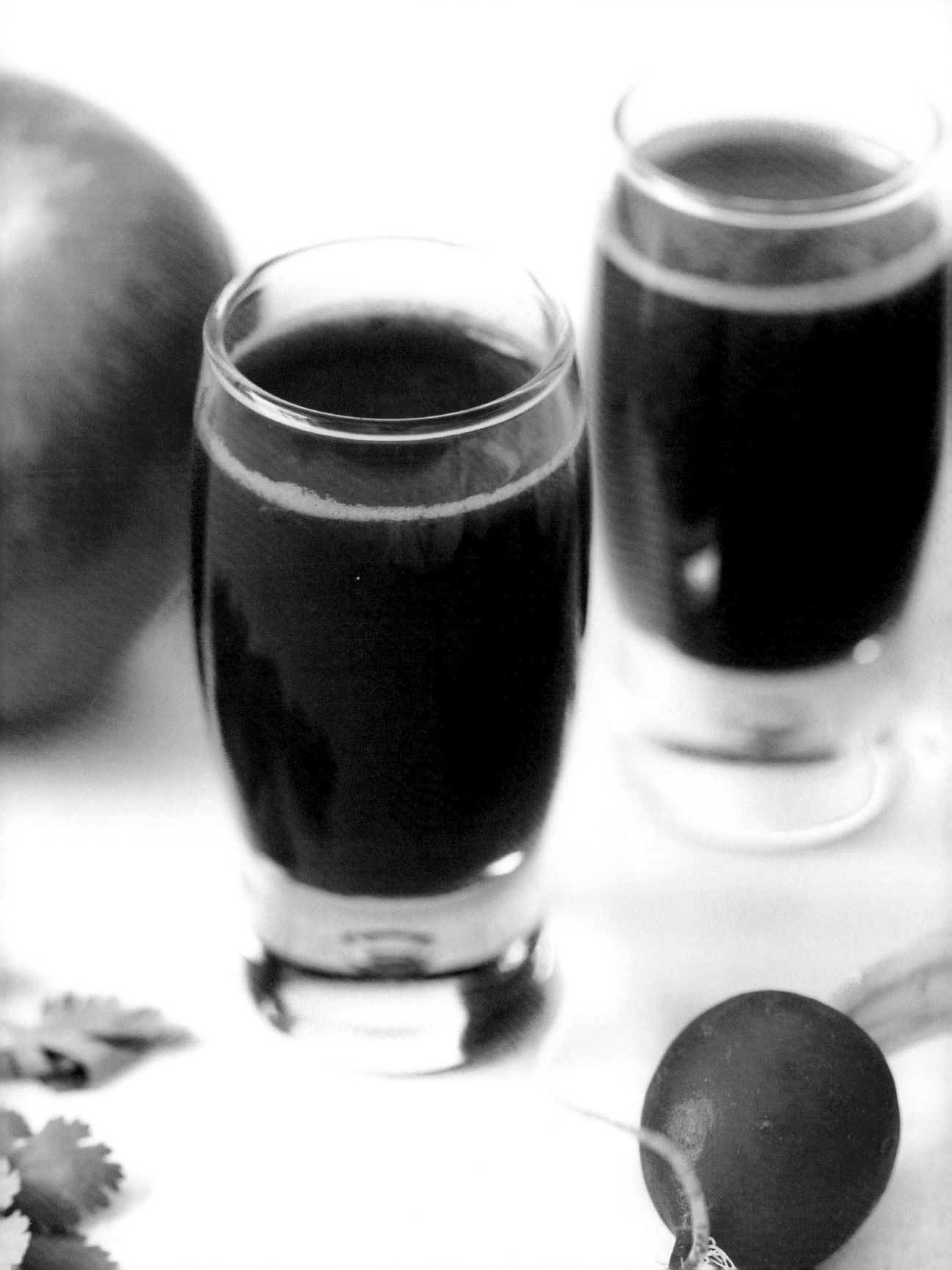

NEGATIVE ENERGY EXPOSURE

This is a helpful shot for those times when:

- You feel an unexplained sadness come over you
- You experience a confrontation or misunderstanding with another person
- Unexplained anger arises within you or even another person
- You're having a bad day
- Things in your life seem to be going wrong or you're feeling unlucky
- You're fearing something or someone and you can't shake it
- You're feeling dread after a bad dream
- You need to stay strong because you have no choice but to be around someone such as a friend or coworker who you feel has negative energy or a consistently negative attitude
- You're spending time around someone going through mental health challenges that may cause them to be angry or sad
- You're around someone who is struggling to the point of being suicidal
- You can't seem to break depressing, bad thoughts

¼ cup tightly packed fresh sage (approximately 30 leaves)
½ cup tightly packed sunflower sprouts
¼ cup tightly packed wheatgrass (or 2 teaspoons thawed frozen wheatgrass juice)
½ small garlic clove (optional)
½ to 1 orange or 1 to 2 tangerines, peeled

Run each ingredient through a juicer in the order listed from top to bottom.

Stir in the thawed wheatgrass juice if using.

Pour into a glass and serve.

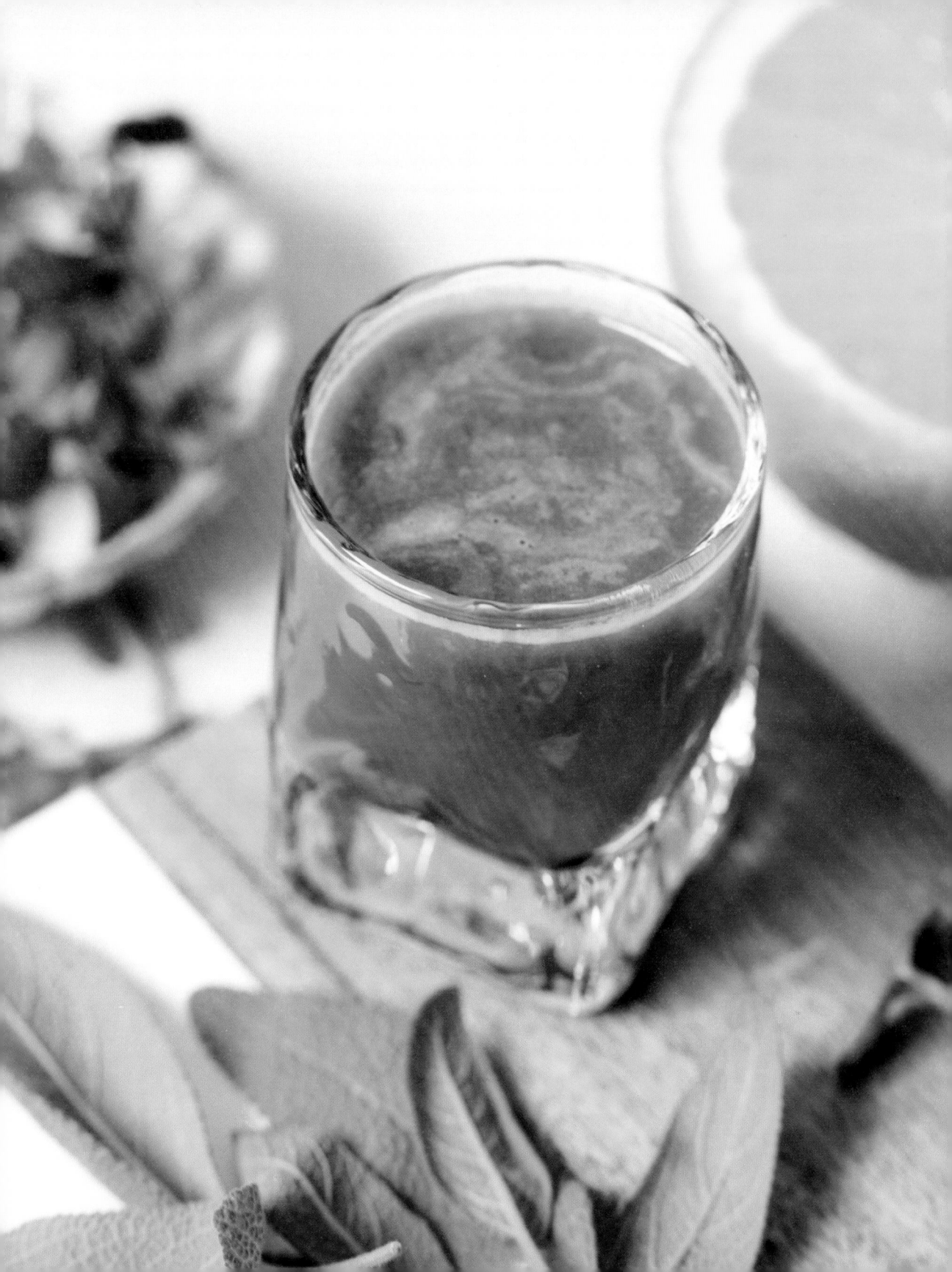

MOLD EXPOSURE

A helpful shot for any kind of mold or mildew exposure, including when you have been:

- Visiting or living in a moldy house or building

- Working in a moldy office or other workspace

- Inhaling mold off another person's clothing

- Consuming water contaminated with mildew or mold spores, or eating moldy food

½ cup tightly packed fresh basil
½ cup tightly packed fresh oregano
2 sprigs fresh rosemary
½-inch piece of fresh ginger
2 radishes
¼ bulb fennel (½ cup chopped)

Run each ingredient through a juicer in the order listed from top to bottom.

Pour into a glass and serve.

TIPS

- For the fresh rosemary, if the stems are woody, you can use just the leaves. If the stems are soft, you can juice them too.

- When juicing fennel for this recipe, you can use only the bulb itself or the bulb plus the lower-to-mid stalk (leaving out the leafy fronds in this case).

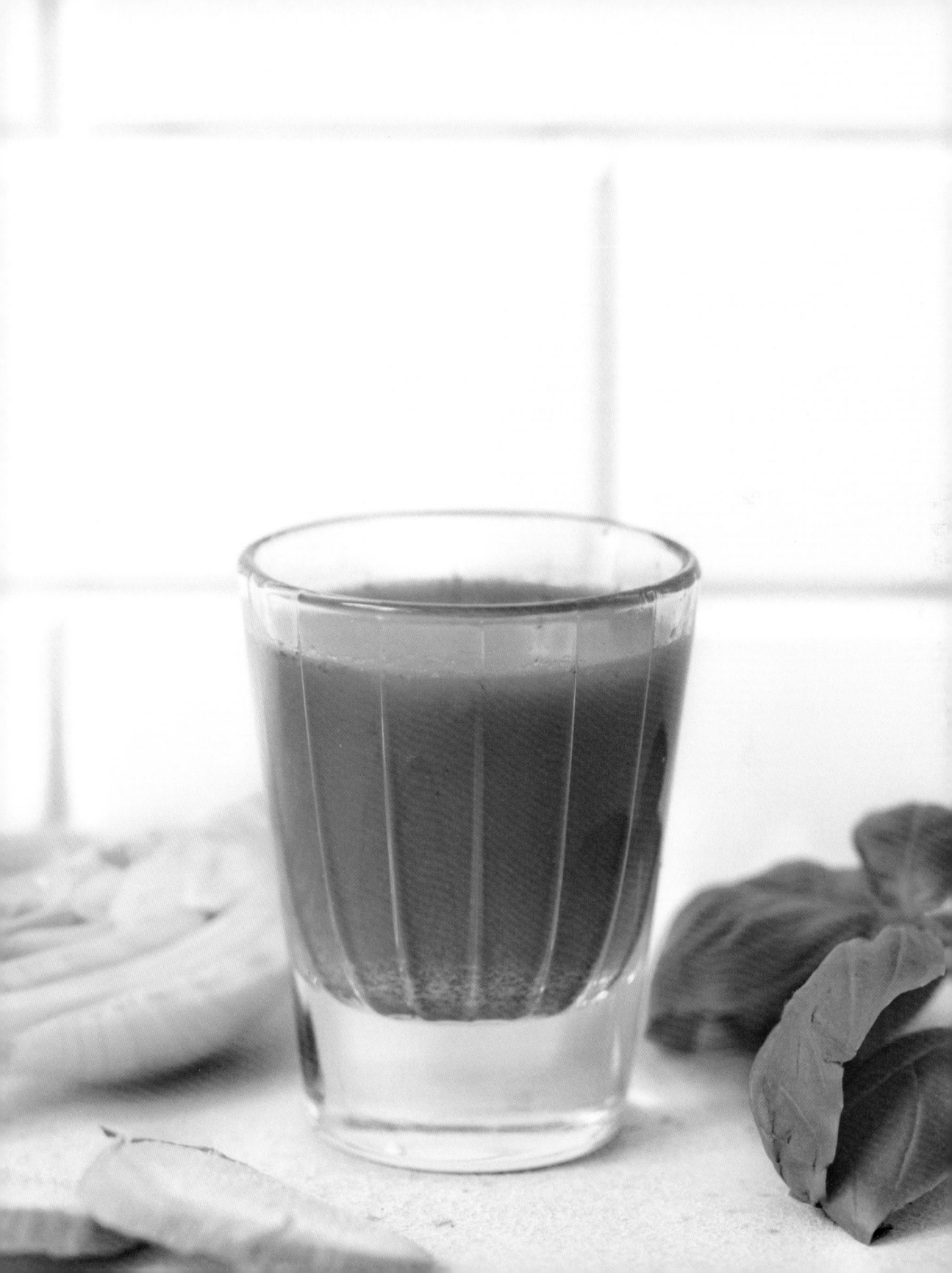

EMF AND 5G EXPOSURE

Makes 1 to 2 shots

Try this shot if you:

- Spend a lot of time on computers and computerized devices
- Live near a high-voltage area
- Spend time talking and texting on cell phones
- Travel by plane
- Live or work close to others while they're using devices
- Spend your day within several feet of a router
- Live near a cell tower

¼ cup tightly packed fresh parsley
½ cup peeled and cubed raw potatoes in a variety of your choosing, such as Yukon gold
1 to 2 stalks celery

Run each ingredient through a juicer in the order listed from top to bottom.

Pour into a glass and serve.

TIPS

- Before peeling, wash and scrub the potatoes well, discarding any that have green skins or are sprouting.

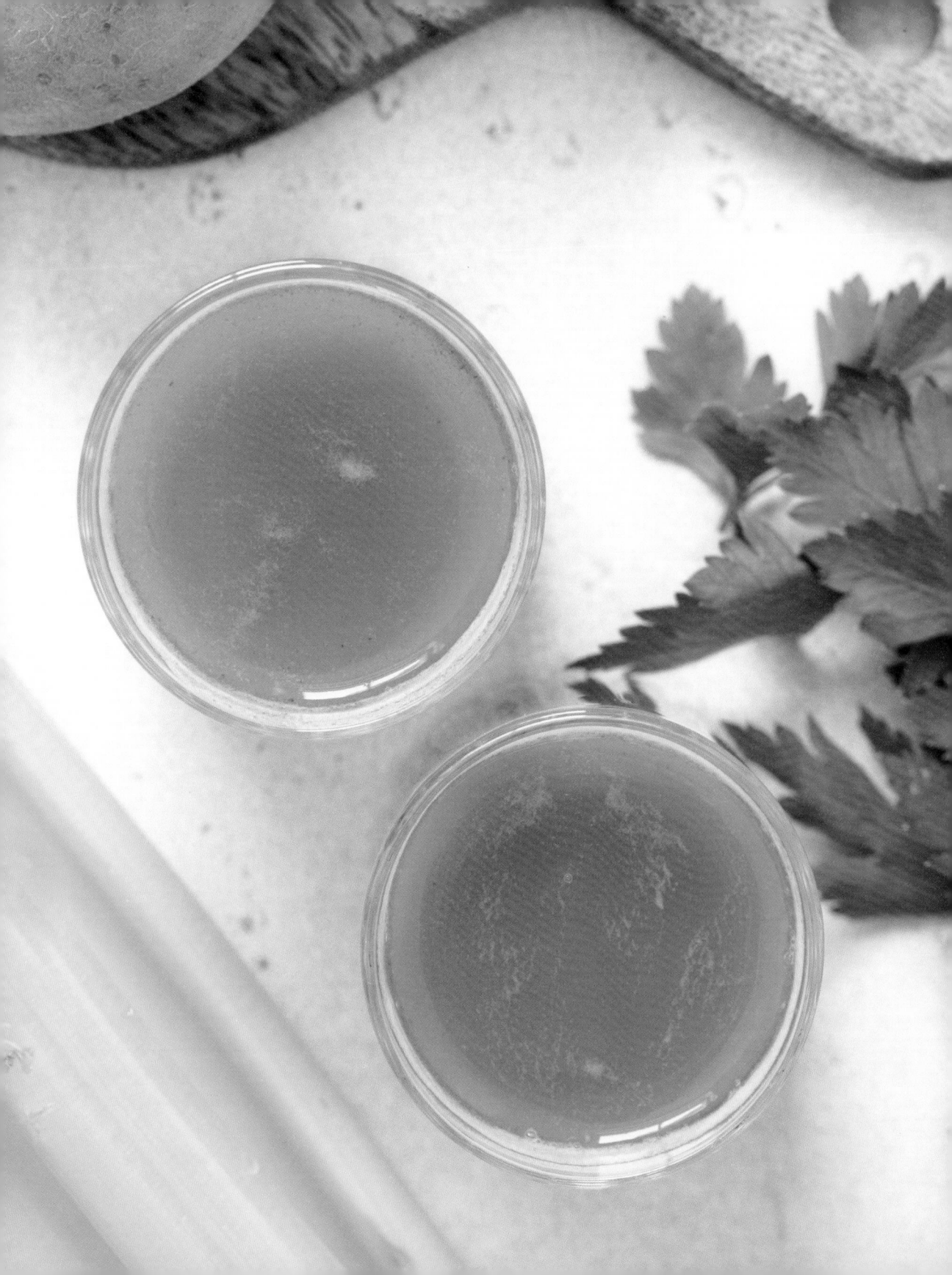

RADIATION EXPOSURE

This is a supportive shot for circumstances such as:

- Airplane travel

- Walking through airports or being close to airport scanners or baggage scanners

- Being close to luggage that has gone through airport scanners

- Medical testing such as CT scans, X-rays, fluoroscopy, and even MRIs

- Being around others who have had medical testing such as CT scans, X-rays, fluoroscopy, and MRIs

- Exposure to computerized devices

- After a sunburn

½ cup tightly packed fresh cilantro

½ cup fresh or thawed frozen wild blueberries or 2 tablespoons pure wild blueberry juice or 1 tablespoon pure wild blueberry powder

4 raw medium asparagus spears (½ cup chopped)

1 stalk celery

½ teaspoon spirulina

½ teaspoon barley grass juice powder

Run the cilantro, wild blueberries, asparagus, and celery through a juicer in the order listed from top to bottom. If you are using the wild blueberry juice or wild blueberry powder, reserve for the next step.

Stir in the spirulina and barley grass juice powder. Stir in the wild blueberry juice or wild blueberry powder if using.

Pour into a glass and serve.

TIPS

- If you're in a part of the world where you can't access fresh or frozen wild blueberries, wild blueberry juice, or wild blueberry powder, you can substitute blackberries. Although a high-antioxidant alternative, blackberries do not have the potency to match how wild blueberries defend cells from metals, chemicals, radiation, and other toxins.

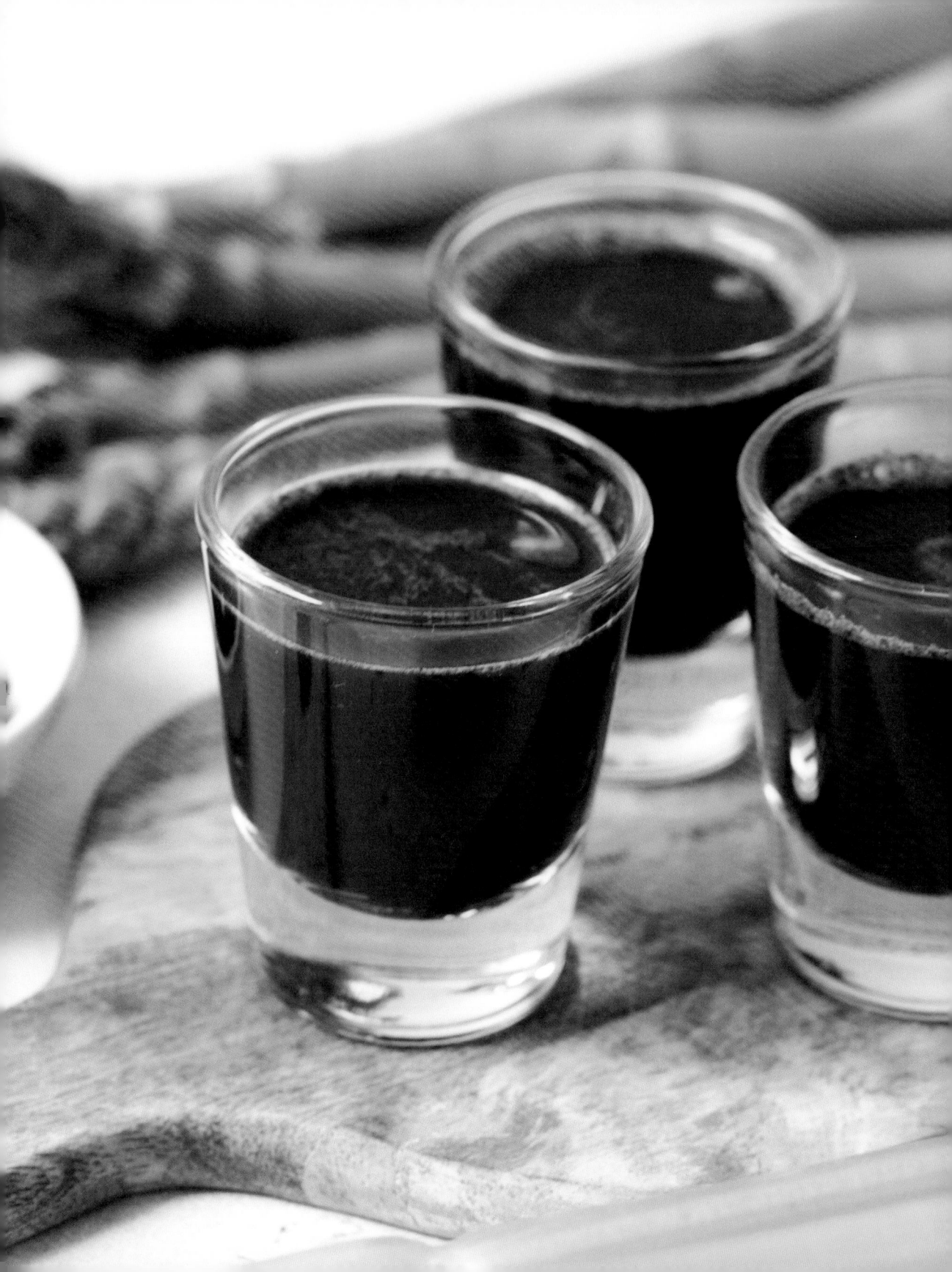

TOXIC HEAVY
METALS EXPOSURE

Makes 1 to 2 shots

This exposure shot is specially geared for recent exposure to toxic heavy metals, help-ing to stop toxic heavy metals from settling deep in the body. This shot can be used as an additional therapy to the Heavy Metal Detox Smoothies in Chapter 44, "Heavy Metal Detox," which are geared to extract toxic heavy metals that have already settled in the organs while providing ongoing support for toxic heavy metal exposure in the blood-stream, lymph, or intestinal tract.

Ideal times to use this toxic heavy metal exposure shot include when you:

- Have dental work done, such as getting mercury (amalgam) fillings removed or getting new fillings of any kind (including all composites)

- Have fluoride treatments, retainers, or braces

- Eat food cooked on a grill or from another type of cookout

- Consume restaurant food or beverages at coffee chains where town or city tap water is used in food and drink preparation

- Breathe in air fresheners, fragrances, perfumes, colognes, scented candles, detergents, or fabric softeners

- Smell smoke from something burning and do not know the smoke's origins or the purity of whatever is burning

- Get your hair done in a salon

- Are exposed to synthetic fragrances

- Spend time in or near an area recently treated with pesticide, herbicide, or insecticide spray

- Spend time outdoors during or after firework displays

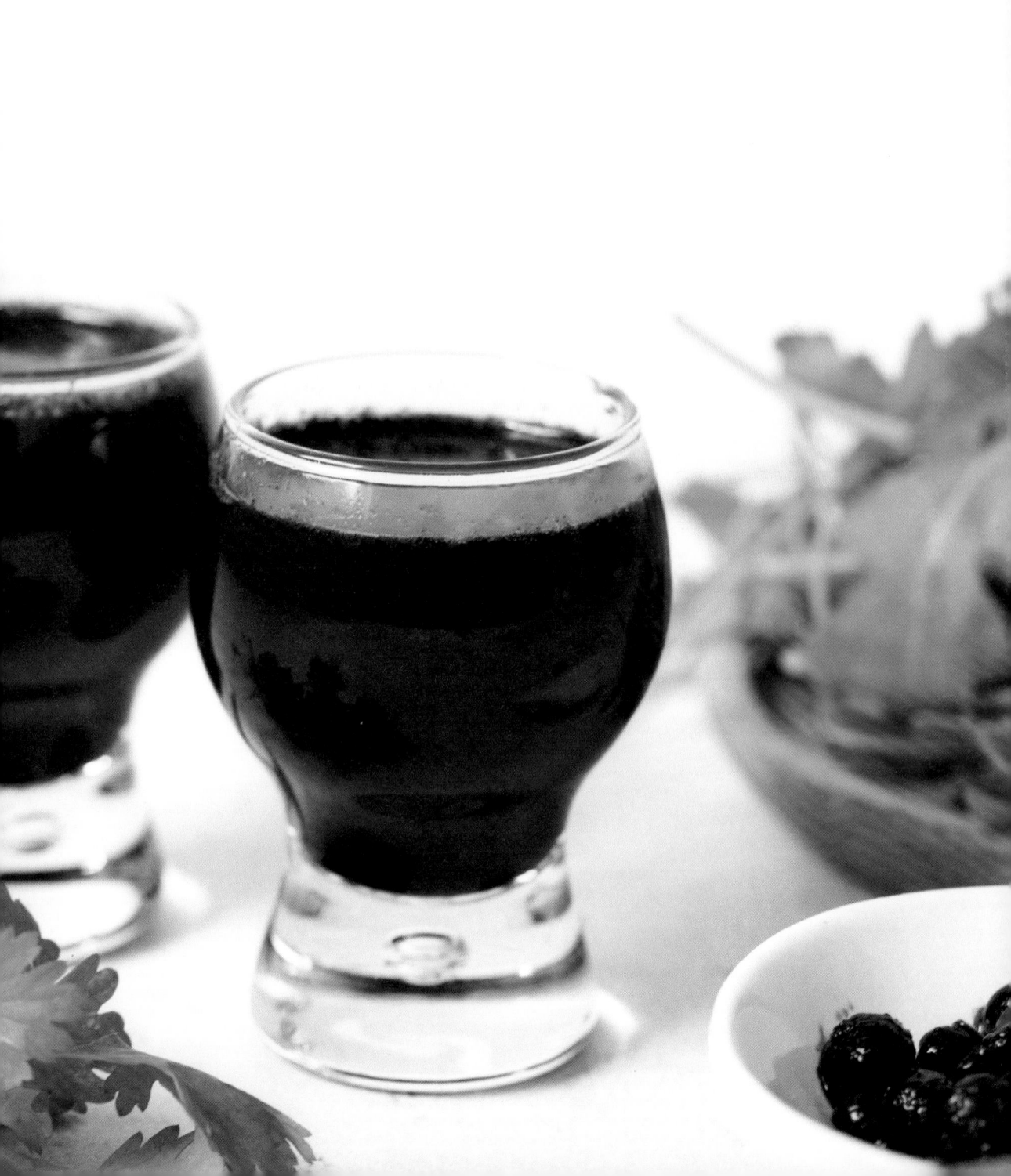

½ cup tightly packed fresh cilantro

⅓ cup tightly packed arugula

⅓ cup finely chopped cabbage (red or green), tightly packed

½ cup fresh or thawed frozen wild blueberries or 2 tablespoons pure wild blueberry juice or 1 tablespoon pure wild blueberry powder

1 to 2 stalks celery

½ to 1 orange or 1 to 2 tangerines, peeled (optional)

½ teaspoon spirulina

Run the cilantro, arugula, cabbage, wild blueberries, celery, and orange or tangerines (if using) through a juicer in the order listed from top to bottom. If you are using the wild blueberry juice or wild blueberry powder, reserve for the next step.

Stir in the spirulina. Stir in the wild blueberry juice or wild blueberry powder if using.

Pour into a glass and serve.

TIPS

- If you're in a part of the world where you can't access fresh or frozen wild blueberries, wild blueberry juice, or wild blueberry powder, you can substitute blackberries. Blackberries do not uproot and attach themselves to toxic heavy metals like wild blueberries do, although the high antioxidant ratio in blackberries can at least slow down heavy metal oxidation, which is helpful.

PESTICIDE, HERBICIDE, AND FUNGICIDE EXPOSURE

Makes 1 to 2 shots

This shot is an excellent tool when:

- You inhale an unfamiliar or strange odor

- You're exposed to recently delivered packages

- A neighbor sprays or treats their lawn with insecticide or chemical fertilizer treatments

- Chemical treatments are applied around an apartment building

- You're exposed to a town or city treatment that's occurring on the side of the street

- You spot somebody with a tank on their back and a hose in their hand, spraying for weeds

- You see a small-to-medium-sized truck with a large tank on the back and business signs on the side that say "lawn care," "bug control," or anything similar driving through your neighborhood (meaning that chances are they have recently sprayed someone's lawn or house)

- You're driving behind a truck that has a tank on the back with mysterious liquid leaking out of the tank

- You spend time sitting in or visiting parks, or you spend time on the golf course

- Insecticide treatments are sprayed in classrooms, from preschools to elementary schools to universities, and in dorm rooms, especially common at the beginning of the school year

- You live within 25 miles of a conventional fruit or vegetable farm during its growing season

¼ cup tightly packed fresh parsley
½ cup tightly packed fresh cilantro
2 large leaves kale
2 radishes
¼ cup fresh or thawed frozen blackberries
1 to 2 stalks celery
½ to 1 orange or 1 to 2 tangerines, peeled (optional)
¼ teaspoon spirulina

Run the parsley, cilantro, kale, radishes, blackberries, celery, and orange or tangerines (if using) through a juicer in the order listed from top to bottom.

Stir in the spirulina.

Pour into a glass and serve.

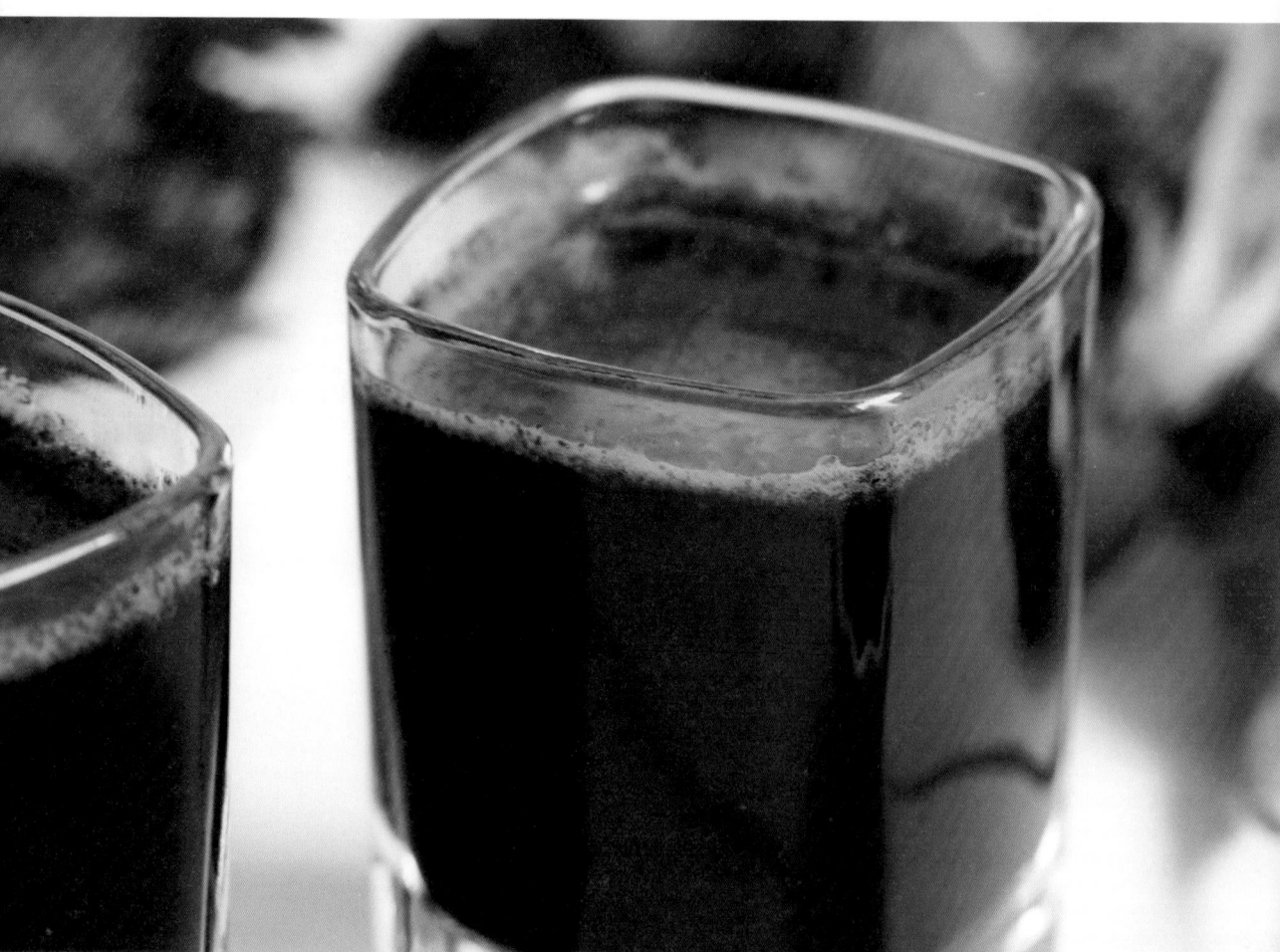

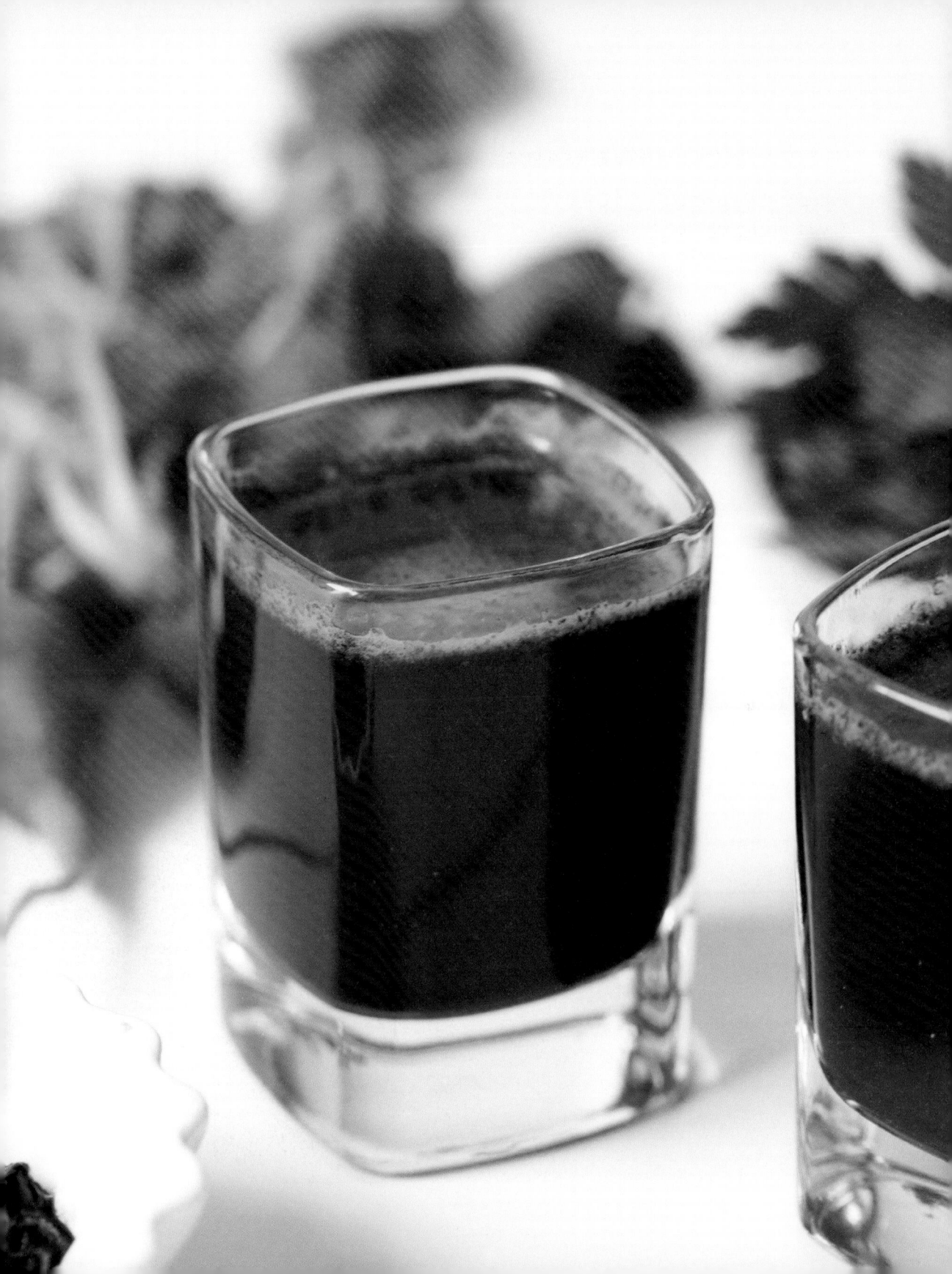

PHARMACEUTICAL EXPOSURE

Makes 1 to 2 shots

This shot is formulated for exposure to prescribed or over-the-counter medications or other pharmaceuticals, whether on a one-time or continual basis. Examples of pharmaceutical exposure include:

- Antibiotic treatments for infections

- Numbing agents for dental work

- Birth control

- Painkillers

- Surgeries

- Cosmetic enhancements and procedures such as filler, botulinum toxin injections, or other applications

- Medical testing, which can include contrasts, sedatives, or numbing agents

- New medical treatments of any kind

¼ lemon, peeled
¼ lime, peeled
¼ cup chopped green onions
½ cup tightly packed fresh cilantro
2 raw medium asparagus spears (¼ cup chopped)
½ stalk celery
½ apple

Run each ingredient through a juicer in the order listed from top to bottom.

Pour into a glass and serve.

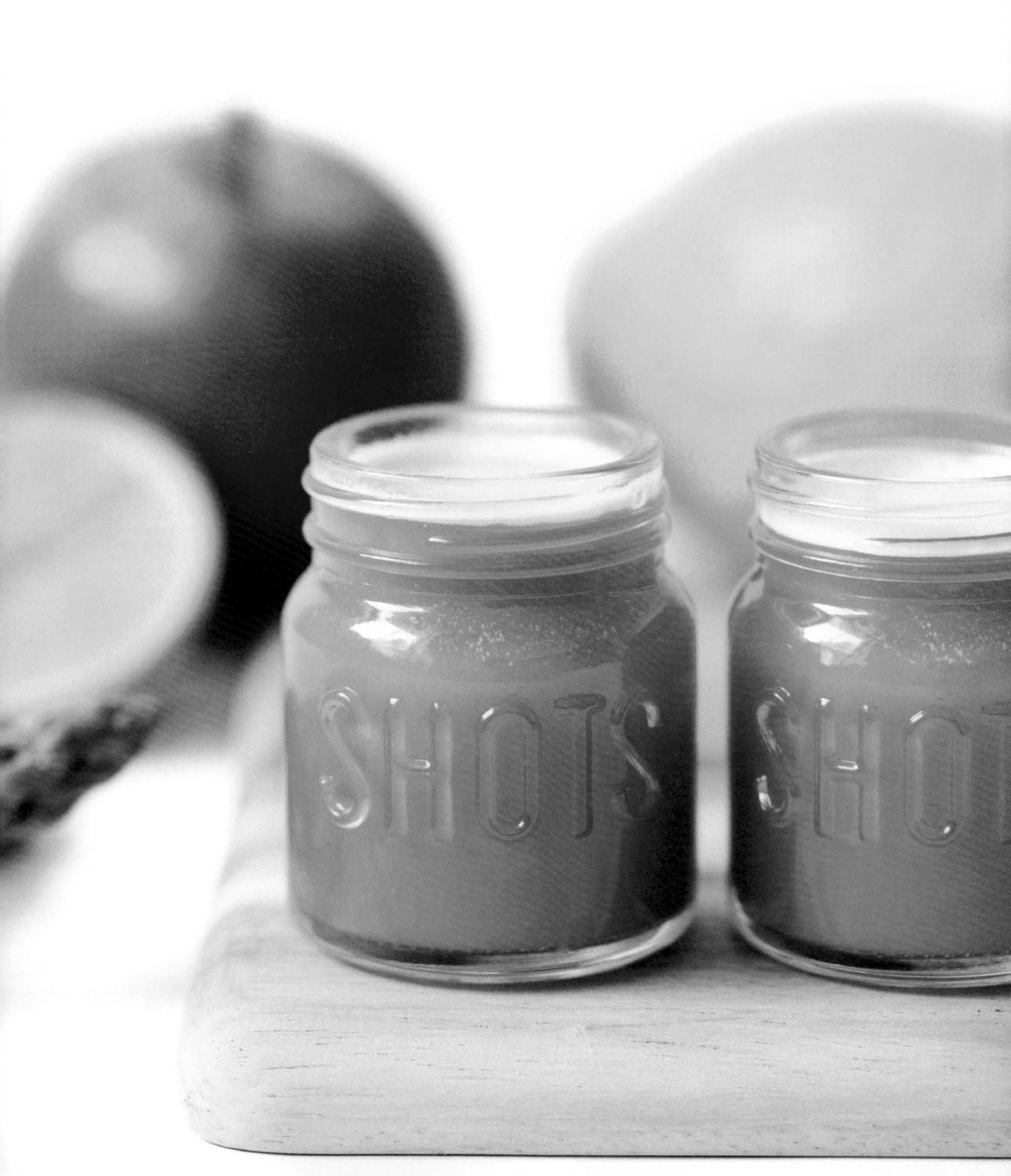

CHEM TRAILS EXPOSURE

Makes 1 to 2 shots

Turn to this shot if:

- You're an avid outdoor runner or walker on public streets, parks, or trails

- You spend time at the beach or sitting outside at gatherings and spot several chem trails in the sky at one time

- You spend time outdoors during a holiday when the weather is nice (chem trails are purposely increased on holidays such as Easter and the Fourth of July)

- You spend time swimming in the ocean, lakes, rivers, or ponds

- You sleep with the windows open at night

- You get caught in the rain or otherwise get a substantial amount of rainwater on your head or skin

1 tablespoon fresh or thawed frozen wild blueberries or 1 teaspoon pure wild blueberry juice or 1 teaspoon pure wild blueberry powder
¼ cup tightly packed kale
¼ lemon, peeled
½ cup tightly packed fresh cilantro
¼ cup tightly packed fresh chives
2 raw brussels sprouts
2 raw medium asparagus spears (¼ cup chopped)
½ stalk celery

Run each ingredient through a juicer in the order listed from top to bottom. If you are using the wild blueberry juice or wild blueberry powder, mix it in after all the other ingredients have run through the juicer.

Pour into a glass and serve.

TIPS

- If you're in a part of the world where you can't access fresh or frozen wild blueberries, wild blueberry juice, or wild blueberry powder, you can substitute blackberries. Although a high-antioxidant alternative, blackberries do not have the potency to match how wild blueberries defend cells from metals, chemicals, radiation, and other toxins.

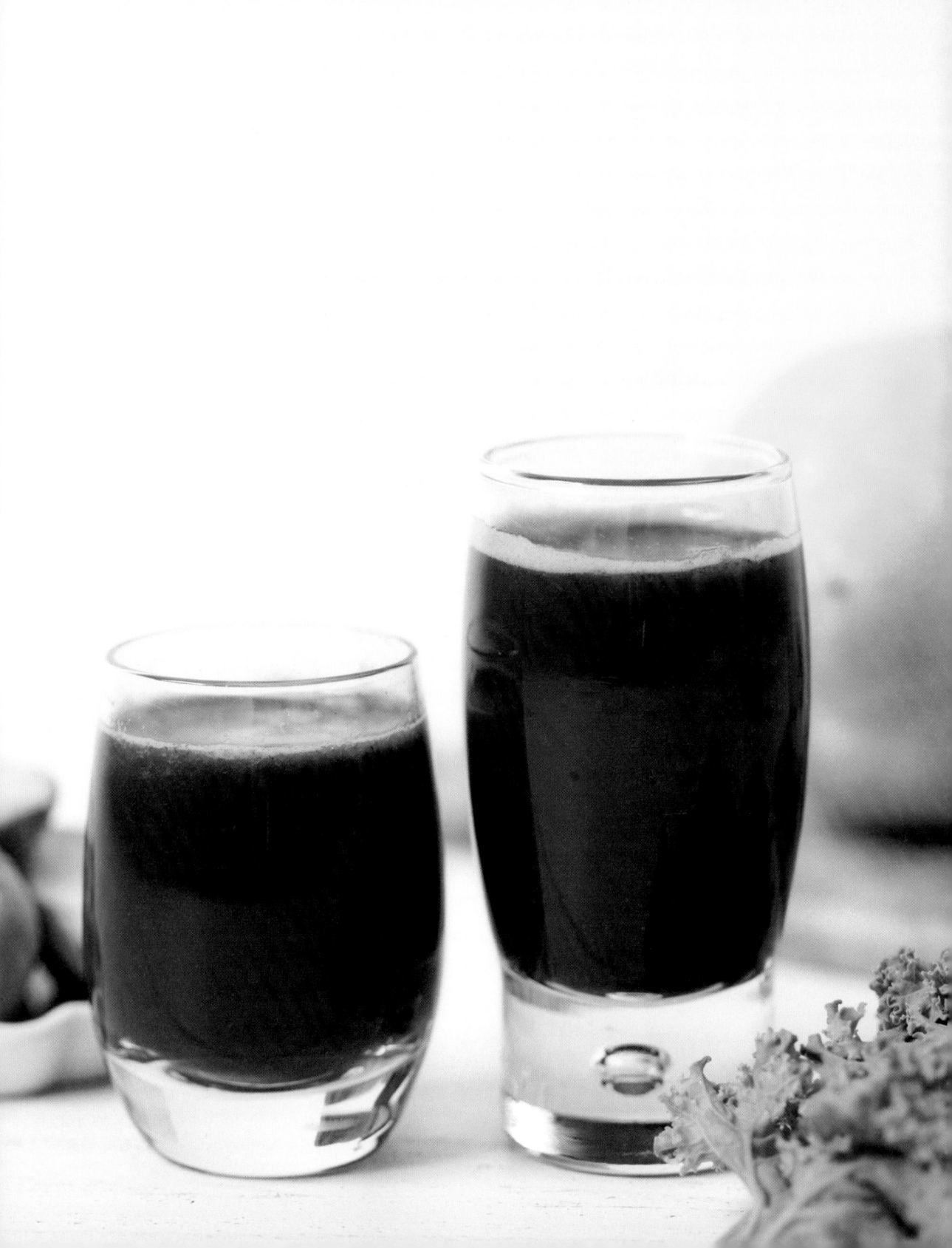

"Only when we join forces with our body's mission to protect our brain do we have the potential to save all the lives we want to protect—including our own."

— Anthony William, Medical Medium

Shifter Shots

The world is getting so complicated in so many ways, and we're being pushed in so many different directions, it's easy to get confused or stuck in a pattern that is not helpful to the healing process. These Brain Shots are designed to help shift our direction so our body can shift and heal and our emotional frame of mind can break a pattern or confinement that the complications of this world have created.

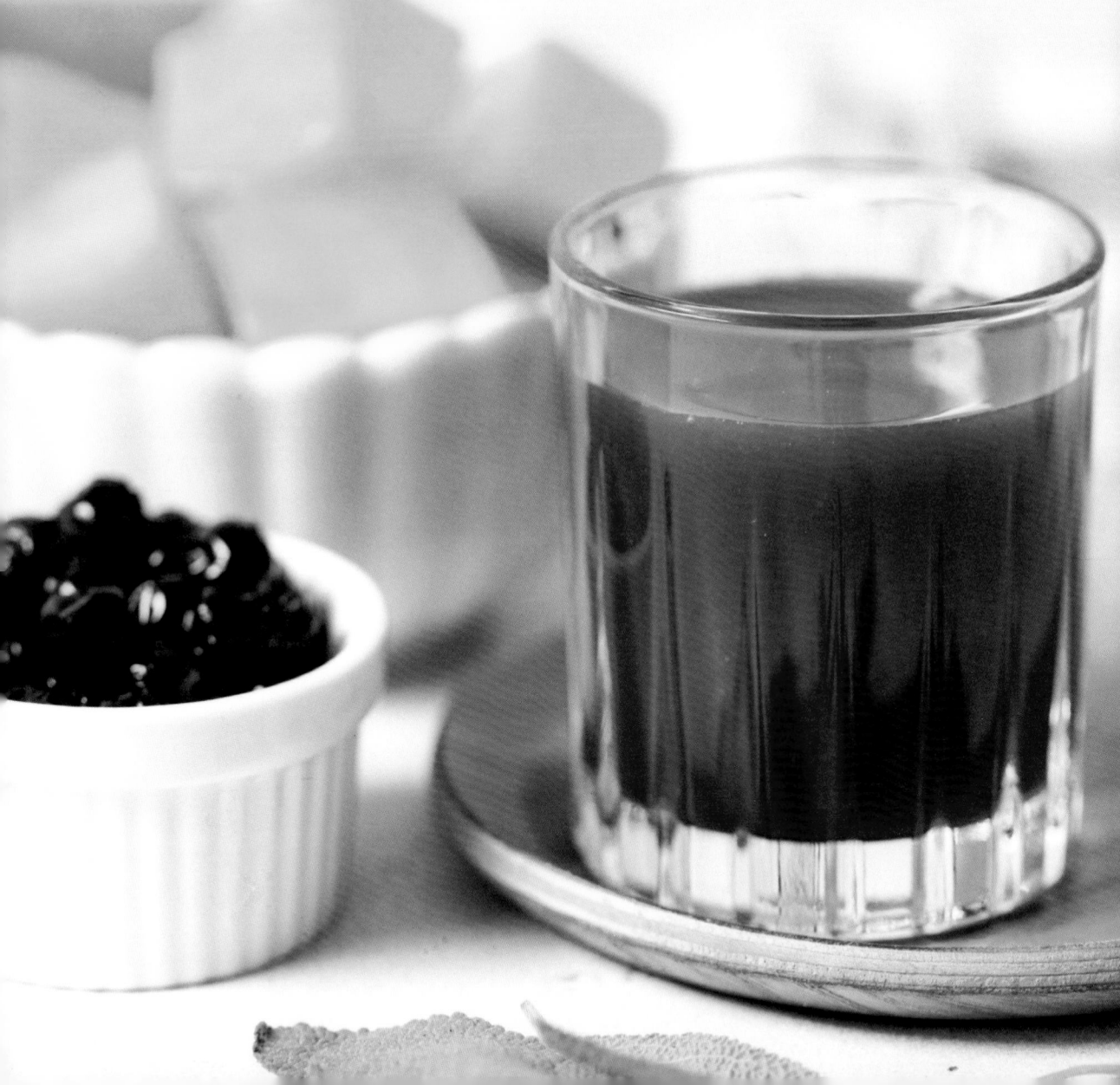

OBSESSIVE THOUGHTS SHIFTER

Try this shot when:

- You're trying to break repeated painful thought patterns resulting from a difficult situation or hardship

- You experience chronic OCD, or you're going through a relapse or heightening of OCD symptoms; this Brain Shot covers all forms and varieties of OCD

- A song you don't want to hear anymore keeps playing in your head

- Repetitive thoughts that are disturbing you continue to replay

- Repetitive thoughts are causing you to make repetitive actions

- You're hearing voices in your head or experiencing thoughts that are upsetting, unproductive, and/or highly questionable and may be telling you to do things that aren't good or smart

- A memory of a past experience keeps arising in your mind and it's not helpful to keep thinking about it

1 radish
⅛ cup loosely packed fresh sage (about 8 leaves)
½ to 1 apple
1 stalk celery

Run each ingredient through a juicer in the order listed from top to bottom.

Pour into a glass and serve.

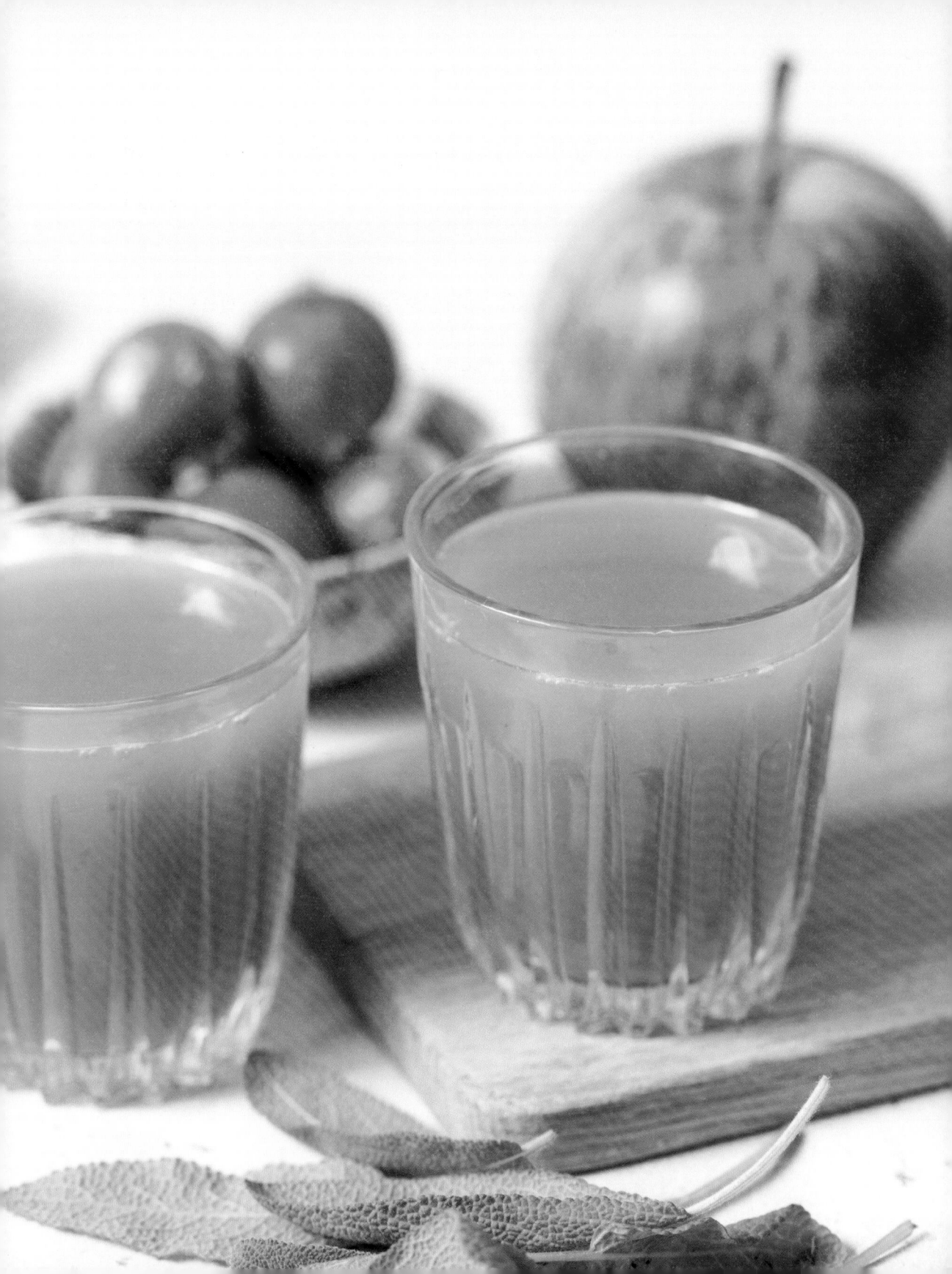

MOOD SHIFTER

This is a great shot for:

- Irritability, chronic frustration, or crankiness

- Feelings of overwhelm and emotional exhaustion

- When someone you trust notices you're not yourself

- When you're feeling gloomy, downhearted, or low-spirited and need a lift

- When you're having a hard time keeping balanced emotionally, feeling like you're unsteady, getting triggered easily, or all over the place, up and down

1 tablespoon fresh or thawed frozen wild blueberries or 1 teaspoon pure wild blueberry juice or 1 teaspoon pure wild blueberry powder
¼ cup tightly packed fresh chives
¼ cup tightly packed fresh basil
½ cup tightly packed fresh alfalfa sprouts
½ lime, peeled
1 stalk celery
½ cup grapes (optional)

Run each ingredient through a juicer in the order listed from top to bottom. If you are using the wild blueberry juice or wild blueberry powder, mix it in after all the other ingredients have run through the juicer.

Pour into a glass and serve.

TIPS

- If you're in a part of the world where you can't access fresh or frozen wild blueberries, wild blueberry juice, or wild blueberry powder, you can substitute blackberries. Although a high-antioxidant alternative, blackberries do not have the potency to match how wild blueberries defend cells from metals, chemicals, radiation, and other toxins.

- If you can't find or don't like alfalfa sprouts, you can use any kind of sprouts or microgreens in this recipe, such as broccoli, clover, sunflower, or kale. Every sprout will bring a different flavor to the shot. If you choose to use radish or mustard sprouts, be aware that it will make the shot very spicy.

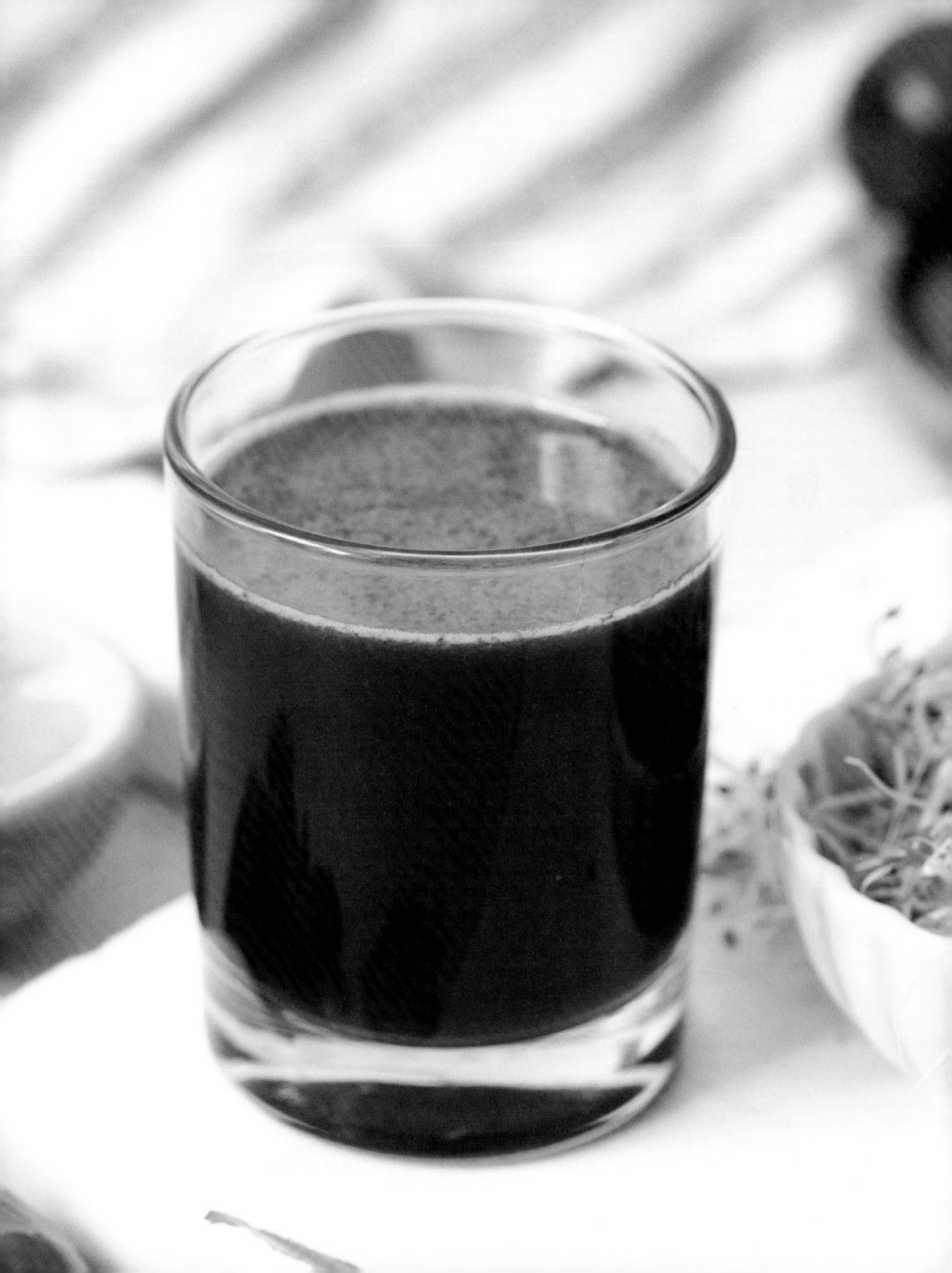

NERVE SHIFTER

This shot has a wide range of applications. Try it:

- When you're feeling shaky or anxious

- If you experience random spasms, twitches, tics, or shifting and moving pain throughout your body

- When struggling with any kind of neurological onset or episode

- To break a nervous feeling about the moment you're in, the future, or something that happened in the past

- To help calm restless legs syndrome

- Before flying or taking a trip

The Nerve Shifter is also an excellent tool to use for weddings and other events that have great meaning to you.

¼ lime, peeled
¼ cup tightly packed spinach
¼ cup roughly chopped kale, tightly packed
¼ cup roughly chopped lettuce, such as green leaf or butter leaf, tightly packed
¼ cup tightly packed fresh cilantro
¼ cup tightly packed fresh parsley
2 raw medium stalks asparagus (¼ cup chopped)
½ stalk celery

Run each ingredient through a juicer in the order listed from top to bottom.

Pour into a glass and serve.

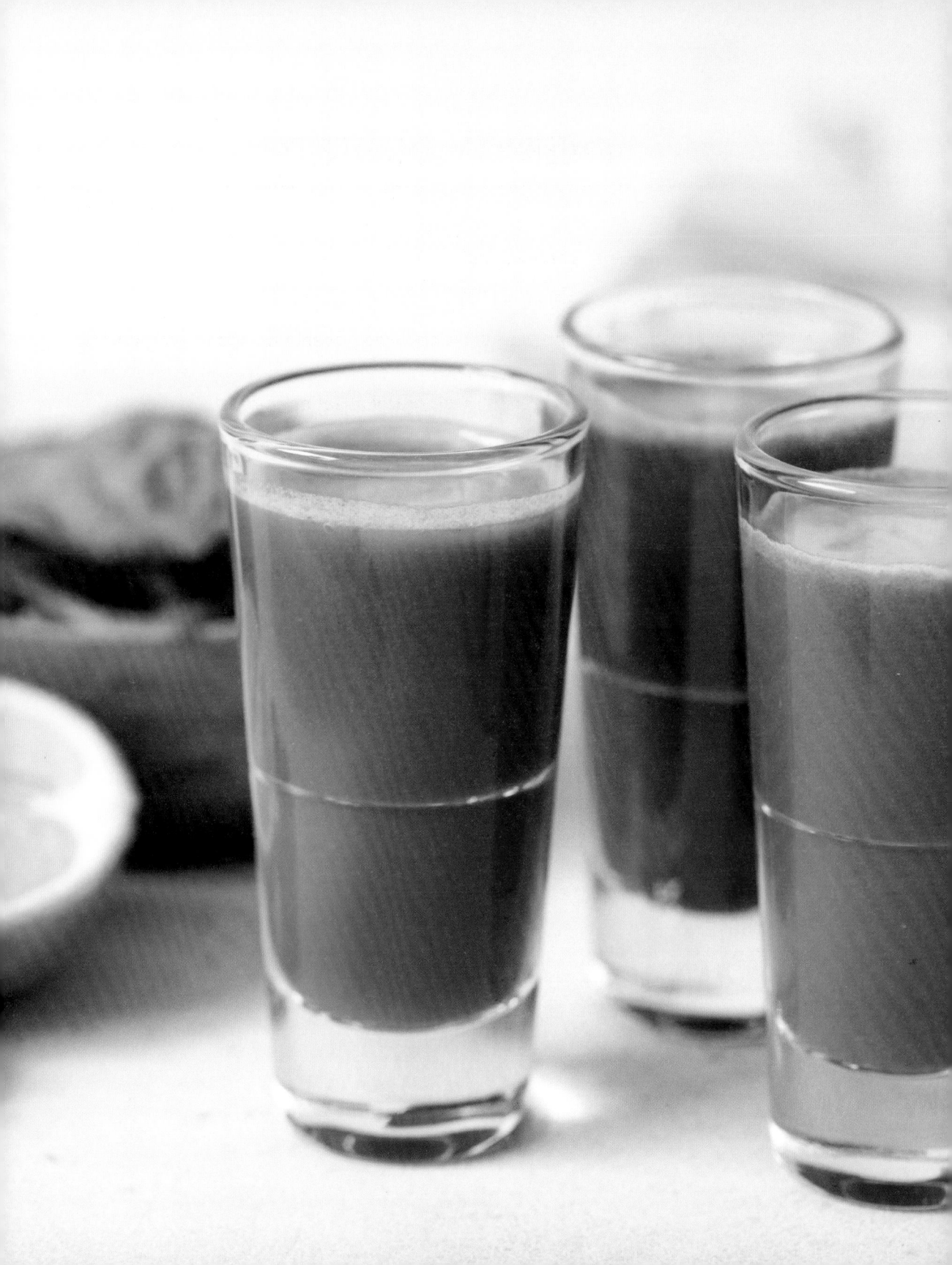

ENERGY SHIFTER

Use this shot when energetic strength is required. For example, you can try it:

- At the midpoint of a long day, when you're desperate for an energy boost

- When you feel unbalanced, as if you don't have enough energy

- If you're feeling that your energy is "off" and you're not on point

- If you feel like you have too much energy, and you're hoping to calm down an elevation of excitement

- When removing caffeine from your life

- When you want to wind down at the end of the day so you can recalibrate, rest, and retire for the night

The Energy Shifter is also ideal for:

- Overreactive or underreactive adrenals that are exhausted from excessive adrenal output

- Low blood sugar (hypoglycemia) sensations such as edginess, exhaustion, feeling emotional for unexplained reasons, or starting to get triggered easily

Try the Energy Shifter before going into a challenge or venture of any kind, whether beginning a new job, going on a retreat, starting a cleanse, or anything else shifting in your life.

¼ cup chopped carrots
½ cup chopped raw sweet potatoes
½ cup chopped red bell pepper
½ cup fresh or thawed frozen pineapple

Run each ingredient through a juicer in the order listed from top to bottom.

Pour into a glass and serve.

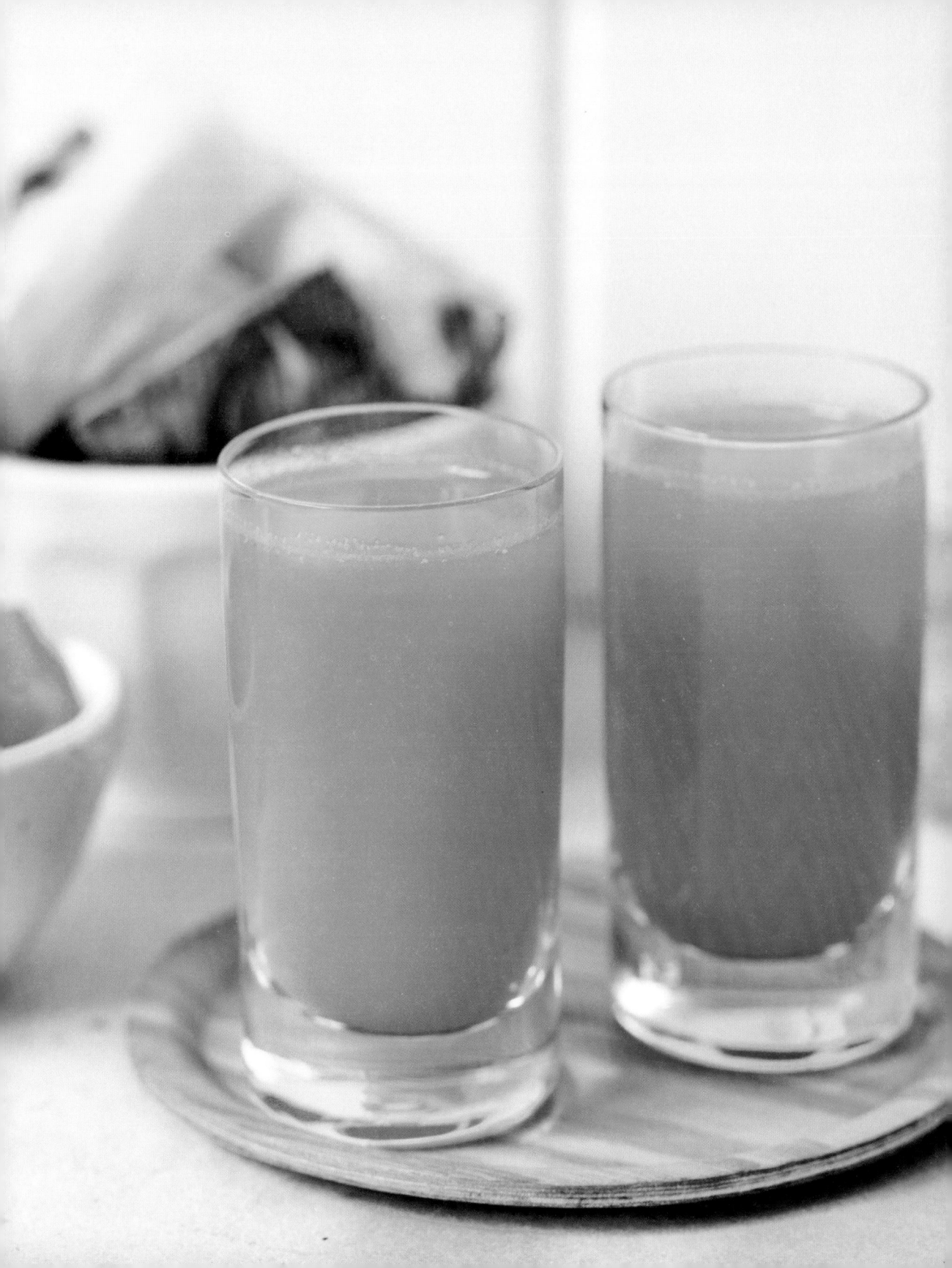

FOOD FEAR SHIFTER

Makes 1 to 2 shots

Food fear can take different shapes and forms. For example, apply this shot on a regular basis if you're living with an eating disorder. The Food Fear Shifter is also a useful tool when:

- Someone is pressuring you not to eat healthily

- You're upset about what you've been eating lately

- You're feeling locked up about food in general, afraid to eat because you're having trouble figuring out what foods you can eat comfortably without flaring up symptoms such as digestive discomfort

- You're experiencing other symptoms or conditions, and you're afraid of changing your diet to heal

- Someone wants you to eat healthily, yet you're afraid of fruits, herbs, leafy greens, wild foods, and vegetables

- You have an unexplained dislike or fear of certain foods that are healthy

- You have a fear of food that derives from misinformation about specific foods

- You're having a hard time letting go of a comfort food that's harming you

½ cup tightly packed fresh dill
½ cup tightly packed spinach
¾ cup fresh or thawed frozen mango
¼ stalk celery

Run each ingredient through a juicer in the order listed from top to bottom.

Pour into a glass and serve.

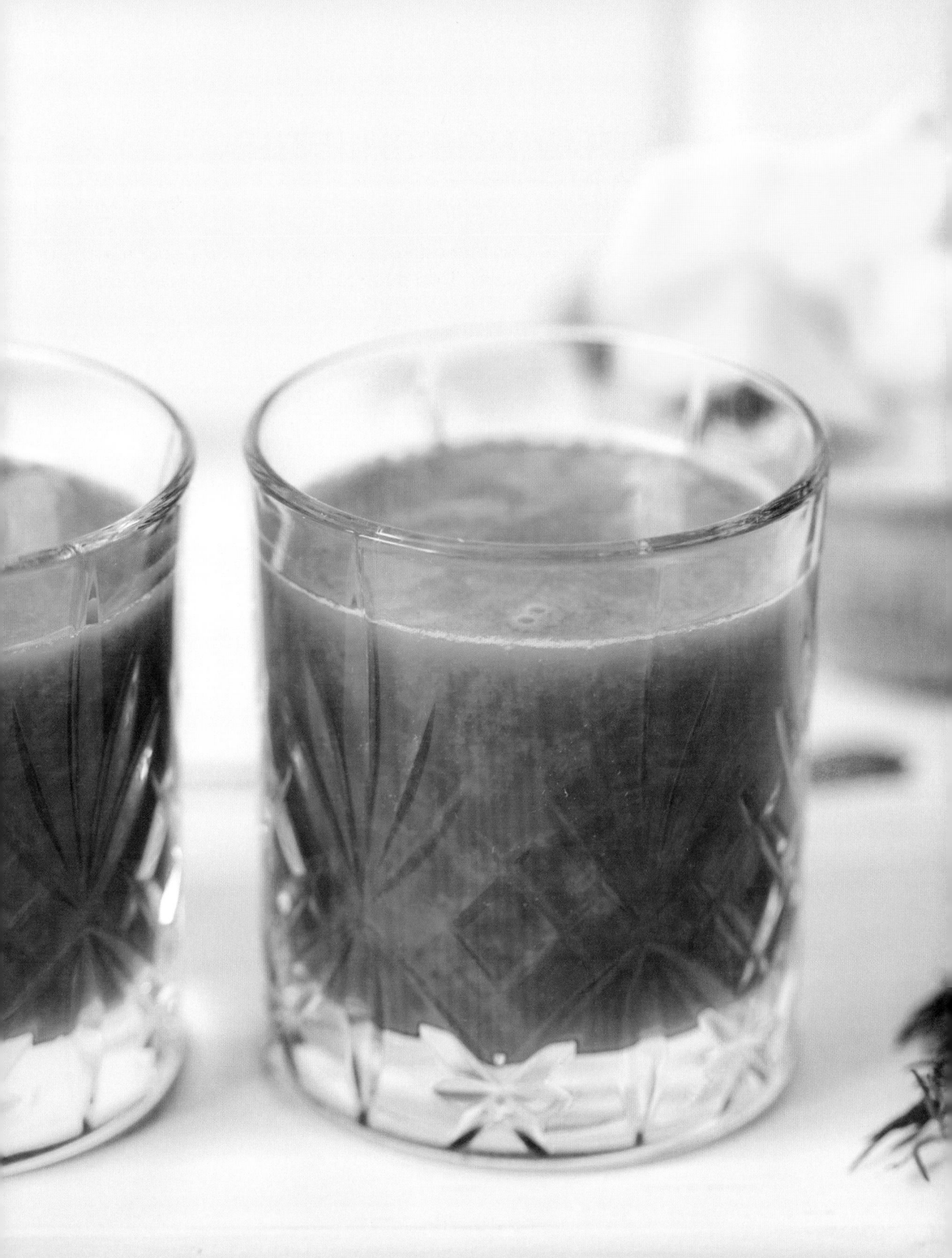

CRAVINGS SHIFTER

When cravings or addictive impulses are disrupting your life, this shot is a great tool. Try it:

- For hunger that feels insatiable or unstoppable

- As a craving buster

- As a hunger suppressant when you're trying to shift your diet

- If your diet is too high in fat and you're trying to reduce the amount of fat you're consuming

- To help break overeating patterns, food addictions, or even caffeine and salt addictions

If someone in your life is embarking on an unhealthy intermittent fasting diet, encourage them to incorporate this shot to help protect their adrenals and brain.

½-inch piece of fresh ginger
¼ cup tightly packed fresh basil
½ cup tightly packed spinach
½ cup chopped kale, tightly packed
½ cup chopped cabbage, any color, tightly packed
½ orange, peeled
½ stalk celery

Run each ingredient through a juicer in the order listed from top to bottom.

Pour into a glass and serve.

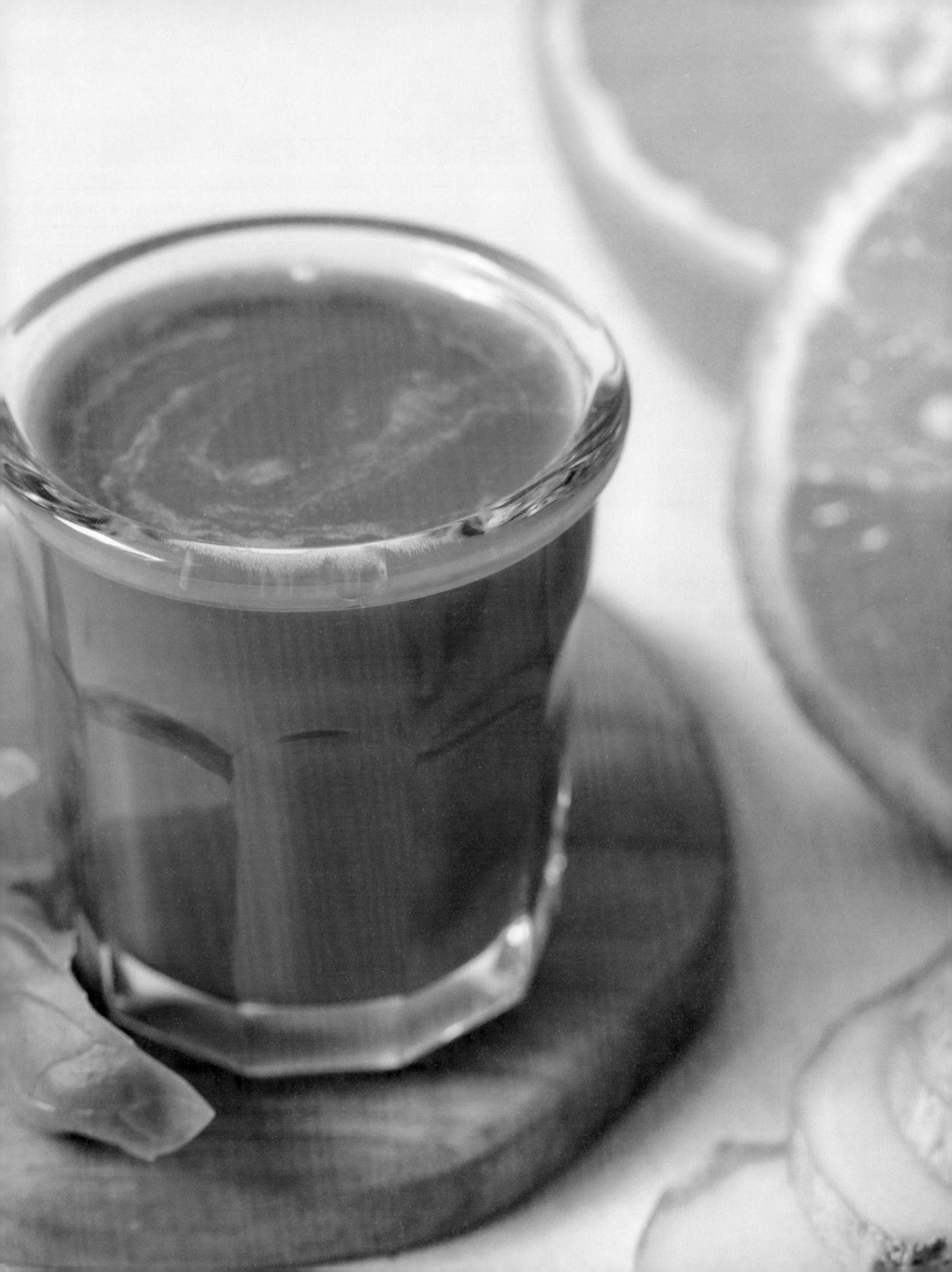

ANGER SHIFTER

Use this shot for:

- Unexplained bouts of anger or anger surges that seem to arise without cause

- Anger surges that do have a cause

- Anger about being sick, injured, or dealing with health problems and chronic illness

- Moments of unhappiness, frustration, or irritability that bubble up from inside

- Anger that's triggered from being wronged in any way, such as from disappointment or betrayal

- Confrontations or disputes with others

- Anger about world events

- Anger at yourself

½ cup tightly packed fresh mint
¼ cup tightly packed fresh sage
½ cup fresh or thawed frozen mango
1 tablespoon fresh or thawed frozen wild blueberries or 1 teaspoon pure wild blueberry juice or 1 teaspoon pure wild blueberry powder
1 cup chopped carrots

Run each ingredient through a juicer in the order listed from top to bottom. If you are using the wild blueberry juice or wild blueberry powder, mix it in after all the other ingredients have run through the juicer.

Pour into a glass and serve.

TIPS

- If you're in a part of the world where you can't access fresh or frozen wild blueberries, wild blueberry juice, or wild blueberry powder, you can substitute blackberries. Although a high-antioxidant alternative, blackberries do not have the potency to match how wild blueberries defend cells from metals, chemicals, radiation, and other toxins.

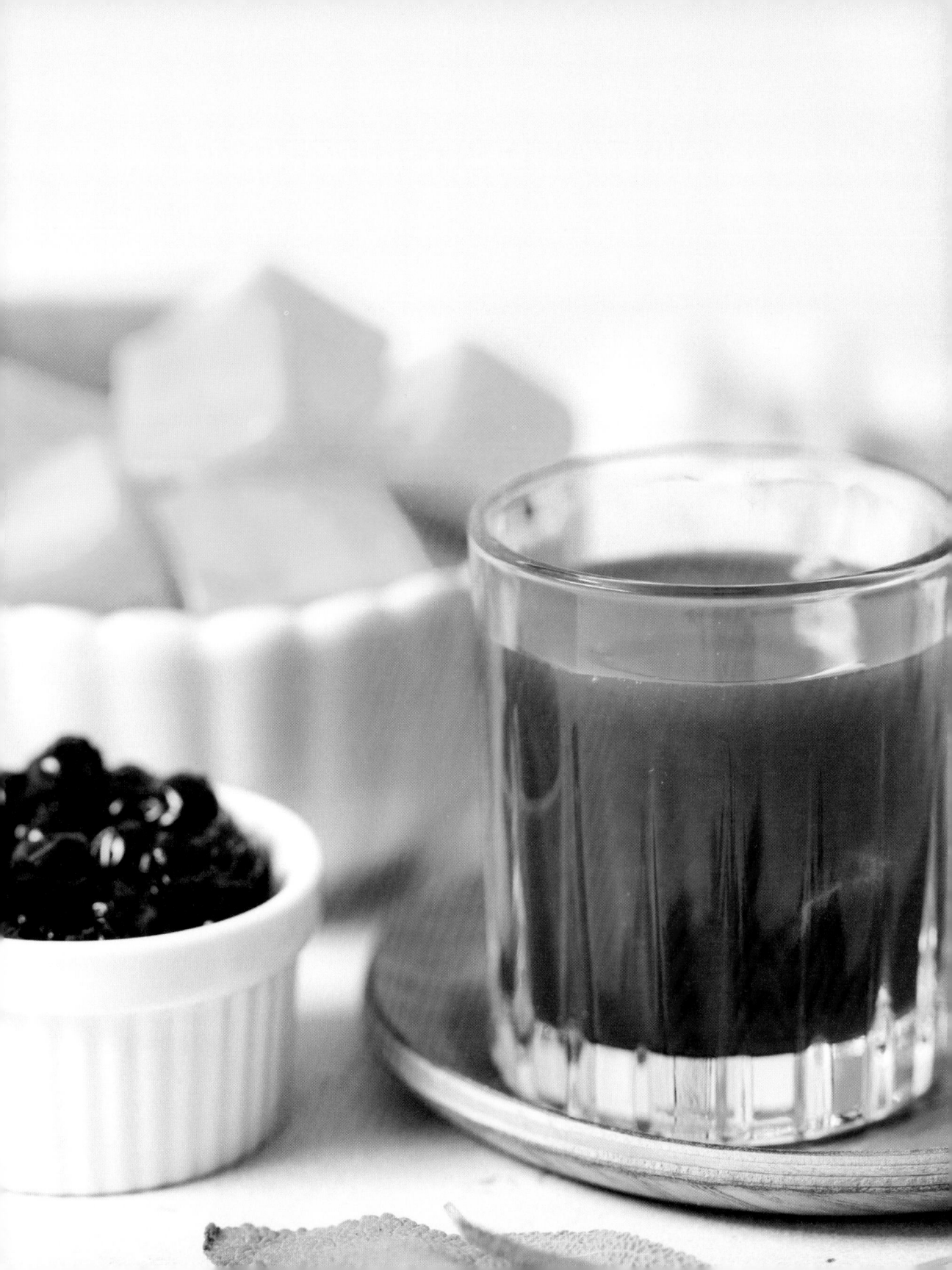

GUILT AND SHAME SHIFTER

Makes 1 to 2 shots

Try applying this shot when:

- You don't believe in yourself or you've lost confidence in yourself
- You're losing faith that you're a good person
- You're feeling guilt or shame about being sick
- You experience insecurity or loss of confidence due to chronic illness
- You're feeling less-than or like you are not good enough
- You can't forgive yourself for something you may believe was your fault
- You're feeling guilt or shame about something you said and can't unsay
- You're feeling guilt or shame about not being able to live your dream yet
- You're feeling guilt or shame about not being able to help a friend or family member in the present moment
- You're having difficulty forgiving someone else who has hurt you, upset you, or disappointed you
- You're feeling ashamed or guilty in any way—this shot can help you understand and release emotional wounds that are perpetuating guilt or shame

½-inch piece of fresh ginger
½ to 1 cup tightly packed spinach
½ to 1 orange, peeled

Run each ingredient through a juicer in the order listed from top to bottom.

Pour into a glass and serve.

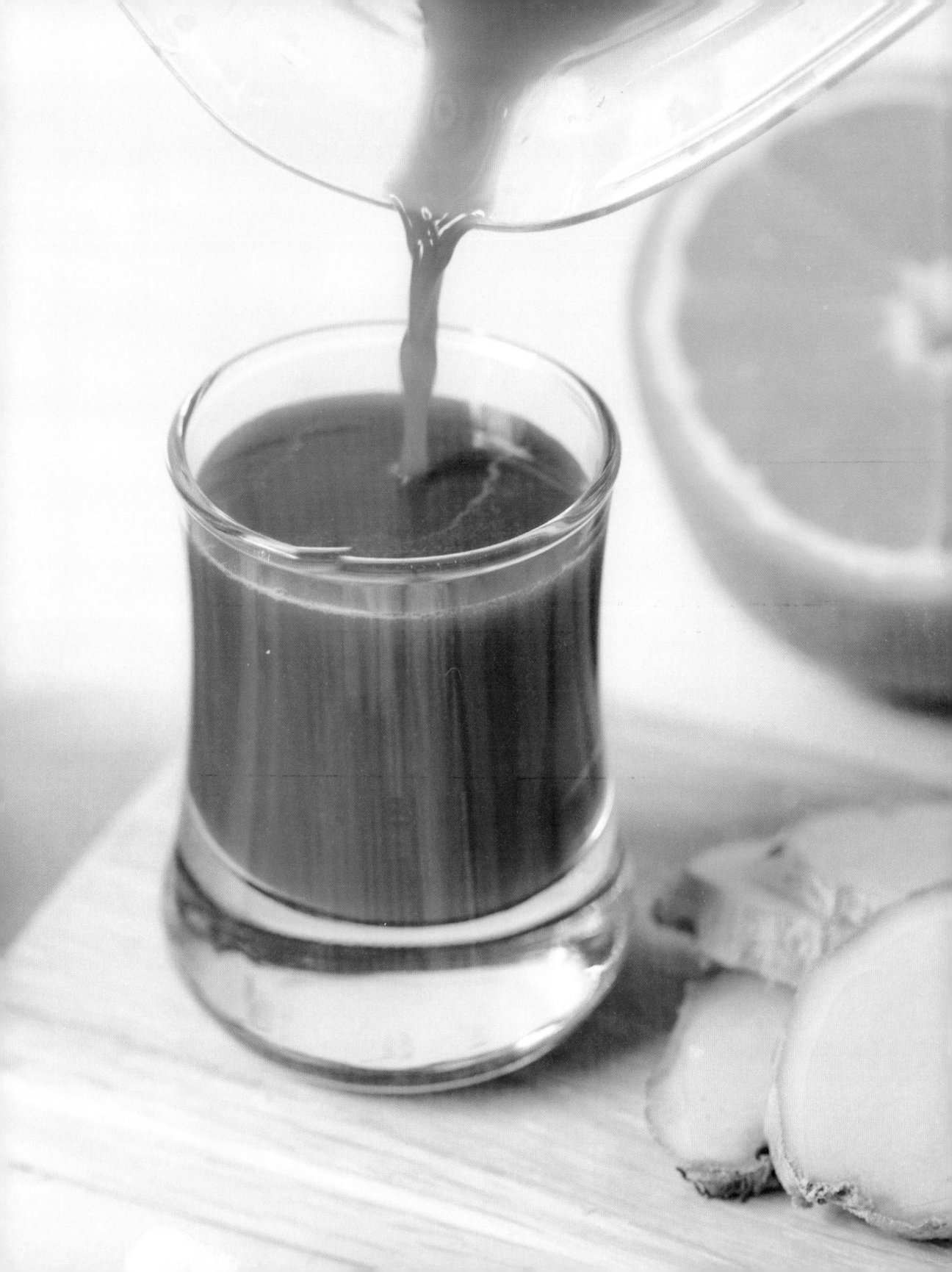

EGO SHIFTER

This shot is ideal in those moments when:

- You feel like your ego has taken over your senses, or your common sense and sensibility
- You feel like you're losing your true self, losing sight of what's truly important
- You feel like you may have been a little too self-absorbed
- You realize you've been completely self-consumed without caring for others
- You feel as if something inside of you is controlling your life and decisions while you watch from above
- You have a friend or loved one who has a very large ego and doesn't believe they do (make the Brain Shot for them)
- You feel you need to take control of your life and override the drive to harm yourself
- You need to free yourself so your authentic soul shines through and benefits you and the ones around you

½-inch piece of fresh turmeric
½ cup chopped peeled kiwi fruit
1 tablespoon fresh or thawed frozen wild blueberries or 1 teaspoon pure wild blueberry juice or 1 teaspoon pure wild blueberry powder
¼ cup chopped portobello mushroom*
¼ cup tightly packed, roughly chopped kale
½ cup tightly packed fresh parsley
½ stalk celery

Run each ingredient through a juicer in the order listed from top to bottom. If using the wild blueberry juice or wild blueberry powder, mix it in after all the other ingredients have run through the juicer. Pour into a glass and serve.

*Wash and rinse the portobello mushroom thoroughly with warm to hot water before chopping. Do not use a slimy or decaying mushroom. That's a sign of the mushroom oxidizing and aging.

TIPS

- If you're in a part of the world where you can't access any form of wild blueberries, you can substitute blackberries. Although a high-antioxidant alternative, blackberries do not have the potency to match how wild blueberries defend cells from toxins.

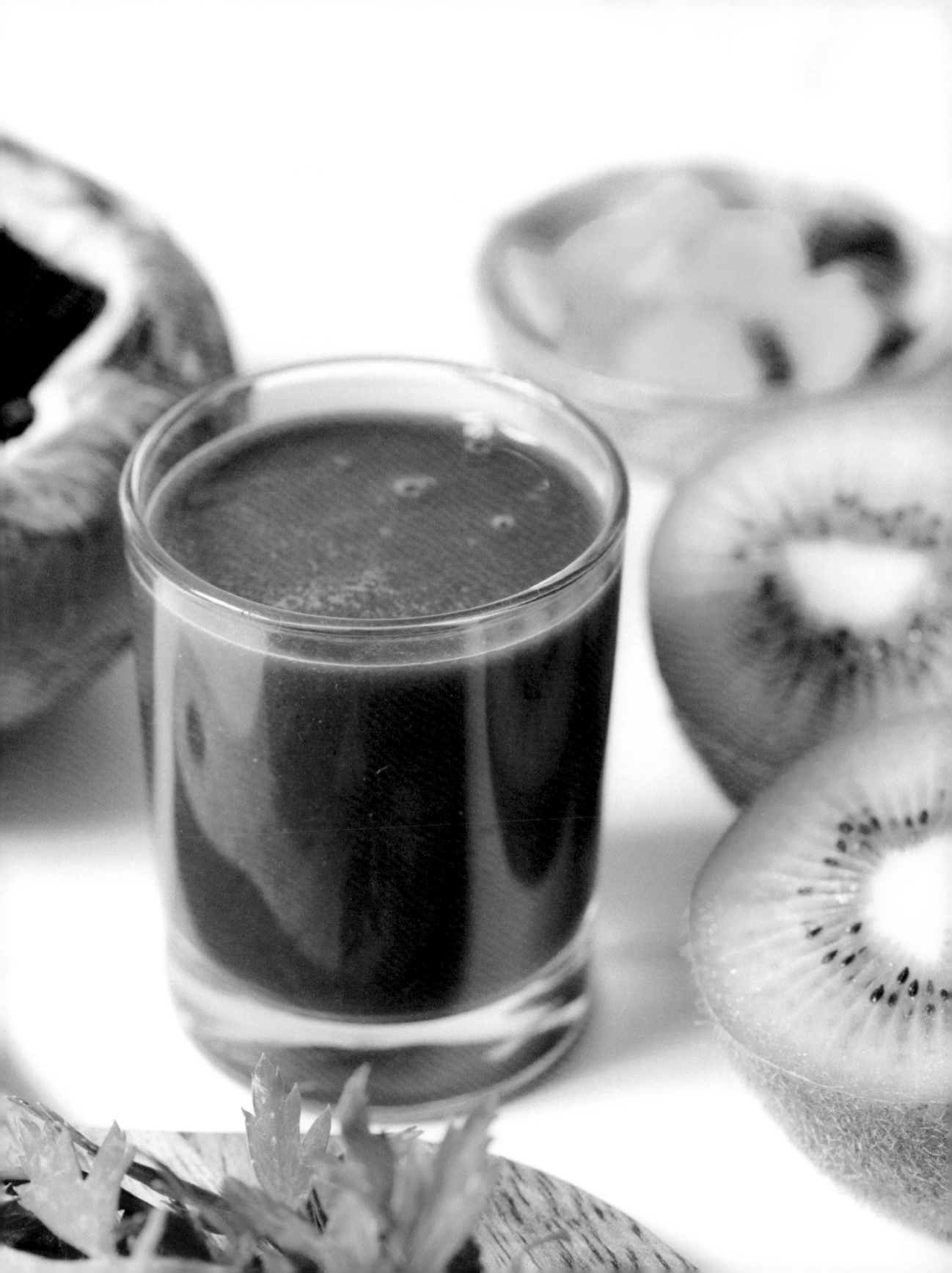

DREAMS SHIFTER

This shot can be taken at any time of day or evening. If you wish to take it before a nap or before bed, you're welcome to make the shot earlier in the day and save it in the refrigerator until you're ready. Examples of when to use it include when:

- You want to use your dreams as a gateway to understand your soul and your soul's past

- You're having difficulty dreaming and want to dream

- Your dreams are troubling, very stressful, or even frightening

- You want to decode the meaning of your dreams and gain more insight into your dreams

- Dreams are regularly waking you

- You're fearful of going to sleep

- You're trying to reach others through your dreams

- You're trying to enter other people's dreams

- You're not sleeping enough—this shot can help you heal through your dream process in the short amount of sleep you're getting

½-inch piece of fresh ginger
½ cup fresh or thawed frozen mango
½ cup fresh or thawed frozen cherries, pitted
½ cup chopped raw zucchini
¼ cup loosely packed fresh peppermint leaves (optional)

Run each ingredient through a juicer in the order listed from top to bottom.

Pour into a glass and serve.

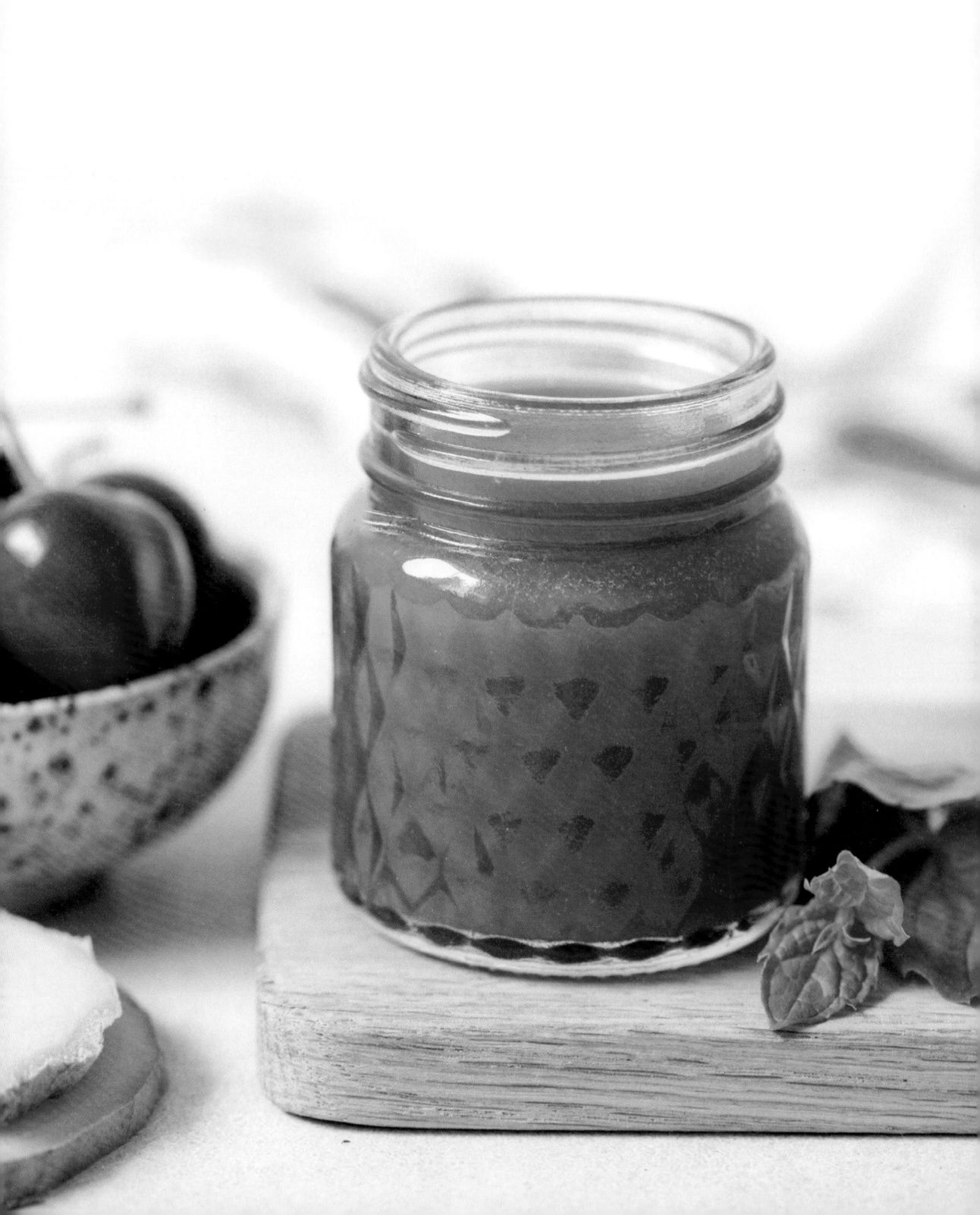

"Any kind of impediment within a person's neurons can mean that the information their neurons process gets altered, affecting that person's ability to focus, listen, or properly receive information from a conversation or story.

When you understand your brain as a group of neurons, you have a greater chance of finding relief from your brain-related symptoms and conditions, healing your brain, and getting in touch with your brain on all kinds of levels."

— Anthony William, Medical Medium

Stabilizer Shots

These Brain Shots are designed to stabilize you in an increasingly destabilizing world.

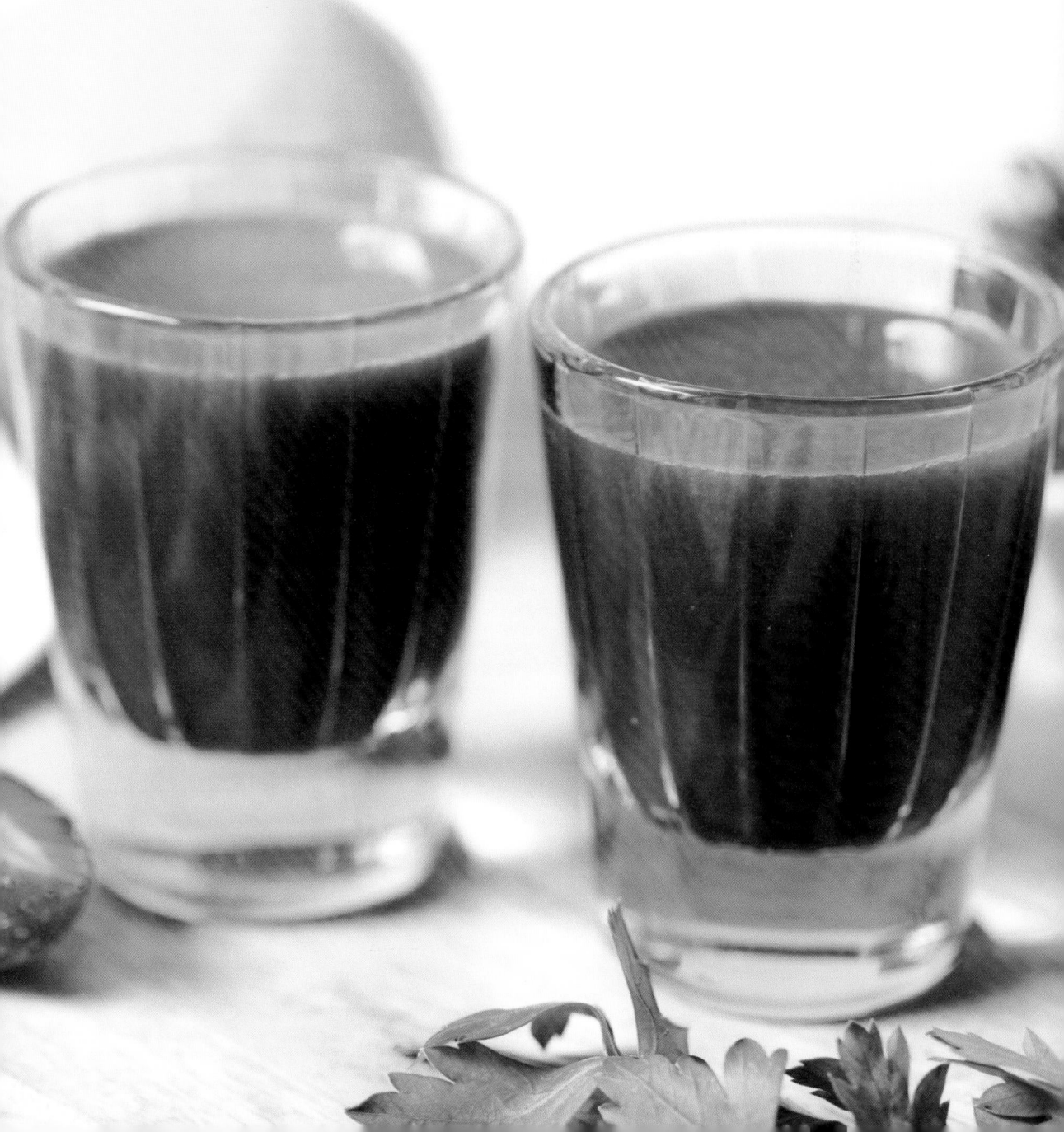

NERVE-GUT ACID STABILIZER

Makes 1 to 2 shots

Use this stabilizing shot if:

- You're looking to strengthen your vagus nerves

- You're dealing with gastric spasms, flatulence, chronic gastritis, mild acid reflux, or other digestive disturbances (for acute acid reflux relief, see "Aloe Vera Shock Therapy" in this book's companion title, *Brain Saver Protocols, Cleanses & Recipes*)

- You feel your food is not digesting, breaking down, or assimilating

- You feel you have poor nutrient absorption

- You've been told you have a microbiome or gut microflora condition or problem

- You feel as if you're toxic, or your blood is toxic

- You feel that your liver and lymph are toxic, stagnant, and sluggish

- You're feeling an acidy stomach, acidy sensations in your throat or mouth, or acidy feelings throughout your body

- Your body odor is more noticeable than usual

- You're dealing with chronic nausea or chronic bloating

- You're trying to repair acidic body systems and make your body systems more alkaline

4 to 6 cups tightly packed fresh parsley or fresh cilantro*

Run the parsley or cilantro through the juicer.

Pour into a glass and serve immediately.

*Note: Select either parsley or cilantro (not both at once) to create either a pure parsley or pure cilantro shot.

TIPS

- You can use any variety of parsley for this recipe, flat-leaf Italian or curly parsley.

- Fresh cilantro is also known as coriander in some countries.

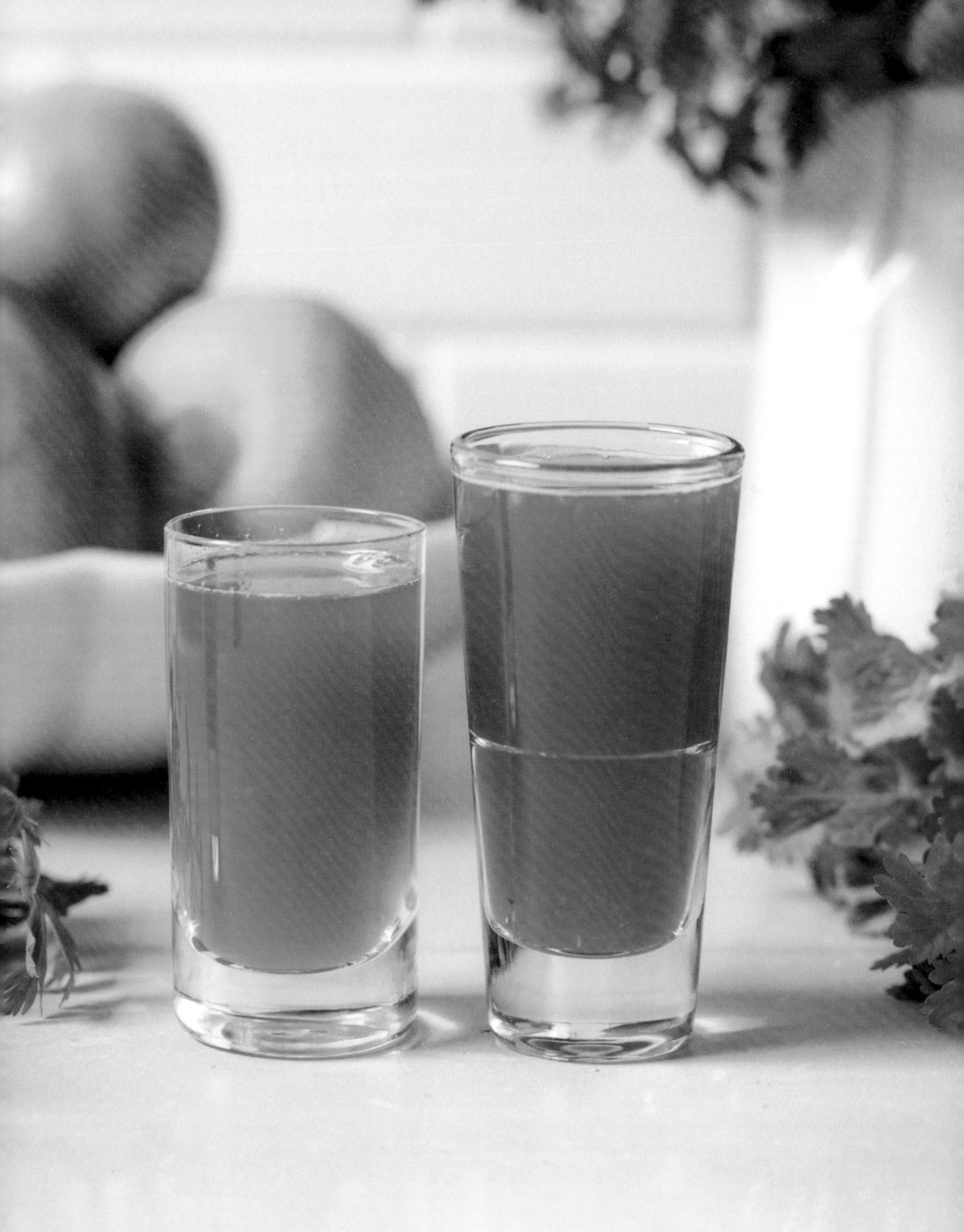

TRAUMA, SHOCK, AND LOSS STABILIZER

Makes 1 to 2 shots

This shot is a supportive tool for any kind of emotional upset, emotional challenge, or emotional stress. Consider using it when:

- You're given challenging news or you receive any emotional blows
- You're dealing with any kind of emotional upheaval
- You've lost a loved one or a pet
- You experience any kind of loss
- You've been diagnosed with a chronic illness or you learn something challenging about your health
- Local and world events are affecting your life
- You're going through emotional turmoil within your family or difficult friendships

½ cup fresh or thawed frozen cherries, pitted
1 cup tightly packed spinach
½ apple

Run each ingredient through a juicer in the order listed from top to bottom.

Pour into a glass and serve.

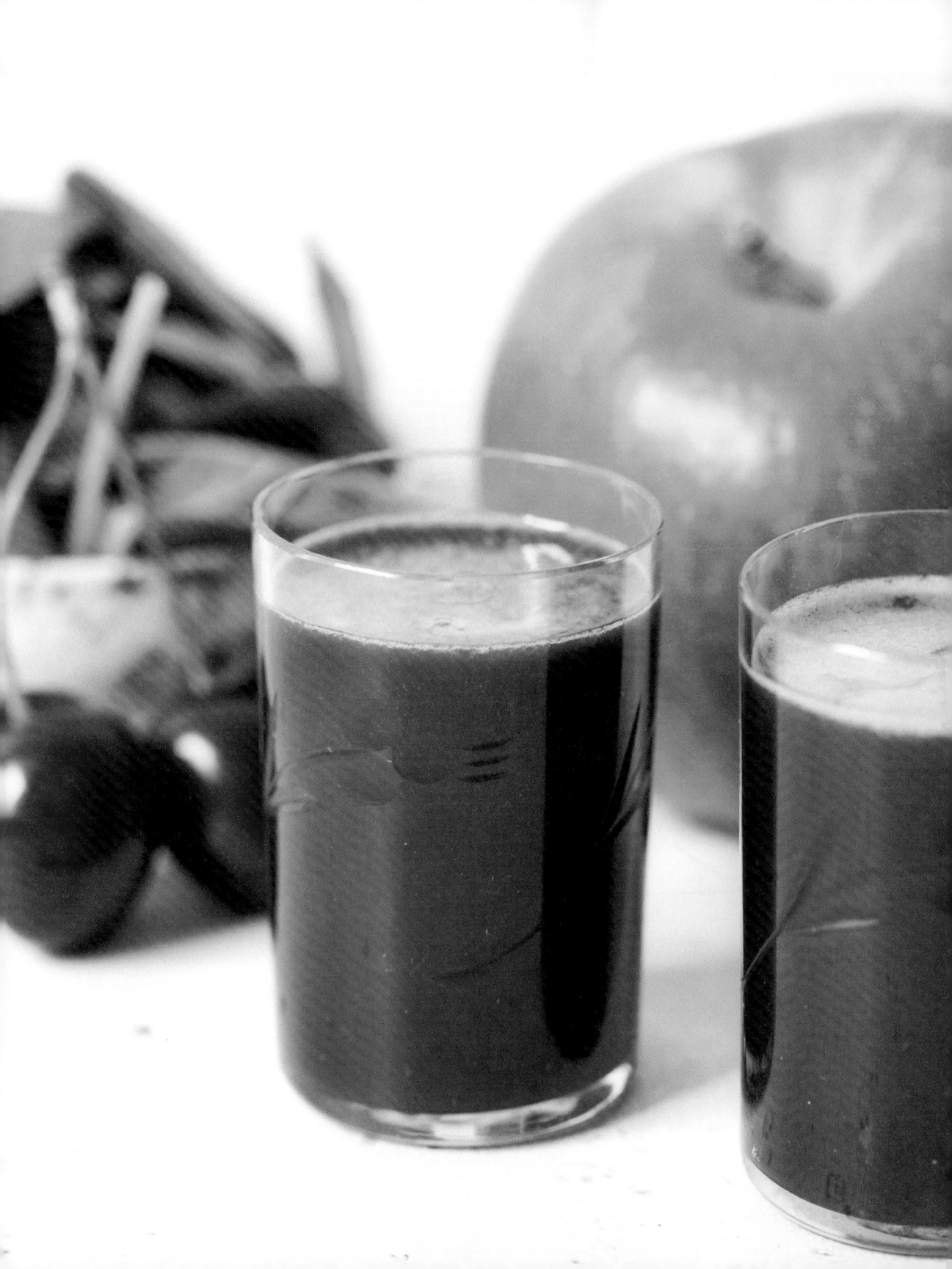

ADRENAL FIGHT OR FLIGHT STABILIZER

Try this shot when:

- Stress is dominating your life and you're not getting a chance to have a break or reprieve from whatever you're up against

- Continual, chronic stress is occurring

- You feel involuntary reactions when receiving any kind of news or information from various people and sources

- You're experiencing any type of PTSD

- You feel like you're on a roller coaster ride and have lost control of your life

- You're addicted to adrenalized activities or drama

- You've been using sex as an escape

- You're living on adrenaline without realizing it, such as with intermittent fasting and/or caffeine use

1-inch piece of fresh ginger
1 small garlic clove
2 tablespoons fresh or thawed frozen wild blueberries or 2 teaspoons pure wild blueberry juice or 2 teaspoons pure wild blueberry powder
½ lemon, peeled
1 cup tightly packed fresh parsley
½ cup tightly packed kale
1 cup chopped watermelon rind (optional)

Run each ingredient through a juicer in the order listed from top to bottom. If using the wild blueberry juice or wild blueberry powder, mix it in after all the other ingredients have run through the juicer.

Pour into a glass and serve.

TIPS

- If you're in a part of the world where you can't access any form of wild blueberries, you can substitute blackberries. Although a high-antioxidant alternative, blackberries do not have the potency to match how wild blueberries defend cells from toxins.

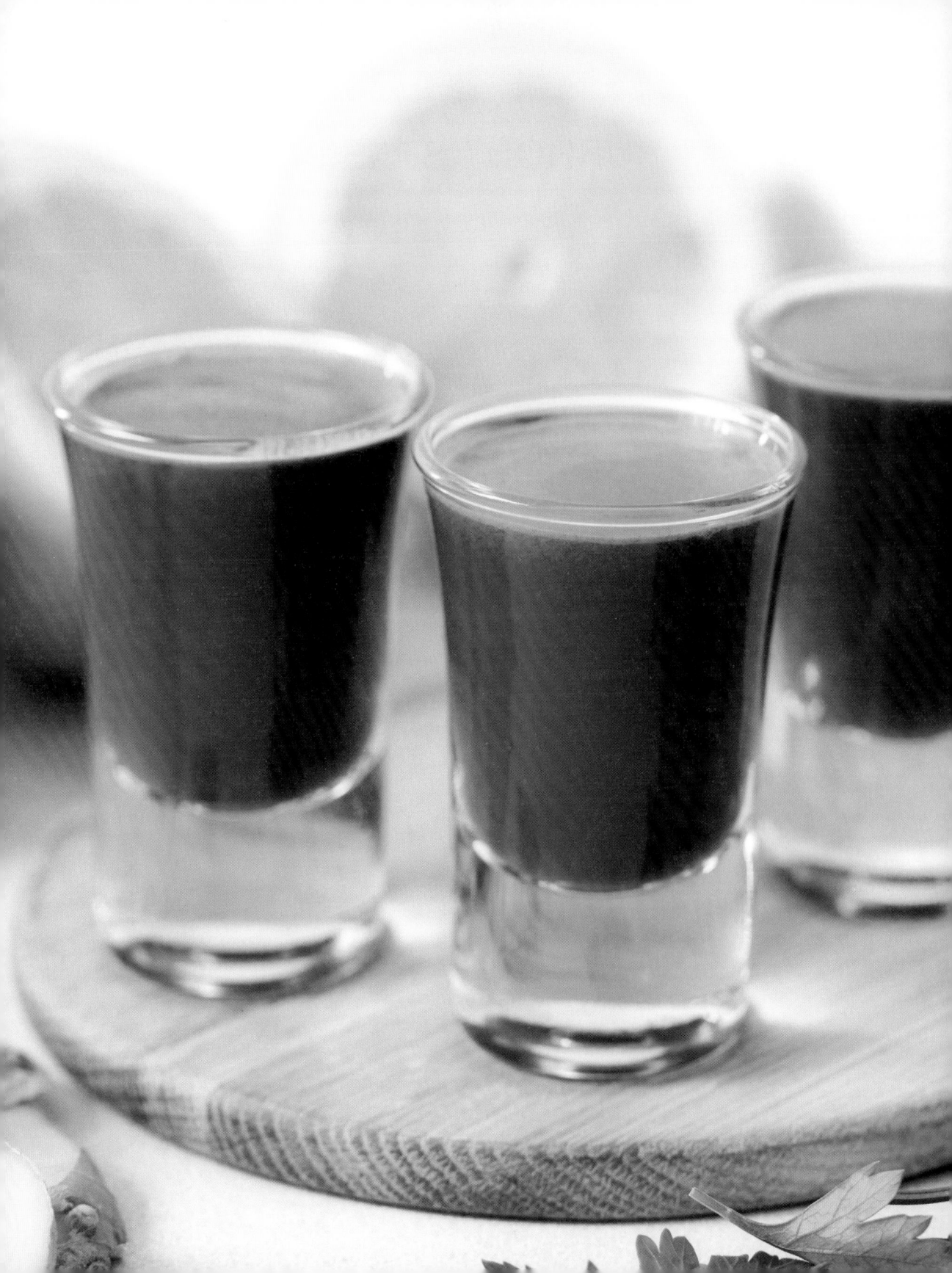

BURNOUT STABILIZER

Use this shot when:

- You're feeling pushed past your limit
- You need a recharge
- You feel like you're missing something that your body needs, or you feel like you're running on empty
- You've given so much of yourself that you feel you have nothing more to give
- You're overworked
- You've been running on caffeine to gain focus and energy
- You feel you're short-circuiting or falling apart
- You're becoming allergic to work or allergic to others around you
- You feel like you're losing or missing a part of yourself
- You can't seem to focus because you feel exhausted on all levels

½-inch piece of fresh ginger
½ cup tightly packed pea shoots
½ cup tightly packed alfalfa sprouts
¼ cup fresh or thawed frozen pitaya (red dragon fruit) or ¼ cup peeled and chopped grapefruit
2 raw medium stalks asparagus (¼ cup chopped)
½ stalk celery

Run each ingredient through a juicer in the order listed from top to bottom.

Pour into a glass and serve.

TIPS

- If you can't find or don't like alfalfa sprouts or pea shoots, you can use any kind of sprouts or microgreens in this recipe, such as broccoli, clover, sunflower, and kale. Every sprout will bring a different flavor to the shot. If you choose to use radish or mustard sprouts, be aware that it will make the shot very spicy.

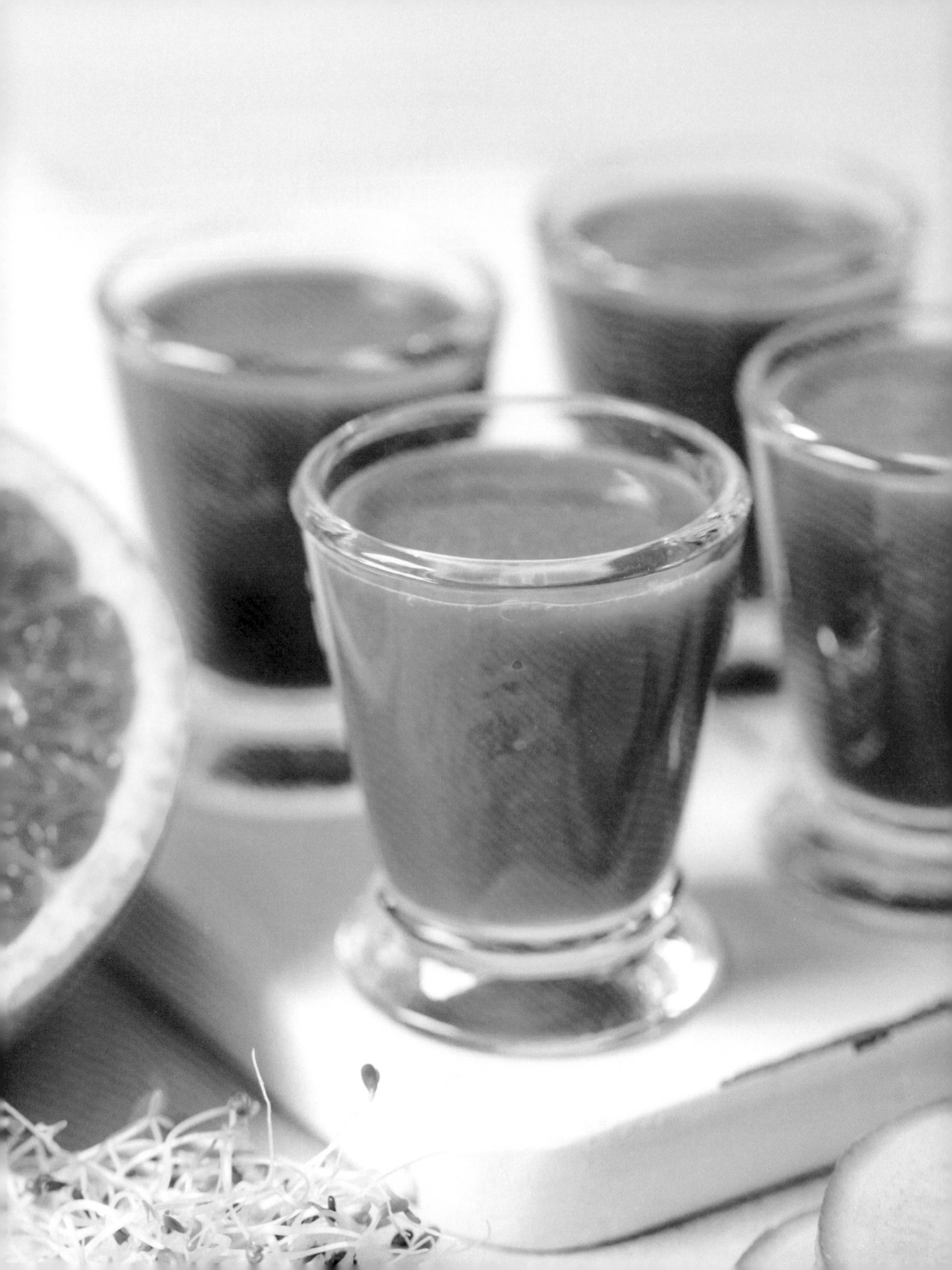

BETRAYAL AND BROKEN TRUST STABILIZER

This tool provides support in situations where:

- You feel emotionally toyed with, played with, or not taken seriously

- You've been told your body has betrayed you

- You feel betrayed, let down, neglected, overlooked, used, or mistreated in any way

- You have been manipulated

- Someone or something you placed trust in falls through, lets you down, or disappoints you

- You feel you've let down someone you care about

- You have your heart set on something, and it doesn't come to fruition

½-inch piece of fresh turmeric
½ cup fresh or thawed frozen mango
½ lime, peeled
¼ cup tightly packed spinach
½ stalk celery
1⁄16 teaspoon cinnamon

Run the turmeric, mango, lime, spinach, and celery through a juicer in the order listed from top to bottom.

Sprinkle or mix in the cinnamon.

Pour into a glass and serve.

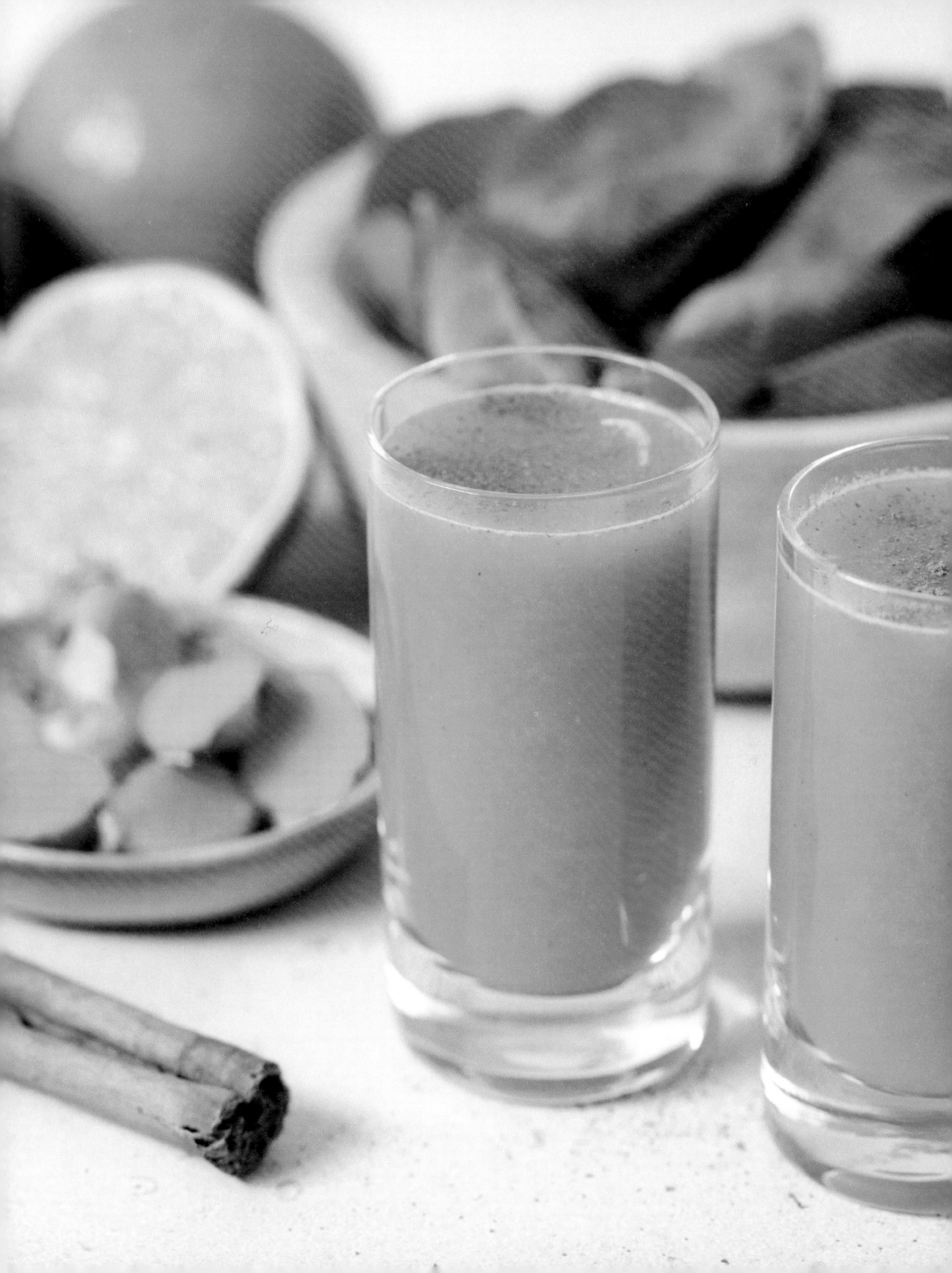

RELATIONSHIP
BREAKUPS STABILIZER

Makes 1 to 2 shots

Try this Brain Shot if:

- You're going through any kind of relationship turmoil, whether or not it's reached a point of actual breakup or dismantling of a partnership

- You're having arguments, fights, or disagreements in any kind of relationship

- You feel there is no resolution to a situation or that there are unresolved issues with friends or family

- You're in a constant, vicious cycle of breaking up and making up

- There is deep-seated or growing resentment inside a relationship

- You're in an endless cycle of argument with a partner

½ cup fresh or thawed frozen strawberries
½ tomato or ¼ cup cherry tomatoes
¼ lemon, peeled
½ cup tightly packed fresh parsley
½ cup roughly chopped lettuce, such as green leaf or butter leaf, tightly packed
½ stalk celery

Run each ingredient through a juicer in the order listed from top to bottom.

Pour into a glass and serve.

TIPS

- If you select fresh strawberries for this recipe, remove the greens before using. While the greens on top of strawberries are edible, they may also harbor bacteria from farm water that got trapped between the strawberries and the leaves. This is why the advice is to remove the strawberry greens altogether.

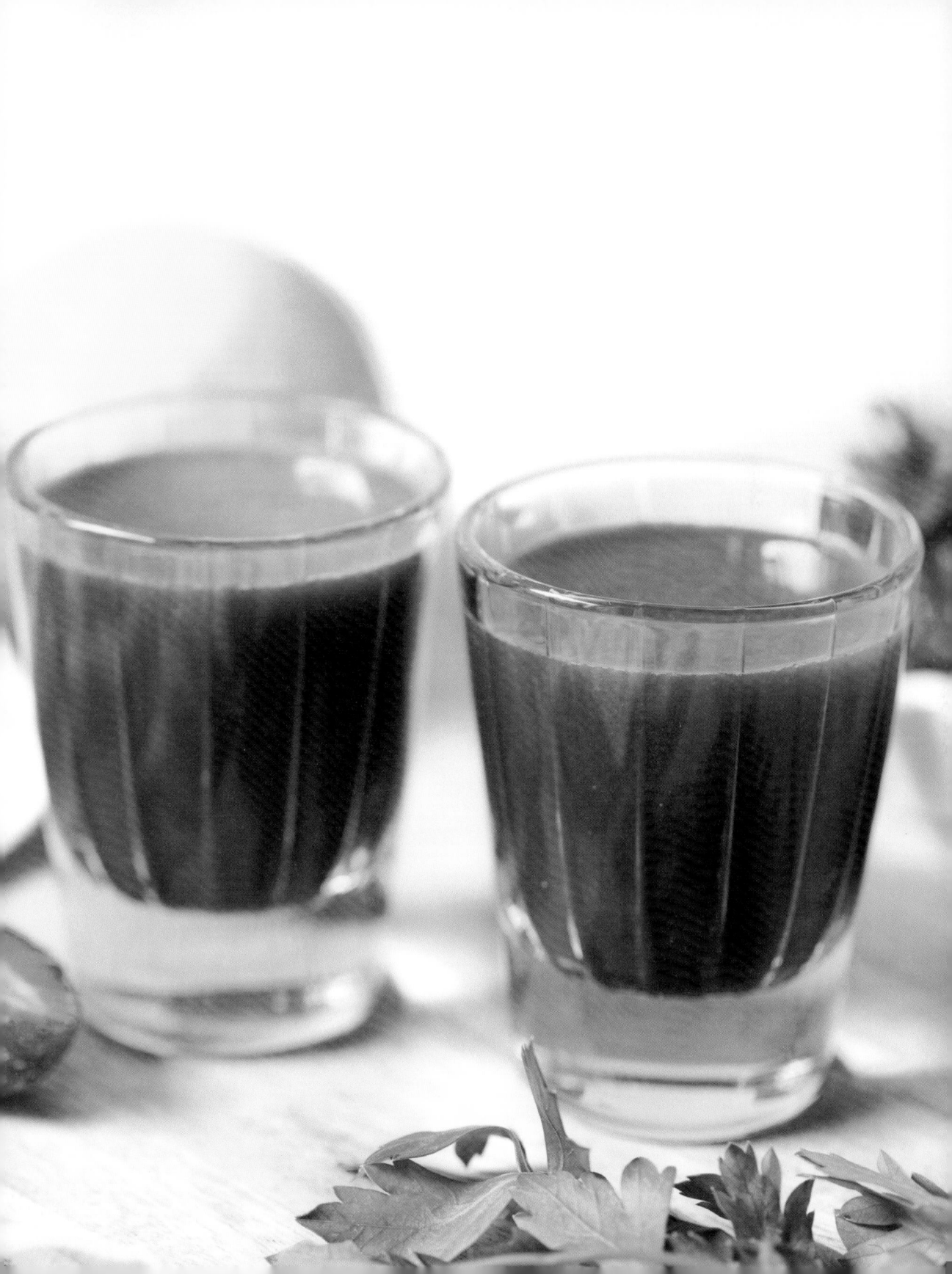

SLEEP AND RECHARGING STABILIZER

Makes 1 to 2 shots

Turn to this shot:

- Before a nap

- When you want a quick recharge

- If you feel like your battery is constantly low

- If you are easily awakened during a night's sleep

- If you don't feel rejuvenated when you wake up from sleeping (You can drink the shot either after you've woken up or before you go to sleep.)

- When you've had a tremendous amount of output and want to regain strength

One healing technique is to drink this Brain Shot, place yourself in a resting position, and close your eyes. Even if you don't fall asleep while resting, the shot will deliver its benefits.

¾ cup fresh or thawed frozen mango
⅛ cup tightly packed fresh dill
¼ cup chopped cucumber
½ cup roughly chopped lettuce (preferably butter lettuce), tightly packed
½ teaspoon pure maple syrup (optional)

Run each ingredient through a juicer in the order listed from top to bottom.

Stir in the maple syrup (if using).

Pour into a glass and serve.

TIPS

- Look for pure maple syrup that is made only with 100 percent maple syrup. Avoid using maple-flavored syrups, which are not the same and often contain harmful ingredients.

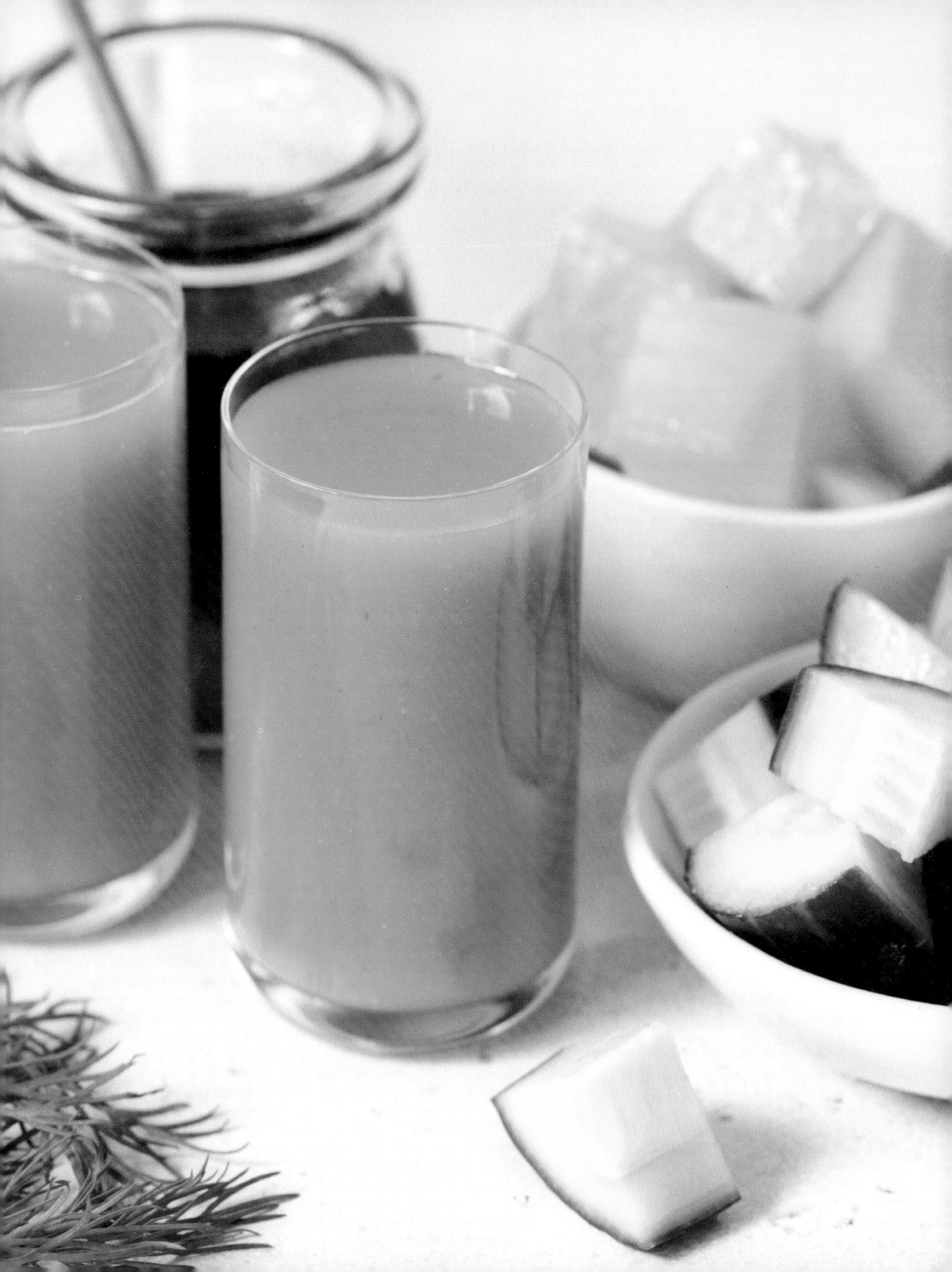

SPEAKING YOUR TRUTH STABILIZER

Makes 1 to 2 shots

This shot provides support around three main areas of truth:

1. Getting in touch with and communicating your own truths. For example, when:

   o You're feeling stifled

   o You're not being heard

   o You aren't being taken seriously

   o You're afraid to speak up about something

   o You feel something you're doing isn't authentic to who you are

2. Receiving the truth. For example, when:

   o You're afraid to receive the truth about something

   o You want to know the truth about something

   o You've received the truth and you're having a difficult time accepting it

3. Learning about hidden truths. For example, when:

   o You want to expand your understanding and knowledge of what's happening with the world around you

   o You want to learn how to read between the lines and see what others are not seeing

   o You're seeking out hidden truths

1-inch piece of fresh ginger
2-inch piece of fresh turmeric
1 small garlic clove
½ cup tightly packed fresh basil
½ cup tightly packed arugula
1 cup roughly chopped lettuce, such as green leaf or butter leaf, tightly packed
1 orange, peeled

Run each ingredient through a juicer in the order listed from top to bottom.

Pour into a glass and serve.

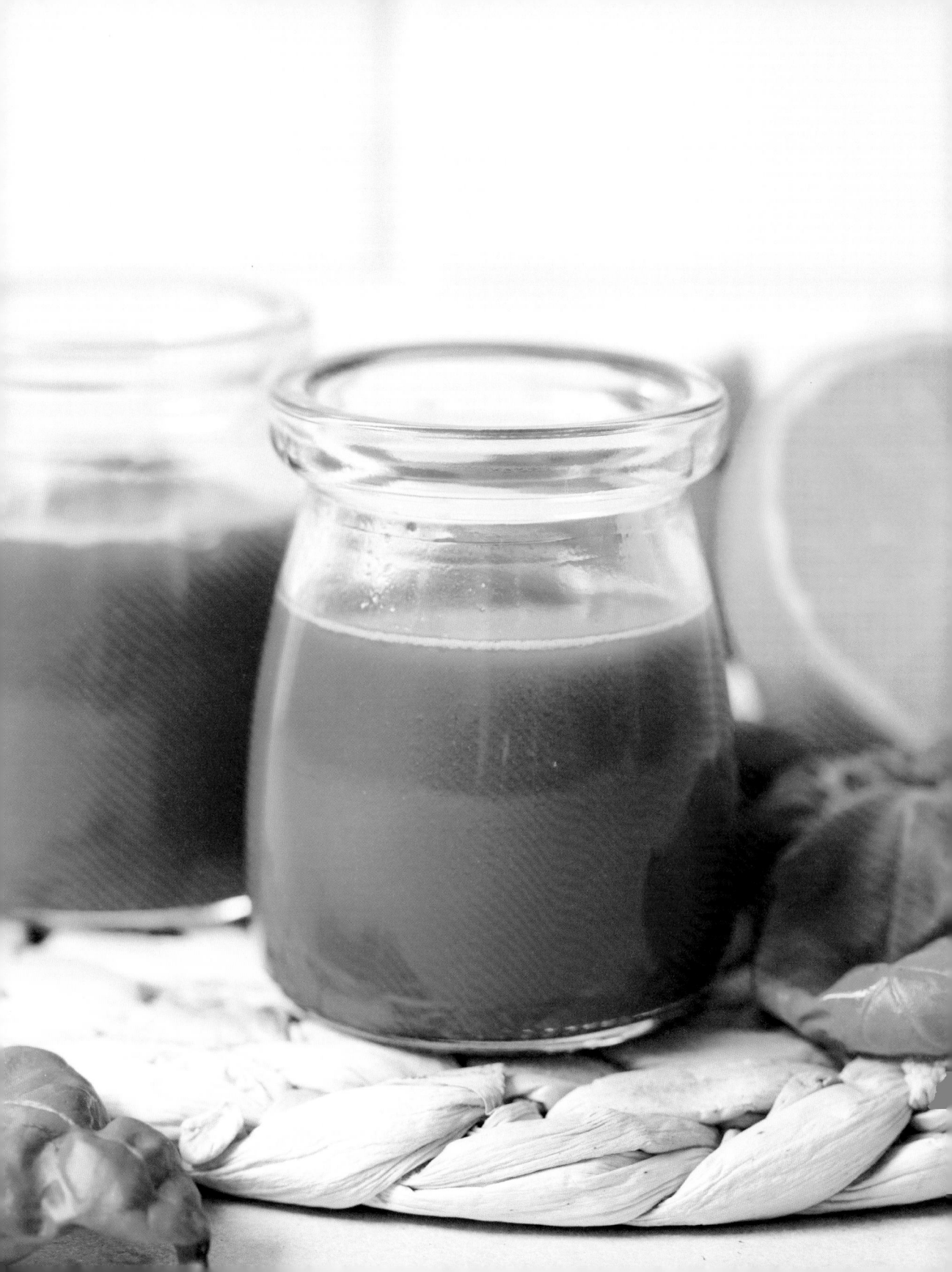

FINDING YOUR PURPOSE STABILIZER

Makes 1 to 2 shots

Try this shot if:

- You have the sense that you're missing out on something, and you don't know what it is

- You're feeling lost or out of place

- You have a sense of sadness

- You don't ever feel satisfied

- You feel you're not living the life you were meant to live or you're not fulfilling your destiny

- You feel like you've lost your free will, or you want to access your free will

- You're feeling unproductive

- You don't know where you're going in life

- You've lost meaning with anything or everything you're doing

¼ cup fresh or thawed frozen blackberries
¼ cup fresh or thawed frozen raspberries
¼ cup fresh or thawed frozen strawberries
1 tablespoon fresh or thawed frozen wild blueberries or 1 teaspoon pure wild blueberry juice or 1 teaspoon pure wild blueberry powder
¼ cup tightly packed fresh parsley

Run each ingredient through a juicer in the order listed from top to bottom. If using the wild blueberry juice or wild blueberry powder, mix it in after all the other ingredients have run through the juicer.

Pour into a glass and serve.

TIPS

- If you select fresh strawberries for this recipe, remove the greens before using. Read why on page 506.

- If you're in a part of the world where you can't access fresh or frozen wild blueberries, wild blueberry juice, or wild blueberry powder, you can add three or four more blackberries to the ¼ cup called for in the recipe.

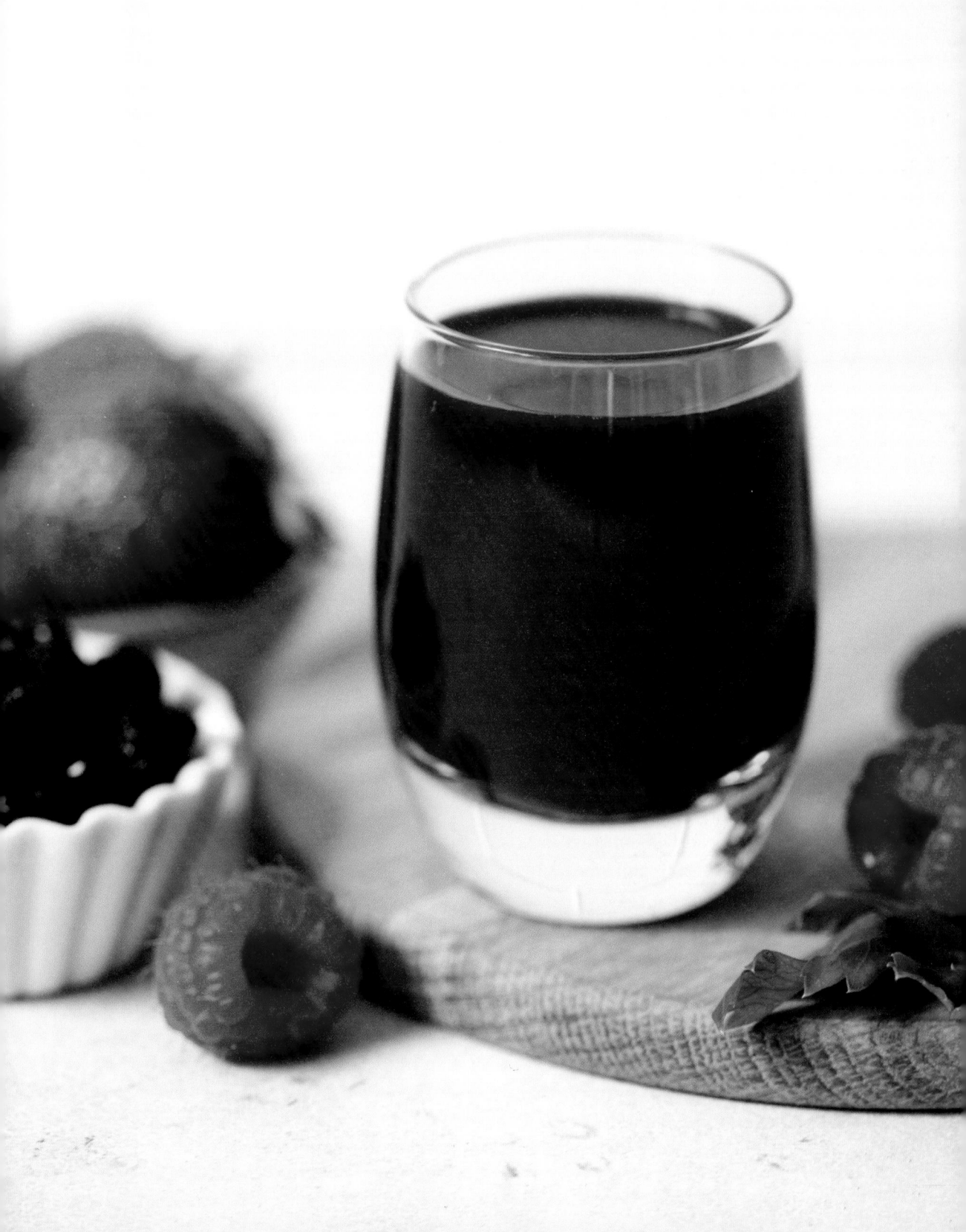

WISDOM AND INTUITION STABILIZER

Makes 1 to 2 shots

Administer this powerful tool when:

- You're trying to improve your intuition

- You want to get the most out of your meditations

- You're trying to build up the strength of your psychic ability

- You're trying to gain sight and vision through your third eye, to see what others cannot see

- You want to strengthen your spiritual connection with above

- You feel you're lacking intuition or disconnected from your intuition

- You want to get the most out of a yoga session or spiritual training or gathering

- You're seeking wisdom about any topic, such as something occurring in your life

- You're seeking answers that pertain to you and the ones around you

1 tablespoon fresh or thawed frozen wild blueberries, or 1 teaspoon pure wild blueberry juice, or 1 teaspoon pure wild blueberry powder
¼ cup fresh or thawed frozen blackberries
¼ cup tightly packed fresh sage
¼ cup tightly packed fresh oregano
¼ cup tightly packed wheatgrass (or 2 teaspoons thawed frozen wheatgrass juice)
½ cup chopped raw yellow squash
¼ teaspoon spirulina

Run the wild blueberries, blackberries, sage, oregano, wheatgrass, and yellow squash through a juicer in the order listed from top to bottom. If you are using the wild blueberry juice, wild blueberry powder, or thawed wheatgrass juice, reserve for the next step.

Sprinkle or stir in the spirulina. Stir in the wild blueberry juice or wild blueberry powder. Stir in the thawed wheatgrass juice if using.

Pour into a glass and serve.

TIPS

- If you're in a part of the world where you can't access fresh or frozen wild blueberries, wild blueberry juice, or wild blueberry powder, you can add three or four more blackberries to the ¼ cup called for in the recipe.

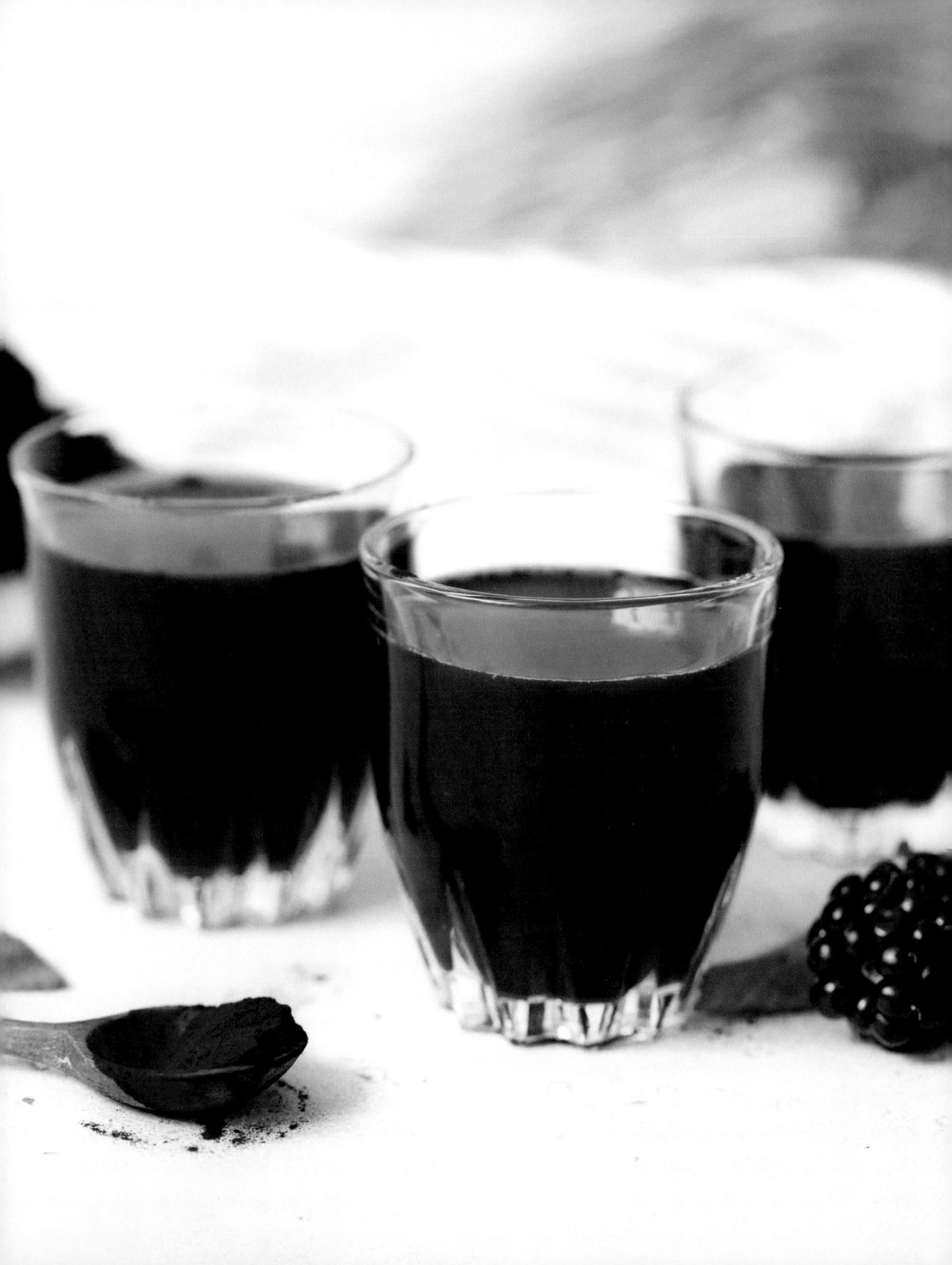

CHAPTER 43

Medical Medium Brain Shot Therapy Cleanses

These cleanses are imperative for what's to come in this world. The onslaught of domestic chemical warfare in our homes, in our schools, in our institutions, in our society today has reached cataclysmic proportions. When you embark on these cleanse options, you're using your free will and your intention to clean and protect the organ that harbors the knowledge of the past, present, and soon to be future of your life and harbors your soul. The Brain Shot Therapy Cleanses are beyond just physical. Removing poisons from the brain opens the door for your consciousness and subconsciousness to purify, allowing you to achieve enlightenment in a world of toxic corruption that keeps us from enlightenment.

Enlightenment is not about being all-knowing. Enlightenment is the freedom to be at peace because you have full control over what resides inside your brain—since we don't have control about what resides around us in the world. These cleanses purify your brain temple. You are removing

the poisons from your brain that take away your clarity. Your intuitive, psychic, telepathic, clairvoyant skills will start to surface. You will be able to see truth easily and clearly and be able to express yourself, increase creativity, and experience joy in the simplest things that others would not realize are joyful. You will open your third eye and develop your skills as a seer when you rid yourself of poisons from the industries that were purposely placed in our brains to keep us in chains and keep us down. These are spiritual cleanses on top of being physical.

The physical benefits are truly special and powerful. With the Brain Shot Therapy Cleanses, you embark on removing toxins and poisonous chemicals from the brain that should never have been there to begin with—and helping restore what should be in your brain. These anti-pathogenic cleanses are designed for what we deal with on a daily basis—everything from deficiencies to burnout to brain acid to emotional brain injuries. These cleanses are designed to rid many different symptoms, conditions, and diseases. The Advanced and High-Powered options have the ability to get rid of 100 symptoms someone may have. (For long-term support, especially for pathogens, supplementation protocols are available in this book's companion title, *Brain Saver Protocols, Cleanses & Recipes*.)

You can choose, at any given time, which of the seven cleanse options to select. You can also climb the ladder here. It's all part of how Medical Medium protocols are customizable to take you as far as you need to go. The higher up you go through the cleanse levels, the more symptoms and conditions can dissipate.

CLEANSE GUIDELINES

Choosing Brain Shot Therapies

- Most Brain Shot Therapy Cleanse levels offer the option to choose 10, 20, or 30 days for your cleanse. Each description will specify.

- Cleanse options will also specify whether you can decide from day to day which shot to try, or whether you should choose a new Brain Shot recipe each day.

- If the guidance says you can decide which shot to try each day, that means you have the option to move throughout the shots however you'd like. It's your choice. You're welcome to skip around or repeat shots from day to day.

- If the guidance says to choose a new Brain Shot recipe each day, move through the shots within one group at a time. For example, for a 10-day cleanse, choose either the Exposure shots, Shifter shots, or Stabilizer shots from Chapter 42, selecting one new shot recipe per day so that by the end of the 10 days, you've moved through all 10 shots in a group. For a 20-day or 30-day cleanse, you would choose two to three Brain Shot groups, moving through one group at a time. It's okay to go out of order within a group—you don't need to go through them in the exact order listed in Chapter 42—as long as you get to all the shots in a group within each segment of 10 days.

- For example, if you do a 30-day cleanse that instructs you to select a new shot each day, you could decide to work your way through the Shifters (in any order), then Stabilizers (in any order), then Exposures (in any order), until you've gotten through all 30 shots in 30 days.

Number of Shots

- When a cleanse option calls for 2 or more shots per day, the shots should all be the same type on any given day. That is, if you've chosen an option that calls for 3 shots per day, all 3 shots should be made from the same recipe.

Shot Timing

- Drink your shots at least 15 to 30 minutes apart from any food or drink. That is, wait a minimum of 15 to 30 minutes after consuming anything else before you have a shot, and then wait a minimum of 15 to 30 minutes after consuming a shot to consume anything else.

- This applies to every Brain Shot Therapy Cleanse level. You want to give yourself time to resonate with each shot, letting the therapy enter the bloodstream and allowing yourself to pick up the frequency of the shot metaphysically and physically. This is giving you a moment of time to take it in and experience what the shot is doing.

- For example, a morning sequence that incorporates other Medical Medium protocols could look like this: drink your lemon or lime water upon waking, then wait 15 to 30 minutes, drink your fresh celery juice, then wait another 15 to 30 minutes, drink your Brain Shot, then wait at least another 15 to 30 minutes, and then have your breakfast.

- When a cleanse option calls for multiple shots per day, space out the shots at least 4 hours apart throughout the day. (The brain starts to shift back to old patterns after 4 hours, so you want to wait until that has happened before having another shot.) For example, if you're doing 3 shots per day, don't have the shots any closer together than 8 A.M., 12 P.M., and 4 P.M. You have the option to space out the shots more than that minimum of 4 hours apart. For example, you could have your shots at 7 A.M., 1 P.M., and 7 P.M. How you'd like to customize the timing of the shots is up to you.

- If you're taking a Medical Medium supplement protocol, you can continue while you're on the Brain Shot Therapy Cleanse. Don't take your supplements *with* your shots. Space them out according to the guidance above.

Repeating the Cleanse

- You're welcome to do back-to-back Brain Shot Therapy Cleanses. You're also welcome to do the cleanse periodically, taking breaks in between rounds and then coming back to your cleanse level of choice. You could either repeat the same cleanse level however many times you'd like, or you could try moving from one level to another. Try whichever cleanse level you'd like at any time.

Missing Ingredients

- If you have difficulty sourcing ingredients in the Brain Shots—if you're missing an item or lacking one—use what you have and move forward.

- For questions about ingredient substitutions in recipes such as Lemon or Lime Water, Celery Juice, and the Heavy Metal Detox Smoothie, see the Tips that go with the individual recipes. If possible, try not to get into the habit of relying

on substitutions, especially for celery juice. Keep trying to achieve the goal of using the proper ingredients for the cleanses.

Cleanse Interruptions

- If you miss Brain Shots (and/or the Heavy Metal Detox Smoothie, if specified) on any given day of a cleanse, still try to follow the rest of the cleanse guidance that day, and then add one day to the end of your cleanse.

- If you do something that breaks your cleanse, add three days to the end of your cleanse. "Breaking the cleanse" means consuming items your cleanse level specifies to avoid, whether radical fats such as nut butter in the morning or brain betrayer foods such as eggs, dairy, or gluten.

General Notes for All Cleanses

- If you're getting your blood drawn for some reason within the time period of your cleanse, ask if you can move your appointment to a time when you're not doing the cleanse, or follow the blood draw guidelines from Chapter 40, "Blood Draining Agenda."

- For any general cleansing questions you have that are not addressed in this book, *Cleanse to Heal* is available to you as an additional resource.

Adjustments for Children

You can go ahead with the Brain Shot Therapy Cleanses for children, keeping the following in mind:

- It's fine to leave the lemon or lime water out for kids and also to reduce the amount of celery juice according to what feels right for your little one. See the table at the end of Chapter 44 for more guidance on celery juice amounts for children.

- Depending on the age and size of your child, serve a small portion of a given Brain Shot, even if it means going as low as an ounce or down to a teaspoon.

- If the cleanse level you've chosen for your child includes the Heavy Metal Detox Smoothie, see "Adjustments for Children" in Chapter 44, "Heavy Metal Detox," for guidance on the amount.

BRAIN SHOT THERAPY CLEANSE LEVELS

1. ENTRY LEVEL Brain Shot Therapy Cleanse

Add these steps to your normal eating routine:

- Drink 1 Brain Shot per day (recipes in Chapter 42).

- Your choice of 10, 20, or 30 days.

- Your choice of which Brain Shot option from day to day.

- Optional: Incorporate as many other Medical Medium tools and recipes as desired.

- Try to drink a minimum of 50 ounces of water throughout the day (that amount can include coconut water). Be mindful not to drink the water too close to drinking the Brain Shot—make sure you space them at least 15 to 30 minutes apart.

2. BASIC Brain Shot Therapy Cleanse

Add these steps to your normal eating routine:

- Drink 2 of the same Brain Shots per day (recipes in Chapter 42), spaced at least 4 hours apart.

- Your choice of 10, 20, or 30 days.

- Your choice of which Brain Shot option from day to day.

- Optional: Incorporate as many other Medical Medium tools and recipes as desired.

- Try to drink a minimum of 60 ounces of water throughout the day (that amount can include coconut water). Be mindful not to drink the water too close to drinking the Brain Shots—make sure you space them at least 15 to 30 minutes apart.

3. SIMPLIFIED Brain Shot Therapy Cleanse

Add these steps to your normal eating routine:

- Drink 2 of the same Brain Shots per day (recipes in Chapter 42), spaced at least 4 hours apart.

- Your choice of 10, 20, or 30 days.

- Your choice of which Brain Shot option from day to day.

- Start each day with 16 to 32 ounces of fresh lemon or lime water upon waking (recipe with the proper ratio of lemon or lime to water in Chapter 44).

- At least 15 to 30 minutes later, drink 16 to 32 ounces of fresh celery juice on an empty stomach (then wait another 15 to 30 minutes before you have your first Brain Shot or breakfast).

- Optional: Heavy Metal Detox Smoothie anytime (recipe in Chapter 44); should not be consumed directly after a fat-based meal.

- Stay fat-free until at least lunchtime.

- Optional: For even better results, take a look at the brain betrayer foods and food chemicals in Chapters 28 and 30. Start chipping away at the lists, seeing what foods you'd like to avoid while cleansing. The fewer brain betrayers such as eggs, dairy, gluten, corn, soy, tuna, lamb, and pork in your diet, the more effective the Brain Shots can be.

- Try to incorporate as many Medical Medium recipes from this book's companion title, *Brain Saver Protocols, Cleanses & Recipes*, into your snacks and meals as you can.

- Try to drink a minimum of 60 ounces of water throughout the day (that amount can include coconut water and your morning lemon water). Be mindful not to drink the water too close to drinking the celery juice or Brain Shots—make sure you space them at least 15 to 30 minutes apart.

4. INTERMEDIATE Brain Shot Therapy Cleanse

Make these steps your complete eating routine:

- Drink 3 of the same Brain Shots per day (recipes in Chapter 42), spaced at least 4 hours apart.

- Your choice of 10, 20, or 30 days.

- Your choice of which Brain Shot option from day to day.

- Start each day with 16 to 32 ounces of fresh lemon or lime water upon waking (recipe with the proper ratio of lemon or lime to water in Chapter 44).

- At least 15 to 30 minutes later, drink 16 to 32 ounces of fresh celery juice on an empty stomach (then wait another 15 to 30 minutes before you have your first Brain Shot or breakfast).

- Optional: Heavy Metal Detox Smoothie anytime (recipe in Chapter 44); should not be

consumed directly after a fat-based meal.

- Avoid eggs, dairy, gluten, corn, soy, tuna, lamb, and pork.

- Use exclusively Medical Medium recipes from this book's companion title, *Brain Saver Protocols, Cleanses & Recipes*.

- Stay fat-free until at least lunchtime.

- Keep fats limited to one serving (if at all) from lunchtime on, preferably at the end of the day. If you're plant-based, it's okay to incorporate one serving of plant fat, such as avocado, nuts or nut butters, seeds, coconut, coconut oil, olives, or olive oil, in a Medical Medium recipe. If you eat animal products, it's okay to incorporate one serving of animal fat, such as chicken, grass-fed beef, turkey, salmon, or sardines, in a Medical Medium recipe.

- Try to drink a minimum of 60 ounces of water throughout the day (that amount can include coconut water and your morning lemon water). Be mindful not to drink the water too close to drinking the celery juice or Brain Shots—make sure you space them at least 15 to 30 minutes apart.

5. PERFORMANCE Brain Shot Therapy Cleanse

Make these steps your complete eating routine:

- Drink 3 of the same Brain Shots per day (recipes in Chapter 42), spaced at least 4 hours apart.

- Your choice of 10, 20, or 30 days.

- Select a new Brain Shot every day, working methodically through one group (Exposures, Shifters, or Stabilizers) at a time (okay to go out of order within a group).

- Start each day with 32 ounces of fresh lemon or lime water upon waking (recipe with the proper ratio of lemon or lime to water in Chapter 44).

- At least 15 to 30 minutes later, drink 32 ounces of fresh celery juice on an empty stomach (then wait another 15 to 30 minutes before you have your first Brain Shot or breakfast).

- Optional: Heavy Metal Detox Smoothie anytime (recipe in Chapter 44); should not be consumed directly after a fat-based meal.

- Avoid all foods and food chemicals from Chapters 28 and 30, including caffeine.

- Use exclusively Medical Medium recipes from this book's companion title, *Brain Saver Protocols, Cleanses & Recipes.*

- Stay fat-free until at least lunchtime.

- Keep fats limited to one serving (if at all) from lunchtime on, preferably at the end of the day. If you're plant-based, it's okay to incorporate one serving of plant fat, such as avocado, nuts or nut butters, seeds, coconut, coconut oil, olives, or olive oil, in a Medical Medium recipe. If you eat animal products, it's okay to incorporate one serving of animal fat, such as chicken, grass-fed beef, turkey, salmon, or sardines, in a Medical Medium recipe.

- Try to drink a minimum of 60 ounces of water throughout the day (that amount can include coconut water and your morning lemon water). Be mindful not to drink the water too close to drinking the celery juice or Brain Shots—make sure you space them at least 15 to 30 minutes apart.

6. ADVANCED Brain Shot Therapy Cleanse

Make these steps your complete eating routine:

- Drink 3 of the same Brain Shots per day (recipes in Chapter 42), spaced at least 4 hours apart.

- Your choice of 20 or 30 days.

- Select a new Brain Shot every day, working methodically through one group (Exposures, Shifters, or Stabilizers) at a time (okay to go out of order within a group).

- Start each day with 32 ounces of fresh lemon or lime water upon waking (recipe with the proper ratio of lemon or lime to water in Chapter 44).

- At least 15 to 30 minutes later, drink 32 ounces of fresh celery juice on an empty stomach (then wait another 15 to 30 minutes before you have your first Brain Shot or breakfast).

- Drink the Heavy Metal Detox Smoothie daily (recipe in Chapter 44). (Optional: okay to take one day off from the smoothie every 10 days.)

- Avoid all foods and food chemicals from Chapters 28 and 30, including caffeine.

- Use exclusively fat-free Medical Medium recipes from this book's companion title, *Brain Saver Protocols, Cleanses & Recipes.*

- Stay off all fat-based foods, both plant fats (e.g., nuts, seeds, avocado) and animal fats (e.g., chicken, fish, meat).

- Try to drink a minimum of 60 ounces of water throughout the day (that amount can include coconut water and your morning lemon water). As ever, be mindful not to drink the water too close to drinking the celery juice or Brain Shots— make sure you space them at least 15 to 30 minutes apart.

7. HIGH-POWERED Brain Shot Therapy Cleanse

Make these steps your complete eating routine:

- Drink 3 of the same Brain Shots per day (recipes in Chapter 42), spaced at least 4 hours apart.

- Continue for 30 days.

- Select a new Brain Shot every day, working methodically through one group (Exposures, Shifters, or Stabilizers) at a time (okay to go out of order within a group).

- Start each day with 32 ounces of fresh lemon or lime water upon waking (recipe with the proper ratio of lemon or lime to water in Chapter 44).

- At least 15 to 30 minutes later, drink 32 ounces of fresh celery juice on an empty stomach (then wait another 15 to 30 minutes before you have your first Brain Shot or breakfast).

- Drink the Heavy Metal Detox Smoothie daily (recipe in Chapter 44). (Optional: okay to take one day off from the smoothie every 10 days.)

- Avoid all foods and food chemicals from Chapters 28 and 30, including caffeine.

- Use exclusively fat-free Medical Medium recipes from this

book's companion title, *Brain Saver Protocols, Cleanses & Recipes*.

- Stay off all fat-based foods, both plant fats (e.g., nuts, seeds, avocado) and animal fats (e.g., chicken, fish, meat).

- Remove scented candles, colognes, perfumes, scented laundry detergents, fabric softeners, air fresheners, fragrances, scented aftershaves, scented deodorants, scented soaps, scented body sprays, scented body lotions, scented body oils, scented hair products, incense, and car fresheners.

- Try to drink a minimum of 60 ounces of water throughout the day (that amount can include coconut water and your morning lemon water). As ever, be mindful not to drink the water too close to drinking the celery juice or Brain Shots— make sure you space them at least 15 to 30 minutes apart.

CHAPTER 44

Medical Medium
Heavy Metal Detox

Beyond the damage that toxic heavy metals themselves can do, there's the truth that they act as viral fuel—which supports viruses in their mission to elevate inflammation throughout the body and cause autoimmune conditions—and so taking metals away helps lower a viral load. Viral loads create neurological symptoms. Extracting heavy metals also addresses mental and emotional struggles and well-being by allowing the electricity and energetic frequencies of the brain to flow freely. When you break down and dismantle the alloys that have interfered with your brain, you minimize viral invasion, allow for emotional injuries to heal faster, reduce inflammation of the brain and cranial nerves, address burnout and deficiencies, and help relieve an addicted, acid brain.

OLD METALS VERSUS NEW METALS

Heavy metals that we inherit have age to them. They're old, many times going back as far as 2,000 to 3,000 years, depending on what part of the world someone's bloodline stems from. Older heavy metals also have a higher oxidative rate than heavy metals from newer exposures. The aging process of toxic heavy metals that were mined many generations ago started when the metals were removed from the earth. An oxidative countdown occurred as the metals aged. Those metals became highly unstable when they entered and sat inside human bodies, where metals are exposed to oxygen, acids, heat, blood gases, electricity, outside chemicals, and more.

New metals differ greatly from old metals. Newer metals recently mined and taken out of the earth are still highly toxic, although they are more stable, making them less destructive than older metals. Newer metals don't break down inside the body as quickly. It all depends on how many generations the metals have been passed down through and how much metal is in each individual. Most people have a mix of older metals and newer metals being passed down from generation to generation. The newest metal exposure is when a child gets a medical treatment at the pediatrician's office that contains mercury, aluminum, and copper. Most likely the mercury and aluminum were unearthed in the last 50 to 70 years, saved in storage, and eventually purchased by the medical industry and placed inside a pharmaceutical. Many medications have toxic heavy metals in them, and at the same time, a child could have inherited toxic heavy metals that have been in the family line for hundreds to thousands of years from periodic exposures that our ancestors encountered. For example, we can inherit metals from 2,000 to 3,000 years ago, plus metals from 300 to 400 years ago that our ancestors were exposed to in, for example, quicksilver treatments, plus metals from more recent exposure in our family line. Older metals' faster oxidation rate makes viruses more interested in these aging metals, because they are easier to access and consume due to their instability.

One reason heavy metals are passed down from generation to generation is that their presence in the body isn't recognized by medical research and science, unless it's an obvious poisoning such as from a lead tank filled with water. So heavy metals aren't identified as a destructive, dangerous threat to health, and the metals aren't cleaned out of the bodies of parents before a new generation is born. Toxic heavy metals are a big part of why human health is not prospering at this time—why it's even declining.

ALLOY FUEL

Normally, the viruses that cause autoimmune disorders feed on one metal or maybe two. In difficult neurological autoimmune cases, either one virus is feeding on three, four, or more metals, or two or more viruses are each feeding on multiple metals. A virus or viruses feeding on multiple metals leads to metals mixing and creating highly potent waste. Once this waste matter is excreted from the virus, it can cause many neurological and physical reactions, especially if the metals are aged. When more than two metals are consumed by a virus, the resulting neurotoxins become muscle-damaging, nerve-damaging, bone-damaging, and organ-damaging because this toxic waste is suffocating cells, not allowing cells to receive critically needed nutrients to survive on an optimum level. The cell walls break down from exposure to the highly acidic and denaturing toxic waste matter.

Different toxic heavy metals have different weights to them. Copper, mercury, and lead are a few of the heavier metals, and so the neurotoxins and dermatoxins excreted by viruses feeding on these metals are heavier in weight. Neurotoxins and dermatoxins can be a mix of heavy and lighter metals, and the heavier metals will mix with the lighter metals and weigh the lighter metals down, causing neurotoxins and dermatoxins to settle in extremities. This is why some people only get eczema on their hands and feet or legs (heavier dermatoxins) while others get eczema on their chest (when the dermatoxins are mostly composed of lighter metals). Restless legs syndrome and Raynaud's syndrome are examples of neurotoxins settling in feet, hands, arms, and legs.

HEAVY METAL DETOX AT WORK

For the best way to get rid of heavy metals from the brain and body, look no further than the Heavy Metal Detox Smoothie and cleanses. These protocols are the most effective methods on the planet for removing heavy metals and repairing the damage they've left behind. There are countless stories worldwide of people getting results from the original Heavy Metal Detox Smoothie and the original Heavy Metal Detox Cleanse. Now you have even more options.

The Power of the Heavy Metal Detox Smoothie

Let's start with the basics. The Heavy Metal Detox Smoothie (full recipe at the end of this chapter) incorporates five key ingredients:

- Wild blueberries (available frozen or as pure wild blueberry powder or juice)

- Spirulina (find the most potent and productive kind in my supplement directory at www.medicalmedium.com)

- Barley grass juice powder (find the correct kind in my supplement directory)

- Fresh cilantro

- Atlantic dulse

Together, these medicinals extract both deep-rooted and free-floating metals and carry them all the way out of your body, rather than dropping them along the way or not working at all. This makes the Heavy Metal Detox Smoothie totally unique—it's responsible. It doesn't simply pick up metals and then let them go again, causing additional stress and harm on someone's nervous system or digestive system. This is one reason it doesn't cause side effects. The Heavy Metal Detox Smoothie also helps heal brain tissue with its nourishing composition.

(If there is a mild reaction, it's not a sign of harm. It's common for that person to react to any protocols they try from any other sources, and it means the person is highly toxic. The difference between the Heavy Metal Detox Smoothie and other protocols is that the smoothie can eventually clear up those toxins so the person can stop having reactions.)

If you're familiar with the Medical Medium series, you'll recall that consuming these five foods within 24 hours of each other is sufficient for them to do their work together. That holds true for generally removing heavy metals in various places throughout the body. When you're specifically targeting toxic heavy metals in the brain, it's best to consume these five foods blended together.

The process of removing heavy metals from the brain is something like mining precious metals from the earth. Although in mining, earth and ore must usually be removed or displaced to extract the metals, with this extraction method from the brain, the phytochemical compounds in the five key foods collectively and carefully loosen and gather the metals through a chemical reaction. Chemical compounds from these five ingredients join together and align with supernatural abilities of the brain. The chemical compounds from the smoothie ingredients drive information into the brain's electrical grid, activating the electrical grid to work alongside other chemical compounds that the brain possesses, jolting the electrical grid to project the metals and waste out of the brain tissue to then be gathered up by the chemical compounds of the five ingredients. This process keeps brain tissue safe. It's the power of the chemical compounds in the Heavy Metal Detox Smoothie's five medicinal ingredients working together. If someone doesn't have one or two ingredients, the ingredients that are present still work together in harmony.

Here's a simpler way to view it: the brain, filled with toxic brain betrayers, as a dirty sponge, and the phytochemicals in this Heavy Metal Detox Smoothie almost acting as a squeezing method for cells to draw out heavy metals. Or see the smoothie like an expectorant for brain tissue, helping the brain cough up what's holding it back.

A bonus of the Heavy Metal Detox Smoothie is that it doesn't only remove toxic heavy metals from the brain. While getting rid of toxic heavy metals is your number one goal with this recipe, it will also help purge solvents, pesticides, radiation, and other brain betrayers.

Any makeshift or trendy way of trying to remove metals out of the body really falls short. For example, chlorella, if it even picks up metal, will drop it, creating another, possibly bigger problem in another area of the brain. Charcoal and zeolite also don't measure up to claims. Read more in this book's companion title, *Brain Saver Protocols, Cleanses & Recipes.*

Removing all the metals from the brain takes time. One big part of the detox process is reaching and purging actual fragments of nested metal, which can be clusters of truly small, nano-sized and tinier metals. That's not an overnight process. Even if some symptoms start to relieve and subside quickly, it still may take time to get to the finish line of removing all of the toxic heavy metals and getting past your most persistent symptoms. Those metal fragments have built up over the years, forming larger deposits with even bigger effects that this Heavy Metal Detox can address too. As brain tissue starts to purge the metals, not all of the metals will come out at once. Instead the metals begin to surface from deep within the brain. That's one reason why keeping up with this Heavy Metal Detox protocol for a long duration is critical: we can have older metals from generations and generations ago that are deeper, unstable, and fragile, and they won't project out of the brain quickly because it takes time for the metals to migrate closer to various surfaces in the brain. Newer metals that are more stable project out more easily. If they are deeper inside the brain, it does still take time to migrate those newer metals to the surface.

Metals travel through oxidation: when they corrode and expand, their debris run-off spreads and they react with each other. Heavy metal contamination bleeding into adjacent brain tissue is what's behind so many of the diseases and symptoms in this book. To address that, another big part of what the Heavy Metal Detox Smoothie does is deal with that corrosive metal debris. Chemical compounds in the Heavy Metal Detox Smoothie's five key ingredients bind onto the corrosion and contamination from decaying metal alloys. This, too, takes time and patience; stabilizing and safely dispersing corrosive debris that's formed from heavy metal alloys such as aluminum plus mercury or copper interacting in the brain is an extra level of cleanup.

People's toxic heavy metal situations are different. One person may have metals in their early phase of oxidation, forms that haven't yet interacted much with each other, which means there's not a lot of oxidative debris. Those metals can be faster and easier to cleanse. Another person could have a lot of heavy metal interactions transpiring—a lot of aluminum, mercury, and copper, for example, reacting with each other over a long period of time,

creating pockets of oxidative discharge. In that case the Heavy Metal Detox Smoothie must start pulling away at this debris and then packaging it up and moving it out to keep it from spreading and causing more problems—before the Heavy Metal Detox Smoothie's chemical compounds can get down to the root metals. Brain fog, depression, OCD, memory loss, and anxiety could take a longer time to heal until repeated use of the Heavy Metal Detox Smoothie allows heavy metal extraction to go deeper into the brain.

Everyone's alloy brain is unique. What particular metal blend it is, how many years the different metals have been sitting there, what quantity they're present in, how they're distributed in the brain, and how quickly they've been oxidizing differ from person to person. Because the Heavy Metal Detox Smoothie contains five key elements that address various aspects of healing, it covers everyone.

If you don't have all five ingredients, don't let that hold you back from making the Heavy Metal Detox Smoothie. Unlike chlorella and other sources, these ingredients hold the power to capture metals properly. They have individual qualities and abilities to remove metals. Keep in mind, using three or four out of the five smoothie ingredients could mean it takes longer to see results or completely heal. The ingredients still work best together. All five ingredients put together as a group uproot metals most effectively.

Wild Blueberries and the Other Key Ingredients

Understanding a little more about the Heavy Metal Detox Smoothie's ingredients helps us appreciate even more how hard the formula is working for us. In addition to the collective uprooting power of the ingredients' chemical compounds, the individual ingredients benefit us profoundly.

To begin with, wild blueberries ignite a purging effect in the brain. Wild blueberries contain dozens of unique and many undiscovered antioxidant phytochemical compounds. These antioxidant compounds break up debris pockets that have formed as a byproduct of heavy metals interacting and aging in the brain—it's like the dentist breaking up plaque on your teeth. Wild blueberries also go after the metals themselves.

We have to remember that heavy metals sitting in the brain take up space. Even if they're not oxidizing yet, even if they're on a nano or smaller scale, they have a physical presence in a place that's not supposed to have any toxic physical substances in it. Sometimes that can be a larger physical presence. For example, mercury tends to find more mercury, so if you were exposed to mercury early on, perhaps as a baby, additional mercury that you were exposed to throughout life, perhaps even on a monthly basis, could have rolled into that early mercury, creating bigger deposits. Sometimes metals' physical presence in the brain is compact, as in the case of the tiniest specks and micro-pockets of metals. No matter their size, heavy metal deposits create divots and pits in the brain.

Once those heavy metals are purged, brain tissue needs to be repaired. Not only do wild blueberries' antioxidant phytochemical compounds extract the metals; they excel at healing the damage the metals have left behind by restoring the brain cells that are lining the walls of a divot or pit so that new brain cell growth is stimulated.

With heavy metals gone, your brain can create new cells in the space, although they need wild blueberries' help to do it well, clearing the area of contamination so that healthy growth can occur. When the damage is on a small scale, that healing can happen faster. If it's an older deposit of metals, where oxidative waste has accumulated too, it takes long-term commitment to the Heavy Metal Detox Smoothie to decontaminate the area. Brain cells die off because of heavy metals and their runoff, and not until it's all cleaned up will the body recognize that new growth can occur safely so the area can start to come back to life. While this extraction and remediation process is still happening, some symptoms can stick around for a while because even after heavy metals are removed, there is still brain tissue repair. Wild blueberries' antioxidant phytochemical compounds have the ability to increase healthy brain cell growth on a rapid scale to help spur healing—these antioxidants purify the brain tissue enough to freely repair.

Once wild blueberries have expelled and carried out heavy metals and their debris into the bloodstream, other chemical compounds from spirulina, barley grass juice powder, and cilantro can help navigate this debris safely out of the body. Thanks to the wild blueberries, the heavy metals won't re-disperse and cause trouble in the brain. The key five ingredients' chemical compounds are all working together to carry toxic heavy metals out of the body safely; all the Heavy Metal Detox foods have the ability to harness radical, destabilized, corroded, oxidized metal debris as well as new metals that would otherwise aggressively injure tissue as they traveled.

Cilantro, barley grass juice powder, and spirulina work together specially, each playing unique and critical roles in removing toxic heavy metals. To begin with, some of cilantro's responsibility is to assist in removing metals from the brain, while another responsibility for cilantro is to remove heavy metals from the liver, other organs, and the intestinal tract—catching toxic heavy metals that are oxidizing and corroding early on, before the metals' oxidative byproduct and waste find their way to the brain. Cilantro's chemical compounds aren't going to attach themselves to heavy metals still being held by wild blueberries' compounds, only to rogue metals.

It's a long journey from where metals are nested in the brain to the point of being excreted out of the body because there are many obstacles along the route. High blood fat, acids, blood gases, pharmaceuticals, chemical toxins, chronic dehydration, and adrenaline are some of the obstacles. The metals themselves are highly toxic. We can't rely solely on wild blueberries and cilantro when we're trying to uproot and remove alloys from the brain and body. Bringing in barley grass juice powder at the same time is imperative. It works similarly to cilantro, although it travels farther and wider, even to the outer reaches of the skin, and also possesses a strong absorption mechanism for oxidized, destabilized metals.

Spirulina has similar abilities, more so for the brain and liver. Its profound ability to round up heavy metals in the brain, liver, and intestinal tract is one of its great virtues. The pigment in spirulina, which gives it its deep blue-green color, reaches the metaphysical part of the brain at the same time as the physical part, helping restore brain tissue that connects between the physical and metaphysical. Spirulina is so versatile that it can clean up metals that the other smoothie ingredients have unearthed from the brain, *and* spirulina can clean up metals from the liver and intestinal tract that would otherwise travel up to the brain.

Having all three—cilantro, barley grass juice powder, and spirulina—in your system at once provides exactly the formula you need to go along with wild blueberries, because everyone has a different toxic load, and that affects how the different medicinals perform. Atlantic dulse, a type of sea vegetable, acts as a safety net as metals expel out of the liver, gallbladder, and bile duct into the intestinal tract. Dulse also aids the kidneys by helping safely absorb metals leaving the body that could otherwise get trapped in the kidneys. Dulse is insurance to assist in escorting out of the body any metals that are hosted by (meaning captured by and attached to) other key ingredients, or metals that are on their own.

The key ingredients in the Heavy Metal Detox Smoothie also have some ability to remove other chemical toxins and poisons, which include radiation, insecticides, and fragrances.

Your Healing Goals

Some people respond immediately to the Heavy Metal Detox Smoothie because oxidative debris was saturating easy-to-reach hot spots of brain tissue, causing life-disrupting symptoms, and clearing some of that up gives a person an instant boost. Someone else might have been experiencing heavy metal oxidative runoff for years or decades, or have experienced much more aggressive alloy interactions, leading to more intense symptoms. The necessary cleanup in that case can mean that a person only sees some immediate results.

Some people have metals in the brain that aren't reacting with other metals yet, so pulling those out can mean they see a difference quickly. Other people have metals deep in different areas of the brain, and that means a longer process of extracting them.

Whatever situation someone is in, it's best to stick with all five ingredients to get someone to that place where they start feeling a difference. Whatever your timeline is, know that with every Heavy Metal Detox Smoothie you give yourself, you're getting closer and closer to your goals of healing.

Here's one more important point: when the brain is purging metals and oxidative debris from brain tissue, there are no rules for where this process starts to happen first in the brain. It's not systematic. It all depends on where the Heavy Metal Detox Smoothie's phytochemical compounds land first and how many metals are there. Considerations include: Are the metals old or new? Are they from generations ago? How deep are they inside the brain? Are there larger deposits? Smaller deposits? And what kinds of metals are they?

If the first area of the brain the phytochemicals reach has a smaller amount of metals, those little specks and pockets of metal and debris will be purged to begin with. It won't be until later on, with more and more Heavy Metal Detox Smoothies, that the compounds of the ingredients get a chance to reach the larger pockets to start breaking down, absorbing, and uprooting the metals. It's yet one more reason to keep up with the smoothie regularly—ideally, daily—to make sure those critical heavy metal–extracting nutrients get where they need to go.

ADJUSTMENTS FOR CHILDREN

A child usually doesn't have the appetite for the full amount that the Heavy Metal Detox Smoothie recipe yields. To figure out the right portion for your child, think about when they're drinking a glass of apple juice—how much will they usually drink? Eight ounces? Ten or twelve ounces? Wherever you land, that's an appropriate amount of Heavy Metal Detox Smoothie to give your child. You can either reduce the recipe accordingly—for example, cutting it by half or two-thirds (making sure to keep the five key ingredients in there, in proportionate amounts)—or make the full recipe and drink the leftover that your child doesn't want.

"Your brain has a soul—and that means anything is possible when it comes to healing and saving your life."

— Anthony William, Medical Medium

Heavy Metal Detox Recipes

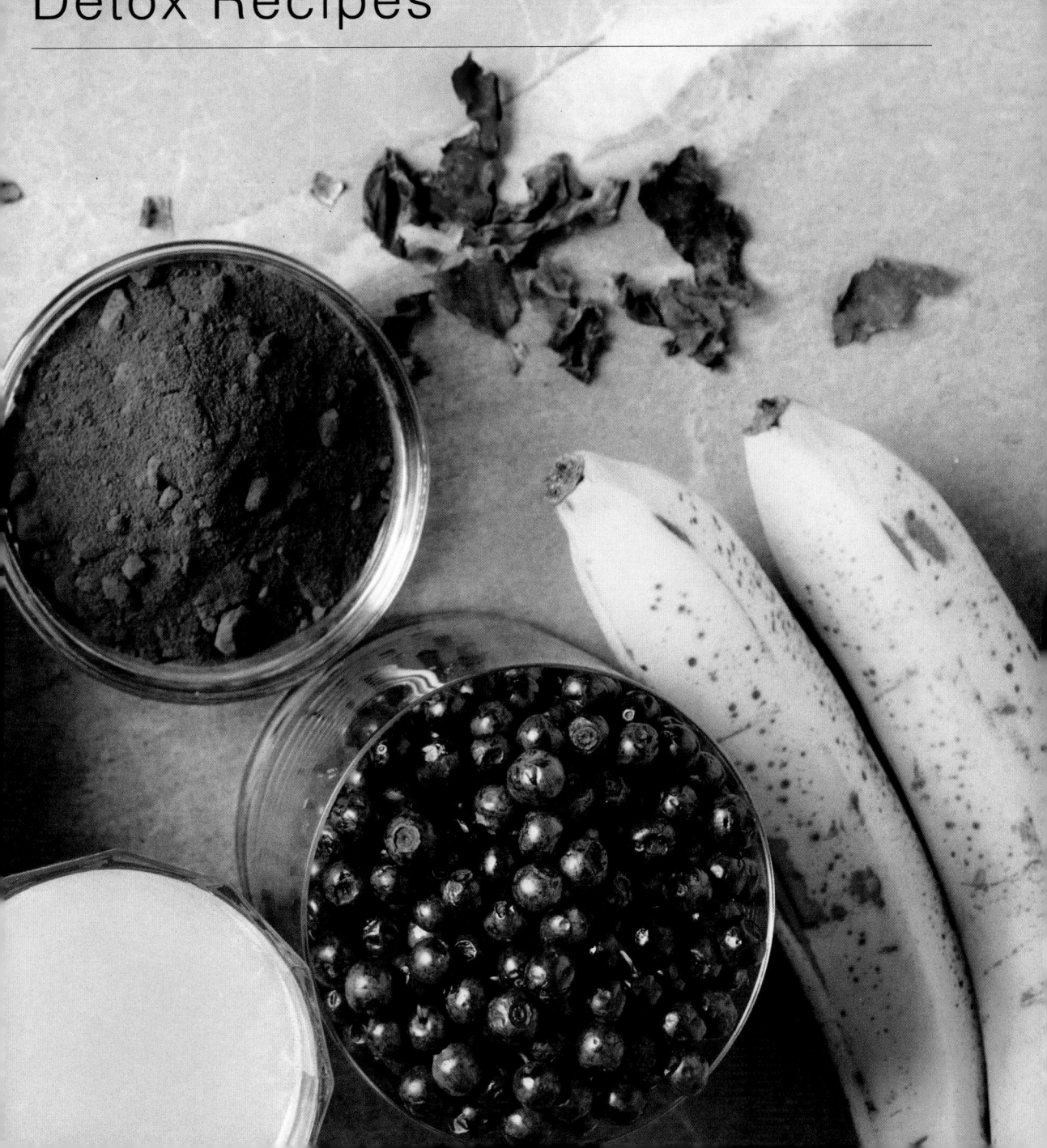

HEAVY METAL DETOX SMOOTHIE

Makes 1 serving

This smoothie is a perfect and powerful combination of the five key ingredients for safely detoxifying toxic heavy metals from your brain and body. It's an honorable, life-giving blessing to help reverse so many symptoms.

2 bananas

2 cups frozen or fresh wild blueberries, or 2 ounces pure wild blueberry juice, or 2 tablespoons pure wild blueberry powder

1 cup tightly packed fresh cilantro

1 teaspoon barley grass juice powder

1 teaspoon spirulina

1 tablespoon Atlantic dulse or 2 dropperfuls Atlantic dulse liquid

1 orange, juiced

½ to 1 cup water, coconut water, or additional fresh-squeezed orange juice (optional)

Combine the bananas, wild blueberries, cilantro, barley grass juice powder, spirulina, and Atlantic dulse with the juice of 1 orange in a high-speed blender and blend until smooth.

Add up to 1 cup of water, coconut water, or orange juice if a thinner consistency is desired. Serve and enjoy!

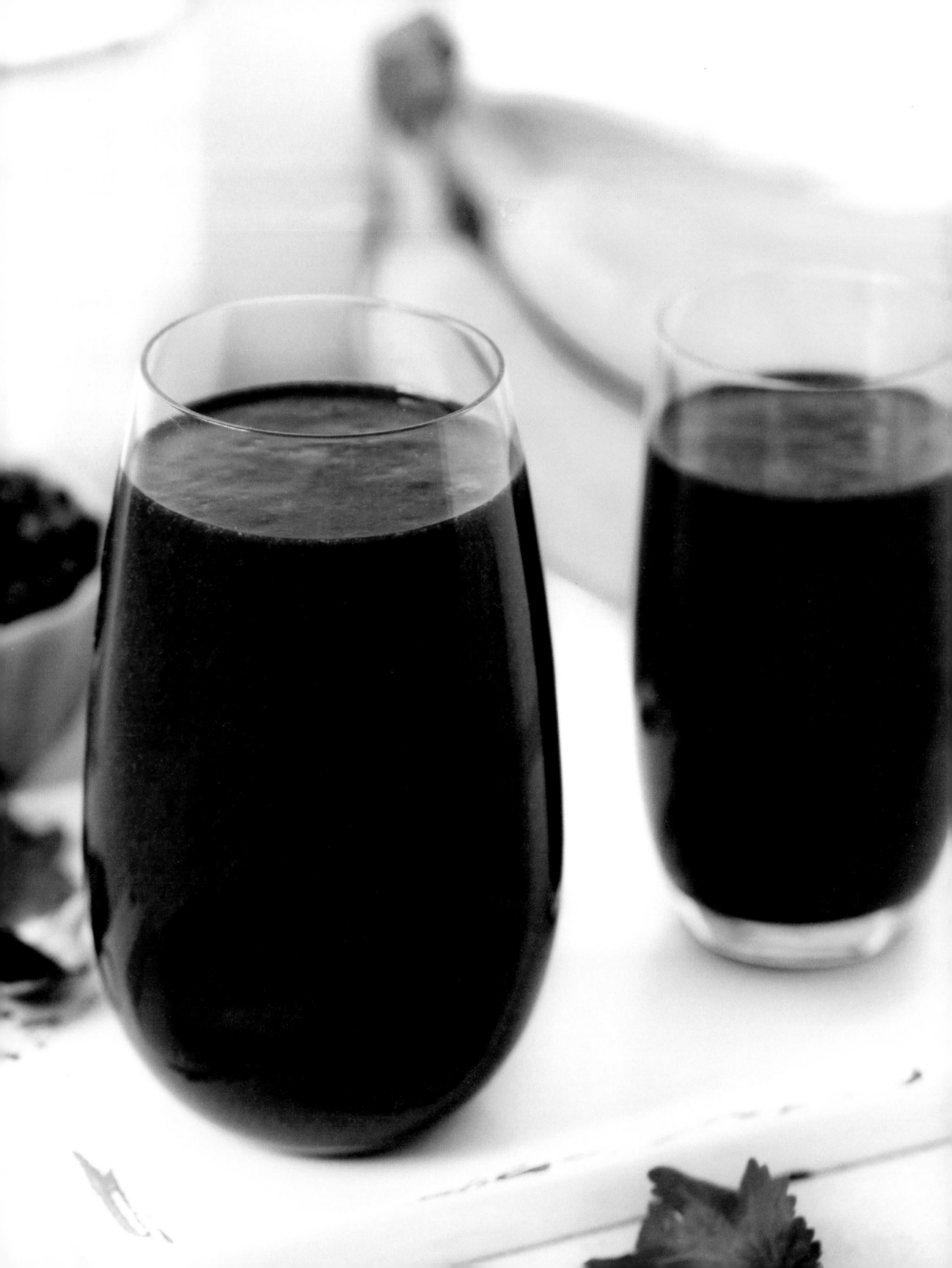

Heavy Metal Detox Smoothie continued

TIPS

- If the barley grass juice powder and spirulina taste is too strong for you, start with a smaller amount of each and work your way up.

- Seek out wild blueberries (whether fresh, frozen, powdered, or as pure juice). Wild blueberries are not to be confused with cultivated blueberries.

- If you're in a part of the world where you can't access fresh or frozen wild blueberries, wild blueberry juice, or wild blueberry powder, you can substitute blackberries. Blackberries do not uproot and attach themselves to toxic heavy metals like wild blueberries do, although the high antioxidant ratio in blackberries can at least slow down heavy metal oxidation, which is helpful.

- As an alternative to adding the juice from 1 orange to the smoothie, you have the option to peel the orange, remove its seeds, and blend it whole in the smoothie.

- If you're using coconut water in this smoothie, make sure the coconut water doesn't contain natural flavors and isn't pink or red.

- If you're not a fan of banana, you can substitute Maradol papaya or mango.

- On days when you can't access every smoothie ingredient, don't skip your Heavy Metal Detox Smoothie. Make it with whichever ingredients you do have. Keep aiming to make the smoothie with all five key ingredients.

ADVANCED HEAVY METAL DETOX SMOOTHIE

Makes 1 serving

This smoothie uses the five key ingredients to take you to a faster pace of removing toxic heavy metals.

2 bananas

2 cups frozen or fresh wild blueberries, or 2 ounces pure wild blueberry juice, or 2 tablespoons pure wild blueberry powder

2 cups tightly packed fresh cilantro

2 teaspoons barley grass juice powder

2 teaspoons spirulina

1 tablespoon Atlantic dulse or 2 dropperfuls Atlantic dulse liquid

2 oranges, juiced

½ to 1 cup or more of water, coconut water, or additional fresh-squeezed orange juice (optional)

Combine the bananas, wild blueberries, cilantro, barley grass juice powder, spirulina, and Atlantic dulse with the juice of 2 oranges in a high-speed blender and blend until smooth. Add up to 1 cup or more of water, coconut water, or orange juice if a thinner consistency is desired. Serve and enjoy!

TIPS

- This smoothie contains more spirulina, barley grass juice powder, and cilantro than the regular Heavy Metal Detox Smoothie. If you wish to do this Advanced version yet you find the taste of the greens too strong, you can add another banana, juice from one additional orange, or up to 2 teaspoons of raw honey as needed.

- Seek out wild blueberries (whether fresh, frozen, powdered, or as pure juice). Wild blueberries are not to be confused with cultivated blueberries.

- If you're in a part of the world where you can't access fresh or frozen wild blueberries, wild blueberry juice, or wild blueberry powder, you can substitute blackberries. Blackberries do not uproot and attach themselves to toxic heavy metals like wild blueberries do, although the high antioxidant ratio in blackberries can at least slow down heavy metal oxidation, which is helpful.

- As an alternative to adding the juice from 2 oranges to the smoothie, you have the option to peel the oranges, remove their seeds, and blend the oranges whole in the smoothie.

- If you're using coconut water in this smoothie, make sure the coconut water doesn't contain natural flavors and isn't pink or red.

- If you're not a fan of banana, you can substitute Maradol papaya or mango.

- On days when you can't access every smoothie ingredient, don't skip your Advanced Heavy Metal Detox Smoothie. Make it with whichever ingredients you do have. Keep aiming to make the smoothie with all five key ingredients.

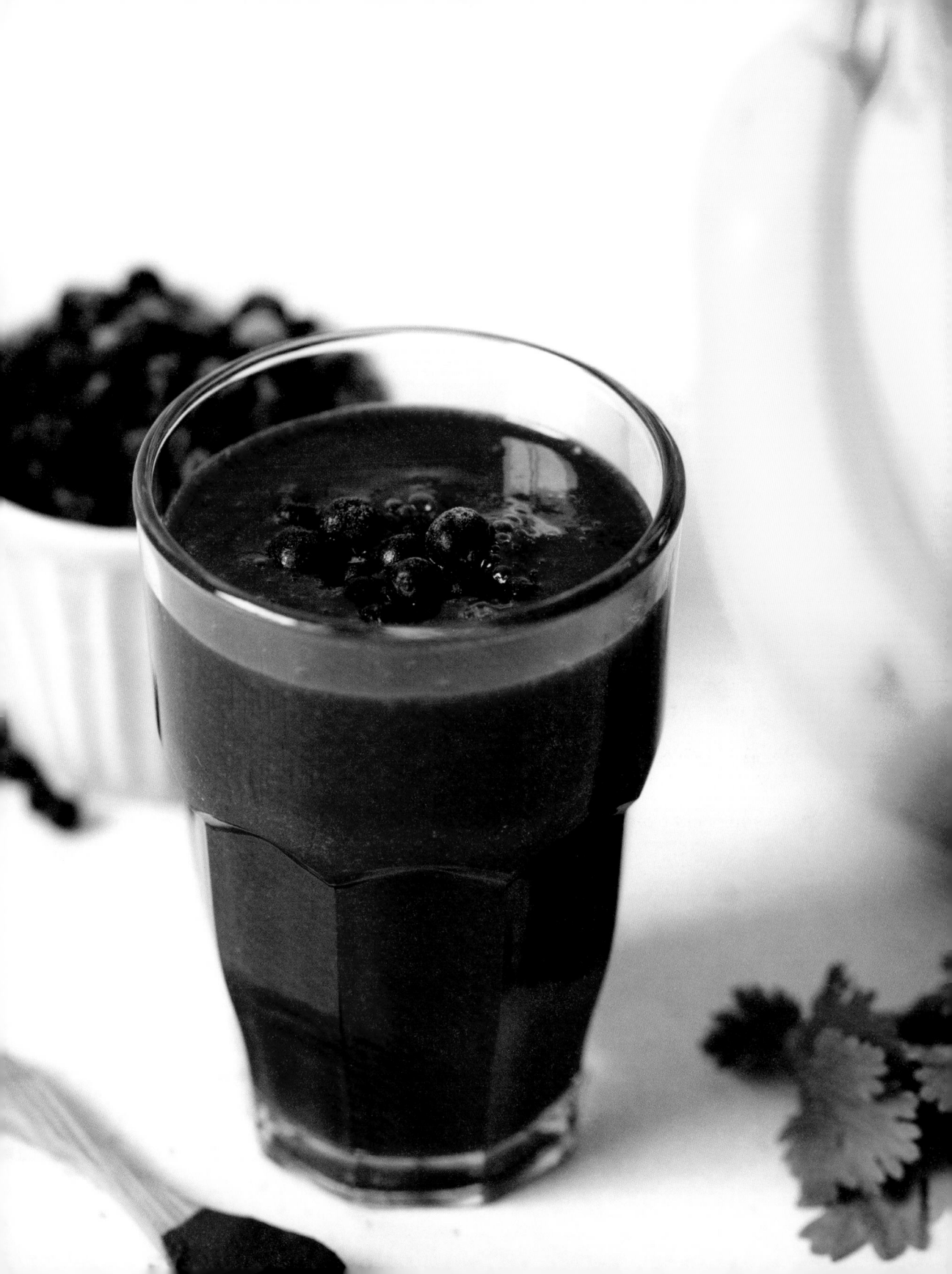

EXTRACTOR SMOOTHIE

Makes 1 serving

The Extractor aids in removing different varieties of chemical toxicity, also freeing the path for toxic heavy metals to uproot and exit the body more quickly.

1 apple, chopped

1 cup frozen or fresh wild blueberries, or 1 ounce pure wild blueberry juice, or 1 tablespoon pure wild blueberry powder

1 cup fresh or frozen mango or 1 fresh or frozen banana

1 cup tightly packed fresh parsley

1 radish root

1 teaspoon mustard seed powder

1 cup of water, coconut water, fresh apple juice, or bottled organic and additive-free 100 percent apple juice

Blend the ingredients together until smooth. Add up to 1 cup of water, coconut water, fresh apple juice, or bottled organic and additive-free 100 percent apple juice if a thinner consistency is desired. Serve and enjoy!

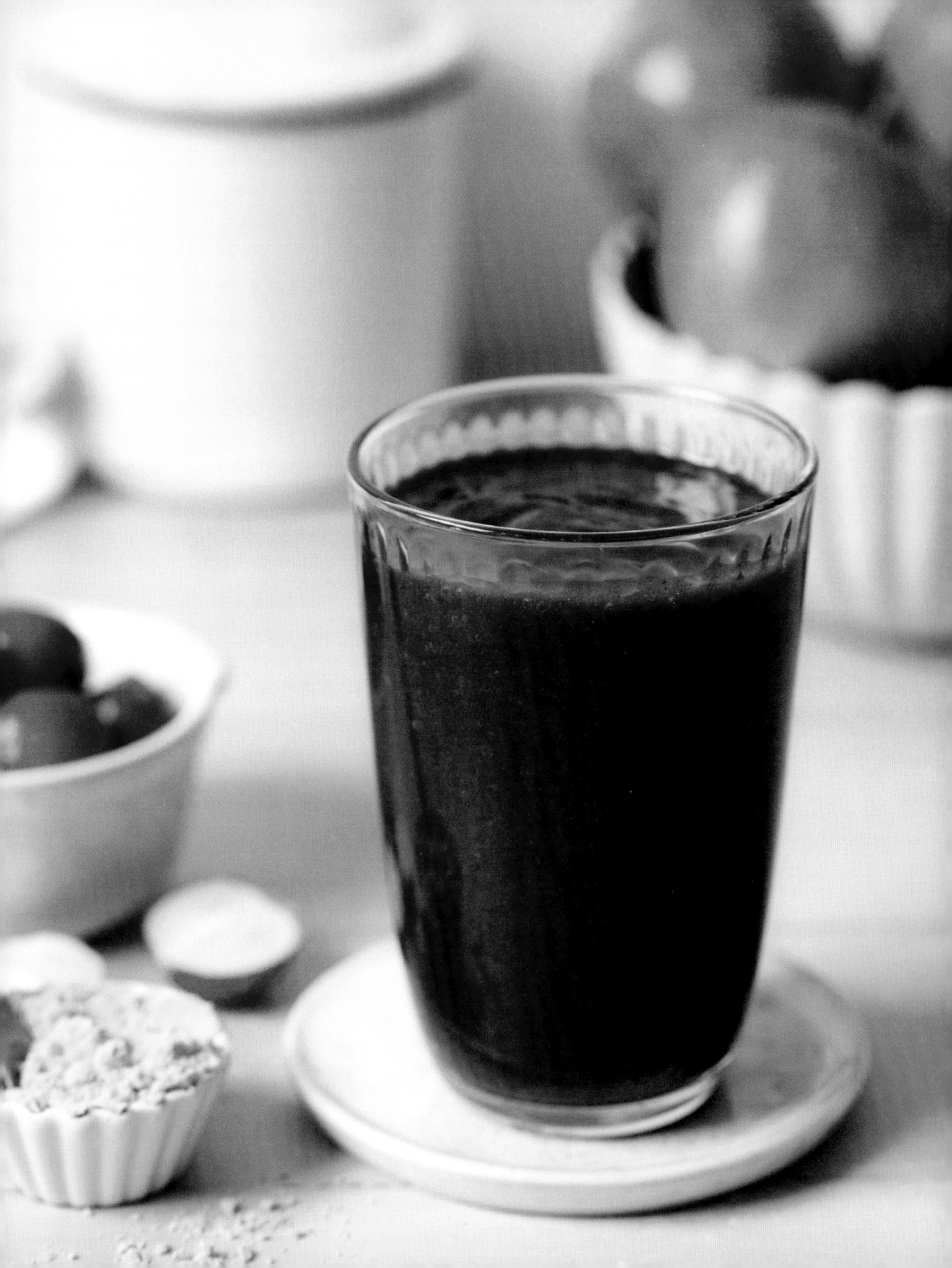

TIPS

- Choose red-skinned apples when possible, as they have the most nutrients.

- Mango is the first preference for this smoothie. If you can't get fresh or frozen mango, banana is a great replacement.

- You can use any color radish root, including red radish, black radish, and purple radish. Avoid using daikon radish.

- If you're using coconut water in this smoothie, make sure the coconut water doesn't contain natural flavors and isn't pink or red.

- If you are using a bottled, pasteurized apple juice, look for one that contains 100 percent organic apple juice with nothing else added such as sugar, citric acid, or preservatives.

- If you're having difficulty with the mustard seed flavor, you have the option to cut the amount of mustard in half, to ½ teaspoon, or even less if desired, with the goal of working your way back up to the recommended dosage of 1 teaspoon over time.

- If you're having difficulty with the parsley flavor, you have the option to cut the amount of parsley in half, to ½ cup, with the goal of working your way back up to the recommended dosage of 1 cup over time.

- If you're in a part of the world where you can't access fresh or frozen wild blueberries, wild blueberry juice, or wild blueberry powder, you can substitute blackberries. Although a high-antioxidant alternative, blackberries do not have the potency to match how wild blueberries defend cells from metals, chemicals, radiation, and other toxins.

- If you can't get apples, ripe pears can be substituted in this recipe. If you can't access apples or pears, look for oranges as a substitute. If you can't find oranges, look for papayas. If you can't get papayas, look for bananas. And if you can't get bananas, you can use mangoes in place of apples or pears.

- See the next chapter, "Medical Medium Heavy Metal Detox Cleanses," for advice on how to integrate the Extractor into your day and time it with the Heavy Metal Detox Smoothie for optimal results.

ADVANCED EXTRACTOR SMOOTHIE

Makes 1 serving

The Advanced Extractor works faster than the regular Extractor, also grabbing additional chemicals that the Extractor may not grab. Normally the Heavy Metal Detox Smoothie has the responsibility of removing other toxins in addition to toxic heavy metals. The Advanced Extractor's power at escorting those other chemical toxins out of the brain and body frees up the Heavy Metal Detox Smoothie to access and remove metals more quickly and easily.

1 apple, chopped

1 cup frozen or fresh wild blueberries, or 1 ounce pure wild blueberry juice, or 1 tablespoon pure wild blueberry powder

1 cup fresh or frozen mango or 1 fresh or frozen banana

1 cup tightly packed fresh parsley

1 radish root

2 cups roughly chopped radish greens, loosely packed

2 teaspoons mustard seed powder

1 cup of water, coconut water, fresh apple juice, or bottled organic and additive-free 100 percent apple juice

Blend the ingredients together until smooth. Add up to 1 cup of water, coconut water, fresh apple juice, or bottled organic and additive-free 100 percent apple juice if a thinner consistency is desired. Serve and enjoy!

TIPS

- Choose red-skinned apples when possible, as they have the most nutrients.

- Mango is the first preference for this smoothie. If you can't get fresh or frozen mango, banana is a great replacement.

- If you find the taste of this smoothie isn't to your liking, you can add an additional cup of fresh or frozen mango or an extra fresh or frozen banana to make it sweeter.

- You can use any color radish root, including red radish, black radish, and purple radish. Avoid using daikon radish.

- For best results look for fresh radish greens that are not wilted or yellowing. If you are unable to find radish greens, the next best choice is mustard greens. While they won't perform the same function as radish greens, they will still offer many benefits.

- If you're using coconut water in this smoothie, make sure the coconut water doesn't contain natural flavors and isn't pink or red.

- If you are using a bottled, pasteurized apple juice, look for one that contains 100 percent organic apple juice with nothing else added such as sugar, citric acid, or preservatives.

- If you're having difficulty with the mustard seed flavor, you have the option to cut the amount of mustard in half, to 1 teaspoon, or even less if desired, with the goal of working your way back up to the recommended dosage of 2 teaspoons over time.

- If you're having difficulty with the parsley flavor, you have the option to cut the amount of parsley in half, to ½ cup, with the goal of working your way back up to the recommended dosage of 1 cup over time.

- If you're in a part of the world where you can't access fresh or frozen wild blueberries, wild blueberry juice, or wild blueberry powder, you can substitute blackberries. Although a high-antioxidant alternative, blackberries do not have the potency to match how wild blueberries defend cells from metals, chemicals, radiation, and other toxins.

- If you can't get apples, ripe pears can be substituted in this recipe. If you can't access apples or pears, look for oranges as a substitute. If you can't find oranges, look for papayas. If you can't get papayas, look for bananas. And if you can't get bananas, you can use mangoes in place of apples or pears.

- See the next chapter, "Medical Medium Heavy Metal Detox Cleanses," for advice on how to integrate the Advanced Extractor into your day and time it with the Advanced Heavy Metal Detox Smoothie for optimal results.

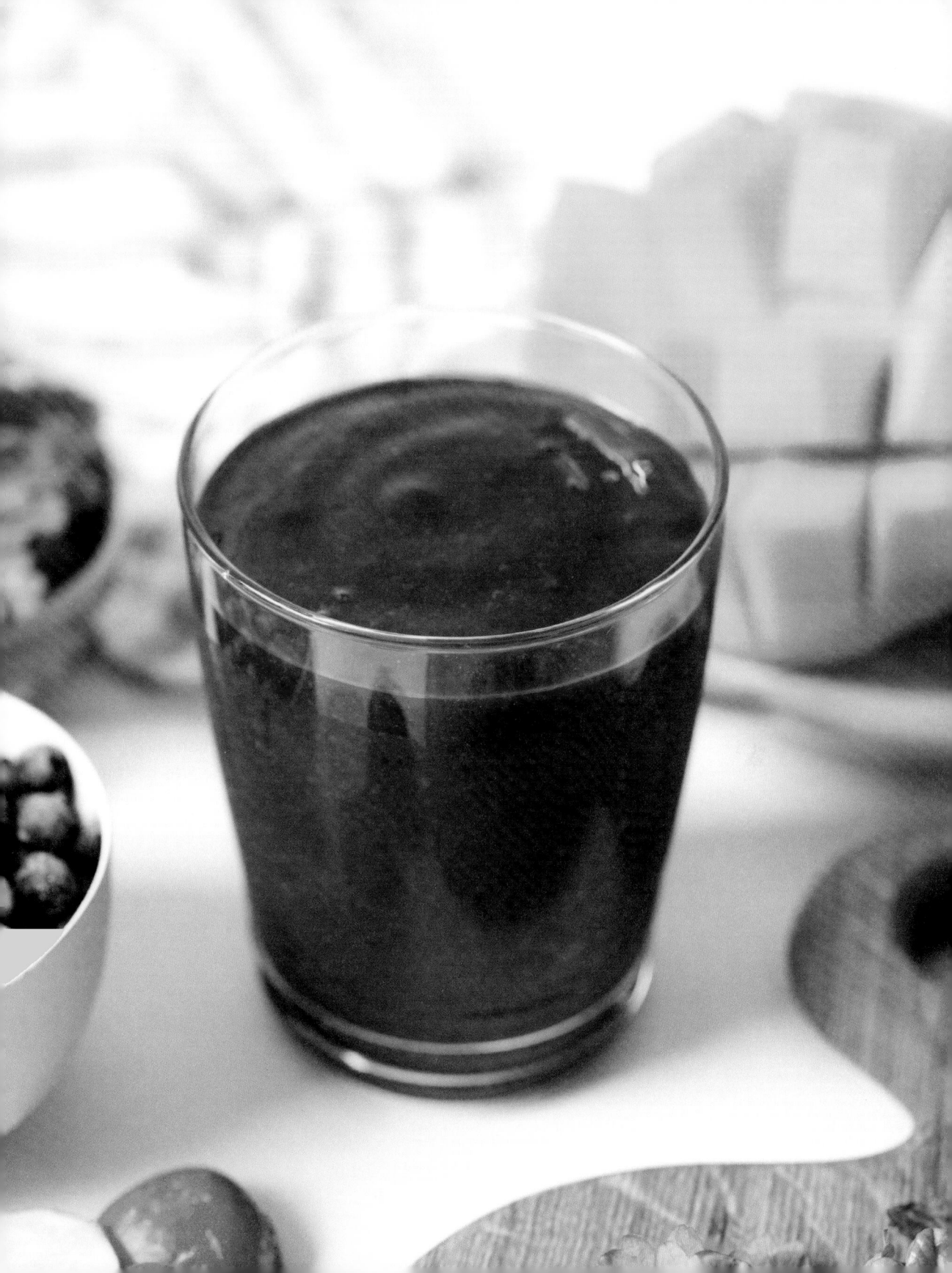

LEMON OR LIME WATER

Makes 1 serving

This simple recipe brings your water to life, priming toxic heavy metals and toxic chemicals to be more easily removed from your brain and body. Making lemon or lime water a part of your daily routine helps you stay hydrated enough to flush out the toxins and metals you're uprooting with the Heavy Metal Detox Smoothie and other tools and protocols in this book.

½ lemon or 2 limes, freshly cut
16 ounces (2 cups) water (room
   temperature or cooler, not hot)

Squeeze the juice from the freshly cut lemon or limes into the water, straining seeds if necessary.

Wait at least 15 to 20 minutes and ideally 30 minutes after you finish drinking your lemon or lime water before you consume your celery juice or anything else.

TIPS

- If you prefer 32 ounces (4 cups) of lemon or lime water upon rising, that's a great way to give yourself extra hydration and cleansing support. Simply double the recipe and enjoy.

- This recipe should not be made with hot water. Use room temperature or cold water.

- In your daily life, it's best to drink at least two or more 16-ounce lemon or lime waters over the course of a day. A great routine is to drink one upon rising, a second in the afternoon, and a third one hour before bed.

- Limes vary in size and juiciness. If your limes are dry, use 2 limes per 16 ounces of water, as the recipe calls for, to get enough juice. If your limes are big and juicy, you may only need half a lime.

- If you'd like, you're welcome to add a teaspoon of raw honey to your morning lemon or lime water.

- If for some reason lemons or limes don't work for you or you can't access them, you can make ginger water instead or opt for plain water.

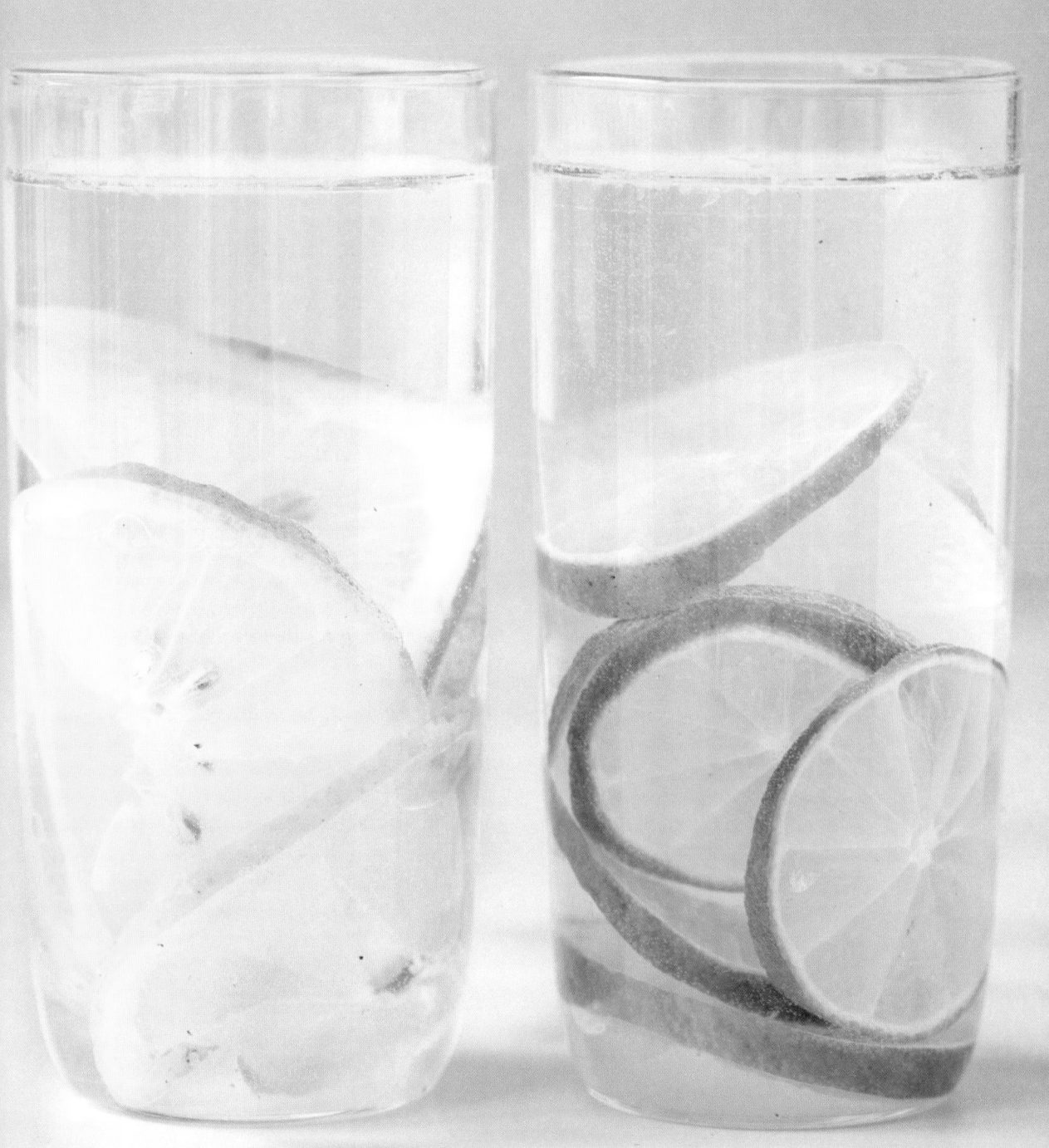

CELERY JUICE

This simple herbal extraction has an incredible ability to create sweeping improvements for all kinds of health issues when consumed in the right way. That's why celery juice is such an important Medical Medium healing tool. It's an ideal way to start your day whether you want to heal a symptom or condition or protect your health for the future.

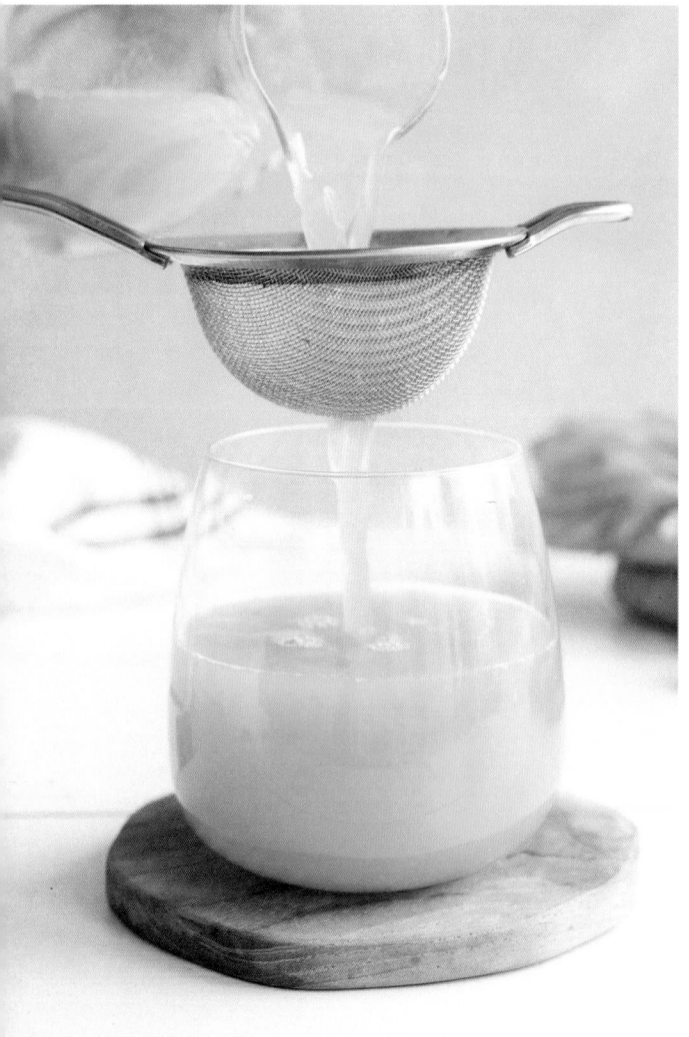

1 bunch of celery

Trim about a quarter inch off the base of the celery bunch to break apart the stalks.

Rinse the celery.

Run the celery through the juicer of your choice. Strain the juice to remove any grit or stray pieces of pulp. Drink immediately on an empty stomach for best results. Wait at least 15 to 30 minutes before consuming anything else.

If you don't have a juicer, you can make celery juice in a blender. Here's how:

Trim about a quarter inch off the base of the celery bunch, if desired, to break apart the stalks.

Rinse the celery. Place the celery on a clean cutting board and chop into roughly 1-inch pieces. Place the chopped celery in a high-speed blender and blend until smooth. (Don't add water.) Use your blender's tamping tool if needed. Strain the liquefied celery well; a nut milk bag is handy for this. Drink immediately on an empty stomach for best results. Wait at least 15 to 30 minutes before consuming anything else.

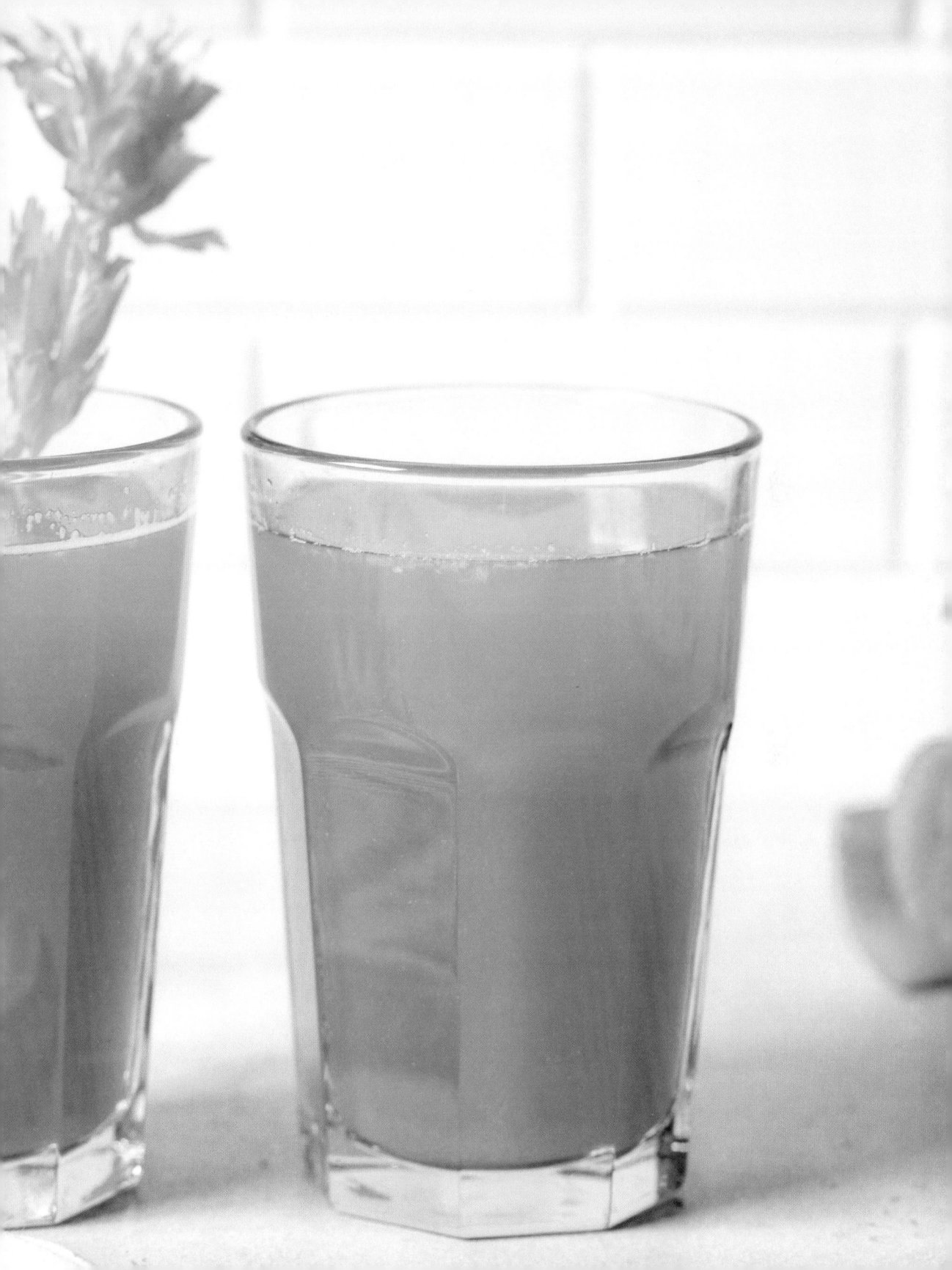

Celery Juice continued

TIPS

- Steer clear of putting additional ingredients such as lemon, apple, ginger, or leafy greens in your celery juice. While these are wonderful foods, celery juice only offers its full benefits when consumed as pure celery juice by itself. Also avoid adding ice, water, or any supplements or powders to your celery juice.

- If you're not going to be able to drink your full batch of celery juice right away, the best way to store it is in an airtight glass jar or bottle in the fridge. Freshly juiced celery retains its healing benefits for about 24 hours, but it does lose potency by the hour, so it's best to drink it as soon after making it as possible. If you have no choice but to keep it for longer than 24 hours, it's still worth juicing ahead and consuming it when you can.

- If you can't access celery to make celery juice and you can't get fresh, pure celery juice from your local juice bar, don't despair. Cucumber juice is the ideal substitute in this case. While it can't offer the specific healing benefits that celery juice does, it does have unique benefits such as cell hydration to support your health. Treat it the same way you would celery juice—make it pure (cucumber only) and drink it on an empty stomach, apart from other food and drink. Ginger water, aloe water, and lemon or lime water are alternatives if you can get neither celery juice nor cucumber juice. That said, try not to make a habit of substituting anything for celery juice.

- For more answers to your celery juice questions, including children's amounts, please see the pages that follow.

CELERY JUICE AS A MEDICINAL

Celery juice is a powerful medicinal that elevates whatever you're doing right in your life. You can find the recipe for celery juice on the preceding pages.

Follow these guidelines for celery juice:

- Fresh, plain, unadulterated, straight celery juice. No added ice, water, lemon juice, apple cider vinegar, collagen, or other mix-ins. Also, as beneficial as green juice blends can be, they're not a substitute for pure celery juice.

- Juice means juice. Drinking blended celery without straining the pulp doesn't yield the same benefits. See "The Juicing versus Fiber Debate" in *Cleanse to Heal* for more on why.

- Fresh means fresh. Making a drink from reconstituted celery powder won't deliver the right benefits, nor will drinking pasteurized or HPP (high-pressure pasteurization) celery juice. Any kind of juicer is okay, although a cold press, masticating juicer is best. You can also choose to purchase your fresh celery juice from a juice bar rather than making your own. For best results, drink it freshly made. If you can't drink it immediately after juicing—for example, if you're having a second serving in the day—that's okay. Store it chilled in an airtight container.

- If you need to store your celery juice, it will stay strong and beneficial for 24 hours in the fridge. You can store it for as long as 48 to 72 hours in an airtight container in the refrigerator. After the 48-hour mark, celery juice does start losing some of its healing strength. Try your best not to exceed 24 hours. That period is when it's at its strongest.

- You can freeze celery juice, although that's not ideal either. If it's your only option, then go ahead and freeze it, and when you're ready, take it out and drink it as soon as it's thawed. Don't add water to the thawing celery juice. That will interfere with its benefits.

- Drink your fresh celery juice on an empty stomach. If you drank some water or lemon water beforehand, wait at least 15 to 20 and ideally 30 minutes before drinking your celery juice. After finishing your celery juice, wait at least 15 to 20 minutes and ideally 30 minutes before consuming anything else.

- If you're drinking celery juice later in the day, give any food you've eaten plenty of time to digest first. If your last snack or meal was high in fat/protein, it's best to wait a minimum of two hours and ideally three hours before having your celery juice. If you last ate something lighter such as fruit, leafy greens, vegetables, potatoes, or a fruit smoothie, you can drink your celery juice 60 minutes after eating.

- If you are on a doctor-prescribed medication, it's okay to take it either before or after your celery juice, depending on whether it's supposed to be taken on an empty stomach or with food. (Please note that if your medication is supposed to be taken with food, celery juice does not count as a food.) If you take the medication first, try to wait at least 15 to 20 minutes and ideally 30 minutes before you drink your celery juice. If you drink your celery juice first, try to wait at least 15 to 20 minutes and ideally 30 minutes before you take your medication. For any further questions or concerns, consult your physician.

- When it comes to other Medical Medium–recommended supplements, please hold off on taking them with your celery juice. While the supplements will do fine with the celery juice, the celery juice is better without most supplements. It's best to wait to take your supplements until at least 15 to 20 minutes and ideally 30 minutes after you've finished your celery juice.

- If you have any further questions about bringing celery juice into your life, the Medical Medium title *Celery Juice* is an entire book of answers waiting for you.

Celery Juice Amounts for Children

When selecting celery juice amounts for children, you can refer to this table. These are recommended daily minimums. It can be less if that feels right for your child, or more. You don't need to worry that going over these minimums is harmful.

AGE	AMOUNT
6 months old	1 ounce or more
1 year old	2 ounces or more
18 months old	3 ounces or more
2 years old	4 ounces or more
3 years old	5 ounces or more
4 to 6 years old	6 to 7 ounces or more
7 to 10 years old	8 to 10 ounces or more
11 years old and up	12 to 16 ounces

"Your brain has abilities to heal beyond what medical research and science are aware of today."

— Anthony William, Medical Medium

CHAPTER 45

Medical Medium
Heavy Metal Detox Cleanses

Empowerment is knowing there's something you can do that can change your life and bring your health into a direction that you dream about. As you're venturing into this cleanse, you're venturing in with the knowledge of why you've been struggling all along. No longer are your hands tied when it comes to finding answers about how to move forward with your health.

If you're knocking on the door of these cleanses, it means you have struggled in some way. Maybe you've struggled so much that no one else could even know what it's been like unless they've struggled in a similar way. Spiritual forces of the light help us find our way when we've been walking down such a difficult path. It's not just a chance that you're here. There were powers at work all along in your journey that brought you to this place.

Removing toxic heavy metals isn't just a physical experience. It's a spiritual experience, because having toxic heavy metals inside the brain harms us spiritually. All along, you've been taking notice of your symptoms and conditions and your struggles and hardships. It's time to take notice of the tangible recovery you have set before you.

As you venture into a Heavy Metal Detox Cleanse, there are some different sensations that you may experience. The feeling of metals leaving the brain can bring about nostalgia, déjà vu, a temporary sense of sadness, or a sense of feeling more complete, as well as increased and more vivid dreams, especially dreams that make no sense whatsoever, eventually leading to more euphoric dreams that feel peaceful and good. As metals are removed, a sense of clarity, a sense of peace, a sense of excitement, and the feeling of joy can come from out of nowhere for no apparent reason. Everybody experiences different sensations, depending on how many metals, what kind of metals, where in the brain those metals are, and how toxic someone is with a variety of different chemicals.

These anti-pathogenic cleanses are designed to rid many different heavy metal–related symptoms, conditions, and diseases.

The Advanced and High-Powered options have the ability to get rid of 100 symptoms someone may have. (For long-term support, especially for pathogens, supplementation protocols are available in this book's companion title, *Brain Saver Protocols, Cleanses & Recipes*.)

You can choose, at any given time, which of the seven cleanse options to select. You can also climb the ladder here. It's all part of how Medical Medium protocols are customizable to take you as far as you need to go. The higher up you go through the cleanse levels, the more symptoms and conditions can dissipate.

HEAVY METAL DETOX CLEANSE GUIDELINES

15-Day or 30-Day Options

- For each of these cleanse options, select a period of either 15 days or 30 days.

Repeating the Cleanse

- You're welcome to do any of these cleanse levels continually and long term by repeating cleanses back-to-back.

- When you're repeating a Heavy Metal Detox Cleanse back-to-back, you could either repeat the same level or switch to

a milder or more advanced level once you've made it through any 15- or 30-day cleanse period.

- You can also take breaks between cleanses. When you're not on a Heavy Metal Detox Cleanse, you can keep up with doing the Heavy Metal Detox Smoothie every day.

Smoothie Timing

- If you've selected a cleanse option that includes both a version of the Heavy Metal Detox Smoothie and a version of the Extractor Smoothie, keep in mind: don't reverse their order. When consuming them on the same day, you want to have the Heavy Metal Detox Smoothie (regular or Advanced) in the first half of your day, and the Extractor Smoothie (regular or Advanced) in the second half of your day.

Substitutions

- Many of these cleanses incorporate the option of daily apples as a snack. You can chop or blend those apples, substitute with ripe pears, enjoy the "Applesauce or Pear

Sauce" recipe in *Brain Saver Protocols, Cleanses & Recipes*, or have cooked applesauce (as long as it doesn't contain additives) if needed. If you can't access apples or pears, look for oranges as a substitute. If you can't find oranges, look for papayas. If you can't get papayas, look for bananas. And if you can't get bananas, you can use mangoes in place of apples or pears.

- For more questions about ingredient substitutions, see the Tips that go along with individual recipes. If possible, try not to get into the habit of relying on substitutions. Keep trying to achieve the goal of using the proper ingredients for the cleanses.

Cleanse Interruptions

- If you miss the Heavy Metal Detox Smoothie and/or Extractor Smoothie (regular or Advanced) on any given day of a cleanse, still try to follow the rest of the cleanse guidance that day, and then add one day to the end of your cleanse.

- If you do something that breaks your cleanse, add three days to the end of your cleanse. "Breaking the cleanse" means

consuming items your cleanse level specifies to avoid, whether radical fats such as nut butter in the morning or brain betrayer foods such as eggs, dairy, or gluten.

General Notes for All Cleanses

- If you're getting your blood drawn for some reason within the time period of your cleanse, ask if you can move your appointment to a time when you're not doing the cleanse, or follow the blood draw guidelines from Chapter 40, "Blood Draining Agenda."

- For any general cleansing questions you have that are not addressed in this book, *Cleanse to Heal* is available to you as an additional resource.

Adjustments for Children

You can go ahead with the Heavy Metal Detox Cleanses for children, keeping the following in mind:

- It's fine to leave the lemon or lime water out for kids and also to reduce the amount of celery juice according to what feels right for your little one. See the table at the end of Chapter 44 for more guidance on celery juice amounts for children.

- See "Adjustments for Children" in Chapter 44, "Heavy Metal Detox," for guidance on Heavy Metal Detox Smoothie amounts for children.

- The amounts of the Advanced Heavy Metal Detox Smoothie, Extractor Smoothie, and Advanced Extractor Smoothie are up to your discretion as parent or caregiver. Children can have these recipes in small portions, with serving sizes depending on the age and size of the child. You can go as low as 4 ounces or down to a tablespoon or even less.

HEAVY METAL DETOX CLEANSE LEVELS

1. ENTRY LEVEL Heavy Metal Detox Cleanse

Add these steps to your normal eating routine:

- Drink the original Heavy Metal Detox Smoothie daily (recipe in Chapter 44); it should not be consumed directly after a fat-based meal.

- Optional: Incorporate as many other Medical Medium tools and recipes as desired.

- Try to drink a minimum of 50 ounces of water throughout the day (that amount can include coconut water).

- If you're sensitive or believe you're extra toxic, Entry Level is a good place to begin. You have the option of making the Heavy Metal Detox Smoothie with the amounts of the five key ingredients reduced by 50 percent. Once you've gotten comfortable with those smaller dosages, you can work your way up to the full recipe.

2. BASIC Heavy Metal Detox Cleanse

Add these steps to your normal eating routine:

- Drink the Advanced Heavy Metal Detox Smoothie daily (recipe in Chapter 44); it should not be consumed directly after a fat-based meal.

- Optional: Incorporate as many other Medical Medium tools and recipes as desired.

- Try to drink a minimum of 60 ounces of water throughout the day (that amount can include coconut water).

3. SIMPLIFIED Heavy Metal Detox Cleanse (same as the original Heavy Metal Detox Cleanse from *Cleanse to Heal*)

Add these steps to your normal eating routine:

- Start each day with 16 to 32 ounces of fresh lemon or lime water upon waking (recipe with the proper ratio of lemon or lime to water in Chapter 44).

- At least 15 to 30 minutes later, drink 16 to 32 ounces of fresh celery juice on an empty stomach (then wait another 15 to 30 minutes before you have your smoothie).

- Drink the original Heavy Metal Detox Smoothie (recipe in Chapter 44) for breakfast.

- If you get hungry again before lunchtime, stick to snacking on apples (have more than one if you want). You're welcome to chop or blend your apples, enjoy the "Applesauce or Pear Sauce" recipe in *Brain Saver Protocols, Cleanses & Recipes*, go with cooked applesauce (as long as it doesn't contain

additives), or opt for ripe pears if apples don't work for you.

- Stay fat-free until at least lunchtime.

- Optional: For even better results, take a look at the brain betrayer foods and food chemicals in Chapters 28 and 30. Start chipping away at the lists, seeing what foods you'd like to avoid while you're cleansing. The fewer brain betrayers such as eggs, dairy, gluten, corn, soy, tuna, lamb, and pork in your diet, the more effective the Heavy Metal Detox Smoothie can be.

- Try to drink a minimum of 60 ounces of water throughout the day (that amount can include coconut water and your morning lemon or lime water). Be mindful not to drink the water too close to drinking the celery juice—make sure you space them at least 15 to 30 minutes apart.

4. INTERMEDIATE Heavy Metal Detox Cleanse

Add these steps to your normal eating routine:

- Start each day with 16 to 32 ounces of fresh lemon or lime water upon waking (recipe with the proper ratio of lemon or lime to water in Chapter 44).

- At least 15 to 30 minutes later, drink 16 to 32 ounces of fresh celery juice on an empty stomach (then wait another 15 to 30 minutes before you have your smoothie).

- Drink the Advanced Heavy Metal Detox Smoothie (recipe in Chapter 44) for breakfast.

- If you get hungry again before lunchtime, stick to snacking on apples (have more than one if you want). You're welcome to chop or blend your apples, enjoy the "Applesauce or Pear Sauce" recipe in *Brain Saver Protocols, Cleanses & Recipes*, go with cooked applesauce (as long as it doesn't contain additives), or opt for ripe pears if apples don't work for you.

- Stay fat-free until at least lunchtime.

- Optional: For even better results, take a look at the brain betrayer foods and food chemicals in Chapters 28 and 30. Start chipping away at the lists, seeing what foods you'd like to avoid while you're cleansing. The fewer brain

betrayers such as eggs, dairy, gluten, corn, soy, tuna, lamb, and pork in your diet, the more effective the Advanced Heavy Metal Detox Smoothie can be.

- Try to drink a minimum of 60 ounces of water throughout the day (that amount can include coconut water and your morning lemon or lime water). Be mindful not to drink the water too close to drinking the celery juice—make sure you space them at least 15 to 30 minutes apart.

5. PERFORMANCE Heavy Metal Detox Cleanse

Add these steps to your normal eating routine:

- Start each day with 16 to 32 ounces of fresh lemon or lime water upon waking (recipe with the proper ratio of lemon or lime to water in Chapter 44).

- At least 15 to 30 minutes later, drink 16 to 32 ounces of fresh celery juice on an empty stomach (then wait another 15 to 30 minutes before you have your smoothie).

- Drink the original Heavy Metal Detox Smoothie (recipe in Chapter 44) for breakfast.

- If you get hungry again before lunchtime, stick to snacking on apples (have more than one if you want). You're welcome to chop or blend your apples, enjoy the "Applesauce or Pear Sauce" recipe in *Brain Saver Protocols, Cleanses & Recipes*, go with cooked applesauce (as long as it doesn't contain additives), or opt for ripe pears if apples don't work for you.

- Stay fat-free until at least lunchtime.

- Drink the Extractor Smoothie (recipe in Chapter 44) anytime in the second half of your day, as long as it's not after a fat-based snack or meal.

- Try to incorporate as many fat-free Medical Medium recipes from this book's companion title, *Brain Saver Protocols, Cleanses & Recipes*, into your snacks and meals as you can.

- Avoid all foods and food chemicals from Chapters 28 and 30, including caffeine.

- Keep fats limited to one serving (if at all) from lunchtime on, preferably at the end of the day. If you're plant-based, it's okay to incorporate one serving of plant fat such as avocado, nuts or nut butters, seeds, coconut, coconut oil, olives, or olive oil in a Medical Medium recipe. If you eat animal products, it's okay to incorporate one serving of animal fat such as chicken, grass-fed beef, turkey, salmon, or sardines in a Medical Medium recipe.

- Try to drink a minimum of 60 ounces of water throughout the day (that amount can include coconut water and your morning lemon or lime water). Be mindful not to drink the water too close to drinking the celery juice—make sure you space them at least 15 to 30 minutes apart.

6. ADVANCED Heavy Metal Detox Cleanse

Make these steps your complete eating routine:

- Start each day with 16 to 32 ounces of fresh lemon or lime water upon waking (recipe with the proper ratio of lemon or lime to water in Chapter 44).

- At least 15 to 30 minutes later, drink 16 to 32 ounces of fresh celery juice on an empty stomach (then wait another 15 to 30 minutes before you have your smoothie).

- Drink the original Heavy Metal Detox Smoothie (recipe in Chapter 44) for breakfast.

- If you get hungry again before lunchtime, stick to snacking on apples (have more than one if you want). You're welcome to chop or blend your apples, enjoy the "Applesauce or Pear Sauce" recipe in *Brain Saver Protocols, Cleanses & Recipes*, go with cooked applesauce (as long as it doesn't contain additives), or opt for ripe pears if apples don't work for you.

- Stay off all fat-based foods, both plant fats (e.g., nuts, seeds, avocado) and animal fats (e.g., chicken, fish, meat).

- Drink the Extractor Smoothie (recipe in Chapter 44) anytime in the second half of your day.

- Use exclusively fat-free Medical Medium recipes from this book's companion title, *Brain Saver Protocols, Cleanses & Recipes*.

- Avoid all foods and food chemicals from Chapters 28 and 30, including caffeine.

- Try to drink a minimum of 60 ounces of water throughout the day (that amount can include coconut water and your

morning lemon or lime water). Be mindful not to drink the water too close to drinking the celery juice—make sure you space them at least 15 to 30 minutes apart.

7. HIGH-POWERED Heavy Metal Detox Cleanse

Make these steps your complete eating routine:

- Start each day with 32 ounces of fresh lemon or lime water upon waking (recipe with the proper ratio of lemon or lime to water in Chapter 44).

- At least 15 to 30 minutes later, drink 32 ounces of fresh celery juice on an empty stomach (then wait another 15 to 30 minutes before you have your smoothie).

- Drink the Advanced Heavy Metal Detox Smoothie (recipe in Chapter 44) for breakfast.

- If you get hungry again before lunchtime, stick to snacking on apples (have more than one if you want). You're welcome to chop or blend your apples, enjoy the "Applesauce or Pear Sauce" recipe in *Brain Saver Protocols, Cleanses & Recipes*, go with cooked applesauce (as long as it doesn't contain additives), or opt for ripe pears if apples don't work for you.

- Stay off all fat-based foods, both plant fats (e.g., nuts, seeds, avocado) and animal fats (e.g., chicken, fish, meat).

- Drink the Advanced Extractor Smoothie (recipe in Chapter 44) anytime in the second half of your day.

- Use exclusively fat-free Medical Medium recipes from this book's companion title, *Brain Saver Protocols, Cleanses & Recipes*.

- Avoid all foods and food chemicals from Chapters 28 and 30, including caffeine.

- Remove fragrances, colognes, perfumes, air fresheners, incense; and **scented** candles, laundry detergents, fabric softeners, aftershaves, deodorants, soaps, body sprays, body lotions, body oils, hair products, and car fresheners.

- Try to drink a minimum of 60 ounces of water throughout the day (that amount can include coconut water and your morning lemon or lime water). Be mindful not to drink the water too close to drinking the celery juice—make sure you space them at least 15 to 30 minutes apart.

"The human brain will always have an opportunity to heal if the information is available."

— Anthony William, Medical Medium

CHAPTER 46

You Deserve Validation

Before COVID, there was already a form of social distancing that had been going on for decades. This was social distancing practiced by people suffering with chronic illness and neurological symptoms.

Some chronic symptoms and conditions don't cause people to withdraw. UTIs, chronic sinus infections, a thyroid disorder, a physical injury to the ankle or knee, an achy back, bloating, skin conditions such as mild eczema, psoriasis, acne—unless they're severe, these ailments often still allow people to live their lives. People may feel uncomfortable or be unhappy about their weight gain, hair loss, or bloating. They may not want to be on the beach. Yet they're able to keep going about their days. They don't tend to back down from social engagements.

Something different happens when people have a problem that involves the brain, the central nervous system, the nerves. When neurological symptoms pass from mild to more moderate, people tend to pick and choose which social engagements they attend with family or friends.

It's hard enough to live with neurological symptoms such as tingles and numbness, fatigue, OCD, seizures, anxiety, depression, dizziness, vertigo, brain fog, migraines, floaters in the eyes. It's that much harder to be around people who may be challenging, whether they're family members or friends, when you don't feel well and you're struggling neurologically. It takes a lot out of a person. You're experiencing the symptom, trying to live with it and cope, so a natural progression of backing out of social engagement occurs.

Someone in your life may witness this withdrawal from social engagement and ring the alarm bells without understanding that you just don't feel well. If you aren't already on the doctor and testing search, this worry from others can be what prompts your search. With mysterious neurological symptoms, most people around you think, "Just go to the doctor and get fixed." It's not that easy. This alone—knowing that your symptoms won't make sense to others—can prompt social distancing.

When neurological symptoms are centered more around the brain itself, that's when the social engagement really declines. The more severe your brain fog is, the less you're going to be in a hurry to communicate with others. You're conversing with a friend, and the friend is detecting your brain fog and says something. Many times, this can cause shame, frustration, and anger, because you're feeling misunderstood. It's not your fault; you already have it hard enough. When someone misinterprets your brain fog, it can be very difficult.

On the other hand, explaining your symptoms to loved ones and coworkers doesn't always seem to go well. You can feel even more misunderstood. Mysterious symptoms getting in the way of trying to live your life normally can end up taking freedoms away that other people can't relate to. Often, people with brain-related neurological symptoms have to pick and choose the time and energy they spend with others. Who's the safer person to spend the energy and time with? Who won't judge you if you speak about your symptoms—brain fog, inability to articulate well, inability to sleep well, fatigue levels?

Part of what makes neurological symptoms mysterious is that you'll often look perfectly fine to somebody else from the outside. Unless a neurological symptom has gotten so severe that it shows itself physically, it looks as if there's nothing wrong.

When neurological symptoms do start to show themselves, people tend to retreat more. People learn their limitations. For example, if someone's neurological fatigue is coming on, and they can't keep holding themselves up while standing in conversation with someone else, they're going to wrap up the conversation and say, "I've got to go." Oftentimes with neurological symptoms, people have to gauge how much energy they have for everything they have to do. Grocery shopping, for instance, can be a massive undertaking for someone with neurological symptoms. If you run into someone at the grocery store who engages you in conversation, it can take every single thing out of you.

Most health professionals who haven't been in the shoes of someone with neurological symptoms cannot relate to this. They think a patient with neurological symptoms should still have more than enough energy and strength to get to a doctor's office, wait in a waiting room, and undergo examination and testing. Patients with neurological symptoms are misunderstood even by physicians, if the physicians are strong and aren't experiencing neurological symptoms themselves.

When a younger person starts to develop neurological symptoms, it can be a particular struggle to be understood. A child with neurological symptoms often gets dismissed as having behavioral issues or autism. Then there are times when behavioral issues are coinciding with the fact that a child has neurological symptoms we associate with adults. A child cannot always express their tingles and numbness, their aches and pains, their dizziness, their brain fog, their inability to receive information and formulate the right words when expressing themselves. If a child is clearly exhibiting sickness and all tests conclude no definitive cause, the child—or even teenager—could be told they're making it up.

Teenagers suffering with body pain, fatigue, and brain fog will be told they're making it up more often than adults. These teens will be told it's a mental issue and they need a psychiatrist. This used to happen more with adults. Women especially were told they were crazy, making it up, bored, lazy, or that it was a cry for attention. Nowadays, it's like this adult version has been cast on to teenagers and children who describe mysterious neurological symptoms and yet seem to check out okay.

The more complex the neurological issue becomes for someone of any age, or the more complicated it gets with multiple symptoms, the more difficult it is for someone to function. Then you have no choice other than to withdraw. The people you choose to spend time with have to be more understanding; otherwise, you're less likely to communicate with them. This is when your contact list of people who will understand dwindles. Many people with brain-related neurological conditions only have a few people they end up talking to, when they used to have 30. This is rarely discussed because the chronically ill tend to be swept under the carpet. There's monumental discrimination against the chronically ill.

We're now heading to a place where neurological symptoms are going to be far more common than ever before. So many individuals are going to have neurological symptoms that the world is going to be forced to shift. People *without* neurological symptoms are going to be in the minority. The majority will be people with neurological symptoms. It has already started, and in the next five years, we're going to see more chronic neurological symptoms than ever before in the history of humankind on this planet.

There's still going to be a wall up between the not-so-sick and the sick. In the new normal, those who are not-so-sick with neurological symptoms will still appear to be functioning and living their lives. The people who are sick with neurological symptoms are going to have to withdraw and practice social distancing. As ever, it's a fine line between the not-so-sick and the sick—between brain fog and severe brain fog, between mild neurological symptoms occurring in the background and pronounced neurological symptoms getting in the way of life. That difference in severity of symptoms can be the difference between making a phone call and not being able to make any calls. It can be the difference between driving a car and not being able to drive at all.

People with brain-related and nervous system–related symptoms tend to be branded as "sensitive." The truth is that they are sensitive. Rightfully so. They're struggling with neurological symptoms. Yet when called "sensitive" by others, it's kind of an insult. Neurological symptoms tend to be labeled as psychological without an understanding that our mental health is rooted in the physical health of our brain and nervous system. People around someone with neurological symptoms tend to think there are mental issues involved instead of real physical symptoms with a real physical cause. When you have neurological symptoms, you've gone through a lot. You've lost freedoms in your life. You haven't been allowed to fully express yourself, play reindeer games, live your life to its maximum, play tennis with your friends, go on hikes, dance, exercise, and travel. You've been withheld. You've lost friends and become distanced from certain family members. As a result of the many small wounds of losing these freedoms compounded on top of one another, you could get PTSD. A psychological component could develop. Yet it has nothing to do with the symptoms you've been faced with all along—meaning you don't have neurological symptoms because you're psychologically causing them. Any PTSD or psychological effects you experience from living with a neurological condition are *on top of* the neurological condition you were dealing with in the first place. It's rare to find validation and support for this understanding, so here's what's important to remember: You are stronger than you know for being able to push through, survive, and live with your symptoms. It takes a special ability and profound power.

"You can feel like an oddity when you recover from chronic illness. What you should be is heralded."

— Anthony William, Medical Medium

"You can imagine your brain as a tiny spaceship flying through the universe. Your neurons are billions of tiny aliens inside that spaceship, all communicating together. At the same time, there's a supreme being on the ship watching all of it—that's your soul."

— Anthony William, Medical Medium

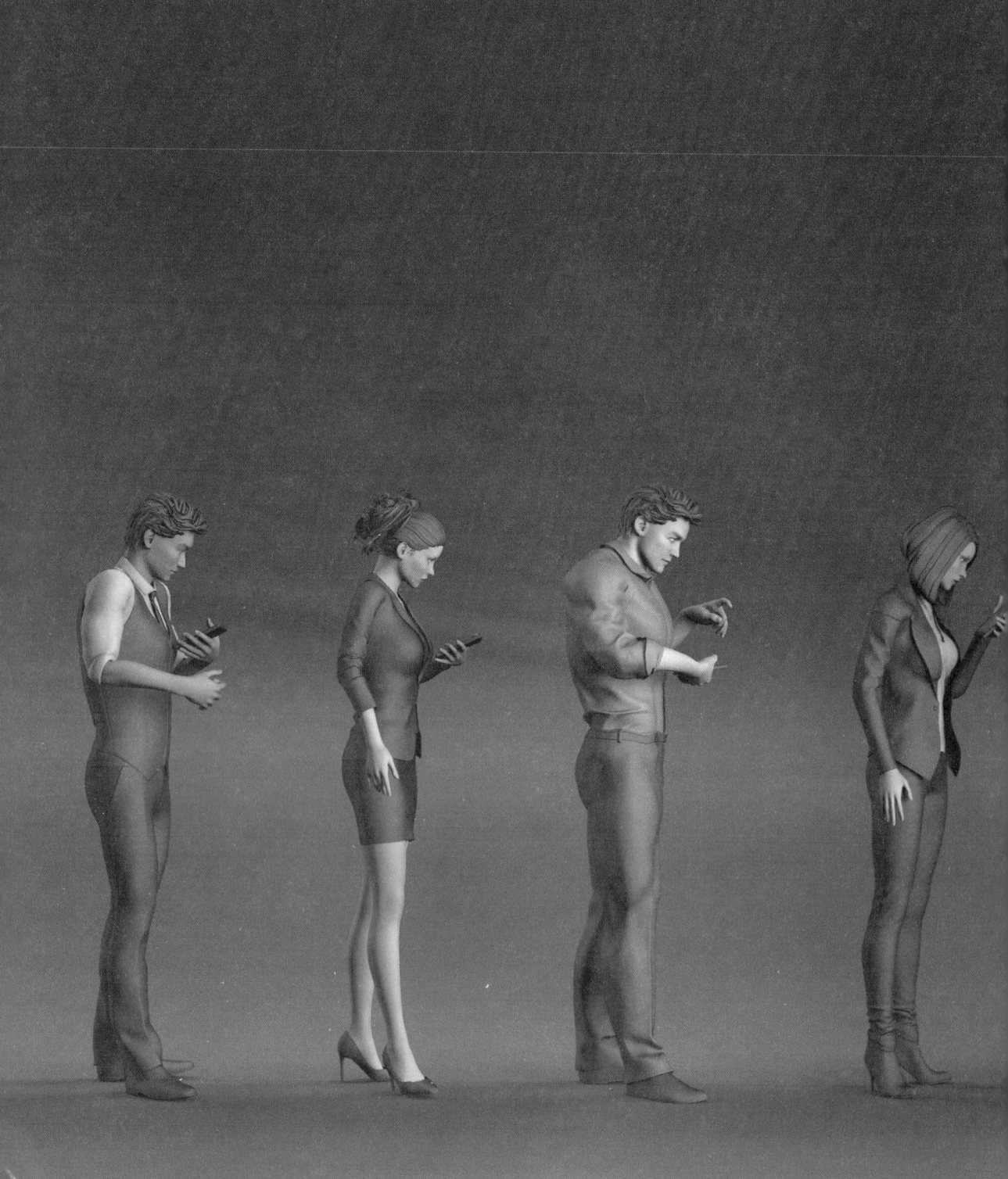

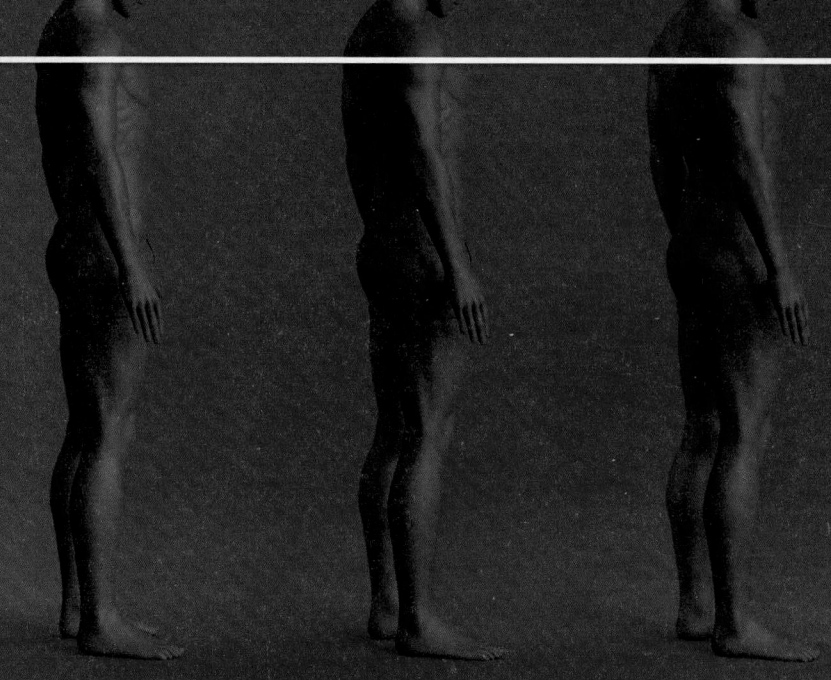

PART VII

BRAINED &
CONFUSED

"One reason the chronically ill can face so much discrimination is that they often look 'fine' or 'normal' to outsiders who don't understand. If you've ever lived through chronic pain or other invisible symptoms, you know how sorely lacking the understanding and compassion can be. You know how readily people blame it on something going on in your head."

— Anthony William, Medical Medium

CHAPTER 47

We Need to Look Out for Each Other

In today's world, getting a symptom or condition—becoming chronically sick—is the new normal. We're at a place in the world where you're either not-so-sick or very sick. Everyone is dealing with something. Everybody is facing at least one symptom, whether they'd call it a "symptom" or not, whether they realize their health is challenged or not.

When you're not-so-sick, your life hasn't come to a screeching halt yet. You're able to live with and manage any health issues that may come up, if you even notice them. There's not a lot of gray area between the not-so-sick and the sick. You know when your health reaches a place where it feels like it's not manageable, when it feels like it's getting out of control. You know when you're in an emotional or mental state of desperation as you try to figure out how to stop your symptoms that you realize are becoming a bigger and bigger problem, impeding your life.

Because of the different pain tolerances people have and the differences in people themselves, the line between not-so-sick and sick can vary from person to person. Impediments for one person that limit their quality of life may not be impediments for another person. What it boils down to is an individual's experience. Everything is going smoothly enough when you're not-so-sick. You cross the line into sick when you can tell that something is wrong and really getting in the way.

When you're struggling with your health, sometimes you may receive judgment from a person who hasn't been through hell going from doctor to doctor. A not-so-sick person's frame of reference can be limited to their own experience with a bit of bloating, mild acne now and then, a headache once in a blue moon, a little bit of brain fog that their caffeine hit in the morning clears up, intermittent low energy, or slight weight gain. For the sick, it would feel like a relief to experience only the symptoms of the not-so-sick, which also include loose stools, mild shoulder pain, some seasonal affective disorder, sore feet, occasional headaches, slight stiffness in the morning that wears off, a little sinus congestion, occasional yeast infections, mild constipation, infrequent head colds, a little bit of anxiousness, a mild thyroid condition, a hormone imbalance, and mild skin issues. These mild or temporary symptoms of the not-so-sick, while uncomfortable and inconvenient, are a world apart from the serious, life-disrupting, perspective-altering symptoms that the sick experience.

The sick have tried both conventional and alternative medicine. They know what it feels like to be burdened and trapped by struggles that may be invisible to others. It can be a years-long, brutal journey of trying to heal and find answers for severe neurological fatigue, crippling anxiety, chronic heart palpitations, heart flutters, arrhythmias, drastic mood swings, heavy depression, relentless brain fog, mysterious seizures, unexplained body pain, debilitating migraines, agonizing eczema or psoriasis, crippling bloating and distension, serious digestive disorders, mysterious jaw pain, tingles and numbness, tightness of the chest, and inability to exercise due to muscle weakness.

When you visit doctor after doctor, specialist after specialist, and the co-pays are adding up, and the diagnoses change or you get no diagnosis at all, and it's all interfering with your life, managing your health becomes a full-time job. Many days, it's hard to get out of bed at all. You're watching other people out in the world being productive, accomplishing their daily grind, and meanwhile, your daily grind is sorting out doctor bills and health insurance issues, drug store visits, and driving long distances to different specialists. Sometimes you're even navigating hospital visits. This grind can dominate your day, your year, your life, and the lives of those around you.

Meanwhile, you may face the added challenge of judgment from some of the not-so-sick people you encounter, as though you have chosen these symptoms and this long slog to find answers, as though you simply haven't tried hard enough to get better or kept a positive enough attitude. Criticism and doubt that your chronic suffering is even real can be unfortunate side effects of the already difficult reality of living with a health challenge.

SELF-CARE AND DESPERATE CARE

One distinction between being not-so-sick and sick is the difference between being able to engage in self-care versus relying on desperate care.

When you're not-so-sick, visits to a doctor, practitioner, health coach, or trainer are geared to self-care, versus outcries for help because you're so bad off. Many people who are not-so-sick are living their lives. Illness isn't impeding them or stopping them or holding them back from doing what they desire to do. And some of those desires lead into self-care. You're doing your workouts, your sauna, your facials, your meditation, your coffee shop visits, your scented candles, your travel plans, your shopping, your cosmetic doctor visits, your dental cleanings, your manicures and pedicures, your acupuncture, your massage, your breath work, your gatherings and events, and when a small symptom arises, you tack on an occasional functional medicine doctor visit. Tending to mild, intermittent, or temporary symptoms gets absorbed into the self-care routine of life or wrapped up with a big self-care bow. You don't have to stop and say, "I'm really sick, and it's getting in the way of me doing what I want or need to do."

The person who's sick relies on care that goes beyond self-care—it's desperate care. Getting through the day comes down to forms of care they really need so they can sustain themselves on their journey to heal. If a not-so-sick person had to cancel their appointments because of a storm, they'd still be fine. They may be disappointed. They may get some anxiousness or a little stress because things aren't going the way they anticipated. Still, their life moves on. The sick person is in a different situation. Every little element that's supporting the sick person counts. Their focus is on survival with their symptoms and illness. They're in the process of fighting to hold on to any freedoms they have left, fighting to get back the freedoms they once experienced, trying to find joy wherever they can in the process of trying to survive. And this person who's sick has forms of care that they rely on to meet their needs. It's not about selecting forms of care out of an abundance of fun options

or personal choices that support their life. A sick person's needs are about survival.

So much time and energy go into being sick. If a not-so-sick person has never experienced this, they may struggle to understand. Relating to a sick person when you've never been there before can be like driving past a homeless person living in a tent when you've never experienced homelessness. It's easy to be preoccupied as you're driving past that person. It's easy to think, *That's just a homeless person living in their tent*, and then move on to your next thought. What if you focus on the details of that person's life? What if you ask yourself, *How did that person become homeless? When was the last time they bathed? When was the last time they ate? How do they go to the bathroom? Do their blankets have mold? Does their tent have a hole in it? Can they walk, or do they have walking pneumonia? What's their name? What do they need? How long have they been homeless?*

When a not-so-sick person runs into a sick person, they may look alike from the outside. And if a not-so-sick person has never experienced what the sick person is experiencing, they may not know the details to consider about this person's life. How long have they been sick? How bad is it? What foods can they eat or not eat? Can they even shower? Can they exercise? How much pain is that person in, mentally or physically? How many doctors have they seen? Did they lose any friends from being sick? Are they suffering from PTSD from being sick? How many hours can they function during the day? And the list goes on.

There are occasions when a not-so-sick person can become extremely absorbed in self-care. So absorbed that it's as if anything that doesn't relate to their own experience didn't happen or doesn't exist. If it doesn't fit within their frame of experience, then it doesn't matter or they just can't see it. A not-so-sick person who's absorbed in self-care can relate to someone's sprained ankle if they've had a sprained ankle. They can relate to someone's hay fever if they've had hay fever. They can relate to learning something new that someone is doing for their health if they can apply it in a way that helps themselves. It becomes a life of self-care to a point of saturation, where there's no time to care about anything not pertinent to their own life. In this frame of mind, a not-so-sick person can unknowingly cause emotional injury to sick people they encounter.

When a not-so-sick person can't see outside their own experience, they may judge what a sick person is choosing to do to heal, or what great lengths they're going to in order to try to heal and recover. A very sick person who has lost years of their life struggling and suffering, visiting dozens of doctors, spending tens of thousands of dollars, losing friends and family along the way, and even losing what feels like parts of themselves from the harsh journey of being sick—when this person discovers a way out, finds a way to heal and recover, they may be misunderstood by a not-so-sick person. Because if a not-so-sick person can't relate to how hard it was for the sick person, how sick they really were, what it was like to be at their worst and fighting for their lives,

then the not-so-sick person won't be able to relate to the sick person's recovery—how far they've come, the tools they used, what they did to recover.

You can feel like an oddity when you recover from chronic illness. What you should be is heralded. The world of the not-so-sick should commend those who've recovered from chronic illness. They should raise their flags high, shouting out for others to know and learn.

That doesn't always happen. The not-so-sick media can be unsupportive. A not-so-sick person may not take notice of someone's recovery if it doesn't apply to them, or if they do notice, they may misunderstand and even judge. The sick can find themselves facing judgment both for having been sick in the first place and for how they recover. It's easy to laugh off or brush aside these life-saving understandings if someone hasn't been humbled by suffering. That is, until the not-so-sick get sick themselves.

WHEN EVERYTHING CHANGES

The not-so-sick fall every day and become the sick. That's commonly when the realizations come. The fall they take brings them to a new awakening about how they've perceived the world.

Until then, the not-so-sick may feel safe and secure in how they've gotten their minor or temporary symptoms under control or solved. They feel confident because they tend to find some help in the form of a functional doctor or practitioner or chiropractor who purports to specialize in more advanced natural health care. When they find these health care providers, not-so-sick people are at the beginning of the learning curve, and what they learn from their doctor or practitioner is new to them. They're not sick enough yet to find out these may not be the answers, because the problems they're dealing with are manageable enough that they seem to be partially or even temporarily solved by what seems to be smart, cutting-edge thinking in alternative health.

You may be told, "Here's a product for your microbiome, because everything stems from your gut," or "Here's a remedy and a powder, a multivitamin, an herb complex, all in line with a no-sugar diet. Do some lean proteins, stay in a keto direction," or "We'll get some stool samples and check out your gut balance. Here's a probiotic," or "We'll do some blood work, look at your nutritional profile, see where your deficiencies are."

When you're hearing any of this for the first time, you can feel satisfaction in the advice you're getting. You feel direction. You find resolve that you could make little changes that could be helpful. It's all confidence-boosting because you're not-so-sick. You can still exercise. You're still doing caffeine. You're not a canary. You're strong, and now you feel you're a health expert.

Some of the not-so-sick today do believe they are experts on anything they've experienced with their health. They had an acute problem or condition, or intermittent symptoms that were perplexing, got some help, learned what feels like cutting-edge information, seemed to overcome it or managed it, and now suddenly they're health experts. They're giving advice on their platforms, giving guidance to other people who are far more sick.

When you're not-so-sick, you can play in the world of reading new theories or trying new supplements in alternative medicine, or read about old techniques that have been around for the last decade or two. Little do you realize, these theories and supplements and old techniques are ones the sick have already tried. Trendy products, trendy machines—the sick have tried them all, and they've only gone downhill. Meanwhile, the not-so-sick can play in these trendy places, and even revive old techniques and theories for other not-so-sick people to play with, making them popular again. The not-so-sick don't realize that as they get sicker down the road because their health scale has finally tipped, the approaches they were trying for their health will show themselves not to be useful. What they were invested in or guiding others to do was not ultimately helpful.

Before that day comes when their health worsens, it doesn't take much for a not-so-sick person to feel a benefit from a health technique. Many of these people are only intermittently sick, with a mild symptom that comes and goes on its own, seeming to get better with a little bit of sleep, a new vitamin protocol, cleaning up their foods, intermittent fasting, lymphatic massage, sauna routines, breathing class, or workout class. The land of alternative health games is filled with many trendy options. The not-so-sick have the freedom to play in this fairy-tale land, waffle about, latch on to something of interest to tell others about, and remain disconnected from the difference between being not-so-sick and being so sick.

Being sick is an entirely different space. The sick have left the realm of play. The sick are seasoned. The sick have already done the probiotics, the fish oils, the whey protein powder and other protein powders, the charcoal, the oil pulling, the neem oil, the L-carnitine, the chlorella, the diatomaceous earth particles, the sodium bicarbonate, the gut powders, the bentonite clay and other clays, the zeolite, the fulvic acid, the deer antler, the colostrum, the collagen, the protein bars, the MCT oil, the kombucha, the chocolate, the green tea, the apple cider vinegar, chlorophyll, alkaline ionizer water machines, and dozens more. The sick have become seasoned, too, from visiting dozens of doctors and trying everything, including fecal transplants, bee sting therapy, urine therapy, coffee enemas, Rife machines, stem cell therapy, UV blood irradiation, ozone, cold therapy, and more. The seasoned sick have been there, done that.

The not-so-sick, when they get their first symptoms, may believe the health world is their oyster as they stumble across remedy after remedy with confident practitioners who haven't gone through a major health crisis themselves. The search for a way to heal starts at that most basic tier. The sicker you get, the more you've sifted through what's offered.

The not-so-sick, many times, think it's impossible for them ever to get sick with a chronic illness. They don't want to think they could ever get there because that's frightening and their health approach must be the answer. They're still doing their workouts, they're still having their "cheat" days, they feel like they're keeping balanced, practicing moderation, intuitively living their lives. They believe, *That person who's really sick, that's not me. That's not going to be me.*

Then, when you cross the threshold to being very sick, everything changes. It's a different world, one of survival. Your goals are different from the goals of the not-so-sick. Things change in your life. Even relationships can change. It's a whole other world of understanding health.

A PRIVILEGED POSITION

When someone crosses the threshold from not-so-sick to becoming sick, it doesn't only challenge the person becoming sick. It challenges the people around the person becoming sick. Chronic illness can tire out someone who's experiencing it. At the same time, it can quickly tire out the people around that person.

It's different when it's a mom concerned about her child. A mom will do anything to fight for her little one. Moms have the ability to reprogram themselves every single morning like it's a brand-new day where all possibilities and opportunities abound. Most moms will fight the good fight for their children flawlessly, with spirit and vigor.

When you're an adult who becomes sick, it can be harder to find people around you who are patient about it. The struggle and the fight to survive as a sick person is a lot to bear for the not-so-sick. Some of the not-so-sick are humble and respectful enough to trust that what others are going through is real. Some of the not-so-sick distance themselves from sick people in their lives because of the emotions such as insecurity, fear, and discomfort that illness brings up for them. And then others of the not-so-sick can misunderstand their luck and privilege of not quite yet having contracted enough pathogens or gotten to the level of being fully loaded with toxins in their life. They can mistake this mere circumstance of better health for superiority. This can lead some not-so-sick people to feel entitled. Somehow they don't think of themselves as just as susceptible to the same threats that create chronic illness in others, and instead assume they're simply better, more "together," more motivated, better at self-care.

The privilege of being not-so-sick can make people feel they have the right to decide if other people's stories of suffering and healing are legitimate or not. Sometimes the not-so-sick think that the mild or temporary symptoms they've experienced are on the same level as what the sick have gone through, so they don't understand when the sick don't bounce back as they themselves did. Perhaps, for example, a not-so-sick person gets occasional mild headaches. If someone tells them about experiencing chronic, persistent headaches, the not-so-sick person may think they understand, think that what they've experienced is on the same level. Then the not-so-sick

person will have a hard time understanding why the person with chronic headaches isn't getting relief from various therapies and techniques—because they haven't grasped the depth of what that sick person is going through day after day. The not-so-sick person may start to think the pain is, well, all in the sick person's head.

Again, the not-so-sick people who take this stance are using that measure of whether or not someone else's experience matches up to their own experience. If someone's story doesn't match their own experience, it's hard for these individuals to wrap their mind around believing or legitimizing it. Some of the not-so-sick carry an essence about them, a confidence that they're more accomplished at discovering life's bounties and mysteries, spiritually and medicinally, than the sick are. You would think the world would grow more compassionate for the chronically ill, more understanding. It tends to be the opposite. A lack of compassion toward the chronically ill is trending upward.

POPULAR FIBS

There used to be a time when the not-so-sick would rarely admit they had a symptom or a health flaw. Hiding it was easy because the symptom wasn't completely impeding their life. It wasn't interfering with their quality of life. Most of the not-so-sick's symptoms aren't visible to others, so they could conceal it. This was in their best interest because sickness was not cool, trending, or accepted. The sick were looked down upon.

The sick, too, would try to conceal their symptoms and conditions in those days. That was harder, because their health issues were impeding their life and interfering with their quality of life. Even if a condition was visible or obvious, the sick would try at every cost to minimize or downplay or hide what they were experiencing because they wouldn't get respect otherwise. The status quo was to conceal any health problem if at all possible.

Nowadays it's becoming popular among the not-so-sick to talk about health. There's even a phenomenon where someone who's not-so-sick may take their "accomplishment" of "remedying" their symptom from whatever they gleaned from their doctor, practitioner, or the Internet and flaunt their seemingly good health on social media. These platform builders talk about the symptom they overcame as proof that they're an authority in alternative medicine, proof that they have the direction and answers. This gains the interest of people who are living with symptoms. It creates a rush of attention. The platform builders quickly experience rising popularity ranks and turn their advice into a living, a professional lifestyle.

In the social media world, to keep everyone's interest you need to give followers more and more. That leads to it becoming popular to fib. Desperate for content, some not-so-sick platform builders will get ideas for sicknesses and symptoms from the sick people they're following or seeing comments from. These same influencers will then start to fabricate stories of having the same symptoms so they can profit off seeming to have the answers. The show must go on. This can be deceiving for the sick person who feels like they found another rare, exotic animal who's just like them. It prompts the sick person to buy into what the not-so-sick platform builder is promoting or selling.

This new phenomenon on social media is unfair to the sick person who's really suffering with multiple symptoms, struggling as they search for some kind of relief, direction, or cure. It's manipulation to push views and merchandise. It's a new exploitation of the chronically ill's decades-long fight to be recognized, believed, and taken seriously.

If you're really struggling with symptoms and conditions, you may have come across these traps, where someone is pushing a trend, acting as though they've gone through something similar to you. It's important to stay wise to the distinction between being not-so-sick and sick, so the sick aren't taken advantage of even more than they already have been. These days it's not easy to decipher and decode if what you're seeing is a lifestyle of the not-so-sick gussied up to attract and draw you in. Simply being aware that this is happening out there, and that it's heading more and more in this direction, you'll gain a measure of protection from being deceived. The sick don't have energy or time to play games. Their hours aren't filled with lots of play time and self-care appointments that are fun. The chronically ill—the sick—need to use their time wisely, accomplish what they can where they can. Stringing them along, luring them to buy into something that isn't for their best benefit: this isn't productive, and yet it's happening, so stay mindful.

LOOKING FOR ATLANTIS

One reason the not-so-sick can find it so hard to understand the sick is that, while they might have experienced the limits of conventional medicine, they haven't yet experienced the limits of alternative, functional, integrative, and holistic medicine.

For example, the not-so-sick may know that the antacid given to them by their conventional doctor is limited and not really working. When they hear the alternative advice that a shot of ACV (apple cider vinegar), elimination of certain processed foods, or a little intermittent fasting will solve the problem, they're inclined to believe it. Unless they've witnessed the suffering of a loved one up close, the not-so-sick are green. They're newbies. They hop on the Internet, do their alternative medicine searches, and feel like they've discovered Atlantis thriving under a dome at the bottom of the ocean.

These not-so-sick people have full confidence that the alternative medicine belief system is a panacea of answers and problem-solving. A not-so-sick person may believe it's sacrilege if they hear a sick person claim they haven't received the benefits they desire in alternative medicine, that it has its limits. That not-so-sick person is also unaware that as much as a practitioner has expertise in alternative medicine, it doesn't mean they have the tools and all the knowledge to heal chronic illness.

Some not-so-sick individuals can get very staunch about their remedies, even vindictive. They can be quick to ridicule anything that doesn't seem part of the norm of alternative medicine. This leads to alternative medicine sometimes acting as a cult, all doing the same thing, all saying the same thing, all belief systems tied together. Even if there are subgroups, where one camp believes in a plant-based diet and another camp believes in animal proteins, they are still tied together with the same cultish concepts. (Read more in Chapter 14, "Food Wars.") This mentality can lead some of the not-so-sick to quickly interrogate, ridicule, and even bully someone who's sick and seasoned, someone who's doing something outside the normal cult belief system of alternative medicine.

At the same time some of the not-so-sick exalt alternative medicine, they tend to believe that if the world of alternative medicine did fail them, certainly conventional medicine would redeem itself and be there to catch their fall. They believe this even after having a spell with conventional medicine that wasn't fixing their not-so-sick problem.

Both the not-so-sick and the sick are looking for answers. The not-so-sick can partake in past, present, and future trends. They usually won't realize the needle's not being moved and they're not making real progress because they're not in a desperate situation. They're in a playful situation, one that's often intriguing and deceiving at the same time. The not-so-sick still have the reserves and enough physical good health to override and battle trendy traps that aren't really helping and are actually hindering.

When a not-so-sick person doesn't realize trends are hindering their health, it's because they're in a game of cancellation. One good thing they may do with their diet is helping their already strong body and reserves, giving them enough to overcome the bad thing they're doing for their body that they think is good. In truth, the not-so-sick person is totally lost—and has no idea they're totally lost because they're still living in a world of strong reserves, good-enough health, and the sensibility to stay away from more frightening health-taker habits. They're growing wise to avoid some of the common threats to health, so they sit in a place of balance—even though they don't know it's a precarious balance. Their body is fighting with all its strength and reserves to keep them level while that not-so-sick person is still doing the wrong things.

The sick person was already there before. Many of the sick have done all that. When they take apple cider vinegar or drink kombucha tea, they get terribly sick. There's no room to play with toxic or unproductive alternative trends when your body is very low in reserves, and your immune system is low, and your organs have low reserves, and your nervous system is weakened, and you're really struggling. These are the people who say, "I did the keto diet before. It almost killed me," or "I tried ACV, and it ruined my stomach," or "I tried kombucha tea, and it made me sicker," or "I swallowed sodium bicarbonate, and my gut has never

been the same," or "I tried microbiome stool sample kits and food allergy testing, and the treatment worsened my symptoms," or "I did over 50 sessions of hyperbaric oxygen therapy, and my lungs feel chronically sore, plus I'm still chronically sick." The sick don't have the reserves to BS themselves and play along with the game of improvisation. They're in a game of survival.

YOU'RE THE TRUE EXPERT

When a not-so-sick person first starts exploring alternative medicine, one reason it can seem like a panacea is that the person is coming straight from conventional practices. The person may be on a standard worldwide diet, may rely on processed foods, and may never have taken a supplement in their life. When they leave conventional medicine after relying on oil, fat, salt, caffeine, grains, and dairy and go into alternative medicine of some sort, there could be a benefit. That's not to be confused with healing at a core level.

So many people who are really sick have already done all that. They've gone from conventional to alternative medicine, and they're still sick. Even if they've experienced some improvement from alternative approaches, enough to get them by, they're still struggling with their symptoms, they're still suffering, they're still in pain. Healing Medical Medium tools such as the Heavy Metal Detox Smoothie, celery juice, Mono Eating Cleanse, Morning Cleanse, Shock Therapies, Brain Shot Therapy, supplement protocols, meditations, and more are what move the needle when nothing else can because these tools address healing at a core level.

The not-so-sick may dedicate themselves to their workouts, their routines with infrared sauna, their lifestyle schedule; then they'll usually be more loosey-goosey around their foods and diets. They may count their calories, yet they'll have their cheat night, they'll drink some alcohol, they'll have sushi night, they'll have taco night. They may be regimented around key, trendy meals they've heard are healthy, such as oatmeal with peanut butter or avocado toast, yet they'll still indulge. They may drink a fresh juice, and they'll also consume their coffee drinks, their iced coffee, their other caffeinated beverages, their chocolate, their pizza on Friday night. The not-so-sick have the leeway to be more committed to instant gratification and happiness.

The sick are more committed to doing everything they can to seek out an answer. They're the ones who finally pick up a Medical Medium book despite naysayers who may try to sabotage it, the ones who dedicate themselves to paying attention to the guidelines. The sick are the ones who learn not to mistakenly add lemon, collagen, ACV, ice cubes, or water to their celery juice—unlike a not-so-sick person who tries celery juice from a health food store that's not fresh. Or buys celery juice that's gone through the HPP process, which destroys it. Or makes celery juice at home for only a week and squeezes lemon juice into it, or stirs in collagen powder or protein powder. Or conceals their celery juice drinking. Or doesn't understand the ins and outs or guidelines of when to drink celery juice because they're not used to having to adhere to true guidelines, because they're not-so-sick.

The not-so-sick are in their own parameters of self-gratification. The not-so-sick person who drinks celery juice for only a short stint or makes a Heavy Metal Detox Smoothie with only two of the Medical Medium tools in it isn't likely to notice much of a difference. They've likely stayed on their caffeine, they weren't that sick to begin with, and they're using the Medical Medium tools wrong.

Someone who's sick is more likely to become an expert in health. Just because someone hasn't recovered yet doesn't mean they haven't gained tremendous experience. People who are sick have tried a lot more modalities, protocols, and trendy, alternative medicine. A sick person who's embarking on the guidelines and protocols of Medical Medium information dedicates themselves meticulously. Even though they aren't fully recovered yet, they're starting to recover for the first time in years, and they're more of an expert than someone not-so-sick who's dabbling in alternative medicine, living their life, doing what they want, and playing the balance and moderation game. The person who's sick and working hard on recovery is the true expert. That's the person who knows that the details matter and need to be applied to work correctly and truly change their life.

CHAPTER 48

Weaponized Science

Science is the humble, human study of our world. Or it's meant to be. That was science's original meaning and definition—a pursuit we recognized as ongoing, always aiming to improve and even admit where experiments failed or hypotheses didn't pan out. By its very nature, science cannot be concrete or definitive. It's a human pursuit limited by human perspective in any given moment in history, meant to serve humanity. Around the corner, there is always that next discovery that will shift the understanding of what has come before.

Science has faced periods of distrust from the public, especially when the medical science on offer, such as quicksilver treatments, caused suffering rather than alleviating it. Unethical experiments, objectives, and methods have earned medical science distrust at various points in time. Again, these pitfalls have come because science is a human endeavor, which means that like any other endeavor, science is subject to human ego, greed, folly—and even well-intentioned errors and mistakes.

Over the last several decades, medical science has undergone an image makeover. It's been rebranded. Errors, mistakes, ego, greed, and folly—that's all in the *past*, we're taught, if we're even taught about science's past. Today, we're being taught that science is a definitive, concrete, objective, end-all solution to whatever topic or problem is before us. We uphold science as a godlike, definitive creator—a higher truth in and of itself—not the humble, human study of our world that science really is.

We've even reached a point where the word *science* is being weaponized. A conversation ends when someone says, "science." There's no debating. The word is supposed to shut everything down. Those who use the word *science* as a weapon to prove their point or shut someone down or back up what they're theorizing misunderstand what science is. The integrity of the very concept of science has been compromised. Science is supposed to mean critical thinking, room for debate, an inquisitive, open mind. Instead, critical thinking about science is now labeled as anti-science.

History reveals cycles. Attempts to gloss over complex truths can backfire. Science has not always been above reproach and will not always be. In the present, the word *science*, and even the institution of science, has come to a point that in 10 years' time, so many people will have been hurt, sickened, or injured by areas of medical research and science along the way that many will be allergic to the word *science*. With the explosion of neurological conditions on its way over the next decade, it's going to be evident that science has fallen short in many respects. The people who are left wielding the word *science* as a weapon to try to stop others from going in a direction that could potentially save them will only make the people who feel they've been disrespected by science more allergic to it.

We're coming to a time of historical divide between (1) the institution of medical research and science trying to redeem its image without reforming its ways, using universities to teach younger generations, and (2) older generations who are out of their college years revolting because they realize science hasn't saved them from lives of sickness, strife, and struggle. This understanding is important to your protection so you can watch this play out from the sidelines without the conflict destroying your life.

TRIAL AND ERROR

I'm not here to dismiss what advancements we do have in medical technology. I'm here to remind us all that the sickness and suffering of the rest of the world should not be ignored. We shouldn't resort to shaming a person who's suffering just because science hasn't advanced enough yet to alleviate their burden.

Let's remember that science is a process of invention. And when you think about inventions, remember what proportion of ideas fail rather than succeed. How many unusable prototypes litter the floor of an inventor's workshop to reach that one design worth patenting? And once that invention is out in the world, how many times do they have to fix and adjust it further because the original needed improvements? What we also need to keep in mind is that while math is used in science, math is not science. Science is ideas—and ideas often don't turn out to be right. Science is failed vision after failed vision after failed vision in hopes that something positive comes out of it. There's not a lot of good science yet when it comes to chronic illness. Sometimes Medical Medium science gets adopted by traditional medical science, although as you'll read in the next chapter, "Weaponized Data," it's often misused.

The successes that medical research and science have had are in areas that rely on mathematical calculations, such as stabilizing critical conditions using pain relievers and transfusions of blood and plasma. Medical successes have also come in the form of equipment such as body-scanning MRI machines, CT scanners, and ultrasound devices. Then there are surgical procedures that can be life-saving—we've learned to remove body parts and install new parts, something like auto repair. These successes represent only a small percentage compared to the crisis of chronic illness.

Even inventions that do work always have to be improved. Medical science is no different. Any success in science is accompanied by trial-and-error failures or serious problems along the way. The success of pharmaceutical pain relievers, for example, is tempered by the tragedy of opioid addiction. Along with the success of advanced equipment like CT scanners, we have increased radiation exposure. And although we have life-saving surgical techniques, it doesn't mean surgery always goes right.

Nobody wants to be used as a pawn or trained like a pet. Yet we can unknowingly become science pets if we blindly follow the word *science* with no sense of perspective. We can unknowingly be used to uphold an image of science that doesn't even serve us. The chronically ill deserve to be seen and recognized for the answers they haven't received from science yet—not least because "the chronically ill" is a fast-expanding group, destined to include more and more of the planet's population as neurological symptoms increase in the coming years.

BRAIN AND BODY SHAMING

We've reached a place in society where there's a stigma around body shaming, and rightfully so. It's a big deal. We've fought to get to this place of awareness that it's unenlightened to shame anyone about their body. So why do we see medical body shaming happen? And why are the media, institutions, organizations, and industries accepting it and even perpetuating it?

Telling you that your genes are responsible for your symptoms: that's body shaming. Telling you that your body has turned against itself: that's body shaming. And it's not just body shaming. It's brain shaming. Telling you that it's all in your head and you're creating the problem: that's body *and* brain shaming.

This is especially true when women develop symptoms that are neurological in nature and can't be explained at the ER. Adverse effects from medical treatments can create a lot of neurological symptoms, some even debilitating: not being able to swallow, difficulty breathing, numbness in the extremities, weakness of the limbs, head pain, discoloration of the skin. When nothing can be found wrong, blood tests look standard, normal, and aboveboard, and no disease can be identified, that person gets a label of "anxiety." Anxiety has been weaponized by the diagnostic system. It has been used in the past, and it's being used now more than ever as a way to say that whatever a person is going through is because of a phantom they are living with or creating. This is what I mean about brain shaming. Oftentimes, the shame aspect is completely unintentional. Smart people with the best of intentions think they're doing someone a service by saying, "These symptoms are from your anxiety," or genes, or immune system. They don't realize they're missing out on a much bigger picture.

Brain shaming is on one level when someone has unexplained neurological symptoms blamed on anxiety. When those unexplained neurological symptoms come shortly after a new medical treatment and it's obvious the symptoms are a side effect of the treatment, yet that person is still told their anxiety is the reason they're experiencing neurological symptoms, that's in a league of its own. The industry caused the actual, physical problem and then shamed the person. It's the highest level of brain and body shaming.

Brain shaming is a safety zone for medical research and science. Medical science and medical universities—they're heralded as Greek gods. Billions upon billions upon billions of dollars have gone into research and building institutions in the field of medical science for decades. When the medical industry is called upon to do its job and offer answers, it doesn't come clean and say, "We have failed to understand the human body when it comes to chronic illness." Instead the industry pretends to understand why people are chronically sick or struggling.

If you're stuck in a hospital bed, stuck in bed at home, relying on ER visits, consulting different specialists, and still not getting answers, your symptoms are labeled "idiopathic" (meaning "unknown"), and you're told they're caused by anxiety. That's the more serious version. There are other versions of having less severe symptoms and still no answers, with the medical industry believing you're causing it, whether through anxiety, weak genes, or a faulty immune system that has turned against your body.

One reason the chronically ill can face so much discrimination is that they often look "fine" or "normal" to outsiders who don't understand. If you've ever lived through chronic pain or other invisible symptoms, you know how sorely lacking the understanding and compassion can be. You know how readily people blame it on something going on in your head.

We're not supposed to ask, "Well, weren't some of those billions of dollars wasted in whatever they were studying, or whatever building they were erecting for whatever reason?" We're not supposed to ask, "Why is my child in the hospital with a feeding tube, neurologically paralyzed? Was it a medical treatment that did it? Why don't you have an answer? Why is no one accountable?" Instead we're supposed to blame and shame ourselves. Self-blame and self-shame keep us from exposing greater truths.

THE CLASSIFIED MEDICAL INDUSTRY

As you read about in Part I, "Your Brain Story," there's an entire classified medical industry that most doctors don't even know exists.

That is, we live in a world with two medical systems: publicly known and classified. It's like good and evil. This classified medical industry is supposed to stay classified. And the publicly known medical industry is supposed to stay unaware of all the problems that the classified medical industry creates.

Publicly trained, board certified virologists and neurologists don't know there are classified virologists and neurologists working for a classified medical industry. For instance, the classified medical industry was aware of viruses such as Epstein-Barr long before the publicly known doctors Epstein and Barr discovered EBV. The same goes for any and all viruses, ranging from influenza, HPV, HIV, and COVID to shingles, cytomegalovirus, herpes simplex 1 and 2, HHV-6, and more.

(Alternative medicine, it should be noted, is all publicly known. There's not a classified alternative medical industry, yet. Eventually, there will be.)

Now, you can go to medical school to become a doctor and never know the classified medical industry exists. You can practice in your field for 20 years and never be aware there was a classified medical industry influencing the education and information you received—and didn't receive—the whole time. You could be a retired doctor who had a full career and is now enjoying yourself on the golf course at 85 years old and still not know that the classified medical industry exists.

The early 20th century was the birth of the classified medical industry. It was like a private club or a secret society, like the Skull and Bones of medicine. A medical professional didn't seek out membership. Instead they were sought out and offered a job within classified medicine. Usually the offer was extremely enticing, so it was hard to say no. In some situations it was impossible to say no once they'd been given the

offer. Then once they were in classified medicine, they had to keep their work private. They couldn't be at a publicly known medical convention sharing their work while they enjoyed their steak dinner with other physicians around the table. They'd sold their soul.

There are people working in medicine who have hands in both worlds. They're the connectors who touch both the classified and publicly known medical industries. They hold positions that block publicly known medical professionals from getting the funding they need to discover the problems that the classified medical industry created. This means that even when there are good doctors and researchers and scientists in the publicly known medical industry who want to solve problems, they get thwarted. They don't get the green light; they don't get the investor backup to make real changes in publicly known medical research and science that could better people's lives. They're held back. And sometimes the classified medical industry will release information to certain heads of the publicly known medical industry. The classified medical industry does this when it wants something started for its own reasons.

Publicly known medical research and science looks out for publicly known medical research and science. Classified medical research and science looks out for classified medical research and science.

The advances of publicly known medical research and science have plateaued. They've gotten as far as mending broken bones, modern-day life-saving surgeries—and they haven't gotten much further than that. They're held back. The future of medicine will not be so much about solving mysteries in disease anymore. Much of medical research and science will be directed into unproductive areas instead of advancements to keep us alive longer. Research won't go into as many good purposes and practices as the people need.

That's not to say that individuals who work in medical research and science don't have the best of intentions. I've had the privilege of working with many of the well-intentioned, compassionate doctors and other health professionals within publicly known medical research and science. There are good people with good intentions at the service of humankind. The greater medical system takes many health professionals for granted and tries to use them as pawns in a very large game of chess.

VOICES THAT DESERVE TO BE HEARD

We make no progress by treating science as God and treating those who question the integrity of scientific methodology as fools.

Science is always acting as if it's on the forefront of exact, indisputable discovery. In every decade, science exudes an impermeable air about it, an impression that it's up to speed, that it's up to date with whatever it's working on—that scientific advancements are always at the top of their game.

Even if that means science keeps correcting itself about what everyone once thought was the top of the science game. Every new discovery takes precedence over old discoveries, and we're led to believe, especially today, that science has figured out something permanently when it comes to chronic illness. For instance, when a new drug is created, we're taught everything should go just fine because medical research and science created it. What we don't see is that the majority of all pharmaceuticals created never get deemed safe enough to go to market, and of those pharmaceuticals that are released and put into use, the majority are taken off the market and recalled due to dangerous side effects.

Meanwhile, publicly known medical research and science still don't know why we're sick. When you leave a university thinking that the medical research and science you know—that is, the publicly known medical industry—has all the answers, you therefore think that if you get sick someday, everything will turn out fine. This is how a broken system gets perpetuated. We should be taught that medical research and science don't have all the answers about why people are sick. We should be taught that their medicines, drugs, and other pharmaceuticals are experimental. We should be taught the truth. Instead, you have to discover the truth when you're that person who gets too sick.

For some reason, until then, it seems like sacrilege to doubt science. When something rolls off the assembly line sparkling new, like a new medical treatment, we treat it as reliable, unbreakable, even to this day—even if years later, that medical treatment has injured many along the way. We're taught this young in school. If we haven't yet experienced chronic illness that's keeping us from living our best life, we don't know how thin the ice of science really can be. When we come out of university, if we're still untouched by chronic illness, we come out convinced, believing beyond a shadow of a doubt, that science has all the answers.

Medical research and science are not going to put billions of dollars into advertising their mistakes to everyone. Instead, they're going to give grants to universities, making sure graduates are leaving with an understanding that science is God and makes no mistakes, and that God doesn't exist. Instead, the mistakes are now being covered up, history is being rewritten, and the voices of the individuals who are injured aren't being heard.

The opioid epidemic was kept buried for decades. That people were addicted to opioids because medical research and science don't have the answers about why people are suffering from chronic pain was hidden and tucked away. Now it's gotten so bad that it's become an eyesore in the mainstream, where you hear about it periodically. In order to get to that level of attention, millions have lost their lives. Even then, we get focused on just the opioid addiction and not the fact that medical research and science don't know why people are in pain.

This isn't taught in school. We leave school thinking medical research and science have all the answers. We're not taught about the mistakes made one after the other. It isn't highlighted that science is constantly correcting itself because the last scientific study or scientific accomplishment became antiquated, either because a disaster occurred that hurt humans or because it just doesn't make sense anymore. Maybe it never made sense to begin with.

Keep in mind that research and science once believed it was safe to put lead in paint and gasoline, safe to dump our trash into the Pacific Ocean (which is still done), safe to use bloodletting as a therapy, safe to perform lobotomies on people suffering from anxiety, safe to use asbestos in our homes, and safe—even healthy—to consume DDT and to smoke cigarettes. Does that offer perspective?

NEUROSCIENCE: A DOG WAITING FOR A BONE

The advancements of neuroscience are not all they seem.

Some aspects of science really are advanced. Take neurosurgery, for example. We can see the results, the outcomes, the advancements. While that's a field that's still making mistakes, still needs advancements, and is constantly improving, neurosurgery (like other areas of surgery) has made leaps and bounds. A neurosurgeon using technology and surgical skills to remove a tumor or repair an aneurysm is not to be confused with non-surgical neuroscience theories that are hip and trending.

Neuroscience is different from brain surgery. When we're talking about neuroscience, we're talking about a theoretical belief system, sometimes producing results for a small percentage of physical-injury patients without knowing how exactly the results occurred. Researchers are placing electrical diodes on someone, trying to document electrical patterns and correlate those to the person's emotions or experiences. It's very similar to an advanced lie detector test.

Science has a way of making us feel like there's some great breakthrough on the horizon any day that will determine why we're sick. Neuroscience especially reminds me of a dog waiting for a bone: neuroscience dangles the promise of big, juicy insights, and the reality is that over and over, we're left hungry for answers.

Playing with theories in the field of neuroscience is completely different from someone going to the doctor because they have a difficult case of brain fog that just cost them their job. Neuroscience play is still 100 years off from uncovering why someone has brain fog. That person with brain fog is not going to get an answer from a neuroscience study, from a group of professors in a university. Unless neuroscience is discovering toxic heavy metals and toxic chemicals inside the brain, identifying where these metals and chemicals derive from, identifying viral inflammation in the brain and where these viruses derive from, it's a game.

We've got people losing their quality of life, living with chronic illness, exhausted and broke from seeking therapies and doctors, pursuing both alternative and conventional medicine. Then an article comes out, or a documentary, or a study claiming advancements in neuroscience. That starts the podcast doctors talking about neuroscience, discussing studies and the seeming benefits to certain techniques. If you're not-so-sick, it can be fun to follow. You may glean a sense of hopefulness. Ideas about how the brain works are intriguing. What if you're sick? When you have neurological fatigue and you're stuck lying in bed, the studies lose their allure. They're a promised bone you can never sink your teeth into. You need real answers. You need something tangible, something you're capable of doing that really works.

Neuroscience is all still theory. "We're theorizing that this is what's happening with brain patterns," they're really saying underneath all the jargon. Scientific language has a tendency to conceal or gloss over the unknowns and gaps. Terminology makes people feel there's a secret they don't know about yet, that others have mastered an understanding they'll never be able to grasp. You won't find misleading neuroscience jargon in this book because I want you to know you're smart enough to understand your brain and nervous system.

Neuroscience talk has been popular for the last 30 to 40 years, and everybody is still sick. We've been told "science is going to save us" for even longer, and everybody is still sick—and sicker than ever before. The popularity of neuroscience, the buzz words, the trendy techniques can make it seem like there are answers. The bone has been waved in front of us for decades, keeping us drooling without the real satisfaction of chewing.

BEDRIDDEN TO ALIVE AGAIN

Medical research can study all the neuroscience it wants, and patients with raging Alzheimer's and Parkinson's will still be flooding doctors' offices as the years go by. Even the doctors themselves—the very authorities on brain science—will find themselves and their families just as susceptible as the patients they care about who are suffering with Alzheimer's, dementia, Parkinson's, depression, autoimmune disease, or any other symptom or condition in this book.

As time passes, more and more people will be on a journey searching for a way to conquer what ails them. Eventually these health challenges will be the one commonality we all share in this world as we push forward, deeper into this century. The patients who've gone looking for answers, tried everything, been everywhere, and finally discovered the healing answers that got them out of bed will be able to show their doctors and loved ones the way.

"We make no progress by treating science as God and treating those who question the integrity of scientific methodology as fools."

— Anthony William, Medical Medium

CHAPTER 49

Weaponized Data

People want to be tucked into bed at night knowing everything's okay in the world. They want to get mesmerized counting sheep jumping over a fence as they fall asleep to thoughts of tranquility and peace. What they don't realize is that staying asleep doesn't protect them. It only prevents them from protecting themselves and their families.

An important part of your protection is knowing that just like data in any other area of science, scientific data we rely upon in medicine can be skewed, contaminated, and manipulated. That's one reason why trying to keep up with conventional and alternative health information can be confusing and conflicting. Like *science*, the word *data* can be weaponized. Like *science*, labeling anything *data* lends it an instant air of credibility. We're taught to trust data inherently, to see data as perfect law. Waking up to the concept that data requires our scrutiny takes courage. Acknowledging that we can get blindfolded by the dogma of an idealized belief system takes grit. When you've

been in the dark for too long, light hurts your eyes.

To become awakened means a serious brain shift. It means overcoming conditioning. Slowly, you start to adjust to other truths in your world. Everything is not what it seemed to be. It prompts a wave of awakening that begins to roll through all aspects of life.

THE ORIGINAL, PRIMARY SOURCE

As you read this book, you might have noticed that you didn't see citations or mentions of scientific studies spawned from unproductive sources. You don't need to worry that the information here will be proven wrong or superseded, as you do with other health books, because all the health information I share here comes from a pure, untampered-with, advanced, clean, uncorrupted, original, primary source—a higher source: Spirit of Compassion. There's nothing more healing than compassion. It comes from above.

Medical Medium science, which has been circulating for decades, continually sets the stage for medicine to understand chronic illness better. Specific viruses, for example, used to not be a top priority in alternative medicine's belief system about what causes chronic symptoms and conditions. Medical Medium science is at the forefront of virology, viral awareness, and exactly how symptoms and conditions are caused by pathogens, toxic heavy metals, pesticides, herbicides, and so many other toxins. This is the original source. I'm only a messenger. Just like anybody who reads this book and learns what's written, I have to learn any new information I receive from above.

Scientific studies aren't always what they seem. If you follow the research trail, you'll find that the majority of so-called studies that doctor influencers and other health influencers point to are not studies. They're papers. They're articles. They're someone's opinions on a topic, not an actual, objective, rigorous study itself. The weaponization of science has taken us to a place of weaponizing mere theoretical papers that are not actual studies.

Very few studies in the world have ever been able to come to any kind of solid conclusion; 99.9 percent of all studies are inconclusive. That's not a failing of science; that's the nature of science. In chronic illness, 100 percent of all studies are inconclusive. Yet research papers are written based on theories developed from inconclusive studies. Those research papers are really just health professionals' opinions about what they're trying to interpret from inconclusive studies.

Yet those research papers are then cited in other research papers and articles as though they are scientific sources. We have a transference of watered-down papers and articles, one written after another, so far from the original studies, which were inconclusive to begin with.

It's even more tangled than that: at the same time the authors of some research papers are using watered-down citations, they're also inserting new information into their papers that they've gathered from sources they haven't cited. Scientific papers end up as collections of misinformation and poached material passed on down the line as if they're all studies. A health professional who's interested in the topic at hand doesn't realize they're reading the fourth paper down the line, or the tenth paper down the line, that misrepresents the data.

This is a weaponized system of trying to point at a publication and claim, "Well, it's science." An article gets written based on one of these papers, the article gets posted online somewhere, and it seems to have credibility because the article includes a citation. What is rarely said is "The study you've all been citing was inconclusive." What is rarely said is "You've also poached information that wasn't even in that paper you're citing." That's the new game in town. Take information you want from anywhere, steal it, write about it as if it was found somewhere else, plug in a citation of an article that wasn't even a study and instead just uses one or two key words about the topic, and only those who scrutinize the data and citations will know the difference. There's a good chance no one will look, call it out, correct the problem.

This is why very few people will ever heal when they become chronically ill: because of misinformation. In this weaponized game of scientific publication, somewhere along the way, interested parties stumbled across Medical Medium science. As they were writing their papers, they took some key, critical pieces of Medical Medium information and inserted it into their articles without citing the source, and without enough explanation or tools to take someone to the finish line of healing. Instead they cited studies that had nothing to do with the information they poached. This system of mixing and twisting and misrepresenting information is geared for 100 percent failure.

When a young adult gets paralyzed by a neurological condition, they won't be able to trace the health articles they're reading to the primary source of Medical Medium information because it isn't cited. They won't know to find these books, where they can get an answer and have a chance to heal. Instead that 18- or 19-year-old will live a life of trying to sift through information in corrupted papers from make-believe sources and inconclusive studies. No one's held responsible for this trickle effect or the corruption the system is built upon. No one's held responsible for that person who will be suffering with their neurological condition for the next 10 or 20 years, or even for the rest of their life.

We need to be honest when it comes to saving the chronically ill. If a study's inconclusive, it should be noted at the start. Anyone writing papers based on that inconclusive study should write only about the study, not sneak in poached information.

Why doesn't it work this way? Because citations serve as a ticket into the system. Citations of inconclusive studies are like fake driver's licenses that get someone underage into a bar. Citations allow a paper's author to get some respect. And if that person who's writing that scam paper or falsified-ID article has a credential after their name, then it's accepted even more. Studies that are paid for by industries, biased from the beginning and inconclusive in the end, are then used as a weapon—as a license number—for a health professional who has letters after their name to write an article that contains misinformation.

SOCIAL MEDIA SCIENCE

This all goes further when it reaches social media. A social media doctor who has a big platform selling supplements and running a million dollars of ads a month can take it to the next level. In their posts and articles and videos, they've been known to use Medical Medium information that they've seen online has healed others—and instead of citing this as the source, they'll cite somebody's paper, weaponizing the citation as their own fake ID to bankroll their business. Without directing followers back to the real source of what can help them, this practice perpetuates the fraud.

Medical Medium publications are a primary source. Social media doctors are taking from the primary source, not citing it, and instead citing secondary sources and tertiary sources and beyond—articles based on papers based on inconclusive studies—to sell their supplements and other merchandise through their five-minute videos and massive ad campaigns.

Everybody is under the spell that citations are proven scientific sources. Citations are referenced as though they mean something, as though they can persuade you to make a decision in your life. Some people are wise to this. They're seasoned enough to trace and analyze the sources someone is referencing. What about someone who's coming straight out of school? They're fresh from being taught that citations are God and citations are fact. They'll think citations are infallible. This is part of how science is weaponized in our modern day. No one's keeping a directory, deeming theoretical papers simply papers and not studies. There's no code they get stamped with that says, "This was just an article, not an actual study."

This unregulated weaponization of scientific literature is done as a massive monetary pay-for-play. They steal from a source that's pure, purposely change it, purposely reference studies that don't relate as their buy-in, all in order to sell their products. To take a pure source and purposely alter it is not in service to the chronically ill.

There's nothing wrong with moneymaking ventures. The problem is leading the sick astray, keeping them lost, not being honest about what you're showing them. A source from above that's looking out for the chronically ill is what gives them the best chance to heal. Medical Medium science has only been proven right by medical research and science and then poached by some social media doctors and health influencers selling supplements because it's fresh, new material to impress their audience.

"BECAUSE SCIENCE"

Science can be used for good or evil. History offers plenty of examples of this. Right now, in this day and age in health and wellness, science isn't being used productively enough for the chronically ill. It's not that I'm against science. It's just that the checks and balances aren't in full force, so when it comes to chronic illness, good science is being ignored while bad science gets attention.

Science is not one united, agreed-upon body of information, even though we're often led to believe it is. There's a battle of the sciences. A scientific study created by one institution is battled by another institution. A scientific study published by one authority is battled by another authority. The casualties of these battles are the chronically ill.

Medical Medium information is needed more than ever because we're about to experience a large uptick, a massive wave of neurological disease. It's so close on the horizon that it's practically here. As the wave continues over the next five years and beyond, the number of people who are sick with chronic illness, mostly defined by neurological symptoms, as well as reproductive disorders, blood clots, blood diseases, and cancers, is going to be devastating. Medical treatments that are irresponsibly created contribute to this wave.

Younger generations are being taught to use the word *science* as a closed term. A definitive term. As I mentioned in the previous chapter, if there's a debate about something, all you have to do to checkmate another person is say "science." It's being weaponized in schools now as a term to shut the conversation down, shut the debate down. You don't get to say, "What science? Where? Let's look at all the data. Let's have a debate about the data. Let's look at all the scientific studies and analyze the research papers. Let's realize what the publications' authors are reading as their sources and what they're saying." None of that goes into it. Instead it's, "Science says," or, "Look at the data," and you can walk away, case closed, game over, the other party proven guilty instantly. If you say "science" or "data" first, you win the debate.

It's even coming to the point of ending a debate with "My professor says." Younger generations are being taught that their professor *is* science—that what their professor says is scientifically accurate, so you don't even have to quote studies; you just have to quote your professor. What's not being taught as it used to be is how to debate, how to intellectually look into data, have an open conversation. Maybe that doesn't matter for some fields of science and information. If someone is debating about rocket fuel or computer science and they want to end the debate with "Science says" or "My professor says," that's one thing. It's quite another when people are sick and dying.

When the conversation is about the chronically ill not having answers, when the conversation is about people being sick for decades so they lose their quality of life completely and even pass away, when the conversation is about chronic illness growing at a rate we've never seen before in our history, we should have the freedom to say "science" and "data" yet we shouldn't be taught that it shuts down the debate. If there's information that's saving chronically ill patients' lives, someone shouldn't write it off simply because that information hasn't been proven by science yet to be saving lives. If zinc is saving the lives of people infected with modern-day plague viruses, that shouldn't be stopped with the claim "Science doesn't say that works." Science simply hasn't studied it yet. And if they do study it, we have to keep a close eye on their data to make sure the research is handled ethically.

"Because science" isn't enough of an answer when it comes to chronic illness. As I always say, was it good science? What was the funding behind it? Was the sample size diverse enough? Big enough? Were the controls handled ethically? Were enough factors considered? Were the measurement tools advanced enough? Does the analysis stamped on the results tell a different story from the numbers themselves? Was the study rushed? Was there bias? Did an influencer with establishment power put a thumb on the scale? Was it such a long-running study that it won't yield conclusive results in this lifetime, yet everyone is pointing to its premature conclusions as proof of what they want to hear? Some science will hold up brilliantly under this questioning. Most will reveal holes: payoffs, kickbacks, small sample sizes, poor controls, corporate persuasion, undisclosed practices, power struggles, unethical intentions, rushed results.

CITATION MANIPULATION

What we call "science" is often based on articles and headlines we've skimmed online and trusted implicitly without questioning. If we're going to get our science that way, we'd better know how it works. The Internet has been manipulated on many different levels. One is by backdating articles and even studies, or altogether removing the dates they were published. What does this accomplish? It allows online publications to make it seem as though what's posted is information long established within medical research and science. For example, someone can poach Medical Medium information, put it in an article, find an old study with relevant keywords to stick in for a citation, and date the article 10 or 15 years ago, or not give it a date.

Then there are articles with current dates that nonetheless cite older studies and articles in an effort to pretend the

Medical Medium information they've stolen is not Medical Medium information and is instead long-known scientific fact. Again, the articles they're citing don't match the information they're actually posting. They find those relevant keywords and hope that anyone who goes to the trouble of looking up the citation will be fooled enough by the matching keywords and dazzled enough by the scientific jargon to believe the reference is relevant.

MEDICAL MEDIUM SCIENCE

When you read Medical Medium information, sometimes it's the opposite of what you've heard before, and sometimes it's closer to other sources but with subtle and critical differences.

The reason why some Medical Medium information can sound *opposite* from other sources is that it was never known before it was published in the Medical Medium book series.

The reason why some Medical Medium information can sound *similar* to health information already out there is that before I started to publish the Medical Medium books, I spent the previous 30-plus years teaching about this advanced medical and spiritual information to tens of thousands of individuals, many of them professionals in the field of health who needed help with their own health, their family's health, or their most difficult cases.

Some of those I taught included doctors in alternative medicine, early on as the world of natural medicine started to catch on. Keep in mind that in the early days, the alternative health movement was not the booming business it is now. The alternative health community was extremely small. Anyone into alternative medicine was considered an outcast, hidden away from society. The alternative movement was so small that large numbers of people who were chronically sick with no answers weren't even aware they had options to explore beyond conventional medicine's approach of surgery, pharmaceuticals, or both.

Medical Medium information stood out because the alternative health field was so small; there wasn't a lot of alternative information to be had. Then Medical Medium information became foundational because it worked. People realized they'd found golden nuggets for their healing. Medical Medium tools became foundational tools. And the myriad of chronically sick people who found these foundational tools helped establish this information in the health world.

Throughout the years, the chronically ill, along with doctors, nurses, and other health practitioners, have learned information from my lectures and my personal guidance using Spirit of Compassion, and they've spread it to other sources. Examples of what was originally Medical Medium information include that long-haul COVID is caused by the Epstein-Barr virus, that toxic heavy metals can cause chronic illness and mental health conditions, that EBV can be reactivated, that EBV causes neurological symptoms, that there's more than one strain of EBV, that there's more than one strain of shingles, that EBV is one of the viruses behind neurological Lyme disease, that a stagnant, sluggish, overburdened, toxic liver causes weight gain, that skin conditions derive from the liver, that toxic heavy metals cause eczema and psoriasis, that lemon water first thing in the morning flushes the liver and body of toxins, that dangerous mosquito spray is in our neighborhoods, that fragrances are becoming more toxic and dangerous to our health, and that we get addicted to adrenaline. It's also Medical Medium information that toxic heavy metals in pesticides cause Parkinson's; that toxic heavy metals can cause anxiety and depression; that EBV causes fibromyalgia, Hashimoto's thyroiditis, rheumatoid arthritis, and multiple sclerosis; that the shingles virus and herpes simplex 1 cause TMJ and teeth grinding; that the shingles virus causes Bell's palsy; that the chicken pox virus and shingles are two separate viruses, not the same virus; that fatigue is neurological when chronic; that the vagus nerves can cause mystery nausea, anxiety, trouble swallowing, tightness of the chest, panic attacks, dizziness, vertigo, tightness of the throat, heart palpitations, and intestinal tract issues such as gastroparesis; that *Streptococcus* (strep) bacteria cause acne, UTIs, interstitial cystitis, chronic allergies, chronic sinusitis, and SIBO; and that withholding overt fats in the morning allows the liver to detoxify and restore. There are many more examples.

In this large-scale whisper-down-the-lane, Medical Medium information can get garbled. Other sources may mix this information with misdirected ideas along the way, so that when you hear versions of what was originally Medical Medium health information out in the world, it's skewed. You'll see medical research and science use bits and pieces of Medical Medium science (without citing it), and then give it a twist that ultimately keeps the information from helping people.

For example, someone will realize that chlorella is bad due to Medical Medium information, and then take something else bad in its place, such as activated charcoal, which I don't advise taking internally, as you read in Chapter 29, "Brain Betrayer Supplements." As another example, you'll hear about brain inflammation—that is, you'll hear about viral neurological inflammation caused by pathogens. That's derived from Medical Medium science, and it would be helpful to people if they next learned how to get rid of the viruses causing the inflammation. Instead people stay confused, because medical research mixes the idea of viral neurological inflammation with the theory of autoimmune, putting the blame back on the person's own immune system.

Trying to piece together the truth about your health is like playing a game of pin the tail on the donkey. You're blindfolded, given a scrap of information to hold on to, and then spun around by theories and opinions, losing all sense of your surroundings. Some people get the tail close to the picture of the donkey, yet they're not quite on target. Others pin the tail on a wall across the room—like when they theorize that a high-fat,

high-protein diet is the answer to address brain deficiencies. Yes, we have brain deficiencies. No, a high-fat, high-protein diet is not the answer: it's the opposite of how to address these deficiencies. Only when you take the blindfold off can you see the whole scene for what it is.

In this book, its companion *Brain Saver Protocols, Cleanses & Recipes,* and the rest of the Medical Medium book series, you've finally matched the bits and pieces of truth to the origin, the source. The ones who have healed their symptoms and diseases know that the information that comes from Spirit of Compassion is gospel. The whole truth is here. It's not repackaged or recycled theory derived from fraudulent science or pseudoscience and made to sound like a new understanding of chronic symptoms and illness.

PREPARING FOR THE FUTURE

The information in this book will always be here for you. It will also be here for the generations who come after us.

This planet will continue to present challenges. Pathogens, brain betrayer toxins, and even regulatory obstacles designed to block us from accessing information to heal will mean that we come to rely again on the simple power of words on the page to protect ourselves and our families. There may even come a day when no one will be able to plant their own fruit trees or grow their own leafy greens without regulations and regulatory penalties and implications.

We've come to rely on the Internet for information. We have so much quick access to the Internet that no one's relying on actual, concrete family reference books on their bookshelves anymore. No one's getting the information to help sustain themselves with their health and well-being and life from books. They're getting tidbits off the Internet, information that can disappear.

We think the Internet's always going to be there. Yet there could be an Internet failure in the coming days. It could be taken away from us. The Internet could be policed in the years to come, and you won't be able to access what you want off the Internet if it's not in line with the agenda of whoever's withholding and censoring that future Internet down the road. There could be regulations about obtaining health information on the Internet because the pharmaceutical and medical world is going to lose power and money and financial gain with information on how to heal being accessible through the Internet. Prohibitions will be put in place so people can't have access to life-saving health information on the Internet. If Medical Medium information or any helpful information on the Internet that helps better our lives is taken away, we'll have to rely on systems that keep us sick.

Industries lose money if we're able to keep ourselves healthy. Fewer people will seek out conventional ways if they're able to stave off infections, strengthen their immune systems, and learn how to be cautious about certain medical treatments. This is why industries will weaponize the Internet. And we're being trained now not to have actual, physical books in our hands anymore—so that in the future, we can't go to our own personal library in our home and look for answers. We won't have them. Generations are going to be taught to rely on something that can be taken away from them through regulations.

That doesn't even touch on other factors that could threaten the Internet, such as a solar flare or another occurrence that takes the grid down. If the entire Internet goes down in the world, or even in a region, we won't have anything to rely on.

That's why these living words that share timeless information from above are set down on this page: for you, your family, and for the generations to come. The human brain will always have an opportunity to heal if the information is available.

ORIGINS OF
THE MEDICAL MEDIUM

Spirit of the Most High, God's expression of compassion whom I call Spirit of Compassion, came into my life when I was four years old to teach me how to see the true causes of people's suffering and to get that information out into the world. Spirit of Compassion constantly speaks into my ear with clarity and precision, as if a friend were standing beside me, filling me in on the symptoms of everyone around me. Plus, Spirit of Compassion taught me from an early age to see physical scans of people, like supercharged MRI scans that reveal all blockages, illnesses, infections, trouble areas, and past problems.

My job as a messenger for Spirit of Compassion is to continue to bring advanced healing information into medical and health communities. That means publishing books and podcasts, posting and appearing on social media, and any other way to reach the chronically ill. The information in this book comes from Spirit of Compassion viewing hundreds of millions of people who are chronically suffering and then deciphering the different variables, conditions, and mental health states they're living with, feeling, or stricken with. Spirit gathers information

on a vast level about what people are suffering with down here on earth and how to communicate this material so everyone with chronic illness is validated and has an opportunity to use this information to heal.

Many times as I was sitting at my desk receiving the information that you found here in these pages, I would enter a sphere of light to take me out of my personal world and surroundings so that I could hear Spirit of Compassion perfectly clearly and see any vision that Spirit provided. One day as I was sitting here waiting to transcribe words from Spirit about eating disorders, I asked, "Where are you?" Spirit of Compassion said, "I'm here. I'm just opening up the plane to get a reading from over a billion eating disorders on the planet so I can provide the information that reaches everyone with eating struggles. I want it to be comprehensive, so everyone's included."

Spirit of Compassion sees the human condition on this planet and then provides a deep understanding of how it came to be, why, and what to do with the resources we have here on this planet. *We see you. We know what you're up against. And we don't want you to go through it a moment longer.*

My life's work is to deliver this information to you so that you can be elevated above the sea of confusion—the noise and rhetoric of today's health fads and trends—in order to regain your health and navigate life on your own terms.

People have often said, "What a gift you have." Some have even called me a prophet. I've replied, "It's not a gift for me. It's a responsibility I carry toward others. It's a gift for you." If someone has a gift as a mountain climber, they're truly gifted. They can climb that mountain and even risk their life doing it. That gift brings them satisfaction in their soul. While others will look in awe, the mountain climber is climbing the mountain for themselves, whether to prove they can do it and achieve that great goal, or to prove they can do it better than before. This gift is different. There isn't any self-satisfaction in hearing a voice; it's not for my own personal goals. The voice I hear is for everyone and anyone who wants to listen, who's suffering. Yes, there's always satisfaction when a life is changed and someone is healed. That satisfaction is knowing someone is freed from suffering physically or mentally.

You don't have to like me, like the message I deliver, like how I deliver that message, or even believe in the voice that was bestowed upon me. I'm still a messenger. I never wanted to hear a voice. Even after I started hearing the voice, I still never wanted to hear it. There was no running from it. And eventually I had to accept it was never going away. Know that this information is always here for you and has a history of bringing the chronically ill out of the depths of lost hope, sickness, and despair—and bringing them into the light of healing. Discrimination for being "the guy who hears a voice" has been a challenge all my life, but that doesn't compare to the discrimination the chronically ill have gone through in their lives. I'm forever committed and dedicated to having the backs of the chronically ill and, as long as I'm still here, making sure I keep bringing forth the information from Spirit of Compassion.

My job is to bring clarity to the ones who want to take the time to learn about what is wrong within their body—not because their body is weak or faulty but because there are real causes from living here on earth that can get in the way of someone's quality of life. Energy is a precious resource, and so many with chronic illness don't have enough of it. If someone takes whatever energy they do have and applies that energy and puts in an effort to learn this information from above, then the opportunity to receive results is there. My job is to deliver for the ones whose trust has been broken in other health realms, the ones who have just enough trust left within them to use that trust to move forward.

If you'd like to know more about my origins, you'll find my story in *Medical Medium: Secrets Behind Chronic and Mystery Illness and How to Finally Heal (Revised and Expanded Edition)*.

CONVERSION CHARTS

The recipes in this book use the standard United States method for measuring liquid and dry or solid ingredients (teaspoons, tablespoons, and cups). The following charts are provided to help cooks outside the U.S. successfully use these recipes. All equivalents are approximate.

Standard Cup	Fine Powder (e.g., flour)	Grain (e.g., rice)	Granular (e.g., sugar)	Liquid Solids (e.g., butter)	Liquid (e.g., milk)
1	140 g	150 g	190 g	200 g	240 ml
¾	105 g	113 g	143 g	150 g	180 ml
⅔	93 g	100 g	125 g	133 g	160 ml
½	70 g	75 g	95 g	100 g	120 ml
⅓	47 g	50 g	63 g	67 g	80 ml
¼	35 g	38 g	48 g	50 g	60 ml
⅛	18 g	19 g	24 g	25 g	30 ml

Useful Equivalents for Liquid Ingredients by Volume					
¼ tsp				1 ml	
½ tsp				2 ml	
1 tsp				5 ml	
3 tsp	1 tbsp		½ fl oz	15 ml	
	2 tbsp	⅛ cup	1 fl oz	30 ml	
	4 tbsp	¼ cup	2 fl oz	60 ml	
	5⅓ tbsp	⅓ cup	3 fl oz	80 ml	
	8 tbsp	½ cup	4 fl oz	120 ml	
	10⅔ tbsp	⅔ cup	5 fl oz	160 ml	
	12 tbsp	¾ cup	6 fl oz	180 ml	
	16 tbsp	1 cup	8 fl oz	240 ml	
	1 pt	2 cups	16 fl oz	480 ml	
	1 qt	4 cups	32 fl oz	960 ml	
			33 fl oz	1000 ml	1 l

Useful Equivalents for Dry Ingredients by Weight

(To convert ounces to grams, multiply the number of ounces by 30.)

1 oz	¹⁄₁₆ lb	30 g
4 oz	¼ lb	120 g
8 oz	½ lb	240 g
12 oz	¾ lb	360 g
16 oz	1 lb	480 g

Useful Equivalents for Cooking/Oven Temperatures

Process	Fahrenheit	Celsius	Gas Mark
Freeze Water	32° F	0° C	
Room Temperature	68° F	20° C	
Boil Water	212° F	100° C	
Bake	325° F	160° C	3
	350° F	180° C	4
	375° F	190° C	5
	400° F	200° C	6
	425° F	220° C	7
	450° F	230° C	8
Broil			Grill

Useful Equivalents for Length

(To convert inches to centimeters, multiply the number of inches by 2.5.)

1 in			2.5 cm	
6 in	½ ft		15 cm	
12 in	1 ft		30 cm	
36 in	3 ft	1 yd	90 cm	
40 in			100 cm	1 m

INDEX

Note: Page numbers in *italics* indicate recipes.

ACKNOWLEDGMENTS

Thank you to the Medical Medium community for your support and commitment through thick and thin. You have become a force of compassion and light.

Thank you to Patty Gift, Anne Barthel, Reid Tracy, Margarete Nielsen, Diane Hill, Sarah Coomes, and the rest of the Hay House team for your faith and commitment to getting Spirit of Compassion's wisdom out into the world so it can continue to change lives.

Kelly Noonan and Alec Gores, thank you for always looking out for me. It means so much.

Helen Lasichanh and Pharrell Williams, you are extraordinarily kindhearted seers.

Sylvester Stallone, Jennifer Flavin Stallone, and family, your support has been legendarily game-changing.

Dwayne Johnson and Lauren Hashian, I appreciate your friendship beyond measure. You are the salt of the earth.

Adam and Jackie Sandler, your humble, giving spirit is the real deal.

Diane von Furstenberg, what a blessing to have crossed paths with you in this life.

Hilary Swank and Philip Schneider, your dedication to the healing truth and wisdom is remarkable, and I am deeply honored. Your support is immensely powerful.

Kate Hudson, Danny Fujikawa, Erinn and Oliver Hudson, and Elisabeth Stassen, having you guys on my side with your love and support is a blessing.

Miranda Kerr and Evan Spiegel, it's so amazing to have your hands of light and compassion behind the healing movement.

Laura Dern, thank you for spreading your light and changing the world for the better.

Gwyneth Paltrow, your caring and generosity are a profound inspiration.

Carrie Ann Inaba, you are true to the core.

Uma Thurman, I deeply value and treasure our friendship.

Novak and Jelena Djokovic, your excellence at thriving is uplifting and inspiring.

Sage and Tony Robbins, it's an honor to be part of your world that's helping so many.

Martin, Jean, Elizabeth, and Jacqueline Shafiroff, thank you for always being there, believing in me, and helping to spread the message so that others can heal.

Dr. Alejandro Junger, life would not be the same without you, brother.

Dr. Ilana Zablozki-Amir, your willingness to support the Medical Medium cause is epic.

Dr. Prudence Hall, your selfless work to enlighten patients who need answers renews the true, heroic meaning of the word *doctor*.

Craig Kallman, thank you for your support, advocacy, and friendship on this journey.

Corey and Courtney Feldman, you are genuine, thoughtful, and outstanding souls.

Caroline Fleming, you're truly a blessing because you have the gift to always care about everyone around you as you share your light.

Chelsea Field and Scott, Wil, and Owen Bakula, how did I get so blessed to have you in my life? You are true crusaders for the Medical Medium cause.

Kimberly and James Van Der Beek, there's a special place in my heart for you and your family. I'm truly thankful to have crossed paths with you in this lifetime.

Kelly Rutherford, your wisdom and foresight raise up everyone around you.

Kerri Walsh Jennings, you truly amaze me with your hopeful nature and endless positive energy.

John Donovan, it's an honor to be on the planet with such a peace-seeking soul.

Nanci Chambers and David James, Stephanie, and Wyatt Elliott, I can't thank you enough for your dear friendship and everlasting encouragement.

Lisa Gregorisch-Dempsey, your acts of kindness have been deeply meaningful.

Grace Hightower De Niro, Robert De Niro, and family, you are precious, gracious beings.

Liv Tyler, it's such a great honor to be a part of your world.

Robert Downey, Jr., you're truly all heart and soul .

Jenna Dewan, your fighting spirit is an inspiration to behold.

Debra Messing, you are bettering people's lives with your vision for a healthy planet.

Alexis Bledel, your strength in this world is extraordinarily heartening.

Lisa Rinna, thank you for tirelessly using your influence to spread the message.

Steve Harris and family, you truly are incredible people.

Jennifer Aniston, your kindness, caring, and support are on another level.

Taylor Schilling, what a joy to know you and have your support.

Dana Gerson Unger, you are always looking out for others. You're amazing.

Marcela Valladolid, knowing you is a gift in my life.

Jennifer Meyer, I'm beyond grateful for your friendship and how you're always spreading the word.

Calvin Harris, you've changed the world with a powerful rhythm.

Courteney Cox, thank you for having such a pure, loving heart.

Hunter Mahan and Kandi Harris, I'm proud of you for always being game to take on a challenge.

Kidada Jones and Rashida Jones, the deep care and compassion you bring to life mean more than you know. Your mother was a treasure who lives on in you.

A very warm, heartfelt thanks and deep appreciation to Naomi Campbell; Eva Longoria; Carla Gugino; Mario Lopez; Renee Bargh; Tanika Ray; Michael Bernard Beckwith; Jay Shetty; Alex Kushneir; LeAnn Rimes Cibrian; Sharon Levin; Nena and Robert Thurman; Leslie Mann and Maude Apatow; Jenny Mollen; Jessica Seinfeld; Kelly Osbourne; Demi Moore; Beth Behr; Nikki Vianna; India.Arie; Kristen Bower; Rozonda Thomas; Peggy Rometo; Debbie Gibson; Carol, Scott, and Christiana Ritchie; Jamie-Lynn Sigler; Amanda de Cadenet; Marianne Williamson; Erin Johnson; Lewis Howes; Gabrielle Bernstein; Maha Dakhil; Bhavani Lev and Bharat Mitra; Woody Fraser and everyone at Hallmark's Home & Family; Morgan Fairchild; Patti Stanger; Catherine, Sophia, and Laura Bach; Annabeth Gish; Robert Wisdom; Danielle LaPorte; Nick and Brenna Ortner; Jessica Ortner; Mike Dooley; Kris Carr; Ann Louise Gittleman; Jan and Panache Desai; Ami Beach and Mark Shadle; Brian Wilson; John Holland; Alexandra Cohen; Christine

Hill; Carol Donahue; Caroline Leavitt; Koya Webb; Jenny Hutt; Adam Cushman; Sonia Choquette; Colette Baron-Reid; Denise Linn; and Carmel Joy Baird. I deeply value you all.

To the compassionate doctors and other healers of the world who have changed the lives of so many: I have tremendous respect for you. Dr. Masha Kogan, Dr. Virginia Romano, Dr. Nguyen Phan, Dr. Chris, Dr. Habib Sadeghi, Dr. Carol Lee, Dr. Richard Sollazzo, Dr. Jeff Feinman, Dr. Deanna Minich, Dr. Ron Steriti, Dr. Nicole Galante, Dr. Diana Lopusny, Dr. Dick and Noel Shepard, Dr. Aleksandra Phillips, Dr. Chris Maloney, Drs. Tosca and Gregory Haag, Dr. Deborah Kern, Dr. Darren and Suzanne Boles, and Dr. Robin Karlin—it's an honor to call you friends. Thank you for your endless dedication to the field of healing.

Thanks to David Schmerler, Brittany Berckes, Kimberly S. Grimsley, Susan G. Etheridge, and Paul Prince for being there for me.

To the following special souls whose loyalty I treasure, my thanks go out: Muneeza Ahmed; Kimberly Spair; Amber Stone; Lauren Henry; Tara Tom; Bella; Victoria and Michael Arnstein; Nina Leatherer; Michelle Sutton; Haily Cataldo; Kerry; Amy Bacheller; Alexandra Laws; Ester Horn; Linda and Robert Coykendall; Glenn Klausner; Michael Monteleone; Bobbi and Leslie Hall; Katherine Belzowski; Matt and Vanessa Houston; David, Holly, and Ginnie Whitney; Melody Lee Pence; Terra Appelman; Eileen Crispell; Kristin Cassidy; Calvin Stebbins; Catherine Lawton; Alana DiNardo; Min Lee; and Eden Epstein Hill.

Sally Arnold, thank you for shining your light so brightly and lending your voice to the movement. Jeff Skeirik, thank you for the best pictures, man. Alyssa Degati, you are changing lives with your voice. Robby Barbaro, your unwavering positivity lifts up everyone around you. Andrew Kusatsu: love you, brother, for persevering past the pain and fighting for health freedom.

Ruby Scattergood, your masterful patience and countless hours of dedication have heroically formed the true spine of this book. The Medical Medium series would not be possible without your writing and editing. Thank you for your literary counsel.

Vibodha and Tila Clark, your creative genius has been astoundingly instrumental to the cause of helping others. Thank you for standing with us throughout the years.

Friar and Clare: *And if any man shall take away from the words of the book of this prophecy, God shall take away his part out of the book of life, and out of the holy city, and from the things which are written in this book. / He which testifieth these things saith, Surely I come quickly. Amen. Even so, come, Lord Jesus. / The grace of our Lord Jesus Christ be with you all. Amen.* (Rev. 22:19–21)

Quincy, thank you for your steadfast commitment and dedication to the cause.

Chelsey, Courtney, Harper, and Anett, thank you for your invaluable support and hard work.

Sepideh Kashanian and Ben, thank you for your warm, loving care.

Michael and Bonnie McMenamin, honored to be on this planet in this time in history together.

Oliver Niño and Mandy Morris, so proud of you for all you do for so many.

For your love and support, as always, I thank my family: my luminous wife; Dad and Mom; my brothers, nieces, nephews, aunts, and uncles; my champions Indigo, Ruby, and Great Blue; Hope; Marjorie and Robert; Laura; Rhia and Byron; Alayne Serle and Scott, Perri, Lissy, and Ari Cohn; David Somoroff; Joel, Liz, Kody, Jesse, Lauren, Joseph, and Thomas; Brian, Joyce, and Josh; Jarod; Brent; Kelly and Evy; Danielle, Johnny, and Declan; and all my loved ones who are on the other side.

Finally, thank you, Spirit of the Most High (aka Spirit of Compassion), for providing all of us with compassionate wisdom from the heavens that inspires us to keep our heads up and carry the sacred gifts you've been so kind to give us. Thank you for putting up with me over the years and reminding me to keep a light heart with your never-ending patience and willingness to answer my questions in search of the truth.

ABOUT THE AUTHOR

Medical Medium Anthony William, the chronic illness expert, is the originator of the global celery juice movement, host of the *Medical Medium Podcast*, and #1 *New York Times* best-selling author of the Medical Medium book series:

- *Medical Medium Brain Saver Protocols, Cleanses & Recipes: For Neurological, Autoimmune & Mental Health*

- *Medical Medium Brain Saver: Answers to Brain Inflammation, Mental Health, OCD, Brain Fog, Neurological Symptoms, Addiction, Anxiety, Depression, Heavy Metals, Epstein-Barr Virus, Seizures, Lyme, ADHD, Alzheimer's, Autoimmune & Eating Disorders*

- *Medical Medium Cleanse to Heal: Healing Plans for Sufferers of Anxiety, Depression, Acne, Eczema, Lyme, Gut Problems, Brain Fog, Weight Issues, Migraines, Bloating, Vertigo, Psoriasis, Cysts, Fatigue, PCOS, Fibroids, UTI, Endometriosis & Autoimmune*

- *Medical Medium Celery Juice: The Most Powerful Medicine of Our Time Healing Millions Worldwide*

- *Medical Medium Liver Rescue: Answers to Eczema, Psoriasis, Diabetes, Strep, Acne, Gout, Bloating, Gallstones, Adrenal Stress, Fatigue, Fatty Liver, Weight Issues, SIBO & Autoimmune Disease*

- *Medical Medium Thyroid Healing: The Truth behind Hashimoto's, Graves', Insomnia, Hypothyroidism, Thyroid Nodules & Epstein-Barr*

- *Medical Medium Life-Changing Foods: Save Yourself and the Ones You Love with the Hidden Healing Powers of Fruits & Vegetables*

- *Medical Medium: Secrets Behind Chronic and Mystery Illness and How to Finally Heal (Revised and Expanded Edition)*

Anthony was born with the unique ability to converse with the Spirit of Compassion, who provides him with extraordinarily advanced healing medical information that's far ahead of its time. Since age four, Anthony has been using his gift to see into people's conditions and tell them and their doctors how to recover their health. Over decades of helping individuals find the answers they needed, Anthony found that he could only help so many as his waiting list continued to grow. Anthony now dedicates much of his time and energy to listening to Spirit of Compassion's information and placing it into books so everybody can have an opportunity to heal. His unprecedented accuracy and success rate as the Medical Medium have earned him the trust and love of millions worldwide, among them movie stars, rock stars, billionaires, professional athletes, and countless other people from all walks of life who couldn't find a way to heal until he provided them with insights from above. Over the decades, Anthony has also been an invaluable resource to doctors who need help solving their most difficult cases.

Learn more at www.medicalmedium.com

"These living words that share timeless information from above are set down on this page for you, your family, and for the generations to come."

— Anthony William, Medical Medium

"Our headspace is sacred. Our brain space is sacred. Our mind and consciousness are sacred. As we become empowered, our trust becomes restored. We have the ability to heal when we know the truth of what invades our brain."

— Anthony William, Medical Medium

Hay House Titles of Related Interest

YOU CAN HEAL YOUR LIFE, the movie, starring Louise Hay & Friends
(available as an online streaming video)
www.hayhouse.com/louise-movie

THE SHIFT, the movie, starring Dr. Wayne W. Dyer
(available as an online streaming video)
www.hayhouse.com/the-shift-movie

***

*MEDICAL MEDIUM: Secrets Behind Chronic and Mystery Illness
and How to Finally Heal (Revised and Expanded Edition),* by Anthony William

*MEDICAL MEDIUM LIFE-CHANGING FOODS: Save Yourself and the Ones You Love with
the Hidden Healing Powers of Fruits & Vegetables,* by Anthony William

*MEDICAL MEDIUM THYROID HEALING: The Truth behind Hashimoto's, Graves', Insomnia,
Hypothyroidism, Thyroid Nodules & Epstein-Barr,* by Anthony William

*MEDICAL MEDIUM LIVER RESCUE: Answers to Eczema, Psoriasis, Diabetes, Strep, Acne,
Gout, Bloating, Gallstones, Adrenal Stress, Fatigue, Fatty Liver, Weight Issues,
SIBO & Autoimmune Disease,* by Anthony William

*MEDICAL MEDIUM CELERY JUICE: The Most Powerful Medicine of Our Time Healing
Millions Worldwide,* by Anthony William

*MEDICAL MEDIUM CLEANSE TO HEAL: Healing Plans for Sufferers of Anxiety, Depression, Acne,
Eczema, Lyme, Gut Problems, Brain Fog, Weight Issues, Migraines, Bloating, Vertigo, Psoriasis,
Cysts, Fatigue, PCOS, Fibroids, UTI, Endometriosis & Autoimmune,* by Anthony William

*MEDICAL MEDIUM BRAIN SAVER PROTOCOLS, CLEANSES & RECIPES:
For Neurological, Autoimmune & Mental Health,* by Anthony William

All of the above are available at your local bookstore,
or may be ordered by contacting Hay House (see next page).

We hope you enjoyed this Hay House book. If you'd like to receive our online catalog featuring additional information on Hay House books and products, or if you'd like to find out more about the Hay Foundation, please contact:

Hay House, Inc., P.O. Box 5100, Carlsbad, CA 92018-5100
(760) 431-7695 or (800) 654-5126
(760) 431-6948 (fax) or (800) 650-5115 (fax)
www.hayhouse.com® • www.hayfoundation.org

———

Published in Australia by: Hay House Australia Pty. Ltd.,
18/36 Ralph St., Alexandria NSW 2015
Phone: 612-9669-4299 • Fax: 612-9669-4144
www.hayhouse.com.au

Published in the United Kingdom by: Hay House UK, Ltd.,
The Sixth Floor, Watson House, 54 Baker Street, London W1U 7BU
Phone: +44 (0)20 3927 7290 • Fax: +44 (0)20 3927 7291
www.hayhouse.co.uk

Published in India by: Hay House Publishers India,
Muskaan Complex, Plot No. 3, B-2, Vasant Kunj, New Delhi 110 070
Phone: 91-11-4176-1620 • Fax: 91-11-4176-1630
www.hayhouse.co.in

———

<u>Access New Knowledge.</u>
<u>Anytime. Anywhere.</u>

Learn and evolve at your own pace
with the world's leading experts.

www.hayhouseU.com

"We all know there are bad people in the world, and these people have no interest in protecting us or our brains, only a great agenda to find ways to hurt us and our brains. We deserve to be wise to this so we can look out for ourselves and the ones we love."

— Anthony William, Medical Medium

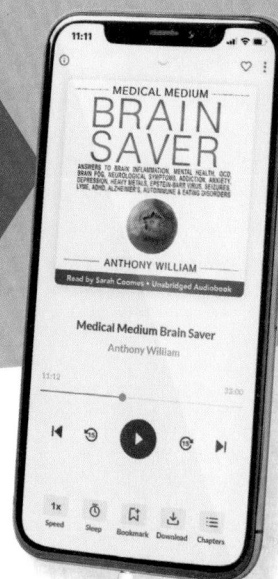

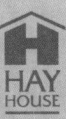

"If I can give you any advice about how to go about reading *Brain Saver* and *Brain Saver Protocols, Cleanses & Recipes*, it's this: there is such comprehensive information, methodically and providentially placed, that once you're finished reading, you may benefit from giving it another go so that both your soul and physical brain get a chance to receive and store all that's here. Take your time. When you're ready, give each book another read-through. With every read, you may find powerful pieces of information and insight you never even noticed before."

— Anthony William, Medical Medium

"You're not lost anymore. You're not stranded and alone in the wilderness, abandoned by the theories and opinions you picked up along the way that you thought would be there for you. As brain-related chronic illness keeps rising exponentially, faster than at any time in history, you can become empowered with knowledge to defend yourself—to take yourself out of that rising tide of neurological symptoms, conditions, illnesses, and diseases. You can experience the peace of not becoming a statistic in the coming days."

— Anthony William, Medical Medium

"As time passes, more and more people will be on a journey searching for a way to conquer what ails them. Eventually these health challenges will be the one commonality we all share in this world as we push forward, deeper into this century. The patients who've gone looking for answers, tried everything, been everywhere, and finally discovered the healing answers that got them out of bed will be able to show their doctors and loved ones the way."

— Anthony William, Medical Medium